MEDICAL HISTORIES OF UNION GENERALS

Medical Histories of Union Generals

By Jack D. Welsh, M.D.

The Kent State University Press
Kent, Ohio, and London, England

© 1996 by The Kent State University Press, Kent, Ohio 44242

All rights reserved

Library of Congress Catalog Card Number 96-13353

ISBN 0-87338-552-7 (cloth)

ISBN-10 0-87338-853-4 (paper)   ISBN-13 978-0-87338-853-5

Manufactured in the United States of America

First paper edition 2005

08 07 06 05   5 4 3 2

LIBRARY OF CONGRESS CATALOGING-IN-PUBLICATION DATA

Welsh, Jack D., 1928–
    Medical histories of Union generals / by Jack D. Welsh
        p.   cm. ⊚
    Includes bibiographical references (p.   ).
        1. United States—History—Civil War, 1861–1865—Medical care. 2. United States—
History—Civil War, 1861–1865—Medical care—Bibliography. 3. Generals—Medical
care—United States. 4. Generals—Medical care—United States—Bibliography.
5. Medicine, Military—United States—History—19th century.   6. Medicine, Military—
United States—History—19th century—Bibliography.   I. Title.
E621.W44 1996   96-13353
973.7′75—dc20   CIP

British Library Cataloging-in-Publication data are available.

Dedicated to

Sylvia Breuchard Mason
March 2, 1932–March 26, 1995

Loved friend and devoted collaborator.
Memories will always keep her near
to all those who knew her.

Contents

Acknowledgments

Three truly professional individuals help made this work possible. Dr. Richard J. Sommers, Archivist-Historian at the U.S. Army Military History Institute at the War College, Carlisle Barracks, Pennsylvania, provided not only the value of his encyclopedic knowledge of the archival material and details of events that occurred during the war but also a wonderful work atmosphere. He always seemed able to find "just one more item." Michael Meier and Michael P. Musick, Military Reference Branch, Textual Reference Division, National Archives, Washington, D.C., helped me through the maze of records and found medical information filed in boxes with titles bearing little relationship to their content.

Robert Denney, author, Springfield, Virginia, and Lt. Col. Warner "Rocky" Farr, M.D., Fort Drum, New York, made helpful and appropriate suggestions.

Many people went out of their way to provide crucial information and missing details: Bonnie Bailey, Ft. Scott, Kansas; Patrick Brophy, Curator, Bushwhacker Museum, Nevada, Missouri; Leslie A. Cade, Reference Archivist, Center for Historical Research, Kansas State Historical Society, Topeka; Nan Card, Research Division, Rutherford B. Hayes Presidential Center, Fremont, Ohio; Suzanne Christoff, Archivist, U.S. Military Academy, West Point, New York; Mary Ann Cleveland, Librarian, Florida Collection, State Library, Tallahassee, Florida; Barbara S. Cook, Reference Librarian, McClung Historical Collection, Knox County Public Library System, Knoxville, Tennessee; Edith Eads, Logan County Genealogical Society, Bellefontaine, Ohio; Adelaide B. Elm, Head, Archives Department, Arizona Historical Society, Tucson; Frank Faulkner, Librarian, San Antonio Public Library, Texas; LeRoy H. Fischer, Oppenheim Professor of History Emeritus, Oklahoma State University, Stillwater; John T. Furlong, Associate Archivist, Missouri Historical Society at St. Louis; John R. Gonzales, Librarian, California Section, California State Library, Sacramento; Gordon O. Hendrickson, State Archivist, State Historical Society of Iowa, Des Moines; George Heerman, Reference Librarian, Illinois State Historical Library, Springfield; Earl J. Hess, Illmo, Missouri; Emily A. Herrick, Maine State Library, Augusta; Beth M. House, Special Collections, Library, Fisk University, Nashville, Tennessee; Roy Jorgensen, Fishkill Historical Society, Fishkill, New York; Marie C. Kalinoski, Secretary, Laurel Hill Cemetery

Co., Philadelphia, Pennsylvania; Norwood A. Kerr, Archival Reference, State of Alabama Department of Archives and History, Montgomery; Chuck Laverty, Irishman/author, Wayne, New Jersey; Alicia Mauldin, Archives Technician, U.S. Military Academy, West Point, New York; Michael Raines, Curatorial Assistant, Harvard University Archives, Cambridge, Massachusetts; John H. Rhodehamel, Curator of American History, The Huntington Library, San Marino, California; Marvene Riss, Archivist, South Dakota State Historical Society, Pierre; David B. Sabine, Hastings-on-Hudson, New York; Ellen L. Sulser, Archives Associate, State Historical Society of Iowa, Des Moines; Thomas P. Sweeney, M.D., Republic, Missouri; William A. Veitch, Lexington, Kentucky; Eric J. Wittenberg, attorney/author, Columbus, Ohio; Martha E. Wright, Reference Librarian, Indiana Division, Indiana State Library, Indianapolis; members of The Kent State University Press, especially John Hubbell, director, who was extremely helpful in supplying battle information; and Linda Cuckovich, editor, and Diana Gordy, designer, both of whom "returned to duty" for this undertaking.

Sylvia B. Mason not only did the tedious work of helping find the causes of the men's deaths but repeatedly reviewed the manuscript, adding the missing commas and correcting strange sentences. She was the major source of support and encouragement and made the work more enjoyable.

Introduction

While reading about the Civil War, I noted the frequent wounds, illness, and accidents that occurred to various officers. Medical events were usually mentioned because they caused an officer to leave the field or prompted a change in command. Such references contain few details, have little documentation, and provide no long-term outcome data. As a physician, I wanted to know more about these men, the details of their medical problems, and the outcome of their conditions. As was the case with the *Medical Histories of the Confederate Generals,* this book was prompted by my difficulties in finding details of such events that occurred during the lives of the Union generals. Only by examining each man's complete medical history can one begin to comprehend the possible effects of such experiences. As a consequence, this compilation of medical events that occurred to the Union generals provides information on a different aspect of their lives and the medicine of the period.

The 583 Union generals included in this volume were those who had met the defined criteria for inclusion by Ezra J. Warner in his book, *Generals in Blue.* As a consequence, they were selected as to who they were and their possible importance to the history of the period rather than because they were known to have been patients.

Since to document only what occurred to them during the Civil War would be incomplete, lifetime medical histories and causes of deaths are presented. Certain information is included because of its possible etiologic importance. For example, attendance at West Point and service in Mexico and Florida along with frontier duties are mentioned because they demonstrate prior exposure to infectious diseases, familiarity with wounds, and possible preexisting conditions. Attention is paid to their degree of being in harm's way at the time they were wounded, the type of projectile, transportation from the field, and treatment, rather than to their location on the battlefield or the units involved. Certain information may appear to be insignificant but is included because it forms part of the man's complete medical history. To put the recorded events in context, a minimal amount of information on their civilian and military careers has been included. I have not speculated how their medical problems might have affected their performance or the war, as this is better left to trained military historians. However, even a brief review of the multiple illnesses and injuries resulting from wounds and accidents would suggest the possible influence poor health had on their field performance.

While there were many reasons why political and military information was retained, there was less impetus to keep or consolidate individual medical records. While available medical data on the Confederate generals was, unfortunately, uniformly sparse, the information on the Union generals was in some cases quite detailed. The best sources were reports of Civil War service, the registers of the Cadet Hospital at West Point, requests for retirement, and pension applications. An ex-officer may write his comrades to help settle an argument as to who captured a cannon, but why else would he write his old surgeon or another to confirm medical details other than for a pension? As a result, such applications contain detailed information from unit surgeons and family physicians not available elsewhere. Equally important, they provide the results of physical examinations and information on the long-term outcome of medical illness, accidents, and wounds. Many men were not treated in a hospital and received their care, even for serious wounds and illness, in camp from the unit's surgeon or at home from their civilian doctors. As a consequence, it was not unusual to find that the individual reviewing records to justify a pension might report that no medical events could be documented from official records, while another source could verify their occurrence. Requests for retirement detailed past events and contained an evaluation of the man's health at the time. They also occasionally include interesting debates. In the case of George Stoneman, there was a question as to whether the injuries sustained by his hemorrhoids and prolapses ani from the saddle qualified as wounds. Other medical details are scattered throughout government records. Clerks were more interested in recording when the men were absent rather than why, so dates of sick or disability leaves were frequently documented but without a diagnosis.

West Point Cadet Hospital registers provided medical data on many who attended the academy. Unfortunately, diagnoses were not recorded prior to December 1831, and records for July 1, 1835, to January 1, 1838, and from August 1, 1840, to October 1846 are not available. (The missing records include the periods that many of these men attended the academy, including the famous class of 1846.) The cadet's last name was listed and a one- to three-word diagnosis was recorded without mention of the type of treatment. Since cadets with the same last name attended at the same time and initials were not always supplied, correct identification of certain individuals was not possible, preventing some data from being included. In the 1830s, common descriptive terms were used for the diagnosis, but by the late 1840s, a headache had become cephalalgia, a corn was clavus, a cold was catarrhus, and a wound was a vulnus.

As was the case with the Confederate officers, autobiographies in some instances were the only source for certain medical facts. The extensive records on Isaac Jones Wistar's multiple medical problems are an example. Letters to families and friends and diaries, when available, provided detailed information. Although some men returned to high positions in business and government, many assumed more obscure positions, and there appears to have been little motivation to keep their wartime papers or letters, which might have provided details concerning their health.

The original archaic words, spellings, and statements used by the surgeons and physicians have been retained throughout, since they provide insight into the actual practices and thinking of the time. To the modern physician, the terms, medical thinking, and diagnoses will seem strange, frequently faulty, and open to various interpretations. In most instances, an analysis of the medical events has not been made. With the limited available data and not knowing the specific criteria used to make the original diagnosis, it is not possible to provide an accurate interpretation of the medical conditions. Obviously, the presence of inflammatory arthritis and the later development of valvular heart disease supports a diagnosis of rheumatic fever. While heart failure attributed to gastritis, is not possible to explain.

A glossary has been included of many of the frequently used terms that may not be familiar to the reader or previously had a different meaning. However, four medical conditions need to be discussed in more detail because of their frequent appearance in these records: *Congestion* was used as a descriptive term, not only of specific organs like the lungs and liver but also of conditions such as chills and fevers. In its strictest usage, it meant too much blood or a fullness of an organ and was considered a primary source of dysfunction and sickness. This pathologic concept was the basis for various forms of depletion therapy. Although there does not always seem to have been a strict criteria for its usage, it usually was used to describe a serious form of the disease. However, it also was used to describe other conditions, such as alterations in brain function supposedly brought on by mental labor and "requiring brain rest" as recommended for Henry Goddard Thomas by Dr. William A. Hammond. After the war, *chronic malaria* or *malarial toxemia* was cited as the cause of otherwise unexplained chronic rheumatism, diarrhea, headaches, fevers, debility, and various neurologic conditions. It appeared to have been a catchall for a number of conditions, and there is little documented evidence that malaria played a role in many of these instances. *Softening of the brain,* which is correctly a pathological term rather than a clinical term, was used when the patient exhibited a variety of unexplained mental changes. Although in most instances there were no localizing signs, some of the described individuals did have paresis. *Fatty degeneration of the heart,* also a pathologic condition and not a clinical term, was considered to be the terminal myocardial change, regardless of the etiology of the patient's heart disease.

Unfortunately, records of the types of medications used are rare. However, evidence that the doctors believed that bad air, abnormal temperatures, changes in altitudes, and certain geographical environs were influential factors in the production and modification of diseases is reflected in their methods of treatment. A frequent recommendation was for the patient to go to a different climate or altitude to improve his health or to use medicinal waters and baths.

The dates of wounds, accidents, and deaths inflicted as well as geographic locations are provided in a sequence section. If the date and/or location of the injury could not be identified, the event was not included in the sequence but was still mentioned in the individual's history. The dates and locations of accidents were the most difficult to accurately identify. However, it was not unusual for more than one date to be officially recorded for a wound. Medical illnesses are not included in the sequence since it was usually impossible to identify their date of onset.

Medical data from before the Civil War was found for almost half of the men. For those who were cadets at West Point, the registers of the Cadet Hospital yielded data for 147. As cadets, the most common diagnoses were respiratory infections, gastrointestinal complaints, toothaches, and headaches. Some contracted childhood diseases while a few had sexually transmitted diseases. A number of the young men sustained injuries, sprains, and wounds that probably were received during artillery and bayonet practice or the mandatory sword drill. Other prewar medical information was primarily derived from military records. No specific diagnosis was available for about half of the medical illness, but the remainder consisted of fever, malaria, dysentery, diarrhea, rheumatism, and respiratory infections. Samuel P. Carter's extensive medical records during his prewar naval service recorded fever, diarrhea, flux, hemoptysis, and intermittent fever among his problems. Some men had medical conditions that affected them the rest of their lives. William T. H. Brooks developed a urethral stricture while in Mexico in 1847 and had recurrent urinary tract infections until his 1870 death from the disease. Sixteen had accidents of all kinds. William W. Averell, for example, fell in December 1858 and sustained a compound fracture of his femur that kept him on crutches until the summer of 1860. Sixty-eight had been wounded; of these, ten were wounded twice. They had been injured by stones, arrows, lances, knives, musket balls, and cannonballs. Unlike the Confederate generals, twelve of whom had received wounds from duels and fights, only two future Union generals suffered such injuries. Cassius Clay had been stabbed, bruised by a bullet, and beaten. Forty-six were wounded in Mexico and fourteen by Indians. Detailed descriptions of these early wounds are sparse, but many were severe and some continued to cause problems. Schuyler Hamilton was wounded in the chest by a Mexican lancer; when the lance was extracted, two ribs were fractured. John Gray Foster was wounded in the leg in Mexico in September 1847. The leg remained painful during the Civil War and was fractured when his horse fell in 1863, disabling him further. Henry Prince's Mexican War wound reopened in 1889 and required further surgery. Four men went into the Civil War minus a limb. Joseph A. Haskin, Phil Kearny, and Tom Sweeny had each lost an arm in Mexico, while Davis Tillson lost a leg as a cadet at West Point.

Nonfatal medical events were identified during the Civil War period for 83 percent of the 583 men. Three quarters of the total group had recorded medical illnesses, usually diarrhea, dysentery, fever, debility, rheumatism, respiratory complaints, typhoid, and malaria. With the field facilities of the time, it is hard to visualize how an officer could be effective when afflicted with dysentery. Darius N. Couch, whose chronic dysentery had started in Mexico, frequently had to command his troops during the Civil War while lying on his back. Henry S. Briggs filled pages and pages of letters to his wife detailing his abdominal pains, sore throat, and headaches and the various forms of treatment and diet he employed.

Today, alcoholism is a specific illness that requires certain criteria for its diagnosis. Although excessive alcohol consumption was not uncommon among the Union generals, it was not possible to label any of them as alcoholics on the basis of the available information. Many were accused of being drunk at various times, but how often the accusations were based on facts or were an attempt to tarnish a reputation is not always clear.

About one-fifth of the men had accidents, which were usually associated with a horse. The horse was frequently shot from under its rider and fell on him, or it fell during a bad jump. Many resulted in injuries serious enough to cause time away from the field and residual.

Nearly half had one or more nonfatal wounds during the war. Of these, twenty-three were wounded on three to five different occasions. Often all that was reported was that an individual was wounded—with no further details. When there was a description of the severity of the injury, it was not always a good indicator of the degree of tissue damage or if there was potential for infection. As a consequence, wounds, bruises, contusions, concussions, and being grazed have all been included. Soft-tissue wounds were usually treated conservatively with the removal of foreign material, the application of water dressings, and immobilization. Although head and chest wounds were usually fatal, such was not always the case. Eight men with recorded wounds of the lung were treated conservatively and survived. John F. Miller lost an eye, and Gabriel Rene Paul lost both eyes. Sixty had a total of sixty-five recorded fractures while a few others had scaling of the bone noted. Pelvic and skull fractures were treated by watchful waiting and responding to developments. At Malvern Hill in 1862, Henry A. Barnum was severely wounded in the abdomen by a ball that exited through the back of the pelvic bone. Despite continuous suppuration and the loss of bone fragments, he continued on the field during the war. He had to wear a drainage tube and had episodes of pyemia until his death. More detailed information was available on the treatment of fractures of the extremities. Conservative treatment was usually administered after determining that there was a fracture and the extent of the wound, even when a joint was involved. Foreign material and bone particles were removed, a water dressing was applied, and the limb was immobilized. Twenty-six individuals had twenty-eight fractures of the upper extremity. Twenty-four of the fractures were from gunshot wounds and four from horse accidents. The one death in this group was not the result of the fracture but rather because the projectile also penetrated the chest. Five had amputations and five had an excision or resection of the bone with no mortality. Twenty-three had a fracture of the lower extremity, with nineteen from gunshot wounds, three from accidents, and one from an unknown cause. Twelve had amputations with three deaths, while one had an excision without mortality. Many with soft-tissue injuries or fractures returned to duty with unhealed wounds that frequently continued to suppurate. Lucius Fairchild had his fractured arm amputated at Gettysburg. Although he had a well-healed stump, he suffered severely with phantom-limb syndrome until his amputated arm was retrieved from its burial site and returned to him.

Sixty-eight men died during the period of the war, with one of these, Louis Blenker, dying in 1863 at his home following his honorable discharge. Twenty were killed in action, with David A. Russell possibly killed by Federal fire. Over half of these died from head or chest wounds. Twenty-eight were mortally wounded or at least died later, supposedly from the effects of their wounds. Some died within a few hours, while E. N. Kirk died after seven months. Stephen G. Champlin died almost twenty-one months later supposedly from the effects of his wound, although anemia, diarrhea, and possibly tuberculosis played a role. Sixteen others died from some medical illness. Almost a third died from typhoid, two from yellow fever, and the majority of the rest died from some form of congestion. Of the three who died from accidents, one shot himself while another was involved in a horse accident. The cause of Michael Corcoran's death is somewhat controversial but was probably due to an accident. The remaining one, William Nelson, was shot by Federal general Jefferson C. Davis during an argument.

Excluding cause of death, postwar information was found for over half of the 515 survivors. Their medical problems consisted of two types: the residual from wartime events and those problems that normally develop in an aging population. Chronic diarrhea, debility, malaria, and rheumatism were some of the most frequently recorded continuing medical problems. In retrospect, it is not possible to provide an etiologic cause or causes for the continued diarrhea. Although amebic colitis could account for some cases, recorded symptoms in many instances do not seem consistent with the diagnosis. Many had residual from their wounds with dysfunctional limbs, pain, and continuous infections and discharge of bone fragments. Joshua L. Chamberlain, mainly remembered for his actions at Gettysburg, was severely wounded in June 1864 at Petersburg. A minié ball had penetrated his right hip, nicked his urinary bladder, fractured the pelvic bones, and exited behind the left hip joint. A urinary catheter produced a urethral fistula, which he had the rest of his life. He returned to Bowdoin College but continued to have recurrent urinary tract infections, which caused his death in 1914. However, the longtime outcome in some instances was good. Egbert B. Brown had an excision of the head, along with part of the shaft of the humerus and a section of the scapula after a gunshot wound in January 1863. Over the next few years the limb shortened and was painful, but by 1870 he was able to chop wood and play billiards. Americus V. Rice served in Congress as a Democrat and Halbert E. Paine as a Republican, each minus a leg. Most postwar medical conditions were those of an older population. Strokes, rheumatism, and heart disease were common as the population aged. Of interest was that about one of twenty displayed signs of rheumatic heart disease and many developed valvular changes.

Half of the survivors had died by 1892, while Adelbert Ames was the last to die on April 13, 1933. The causes of death were obtained from death certificates, burial records, reports by the attending physician, or the results of an autopsy for approximately eighty percent of the survivors. Some recorded causes now seem strange and not the cause of death, such as albuminuria. "Loss of vital forces" or "found dead in bed" are true but not very instructive. A hundred and ten died from an infection, seventy-seven from heart disease, sixty-six from a cerebral vascular accident, and forty-five from renal disease. According to the physicians' statements, in some cases their deaths were related to the conditions of their wartime service. Pneumonia in the area of an old wound and the "breakdown of vital forces" from service in the field are examples. George Custer's death is probably the most often written about and remains a source of continuing debate. President James A. Garfield's lingering death in 1881 due to an assassin's bullet demonstrated that the methods for locating intra-abdominal projectiles had not improved.

Although it has been stated by some that medical practice profited by the Civil War, any such gains did not readily translate into the improvement of general civilian or veteran care. There were improvements in military medicine, particularly in logistics, and in the treatment of trauma, while the experience gained with the use of general anesthetics allowed more complicated surgery. Better prostheses were developed. However, the concept of scientific evaluation of medical therapy had not been developed, and the various treatments were championed or defamed by individual surgeons with little or no evidence. Although the present data is limited and far from scientific, there is little evidence that treatment or concepts in the years after the war were different in actual practice. The single factor preventing true improvement in medical knowledge was that the existence of microorganisms was not recognized.

As was the case with their Confederate counterparts, the medical histories of these Union officers are incomplete but still present a picture of dedication to their beliefs, in spite of suffering from illness or wounds. Men remained on duty or returned to the field with fevers, diarrhea, debility, or suppurating wounds. This probably reflected not only the types of men who became generals but also the attitudes of the time. They did not consider themselves victims but accepted what happened and carried on with their lives.

Abbreviations

CLCO	Record Group 94. Casualty Lists of Commissioned Officers: Civil War, 1861–65, entry 655. National Archives.
CSR	Record Group 94. Records of the Adjutant General's Office. Compiled Service Records.
CV	*Confederate Veteran Magazine*
LR, ACP	Record Group 94, M1395, Letters Received by the Appointment, Commission, and Personal Branch, Adjutant General's Office, 1871–94, National Archives.
LR, CB	Record Group 94, M1064, Letters received by the Commission Branch, Adjutant General's Office, 1863–70, National Archives.
MOLLUS	*Military Order of the Loyal Legion of the United States*
MSHW	*Medical and Surgical History of the War of the Rebellion*
NA	National Archives, Washington, D.C.
RAGO, entry 534	Record Group 94, Records of the Adjutant General's Office, entry 534, carded medical records, volunteers: Mexican and Civil War, 1846–65, National Archives.
RAGO, entry 623, "File D"	Record Group 94, Records of the Adjutant General's Office, entry 623, "File D," 1860s, National Archives.
RVA	Record Group 15. Records of the Veterans' Administration. Pensions. National Archives.
Rx.	Treatment.
U.S. Army, CWS	Record Group 94, M1098, 8 rolls, U.S. Army Generals' Reports of Civil War Service, 1864–87, National Archives.

USAMHI   United States Army Military History Institute. Carlisle Barracks, Pa.

USMA   United States Military Academy, West Point.

UV   University of Virginia.

WPCHR   Record Group 94. New York Hospital Registers. West Point Cadet
             Hospital Registers. U.S. Military Academy, West Point, N.Y. 14 vols.
             Entry 544, National Archives.

A

JOHN JOSEPH ABERCROMBIE • *Born March 4 (or 28), 1798,* in Baltimore, Maryland. Graduated from the USMA in 1822. He served in the Florida and Mexican wars. During the Mexican War, he was wounded at the Battle of Monterey, September 21, 1846. He had duty on the frontier and was a colonel at the start of the Civil War.[1] Abercrombie was appointed brigadier general of volunteers in August 1861. At Fair Oaks Station, Virginia, on May 31, 1862, he was slightly wounded in the head. A ball had passed through his cap and scraped his scalp, frightening his horse so that it threw him to the ground. One of his aides lifted him upon his horse and led him out, without his hat and in a dazed condition. After having the injury dressed at a farmhouse, he returned to command. During the Peninsula campaign he served in garrison and administrative posts. He was brevetted a brigadier general in the Regular Army on March 13, 1865, and retired from active service on June 12. Abercrombie remained on court-martial duty until 1869. He died January 3, 1877, at his home in Roslyn, Long Island, and was initially buried in Jersey City, New Jersey. In 1887 his remains were removed and reburied in Woodlands Cemetery, Philadelphia.[2]

1. Record Group 94, Letters Received by the Commission Branch, Adjutant General's Office, 1863–70, M1064, roll 239, A390, 1866, National Archives, Washington, D.C. (hereafter cited as LR, CB); Francis B. Heitman, *Historical Register and Dictionary of the United States Army* 2:13.

2. LR, CB, roll 239, A390, 1866; RG 94, U.S. Army Generals' Reports of Civil War Service, 1864–87, M1098, roll 2, vol. 3, report 2, pp. 85–93, NA (hereafter cited as U.S. Army, CWS); *Military Order of the Loyal Legion of the United States* 28:460 (hereafter cited as *MOLLUS*); letter from Assistant Superintendent, Woodlands Cemetery, Philadelphia, Pa., to author, July 25, 1994.

ROBERT ALLEN • *Born March 15, 1811,* in West Point, Ohio. Graduated from the USMA in 1836. Allen had routine garrison duties until the start of the Mexican War when he was transferred to the Quartermaster's Department. During the Civil War he rose through the ranks and ended the war as a brevet major general and as chief quartermaster of the Department of Missouri. His health was poor in January 1875 and after a leave to Japan he returned in May in better health. In 1878 he retired from the army as assistant quartermaster general. He died August 5, 1886, in Geneva, Switzerland, and was buried there in the cemetery of Chene-Bugeries.[1]

1. RG 94, Letters Received by the Appointment, Commission, and Personal Branch, Adjutant General's Office, 1871–94, 278, 1875, fiche: 000078, NA (hereafter cited as LR, ACP).

BENJAMIN ALVORD • *Born August 18, 1813,* in Rutland, Vermont. Graduated from the USMA in 1833. While at West Point he was seen at the Cadet Hospital once for sore eyes and twice for a toothache. Served in Florida and Mexican wars. During the Mexican War he first began having trouble with diarrhea, a problem that continued throughout his life. When the Civil War started he was chief paymaster of the Department of Oregon. In April 1862 he was appointed a brigadier general of volunteers and was placed in command of the District of Oregon. Following the Civil War, he remained in the army and served as chief paymaster at various locales. In 1876 he was made a brigadier general in the U.S. Army and retired at his own request in June 1880. The diarrhea that had been intermittent over the years became a more constant feature beginning in 1876. He required the daily use of remedies that, according to his attending physician, led to a feeble action of his heart, general debility and organic disease of his kidneys, and to his death. Another physician attributed his death to albuminuria.[1] He died October 16, 1884, in Washington, D.C., and was buried in Rutland.

1. RG 15, Records of the Veterans Administration, Pensions, Old War 29,366, NA (hereafter cited as RVA); LR, ACP, 3879, 1876, fiche: 000079; RG 94, New York Hospital Registers, West Point Cadet Hospital Registers, U.S. Military Academy, West Point, N.Y., entry 544, vol. 602 (hereafter cited as WPCHR).

ADELBERT AMES • *Born October 31, 1835,* in Rockland, Maine. Graduated from the USMA in 1861. While he was a cadet at West Point, he was treated twice each for contusio, odontalgia, and ophthalmia and once each for tonsillitis and an ingrown nail. In the battle of First Bull Run on July 21, 1861, Ames, a lieutenant of artillery, received a severe wound in the right thigh. He refused to leave the field and, unable to ride a horse, had to be helped on and off the caisson when its position was changed. Ames returned to Washington in an ammunition wagon with the defeated Federal Army. On the first of October he was able to ride a horse and returned to assume command. He was quite sick with diarrhea for a few days in April 1862 and took quinine daily. His appointment as colonel of the 20th Maine ranked from August 1862. In May 1863 he was appointed a brigadier general of volunteers. By the end of the war he had risen to brevet major general of volunteers and brevet brigadier and major general, U.S. Army. He had served on the Peninsula and at Antietam, Fredericksburg, Chancellorsville, Gettysburg, and Fort Fisher. In 1868, Ames, a lieutenant colonel, was appointed provisional governor of Mississippi. He resigned from the army in 1870 to accept election to the U.S. Senate. During the summer of 1870 he was sick and was confined to his bed for a few days. On October 22, 1872, he was staying in a hotel that caught fire, and he had to tie sheets together to get down from the second floor. He injured his hand, which took a few weeks to heal. In 1874, he became governor of Mississippi but resigned the next year when threatened with impeachment. He had diarrhea for more than a week in November 1874 and a bilious attack the following August. During the war with Spain, he served as a brigadier general of volunteers from June 20, 1898, to January 3, 1899. Although most of the troops were afflicted with malaria, slow fever, and diarrhea, Ames's health was quite good at the time. At Montauk Point, Long Island, after his return from Cuba in August 1898, he had a low fever that continued for a while and lost several pounds. A scar at the end of his right middle finger and on his right thigh were noted at the time of his pension examination in December 1915. Ames died April 13, 1933, at Ormond, Florida, the last remaining full-rank general officer on either side of the conflict. He was buried in the Hildreth Family Cemetery, Dracut, Massachusetts.[1]

DEATH CERTIFICATE: Cause of death, septicemia following infection of foot; contributing cause, senile exhaustion.

1. WPCHR, vol. 609; RG 94, Records of the Adjutant General's Office, Compiled Service Record, NA (hereafter cited as CSR); U.S. War Department, *The War of the Rebellion: A Compilation of the Official Records of the Union and Confederate Armies,* vol. 2:386, 394 (hereafter cited as *OR.* Unless otherwise indicated, all references are to series 1); RVA, Pension XC 2,657,412; Harry King Benson, "The Public Career of Adelbert Ames, 1861–1876" (diss.), 24; "Dear mother" from Adelbert, Aug. 28, 1898, Adelbert Ames Papers, Correspondence, U.S. Army Military History Institute, Carlisle Barracks, Pa. (hereafter cited as USAMHI); Blanche Butler Ames, comp., *Chronicles from the Nineteenth Century: Family Letters of Blanche Butler and Adelbert Ames* 1:10, 131–32, 176, 409; 2:55, 138–39; Phil Arnold, ed., "Grave Matters" 5, no. 2 (1995): 3.

JACOB AMMEN • *Born January 7, 1806,* in Botetourt County, Virginia. Graduated from the USMA in 1831. He resigned from the army in 1837 and taught at various colleges until 1861. Ammen reentered the U.S. Army as captain of a company of the 12th Ohio at the start of the war. On the advance from Shiloh, he was sick and absent from the brigade until May 28, 1862, when he joined his command a few miles from Corinth. He was promoted to brigadier general of volunteers in July. On the army's return to Louisville in September 1862 he was confined to his room for more than two weeks because of illness. In October, as soon as he had partially recovered, he returned to duty. He was assigned to the command of the District of Middle Tennessee in December 1863.[1] Ammen resigned from the army in January 1865. Initially, he was a surveyor and civil engineer and then settled on a farm near Beltsville, Maryland, in 1872. He moved to Lockland, Ohio, in 1891 and died there on February 6, 1894. He was buried in Spring Grove Cemetery, Cincinnati. Burial records: Cause of death, paralysis of heart.

1. CSR; *OR,* vol. 10, pt. 1:684; U.S. Army, CWS, roll 1, vol. 1, report 30, pp. 387–93; William B. Hazen, *A Narrative of Military Service,* 53.

Robert Anderson • *Born June 14, 1805,* near Louisville, Kentucky. Graduated from the USMA in 1825. He participated in the Black Hawk, Florida, and Mexican wars. He received a shoulder wound at Molino del Rey on September 8, 1847, and recovered in a Mexican general's house. He was sent home in October, along with other sick or wounded officers. In November 1860 he was sent to Charleston Harbor to command the three United States forts there. Although there were reports that he was in poor health in February 1861, supposedly there was no foundation for such speculation. On April 13, 1861, he was forced to surrender Fort Sumter, South Carolina, to Confederate forces. He took command of the Department of the Cumberland on August 15, 1861, but by October had to be relieved so he could restore his health. In January 1863, Anderson wrote Gen. Lorenzo Thomas that he had been prevented from making a full official report on the final events at Fort Sumter on the strict advice of his physicians. Following a medical examination on September 21, 1863, he was judged to be physically incapacitated. The following month, Anderson was relieved of command and ordered to report to Gen. John A. Dix. At his own request, he was placed on the retired list in October 1863, but until 1870 he was retained on such duties as he could perform. On March 23, 1865, Edwin M. Stanton wanted Anderson to come to Washington, D.C., to discuss his raising the flag over Fort Sumter if his health permitted. Although sick, Anderson was able to help on April 14, 1865: He read the General Order of the War Department, gave a brief speech, and presented the original flag. Seamen attached it to the halyards; too feeble to raise the flag himself, Anderson held on to the rope while it was raised to the masthead. Exhausted and near collapse, he was carried to the waiting steamer. After being sick for some time, he had improved enough by July 1870 to go to Europe in an attempt to regain his health. He died in Nice, France, on October 27, 1871. His remains were returned to the United States and buried at West Point.[1]

1. *OR,* vol. 1:186; vol. 4:254, 296–97; vol. 47, pt. 2:979; LR, CB, roll 1, 1863; LR, ACP, 5135, 1871, fiche: 000001; B. Huger to Wife, Sept. 18, 1847, and General Order no. 324, Headquarters of the Army of Mexico, Oct. 26, 1847, Benjamin Huger Papers, University of Virginia Library, Manuscript Division, Special Collections Department, Charlottesville, Va.; Heitman, *Historical Register and Dictionary* 2:13; *MOLLUS* 5:529.

Christopher Columbus Andrews • *Born October 27, 1829,* at Hillsboro, New Hampshire. At age twelve he had the measles. Andrews was admitted to the Massachusetts bar when he was twenty-one years old and practiced in that state until 1854, when he moved to Kansas. In November, while on a trip back to Washington, D.C., he developed typhoid and had to have a nurse for sixteen days. Three years later he moved to Minnesota and was a state senator when he enlisted as a private in the U.S. Army in 1861. He was soon made a captain of the 3rd Minnesota. Captured near Murfreesboro, Tennessee, on July 13, 1862, he was held as a prisoner for three months. When he was released he ate raw ham and drank his first good coffee, then developed stomach trouble that continued for weeks. Andrews was afflicted with malaria in the winter of 1863–64 and performed his first duties as commander of the post at Little Rock while lying on his back. He rose through grades to be appointed brigadier general of volunteers in January 1864. On May 25, 1865, when the Marshall warehouse at Mobile, Alabama, blew up, Andrews was in a nearby office. He was showered with glass; because of the shock he staggered against the wall, apparently without serious injury. During the war he fell from his horse three times with no injury other than, as later claimed, the production of a hydrocele. He was brevetted major general of volunteers in March 1865. He had a fever throughout June. Mustered out the following January, he returned to St. Cloud, Minnesota. Andrews had a varied postwar career and was United States minister to Sweden and Norway, a newspaper editor, a writer, a warden, and forest commissioner of Minnesota. Because of la grippe, he was confined to his bed for a time in 1897 and unable to attend to his business. A physical examination and urinalysis on April 20, 1904, were not remarkable except for signs of old age, debility, and a right-sided hydrocele.[1] He died at St. Paul, Minnesota, on September 21, 1922, and was buried in that city in Oakland Cemetery.

DEATH CERTIFICATE: Mostly old age and also infection of right kidney.

1. OR, vol. 49, pt. 2:912–13; RVA, Pension XC 2,516,161; MOLLUS 26:364, 29:39; Christopher C. Andrews, Recollections of Christopher C. Andrews: 1829–1922, 29, 103–4, 173, 183, 202, 287.

GEORGE LEONARD ANDREWS • Born August 31, 1828, at Bridgewater, Massachusetts. Graduated from the USMA in 1851. At West Point he was treated three times for cephalalgia and once each for catarrhus, colica, and vulnus punctum. He served in the Engineer Corps until 1855 when he resigned to become a civil engineer. Andrews returned to the army at the start of the Civil War and was made lieutenant colonel of the 2nd Massachusetts Volunteers. On December 1, 1861, his surgeon certified that Andrews had been sick with bilious remittent fever for the previous four weeks. He was given sick leave and went to Washington, D.C. He was listed as present on the muster rolls for January and February 1862. On September 28 he wrote his wife that he had been sick with a very painful colic but was improving. He served at Cedar Mountain and Antietam, and in November 1862 he was appointed brigadier general of volunteers. Andrews was at Port Hudson and Mobile. On April 17, 1864, he was unable to attend to business because of severe indisposition. From May 16 to June 23 he was treated for chronic gastralgia and was at his home on leave. Andrews was mustered out of volunteer service in August 1865 after being brevetted as major general. He remained in the army and taught at the United States Military Academy until he retired in August 1892. There were a number of illnesses recorded during his service: May 7–9, 1886, acute bronchitis; February 4–11, 1890, influenza with a relapse; April 11–15, 1890, acute tonsillitis; January 12–14, 1891, acute diarrhea, and April 27 to May 15, 1891, influenza. The influenza was associated with ulceration of the anterior arch of his soft palate and inflammation of the tongue. He was again diagnosed as having influenza from December 22–23, 1891, and March 1–8, 1892. Four years before his death Andrews had an attack of epidemic influenza. On January 4, 1898, he consulted his physician because of pain in both his cardiac region and his left arm on very slight exertion. The pain was especially marked when he attempted to walk rapidly or go up a slight grade. Exertion also produced some irregularity of his heart. On physical examination his heart sounds were normal. From that time until his death he was never able to walk more than a short distance. He continued having attacks of chest pain, and on March 29, 1899, he had one accompanied by edema of the lungs. He never completely recovered from this last attack. He died April 4, 1899, at Brookline, Massachusetts, and was buried in Mt. Auburn Cemetery, Cambridge, Massachusetts. According to the attending physician, the cause of death was angina pectoris, probably due to calcification of coronary arteries.[1]

1. CSR; *OR*, vol. 34, pt. 3:194; RVA, Pension WC 531,596; WPCHR, vols. 606, 607; George L. Andrews Papers, folder: Correspondence, Jan.–Oct. 1862, USAMHI; RG 94, Records of the Adjutant General's Office, entry 534, carded medical records, volunteers: Mexican and Civil War, 1846–65, NA (hereafter cited as RAGO, entry 534).

LEWIS GOLDING ARNOLD • *Born January 15, 1817,* at Perth Amboy, New Jersey. Graduated from the USMA in 1837. At West Point, he was treated for diarrhea four times and once each for a cold, fever, headache, and influenza. Served in the Florida and Mexican wars. Arnold was wounded on March 11, 1847, at Vera Cruz and again on August 20, 1847, at Churubusco. He engaged in various garrison duties and at the start of the Civil War was commissioned a major in the Regular Army. In January 1862 he was appointed brigadier general of volunteers and served in Florida until autumn, when he was transferred to New Orleans. While reviewing troops in New Orleans on October 18, 1862, he had a stroke that resulted in paralysis. On November 10 he was relieved from duty and sent home to await orders. He remained there until he was retired on February 8, 1864; afterward it became apparent that his paralysis was stable, disabling him permanently. He died as a result of his paralysis on September 22, 1871, in South Boston, Massachusetts. Arnold was buried in St. Mary's Cemetery, Newton Lower Falls, Massachusetts.[1]

1. CSR; *OR*, vol. 15:160; vol. 53:542; WPCHR, vol. 603; Heitman, *Historical Register and Dictionary* 2:14.

RICHARD ARNOLD • *Born April 12, 1828,* in Providence, Rhode Island. Graduated from the USMA in 1850. As a cadet at West Point he was treated six times each for cephalalgia and diarrhea, three times each for catarrhus and contusio, two times each for colica, excoriatio, and nausea, and once each for a burn, subluxatio, and vulnus incisum. He was commissioned into the artillery and served as a captain of the Fifth Artillery at First Bull Run and as a staff officer and chief of artillery on the Peninsula. In July 1862 he contracted typhoid fever and on the seventeenth left for a two- month sick leave. His surgeon reported on August 28 that Arnold had congestion of the liver as a result of the disease. He was able to return to duty in October. In November he was promoted to brigadier general of volunteers and was made chief of artillery, Department of the Gulf. At the end of hostilities he received the brevets through major general in the regular and volunteer service. He remained in the army as a captain. In the middle of 1872 he had chronic albuminuria and enlargement of the left side of his heart. Arnold was granted a sick leave from December 1, 1872, to April 1, 1873. His promotion as major in the Regular Army occurred in 1875. When a surgeon examined him in June 1882, he certified that Arnold had been suffering from repeated attacks of rheumatic gout. Arnold was thus granted a sick leave from July 5 to September 5. In August he was ordered to take command of West Point, but his surgeon claimed that the disease required more treatment, and Arnold did not assume the post. While acting assistant inspector general, Lieutenant Colonel Arnold was admitted to the post hospital, Fort Columbus, New York Harbor, on November 2, 1882, and died suddenly six days later. According to the attending physician, the cause of death was fatty degeneration of the heart.[1]

1. RVA, Pension WC 200,638; WPCHR, vols. 605, 606, 607; U.S. Army, CWS, roll 3, vol. 4, report 14, pp. 463–78; LR, ACP, 4851, 1882, fiche: 000002; RAGO, entry 534.

ALEXANDER SANDOR ASBOTH • *Born on December 18, 1811,* in Keszthely, Hungary. Asboth was an engineer for the Hungarian government until the Hungarian revolt against Austria in 1848. He came to the United States in 1851 and became a citizen. Asboth served as a brigadier general of volunteers early in the war, but his appointment was not made official until March 1862. At Pea Ridge, Arkansas, on March 7, 1862, a musket ball passed through his right arm, fracturing the humerus. In spite of his wound, he was back in the saddle the next day. His surgeons reported in May that the wound had healed, but that there was still pain because of the injured bone and Asboth's continued use of the limb. On May 29 he was given a leave on surgeon's certificate, but he did not take it because Gen. Henry W. Halleck wished him to remain in command. However, because of his feeble health and the continued problems with his wound he was forced to take the leave on August 3. In addition to the limited use of his arm, the warm climate and swampy region around Rienzi, Missouri, was detrimental to his health. Gastric and intestinal catarrh detained him in St. Louis, and he was not able to arrive in New York until the fourteenth. On August 29, he wrote that continued intestinal symptoms prevented him from starting the sea baths believed essential for proper healing of his wounded arm. Asboth did not reassume command until December 15, 1862. While leading a cavalry charge at the battle of Marianna, Florida, on September 27, 1864, he received two severe gunshot wounds: one fractured the middle third of the left humerus in two places and the other fractured his left superior maxillary bone. The latter missile passed through the left antrum of Highmore and lodged upon the palatine bone. Asboth was taken to a private house where his wounds were dressed, and about midnight he was carried off in a carriage. The following night he went to Washington Point, at the head of the Choctawhatchee Bay, and from there by the steamer *Lizzie Davis* to Barrancas. On November 16 he was admitted to the St. Louis U.S. Army General Hospital in New Orleans. Initially the fractured bones of the arm refused to unite. However, after three months, union began slowly, leaving deep and adherent cicatrices that rendered the arm useless. Although Asboth wanted to return to the field in February 1865, he was feeble, weighed only one hundred and forty pounds, and required assistance to mount and dismount his horse. Medical records also report that he had received a flesh wound of the thigh and several saber wounds of the face at some time. By September 1865, the fracture of the maxillary bone had still not united. Spicules of bones were frequently extruded, and pus was constantly discharged from the posterior nares. In addition, he still suffered from the gunshot wound of his right arm, which had left a deep scar. At St. Louis in November, surgery was attempted to remove the ball impacted in the superior maxillary and palate bones but was not completed due to severe hemorrhage. The following February, due to the complicated fracture of the left humerus, the arm was shortened and its muscles were partially paralyzed and contracted. Also, the ball, which was still imbedded in the maxillary and palate bones, continued to produce suppuration and caries of the bones. As a consequence, his senses of smell, sight, and hearing were impaired. The exact location of the ball could not be determined, but another attempt at surgery was reported to be too dangerous. In 1866 Asboth was appointed United States minister to the Argentine Republic and Uruguay. An examination in 1866 revealed that the external cheek wound had healed but there was profuse secretion and interminable exfoliation from the posterior nares. For some reason, by this time the location of the ball was readily detected by passing an index finger about the arch of the soft palate. In addition, Asboth was feeble and steadily losing strength. Although he had resolved to have surgery to remove the ball, he felt his duties in connection with the mission to the Argentine Republic were so urgent that he sailed without the surgery.[1] He died on January 21, 1868, at Buenos Aires and was first buried in the British Cemetery in the Victoria District. Later, when the area became a public park, the cemetery was moved to the Chacarita District. His remains were returned to the United States and reinterred at Arlington National Cemetery on October 23, 1990.

1. *OR*, vol. 8:192, 201, 241; vol. 35, pt. 1:37, 444–45; vol. 39, pt. 1:828–29; vol. 49, pt. 1:653, 790; vol. 53:633; *Medical and Surgical History of the War of the Rebellion*, vol. 2, pt. 1:389 (hereafter cited as *MSHW*); LR, CB, roll 1, A61, 1863; RAGO, entry 534; "Grave Matters" 5, no. 1, (1995): 3.

CHRISTOPHER COLUMBUS AUGUR • *Born July 10, 1821,* at Kendall, New York. Graduated from the USMA in 1843. While serving in the Mexican War, his health was so poor that his transfer to a northern climate was necessary, and in July 1846 he was ordered to New York City. On his arrival there in August, his condition was still so bad that he was authorized to be absent from recruiting service until his health was restored. He reported for duty on April 8, 1847, and was appointed aide-de-camp to Gen. E. D. Hopping. Over the next few years he performed routine garrison and frontier duties. Augur was promoted through grades and commissioned a major in the Regular Army in May 1861. In November 1861 he was ill at West Point, New York, and unable to travel. That same month he was appointed brigadier general of volunteers. His horse was shot at the Battle of Cedar Mountain on August 9, 1862; a moment later he was wounded by a gunshot in his right hip and had to leave the field. He went to Washington, D.C., and then home on leave. In early September, although still suffering from his wound and advised by his surgeon not to travel, he felt he could return to duty. For his conduct at Cedar Mountain he was brevetted a colonel in the Regular Army and commissioned a major general of volunteers to date from that battle. He reported back to Washington in mid-September and was placed on a military commission. In December he was assigned to command in Louisiana. Following the surrender of Port Hudson in July 1863, he went north on sick leave because of diarrhea and dysentery. He was absent until the last of August when he received orders to Washington, D.C., to serve as president of a military commission. Following the war, Augur was brevetted brigadier and major general in the U.S. Army. He was appointed colonel of the 12th Infantry in March 1866 and brigadier general, U.S. Army, in 1869. On February 13, 1879, he was admitted with catarrh to the post hospital at Newport Barracks, Kentucky, and returned to duty thirteen days later.[1] He commanded military departments in the West and South until his retirement in 1885. Augur died at his residence on January 16, 1898, in Georgetown, D.C., and was buried in Arlington National Cemetery.

DEATH CERTIFICATE: Primary cause of death, paresis, softening of the brain. Duration, years.

1. *OR,* vol. 12, pt. 2:157–58; vol. 19, pt. 2:551; vol. 26, pt. 1:642; LR, CB, roll 423, A36, 1869; Ulysses S. Grant, *Personal Memoirs of U. S. Grant* 1:75; U.S. Army, CWS, roll 5,vol. 8, report 8, pp. 589–95; RVA, Pension WC 493,788; RAGO, entry 534.

WILLIAM WOODS AVERELL • *Born November 5, 1832,* in Cameron, New York. He graduated from the USMA in 1855. Averell was treated at the West Point Cadet Hospital for phlegmon eleven times, odontalgia four times, catarrhus three times, and twice each for excoriatio and diarrhea. Before the war he performed garrison and frontier duties. While chasing a wounded deer across the Arkansas River on October 9, 1857, his horse turned a half somersault after it went into a deep hole. Averell was carried under the water and was hit on the head by one of the horse's hooves. A sergeant had to rescue him from drowning. On October 8, 1858, at Rio Puerco, New Mexico, while checking the pickets just before midnight, he was shot through the middle of his left thigh by one of the Navajo Indians. The projectile passed medial to the bone and carried fragments of his clothing into the tissue. The entrance and exit of the bullet were each about two inches in diameter. The wound was dressed by candlelight but the bleeding could not be stopped. The next morning, Averell was taken by wagon to Fort Defiance, Texas, where a surgeon remained with him for three days. Averell convalesced on a ranch, and about three weeks after he was wounded he started getting around on crutches made by the company carpenter. On December 7, he let go of one of his crutches and fell, landing on his injured leg. He sustained a compound oblique fracture of the upper third of the left femur and was placed on an inclined-plane machine with a straight splint reaching from his foot up to under his arm. The end of the splint was fastened to the foot of the bed and he was not allowed to turn or move for ten days. When the building caught fire both he and the bed had to be removed. He was able to sit up after almost two months' time. On February 8, he left in an ambulance drawn by four mules for the 180-mile trip to Albuquerque. A sack made of buffalo hide protected him when the temperature dropped to 20 degrees below zero. Averell returned home and in the summer of 1860 was able to discard one of his crutches. Able to walk using just a cane in February 1861, he presented himself ready for duty on April 16. The next day he was ordered to proceed to Fort Arbuckle, Indian Territory, and deliver a letter to the senior officer present. He took a train from Washington, D.C., to Rolla, Missouri, and from there traveled by stagecoach to Fort Smith, Arkansas. He purchased a horse, which was unbroken to the saddle, and rode the final 260 miles to Fort Arbuckle. At one point where a bridge had been destroyed, he had to swim his horse across the river and was again injured when struck by the horse. He issued his report on May 31 following his return to Washington, D.C. In September 1862 he was appointed brigadier general of volunteers. That same month, while stationed on the Peninsula, he was sick with malarial fever and the "type of typhoid which exhibited itself in congestive headaches and in a general dislocation of all joints." His sister came to nurse him and reported that he was weak and out of his head. She complained that she had had no sleep for five weeks since he would not let her out of his sight. Reporting that bilious diarrhea had set in, she requested that their father send herbs, including red raspberry leaves. Averell was ordered back to duty in October. However, because he was sick, he went to Warrenton, Virginia, on November 9, following the advice of his surgeon. He was in the Chancellorsville campaign but was so sick on March 20, 1864, that his surgeon would not allow him to even read dispatches. By March 22 he was back in command. On May 10, 1864, while at Cove Mountain Gap near Wythesville, Virginia, he received a glancing wound on his forehead from a musket ball. After having his head bandaged, he returned to the fight. In September he requested permission to return home to await orders since his chronic dysentery and malaria attacked him with increased violence. After the war he was breveted brigadier and major general, U.S. Army, and resigned in May 1865. He had atrophy of the left thigh, permanent shortening of the leg, and frequent neuralgic attacks of his scalp due to his old head wound. After serving as a United States consul general until 1869, he took up inventing and proved to be quite successful. Two years before his death he was afflicted with paresis.[1] Averell died February 3, 1900, at Bath, New York, and was buried there.

DEATH CERTIFICATE: Cause of death, cerebral hyperemia.

1. *OR*, vol. 1:648; vol. 19, pt. 2:122, 125–29, 379; vol. 33:704, 710, 719; vol. 37, pt. 1:520; vol. 43, pt. 2:168; vol. 53:488, 493–96; WPCHR, vols. 608, 609; LR, ACP, 305, 1879, fiche: 000003; William W. Averell, *Ten Years in the Saddle: The Memoir of William Woods Averell*, ed. Edward K. Eckert and Nicholas J. Amato, 101, 204–5, 212, 220–21, 223–25, 234, 241, 247, 385, 402; Heitman, *Historical Register and Dictionary* 2:14.

ROMEYN BECK AYRES · *Born December 20, 1825,* in Montgomery County, New York. Graduated from the USMA in 1847. While at West Point he was treated once each for catarrhus and odontalgia. He served on garrison duty in Mexico following the Mexican War and then in garrisons throughout the United States. Ayres was made a captain of the Fifth Artillery in May 1861 and served with distinction at First Bull Run, Antietam, and Fredericksburg. He then led an infantry division from Chancellorsville until the end of the war. From October 15 to November 20, 1862, he was on sick leave. In November he was promoted brigadier general of volunteers. He obtained a leave of absence on January 29, 1863, because of lameness caused by an injury received when his horse fell. After his return in April he was assigned to command. He was wounded on June 19, 1864, during the siege of Petersburg. Following the war, Ayres was given the brevets of brigadier and major general in the Regular Army and in July 1866 was appointed lieutenant colonel of the 28th Infantry. He performed garrison duty at a number of stations and was commissioned colonel of the Second Artillery in July 1879. He had a severe nasal hemorrhage in December 1885, followed by great prostration and anemia. During May 1886 he requested a four-month leave because he had been suffering from chronic diabetes (insipidus) for the last six months. The leave was granted in June. On April 22, 1887, his surgeon reported that Ayres was suffering from congestion of the liver, intense headaches, and vertigo, and if he remained in the Florida climate during the summer it would endanger his life. He recommended that Ayres go to the mountains. In May he was given a sick leave. An extension was requested in September because of debility due to excessive nasal hemorrhage. While at the dinner table on December 28, 1887, he had an attack of incipient paralysis. It affected his eyes, especially his right eye, almost depriving him of sight. The post surgeon was ill at the time, and Ayres refused to have another physician called. On the pretense that she was calling about her own condition, his wife called her doctor when his symptoms continued. The doctor ordered him to bed and had a hospital steward stay with him. About two o'clock in the morning he had a severe convulsion. That day he was in a half stupor and spoke little. He remained sick at the post until April 1888, when he was sent to a sanitarium at Flushing, New York. The Secretary of War regretted it, but he did not allow payment for accommodation of quarters. Ayers died December 4, 1888, at Fort Hamilton, New York Harbor, and was buried in Arlington National Cemetery. The attending physician reported the cause of death was general paresis and cerebral apoplexy.[1]

1. *OR*, vol. 25, pt. 2:190, 250; WPCHR, vol. 605; U.S. Army, CWS, roll 1, vol. 1, report 19, pp. 285–91; ibid., roll 4, vol. 7, report 22, pp. 333–51; LR, ACP, 1304, 1884, fiche: 000039; RVA, Pension WC 260,294.

B

JOSEPH BAILEY • *Born on May 6, 1825,* at Pennsville, Ohio. Bailey studied civil engineering in Illinois, then moved to Wisconsin in 1847 where he became a lumberman. In July 1861, he entered Federal service as a company captain of the 4th Wisconsin Infantry. His proficiency as an engineer earned him the promotion to full brigadier general of volunteers and brevet major general by the end of the war. In December 1862 he stated his health had been quite good except for occasional ague and rheumatism, which had bothered him during the winter. At Mansfield, Louisiana, on April 8, 1864, he received a "rap" on his head from a ball and continued to be sore over the next couple of months. That summer he felt tired and used up, and during September he was having considerable problems with his rheumatism. In April 1865 he was having trouble with his eye, which had been hit with a shell fragment, and expressed the fear that he might lose it. He and his wife were both sick in November 1865. After hostilities were over, Bailey went to Vernon County, Missouri, and was elected sheriff in the fall of 1866. Northwest of Nevada, Missouri, on March 22, 1867, he was shot in the back of the head. (The date he was killed has been reported as March 21, 26, and 27, while his gravestone has the twenty-second.) He had gone out and arrested two brothers for stealing a hog. They agreed to go back with him but refused to give up their arms. When Bailey did not return to town, a search party went out the next morning and found his body in a small stream near the trail. He was buried first in the military graveyard in Fort Scott, Kansas, and was later moved to the Evergreen Cemetery.[1]

1. CSR; RVA, Pension Min. C 538,758; J. Bailey to Stroud, Dec. 5, 1862, June 6, 1864; J. Bailey to Captain, July 30, Sept. 17, 1864, Apr. 16, 1865, Bailey-Stroud Papers, folder 1862, USAMHI; J. B. Johnson, ed., *History of Vernon County Missouri, Past and Present,* 314–19; Mrs. Bonnie Bailey to author, Oct. 23, 1993.

ABSALOM BAIRD • *Born August 20, 1824,* at Washington, Pennsylvania. Graduated from the USMA in 1849. As a cadet he was seen eight times for cephalalgia, three times for catarrhus, twice each for odontalgia and pyrosis, and once each for clavus, excoriatio, luxatio, morbi. varii., obstipatio, and rheumatism. While in Florida during the autumn of 1851 he had fever and recurrence of a liver condition that had bothered him when he was at West Point. In November he had a sick leave and went to Philadelphia where he remained until spring. Still in poor health and suffering from torpidity of the hepatic system, he was granted a leave on March 30, 1852, to go to Europe until the middle of August for the benefit of his health. In October 1853, while an instructor at West Point, he was treated for tonsillitis.[1] He was a staff officer at First Bull Run and on the Peninsula. In April 1862 he was appointed brigadier general of volunteers; as a division commander he took an active part in the fighting in the West—at Chickamauga and in the Atlanta campaign, the March to the Sea, and the Carolinas campaign. In 1866 he was mustered out of volunteer service and reverted to his regular rank of major. Baird served as inspector general of various military departments and finally in 1885 was made army inspector general. He held this position when he retired in 1888. Baird died near Relay, Maryland, on June 14, 1905, and was buried in Arlington National Cemetery.

1. WPCHR, vols. 605, 606, 607, 608; John A. Baird, Jr., *Profile of a Hero,* 36–37, 43.

EDWARD DICKINSON BAKER • *Born on February 24, 1811,* in London, England, and brought to Philadelphia when he was four years old. In 1847, while quelling a mutiny of a regiment on board a transport at Mobile, he was wounded in the throat. Following his recovery, he served until the end of the Mexican War. He had an attack of fever while in Panama on his way to California in 1851 and was near death. Before the Civil War he was a politician in Illinois, a lawyer in California, and a U.S. senator from Oregon. He was made a colonel in June 1861 and in September of that year was appointed major general of volunteers. At the Battle of Ball's Bluff on October 21, 1861, Baker was on foot directing the fire when he was mortally hit by four balls, one of which pierced his brain.[1] Baker was buried at the Presidio, San Francisco, California.

1. *OR,* vol. 5:326–29; Isaac J. Wistar, *The Autobiography of General Isaac J. Wistar,* 304, 368, 377.

LA FAYETTE CURRY BAKER • *Born October 13, 1826,* at Stafford, New York. His life before the war is poorly documented, but he apparently held a number of jobs in New York, Philadelphia, and San Francisco. During the war he served as a special provost marshal of the War Department and was active in counterintelligence. During August 1862 he rode his horse 124 miles in 21 hours without

sleep to deliver a message to Gen. Nathaniel P. Banks. Under pursuit on the return trip, he constantly held the reins of his horse in his left hand and a pistol in
his right. His badly swollen left hand required medical care. He was appointed
colonel of the 1st District of Columbia Cavalry in May 1863. While at Dumfries,
Virginia, in November 1863, he had a severe fainting spell that affected his head,
and he was sent by tugboat to Washington, D.C. His surgeon reported that in
May 1864 he was suffering from cerebral congestion accompanied with "native"
fever, which he believed to have been superinduced by his great mental excitement and exhaustive duties. The surgeon had frequently advised Baker to resign
and admonished him as to the bad results of continued active service. On September 13, 1864, Baker had surgery for a fistula in ano at his own urgent request
because he attributed most of his nervous symptoms to this condition. Apparently, the surgery was successful as far as his anal condition. He was promoted to
brigadier general of volunteers in April 1865. During the fall of 1865, he had two
attacks of congestive chills, one of which came close to being fatal, and urinary
problems. The disease, in part, and for which his surgeon had treated him in 1864,
was diagnosed as meningitis. It continued and progressed to spinal disease and
utimately contributed to his death. Baker was mustered out in January 1866 supposedly because of his continued disability. Following his discharge he was not
fully competent for business and his brain disease made him an invalid. According to his attending physician, he died in Philadelphia on July 3, 1868, of meningitis, the result of cerebral congestion supervening upon and associated with severe
kidney disease.[1] Baker was buried in the Mutual Family Cemetery in Philadelphia. When it was discovered in 1924 that the city needed the land, his remains
were disinterred and put in an unmarked common grave elsewhere in the city.[1]

1. RVA, Pension WC 150,246; Jacob Mogelever, *Death to Traitors,* 136, 419.

NATHANIEL PRENTISS BANKS • *Born on January 30, 1816,* at Waltham, Massachusetts. A prewar politician in Massachusetts, he was governor of the state from
1858 until his appointment as a major general of volunteers in May 1861. He was
ill on July 3, 1862, but able to travel the next day. Banks was severely injured
when a runaway cavalry horse struck his right hip on the evening of August 9,
1862, during the Battle of Cedar Mountain. However, he remained on his mount
and stayed on the field all night. Unable to actively move about, he remained in
command and was conveyed in an ambulance. He sought medical help on August 20 from a surgeon in a large farmhouse in the rear of their lines. His body
was badly swollen and ecchymosed.[1] Banks commanded the movement against
Port Hudson and the thoroughly mishandled Red River campaign. Mustered
out of service in August 1865, he returned to Massachusetts political life. He
died September 1, 1894, at his home in Waltham and was buried in Grove Hill
Cemetery in that city.
DEATH CERTIFICATE: Cause of death, senile dementia.

1. *OR*, vol. 12, pt. 3:451; *Supplement to the Official Records of the Union and Confederate Armies*, vol. 2, pt. 1:522, 529 (hereafter cited as *OR Suppl.*); U.S. Army, CWS, report of A. S. Williams, roll 2, vol. 3, report 17, pp. 461–513; Gwinn Cox Merlin, "John Pope, Fighting General from Illinois" (diss.), 181.

FRANCIS CHANNING BARLOW • *Born October 19, 1834,* in Brooklyn, New York. He was admitted to the New York bar in 1858 and was practicing law at the start of the Civil War. Barlow entered Federal service as a private in the 12th New York, a three-month regiment, and was soon commissioned lieutenant colonel and then colonel of the 61st New York. He was on the Peninsula, and on September 17, 1862, at the close of the Battle of Antietam, he was severely wounded in the left groin by a spherical case shot and in the face by a small piece of shell. The wounds were treated by simple water dressings, and he was given no medications. He was promoted as brigadier general of volunteers from the date of that battle. When examined in October while in New York City, he had, in addition to his wounds, an abscess in the right anterior thoracic region. Barlow returned to his home; when visited by friends he was supposedly on the stretcher that had been used to carry him from Antietam. By the middle of November the wound had not entirely healed and the abscess had not closed. There was numbness of his left leg, and he was emaciated and suffering from the influence of malaria. Although still not fit, the following April he rejoined the army in time for Chancellorsville. At Gettysburg on July 1, 1863, he was wounded by a minié ball in the left side, about halfway between the armpit and the hip. He dismounted and tried to walk but soon became too faint to continue and had to lie down. The story that Confederate general John B. Gordon saw Barlow lying on the field and gave him water is doubtful. Confederate troops carried Barlow into the woods and placed him on a bed of leaves. Later, captured Federal troops carried him in a blanket to the Josiah Benner house. He was in considerable pain and bleeding a good deal. On the evening of July 3, a Confederate surgeon gave him chloroform and probed the wound. Within a day, Barlow was moved to the John S. Crawford house just inside Gettysburg and, under morphia, rested better. Since Barlow was considered to be mortally wounded, the Confederate forces left him when they retreated, and he was rescued by Federal troops. During August the wound suppurated, and he was confined to bed. He still had an unhealed, discharging wound in October. In December, he was ordered to proceed to Springfield, Illinois, for recruiting duty, but his health remained bad and he had not yet attempted to mount a horse. He was back in command in April 1864. He led a division at Spotsylvania but, very sick with diarrhea on August 17, had to go to the corps hospital at City Point. On his release from the hospital he received a twenty-day leave on surgeon's certificate of disability. Another sick leave was granted for the same condition, now considered chronic, from November 5, 1864, until April 1, 1865, and he went to Europe for part of the time. On April 6 he reported for duty and was assigned to command of a division. He was promoted to major general of volunteers in May.[1] Following the war, Barlow returned to New York where he was twice secretary of the state, a United States marshal, and state attorney general. He practiced law until he died in a private home in New York City on January 11, 1896. He was buried in Brookline, Massachusetts.

DEATH CERTIFICATE: Chief cause, chronic Bright's disease; contributing, chronic endarteritis (inflammation inside the artery).

1. CSR; *OR*, vol. 19, pt. 1:282, 286, 290–91; vol. 27, pt. 1:72, 705, 707, 712, 729, pt. 2:445, 469; vol. 33:427; vol. 36, pt. 1:325; vol. 42, pt. 1:249–51, pt. 2:447, pt. 3:518; vol. 51, pt. 1:1007, 1134; U.S. Army, CWS, roll 1, vol. 1, report 21, pp. 297–303; LR, CB, roll 241, B583, 1866; Maria Lydig Daly, *Diary of a Union Lady, 1861–1865,* ed. Harold Earl Hammond, 190, 228; John B. Gordon, *Reminiscences of the Civil War,* 151–53; Gregory A. Coco, *A Vast Sea of Misery,* 121, 124; RG 94, Records of the Adjutant General's Office, entry 623, "File D," 1860s, NA (hereafter cited as RAGO, entry 623, "File D").

JOHN GROSS BARNARD • *Born on May 19, 1815,* at Sheffield, Massachusetts. Graduated from the USMA in 1833. While at West Point he was treated twice each for a cold and a headache and once each for influenza and a sprain. Served in the Mexican War. In December 1850, he went on leave from the army to make a survey of the Tehuantepec Isthmus in Mexico for the Tehuantepec Company. Following his arrival upon the Isthmus in 1851, he started having episodes of serious illness, which debilitated him and made him unfit for travel. Unable to ride on horseback, he was confined to his quarters at El Barrio for long periods. In December he came back to New Orleans and was given a six-month leave of absence. He arrived in Washington in February 1852. No specific diagnosis was recorded for his medical problem, but in March his surgeon reported that he was disabled by general debility and slight melancholia. He was promoted to major in the Regular Army in 1858. In September 1861 Barnard was appointed brigadier general of volunteers and served as chief engineer of the Army of the Potomac throughout the war. He received brevets of major general in both the Regular Army and the volunteers. In December 1865, he was commissioned colonel, Corps of Engineers, and undertook the task of restructuring the coastal defenses and writing about the Civil War. In May 1878 he had a severe inflammation of his eyes. His health began to give way in May 1879, and by July he was suffering from great prostration of his body and mind. His serious illness prompted another officer to be detailed to act in his place on the lighthouse board in October. He was still ill at his station in New York City in November, unable to take his sick leave. In December he went to a sanatorium for treatment. The attending physician stated that Barnard was suffering from the effects of malarial poisoning, which from the evidence he had, was contracted during military service. He further reported that the indications of chronic malaria included a congested liver and spleen. His liver and bowels were inactive and his tongue heavily coated. Nutrition was much affected, and he was sallow and very anemic. In addition, he was suffering from mental depression and delusions in regard to his own character, thinking that he had been selfish and covetous and that he had no right to live. During the next two years he improved in many ways, especially in the quality and quantity of blood and the amount of flesh. His liver and bowels had improved, and a urinalysis showed no evidence of kidney trouble. He retired from the army in 1881. In April 1882, while visiting Detroit, Michigan, he developed acute Bright's disease and died on May 14, 1882. His records contain a number of different possible causes of his death, including an embolism to the brain and chronic nephritis.[1] He was buried at Sheffield, Massachusetts.

DEATH CERTIFICATE: Cause of death, chronic encephalitis.

1. WPCHR, vols. 601, 602; RVA, Pension XC 2,685,332; U.S. Army, CWS, roll 1, vol. 1, report 1, pp. 25–30; LR, ACP, 1745, 1874, fiche: 000043.

JAMES BARNES • *Born December 28, 1801,* in Boston, Massachusetts. Graduated from the USMA in 1829. He served as an instructor at West Point until he resigned in 1836 and became a railroad engineer. Barnes was made colonel of the 18th Massachusetts in July 1861 and was appointed a brigadier general of volunteers in November 1862. After service on the Peninsula he was a brigade commander at Antietam, Fredericksburg, and Chancellorsville. He was wounded in the leg by a large piece of shell at Gettysburg on July 2, 1863; disabled, he had to relinquish command on July 4. The brigade surgeon who examined him in 1864 stated that he was still suffering from his old wound and the effects of malarial poisoning. Barnes spent the rest of war on garrison and prison duty. He was brevetted major general of volunteers in March 1865 and was mustered out the following year. In 1868 he was appointed to a United States commission that was to investigate the construction of the Union Pacific Railroad and telegraph line. Early in 1869 he developed congestion of the liver. His condition initially fluctuated in severity, but finally he became worse and died February 12, 1869, in Springfield, Massachusetts. An autopsy revealed an abscess of the liver accompanied by impaction of gallstones with complete obliteration of the duct. He was buried in Springfield Cemetery.[1]

1. *OR,* vol. 27, pt. 1:605; RVA, Pension WC 157,973; Amos M. Judson, *History of the Eighty-Third Regiment Pennsylvania Volunteers,* 137.

JOSEPH K. BARNES • *Born July 21, 1817,* in Philadelphia. Served in the Florida and Mexican wars. Barnes obtained a medical degree from the University of Pennsylvania in 1838 and joined the army medical corps in 1840. In 1862, Major Barnes was appointed acting surgeon general to replace Surgeon General W. A. Hammond. He advanced to surgeon general in August 1864 and was brevetted major general in the Regular Army in March 1865. Barnes retired in June 1882 and died soon afterward on April 5, 1883, in Washington, D.C. He was buried there in Oak Hill Cemetery. His surgeon reported that the cause of death was cirrhosis of the kidneys.[1]

1. RVA, Pension WC 200,841.

HENRY ALANSON BARNUM • *Born on September 24, 1833,* at Jamesville, New York. Before the Civil War, he was a teacher, member of the bar, and part of a local New York militia company. Enlisting at the beginning of the war, he was elected captain of a company of the 12th New York, which was at First Bull Run. He was wounded in the abdomen at Malvern Hill on July 1, 1862. A conical musket ball had entered midway between his umbilicus and the anterior-superior spinous process of the left ilium; after passing through the middle of the ilium, it emerged posteriorly. The wound was regarded as fatal, and he was left in a field hospital. The following day he was captured and taken in a wagon to Libby Prison. Thinking Barnum was dead, Col. James C. Rice wrote a glowing report about him. After learning that Barnum was alive, he said, "Well, what I lost in fact I made up in rhetoric." On July 17 Barnum was moved to Aikin's Landing in an ambulance and exchanged. He went by water to Albany and finally by rail to Syracuse, New York. At no time did he display any symptoms of peritonitis. On October 1 he went to Albany where the anterior wound was enlarged by an incision. Several fragments of the ilium were extracted from the exit wound and a tent introduced. After a month the anterior wound had healed, and he took to the field in January 1863. About the middle of March, a large abscess formed at the site of the anterior wound and spontaneously evacuated itself. The following month his surgeon again cut down to the ilium and introduced a tent. No loose bone fragments were present. From March to May 1863 he was on leave because of inflammation of his wound. At Gettysburg, although still suffering greatly, Barnum was in command of his regiment until after the close of the fight on the second day. He developed diarrhea on July 24. Emaciated and in broken health, he was taken to a private home in Washington, D.C. In August he was sent to the officers' hospital in Georgetown, D.C., and was then given a sick leave. He returned to duty on October 13. Because of his unhealed wound, he was scarcely able to march with his regiment at Lookout Mountain, Tennessee, on November 24. However, he urged his men on until a musket ball passed through his right forearm. This wound, along with his prior injuries, completely disabled him for duty, and he went on sick leave. In January 1864, another large abscess formed over the anterior abdominal entry site. When Barnum was seen by Dr. Lewis A. Sayre on January 6, he was cadaverous-looking, pale, and anemic. There was an opening above Poupart's ligament and just inside of the left anterior superior spinous process of the ilium, from which a considerable amount of pus escaped. A pocket probe was passed into the opening, which led into a sinus on the inside of the ilium. However, the probe was not long enough to reach the bottom. A zinc and lead-flexible bougie was next passed into the opening, and after a few inches it came in contact with dead bone. An opening in the ilium was detected by the probe tip, and with slight pressure the probe passed inside the opening. Once inside, the probe could not be withdrawn. It was pressed onward until the end could be felt under the gluteal muscles below the posterior superior crest of the ilium. A cut was made down to the tip of the bougie, which when pushed through this opening led to the discharge of a large amount of pus and great relief to Barnum. On his buttock below the old cicatrix at the point of the bullet's exit, there was an unhealed opening of a recent abscess near the newly made incision. Dr. Sayre flattened the end of the bougie and, using his penknife, drilled a hole in it to make an eye through which he threaded a string of oakum. The oakum string was saturated with Peruvian Balsam and drawn back through the entire canal to establish through and through drainage. The complete procedure was performed without any anesthetic per Barnum's insistence. Dr. Sayre's plan was to twist on new oakum saturated with Peruvian Balsam every day and pull it through, then cut off the soiled portion. The following morning Dr. Sayre was called to the Metropolitan Hotel in haste because Barnum was having a severe cutting pain in his buttock. Barnum, wanting to hurry his treatment, had twisted on additional oakum without making it small enough or free of knots and had pulled it forcibly through the tract. This had broken off large pieces of bone, one of which was cutting into his buttock and producing intense pain. The opening was enlarged by a star incision, and several large portions of the ilium were removed with forceps. One of the pieces was an inch and a half in length on one side of the triangle and more than half an inch at the base. This piece was a complete portion of the wing of the ilium, showing the external and internal plate, but perfectly free of its periosteum. Many other smaller pieces of bone were removed, all without their periosteum, and gave evidence of long maceration in pus. The string was worn for several weeks until a seton of candlewick was substituted, which was gradually reduced in size. Finally Dr. M. K. Hogan replaced the seton with a single linen thread. Barnum remained on sick leave and recruiting detail and did not return to command until June 1864. Although the wound continued to discharge slightly and the thread seton was still worn, he was almost continuously in the field for the remainder of the war. Medical records list him as being shot through the right forearm at Kennesaw Mountain in June 1864 and as receiving a shell wound in the side at Peach Tree Creek on July 20, 1864. After the war he received the brevets of brigadier and major general of volunteers and was also appointed full brigadier in May 1865. Barnum was seen by Dr. Sayre at intervals when there was retained pus and the opening had to be enlarged to improve drainage. The surgeon wanted to fully enlarge the openings of the wound and make sure all dead bone was removed. However, the operation was not performed since other surgeons advised that such surgery might weaken the ilium to the degree that it would be broken by even slight trauma. Dr. Sayre did not see Barnum from early 1873 until June 1874, when he was brought back in a dangerous condition because of retained pus. The wound was enlarged, several small pieces of bone were removed, and a large, perforated, india-rubber drainage tube was passed through the tract. In

August 1888 he was still wearing a large-sized, perforated drainage tube that passed clear through the tract of the wound. When the catheter was inserted it was sometimes followed by a copious flow of blood. The distance from the anterior to posterior opening was about eight inches. There was a constant discharge, and the wound had to be kept disinfected and frequently dressed. The clothing and absorbent dressing also indicated a constant discharge from both points. His general health was good but at times he suffered from blood poisoning from absorption of septic matters from the wound.[1] Barnum died January 29, 1892, in a New York City hotel and was buried in Oakwood Cemetery at Syracuse, New York.

DEATH CERTIFICATE: Chief cause, influenza-catarrhal pneumonia of eight days' duration; contributing cause, pulmonary congestion and edema of six hours' duration.

1. CSR; *OR*, vol. 11, pt. 2:321; vol. 27, pt. 1:857, 869; vol. 30, pt. 2:300; vol. 31, pt. 2:437, 448; vol. 38, pt. 2:300; *MSHW*, vol. 2, pt. 2:213, case 619; RVA, Pension SC 78,753; Eugene Arus Nash, *A History of the Forty-Fourth Regiment New York Volunteer Infantry*, 90.

WILLIAM FARQUHAR BARRY • *Born August 18, 1818,* in New York City. Graduated from the USMA in 1838. While a cadet he was treated twice for fever and once each for a headache, a sore foot, and a sore throat. Served in the Mexican and Florida wars. He was sick at Tampico, Mexico, from February to April 1847 and was on sick leave to the middle of December. He was promoted to captain of the Second Artillery in 1852. Barry was chief of artillery for Gen. Irvin McDowell at First Bull Run and then for Gen. George B. McClellan on the Peninsula. He was commissioned brigadier general of volunteers in August 1861. Barry took an active part in the Atlanta campaign (1864) and the North Georgia campaign, and served in the Carolinas until Gen. Joseph E. Johnston's surrender. He received brevet promotions, including that of major general in the volunteers and in the Regular Army. He was absent on sick leave from November 25, 1864, until January 4, 1865. In December 1865 he was commissioned colonel of the Second Artillery. The rest of his military career was spent at various frontier and artillery posts. On July 9, 1879, while at Fort McHenry at Baltimore, Barry was slightly under the weather and stated he should remain indoors to avoid the sun. His illness developed into dysentery, which during the intensely hot weather weakened him so that he failed to rally. He appeared to have improved by July 15, but on July 17 he developed a high fever and became delirious. The physician, who could not be found until the next morning, reported that the general had malarial fever and had no hope of recovery. Barry died July 18, 1879, and was buried in Forest Lawn Cemetery, Buffalo, New York. The cause of death recorded in the hospital register was exhaustion from acute bilious dysentery followed by remittent fever.[1]

1. *OR*, vol. 44:14; WPCHR, vols. 603, 604; RVA, Pension WC 185,250; U.S. Army, CWS, roll 5, vol. 9, report 3, pp. 13–21; LR, ACP 4048, 1879, fiche: 000033.

JOSEPH JACKSON BARTLETT • *Born November 21, 1834,* in Binghamton, New York. He was practicing law at the start of the Civil War and enlisted in May 1861. First elected a company captain in the 27th New York Volunteers, Bartlett was promoted to major and then, in September 1861, to colonel. Early in November he had an attack of bilious fever and obtained a sick leave, which was extended. In October 1862 he was made a brigadier general of volunteers. In November he had a twenty-day sick leave. Bartlett's first appointment as a brigadier expired in March 1863, but he was reappointed and duly confirmed the same month. In November 1863 he had an attack of acute rheumatism and the following month he had an additional sick leave. After yet another sick leave in August 1864, he rejoined his troops in October. During January and February 1865 he was on sick leave and returned to command in April. He obtained the brevet of major general near the close of the war. He had fought in every battle with the Army of the Potomac except Second Bull Run. Following his discharge from the army in January 1866, he had repeated attacks of rheumatism, some quite severe. He served as United States minister to Sweden and deputy commissioner of pensions. During a reunion of his old unit in July 1886, he had such a bad attack of rheumatism that he was confined to his room for a portion of time.[1] He died January 14, 1893, in Baltimore and was buried in the National Cemetery at Arlington, Virginia.

1. CSR; *OR,* vol. 46, pt. 2:193, 519, 741, pt. 3:894; vol. 51, pt. 1:1216; RVA, Pension SC 418,294; Richard J. Sommers, *Richmond Redeemed: Siege at Petersburg,* 356.

WILLIAM FRANCIS BARTLETT • *Born June 6, 1840,* in Haverhill, Massachusetts. A student at Harvard University at the start of the Civil War, Bartlett enlisted as a private. In August 1861, he was made captain of the 20th Massachusetts Volunteers. At Yorktown on April 24, 1862, he received a gunshot wound that destroyed the left patella and shattered the tibia for six inches below. His left thigh was amputated four inches above the knee. The same afternoon he left for Baltimore, where his mother nursed him for some weeks. Although not well enough to return to his unit, he rejoined his Harvard class and received his degree in June. In November 1862 Bartlett returned to duty and was made colonel of the 49th Massachusetts, which was sent to Louisiana. His leg gave him great pain in March 1863. In May, when his regiment was in the advance upon Port Hudson, Bartlett was told by his surgeon that he should not accompany them. However, he obtained a carriage and went anyway. The ground proved to be too rough for his artificial leg during the May 27 Port Hudson assault, and Bartlett had to go into battle on horseback, supposedly the only man on a horse. He was wounded twice. A round ball struck the joint of his left wrist, shattering the bone, while a buckshot struck the outside of his right ankle, glanced down, entered the flesh, and passed through the sole of his foot. Attempting to grasp the reins in his right hand, he fell over the head of his horse. He was taken to the rear where the ball was cut from his wrist. He was then sent to Baton Rouge by steamer. His arm became markedly inflamed and discharged profusely. Many pieces of bone were removed and water from melting ice was dropped on the wrist to decrease inflammation. Almost every day amputation was considered, but the state of Bartlett's health would not allow it. Finally, the wound healed, although the wrist was stiffened and he never fully recovered the use of the hand. He returned to duty with his arm in a sling. During the fighting in the Wilderness on May 6, 1864, he received a gunshot wound of the scalp and was sent to the hospital in the rear. The wound was treated with simple water dressings. He was appointed brigadier general of volunteers in June and returned for duty in late July. In the Battle of the Crater on July 30, 1864, Bartlett's cork and spring leg was shattered as he tried to get out of the hole using two inverted muskets as crutches. He was captured and sent to Libby Prison hospital where he contracted diarrhea, which would remain with him the rest of his life. He was exchanged in September and returned to a division command in June 1865. He received the brevet of major general in March 1865 and was mustered out in July 1866. When he was examined the next month, the left wrist was anchylosed and motion of the hand was limited to flexion and extension. The fingers of the hand could not be flexed upon the palm, and the limb was nearly useless. Following the war, Bartlett conducted business with the Tredegar Iron Works in Richmond, Virginia, before moving to Pittsfield, Massachusetts. His physician, who attended him from 1869 until his death, treated him during that period for his chronic diarrhea and neuralgia of his amputated stump. The neuralgia was very severe and caused marked spasms of the muscles of the thigh, especially of the psoas and iliacus muscles. The muscle contractions sometimes continued for several days and prevented sleep except when he was under the influence of anodynes. Bartlett became emaciated from the neuralgia and disassimilation of food resulting from the chronic diarrhea. Tubercles gradually developed in his mesentery and finally, prior to his death on December 17, 1876, were detected in the apices of both lungs.[1] He was buried in the Pittsfield Cemetery. DEATH CERTIFICATE: Immediate cause of death, consumption.

1. CSR; *OR*, vol. 38, pt. 2:437; vol. 40, pt. 3:371; RVA, Pension WC 180,847; RAGO, entry 623, "File D"; *Confederate Veteran Magazine* 3:69, 14:25 (hereafter cited as *CV*); *Southern Historical Society Papers* 33:365 (hereafter cited as *SHSP*); *MOLLUS* 12:155–71.

HENRY BAXTER • *Born on September 8, 1821,* in Sidney Plains, New York. In 1831 he moved to Jonesville, Michigan. He later spent a three-year period in California, then returned to Jonesville in 1852 where he was involved in the milling business. When the Civil War started he was made captain of a local militia company that was mustered into the 7th Michigan Volunteers. In July 1862 he was appointed a lieutenant colonel. Baxter was wounded at Antietam on September 17, 1862. A ball entered near his right femoral region and passed posteriorly to the right and back of the ilium where it remained until his death. Baxter returned on leave to his home in Michigan, where his physician examined him and reported considerable tumefaction of the parietes and cellular tissues of the abdomen. The opening of the wound was inflamed and ragged but there was no suppuration. The track of the ball passed toward the crest of the right ileum and was distinct to the touch. There was some pain in the right hip and knee and walking was painful. Baxter returned to the service and lead the assaulting boat party at Fredericksburg on December 11, 1862. During this attack a minié ball entered through the top of his left scapula and exited near the spinal column. When he was able, he went home on sick leave. Baxter was appointed brigadier general of volunteers in March, returned to duty in April 1863, and served at Gettysburg. At the Battle of the Wilderness on May 6, 1864, he was wounded by a gunshot in the left leg. The ball entered from the front and came out on the inside of the middle third of the femur. Admitted to the division field hospital, he was transferred within a week to a hospital in Washington, where his condition was complicated by diarrhea. After a leave at home, he returned late the following August and resumed command. He was brevetted major general in April 1865 and was mustered out in August of that year.[1] Except for a few years as minister resident to the Republic of Honduras, Baxter lived in Jonesville, Michigan. He died of pneumonia on December 30, 1873, in that city and was buried in Jonesville Cemetery.

1. CSR; OR, vol. 19, pt. 1:321; vol. 21:221, 262, 265, 282; vol. 25, pt. 2:229; vol. 36, pt. 1:124, 434, 540, 549, 596, 615; vol. 42, pt. 1:511; RVA, Pension WC 189,128; RAGO, entry 534.

GEORGE DASHIELL BAYARD • *Born December 18, 1835,* in Seneca Falls, New York. Graduated from the USMA in 1856. At West Point he was seen seven times for cephalalgia, four times each for catarrhus and nausea, three times for phlegmon, twice for subluxatio, and once each for clavus, odontalgia, influenza, and rheumatism. His service before the Civil War was spent on the frontier. On July 11, 1860, at Blackwater Springs, Nebraska, he was struck in the face by a Kiowa arrow. The arrowhead embedded itself in the bone, and the wound gave him intense pain for months.[1] After the start of the Civil War, he was appointed colonel of the 1st Pennsylvania Cavalry, which he led in the Shenandoah Valley. He was granted a two-week leave of absence on January 30, 1862, for the benefit of his health. The surgeon found that Bayard had an abscess of the superior maxillary bone as a consequence of the arrow injury he had received two years before. The abscess was opened and drained. In April 1862 he was appointed brigadier general of volunteers. During September he was hospitalized for thirteen days in Washington with cystitis. On December 13, 1862, while in front of a stone mansion being used for a hospital in Fredericksburg, Virginia, Bayard was mortally wounded through the thigh by a round shot. He and a friend were just rising from the ground when he was struck by the shot, which had severed a nearby officer's sword belt. The next day Bayard died, apparently from continued bleeding, at the "Mansfield" or Bernard house, which was used as a temporary hospital.[2] He was buried at Princeton, New Jersey.

1. WPCHR, vols. 608, 609; CSR of James Deshler; Averell, *William Woods Averell*, 49; Heitman, *Historical Register and Dictionary* 2:14.

2. CSR; *OR*, vol. 21:61, 92, 142, 221, 451; vol. 25, pt. 2:141, 187; U.S. Army, CWS, report of H. J. Kilpatrick, roll 2, vol. 3, report 25, pp. 677–707; RAGO, entry 534; Robert U. Johnson and Clarence C. Buel, eds., *Battles and Leaders of the Civil War* 3:136–37; George T. Stevens, *Three Years in the Sixth Corps,* 169.

GEORGE LAFAYETTE BEAL • *Born May 21, 1825,* in Norway, Maine. Prior to the war he was an agent of the Canadian Express Company and captain of a militia company, the Norway Light Infantry. Initially mustered in a three-month regiment, he was subsequently appointed colonel of the 10th Maine. During May and June 1862 he was present sick. At Antietam on September 17, 1862, a sharpshooter mortally wounded his horse and then shot Beal. The ball passed through his right thigh and lodged in the left leg. He arrived at Frederick City that afternoon but received a sick leave instead of being treated in the hospital. While on leave, he had diarrhea and, exercising in the saddle, caused the wound to break down. Beal was able to return to command on November 9. In January and February 1863, he was absent in Washington with diarrhea. When his regiment was mustered out in May, he recruited the 29th Maine, which served in the Red River campaign. A cold he contracted on the night of April 10, 1864, produced loss of hearing in his left ear. During October he was unfit for duty because of acute diarrhea. Beal was appointed a brigadier general of volunteers in November 1864 and in December was ordered to report for assignment. He was brevetted major general of volunteers in March 1865 and was mustered out in January 1866. Following the war, he was adjutant general of Maine from 1880 to 1885 and state treasurer from 1888 to 1894. Over the years the weakness and pain in his left leg increased. By October 1888, he was totally deaf in his left ear and partially deaf in the right. He died December 11, 1896, in Norway, Maine, and was buried in South Paris, Maine. Death record: Cause of death, heart disease.[1]

1. CSR; *OR*, vol. 19, pt. 1:488–89; vol. 43, pt. 2:766; RVA, Pension SC 315,923; U.S. Army, CWS, roll 6, vol. 10, report 56, pp. 555–75.

JOHN BEATTY • *Born on December 16, 1828,* near Sandusky, Ohio. Prior to the war he was engaged in banking in Cardington, Ohio, and in April 1861 he raised a company for the 3rd Ohio. He was soon made lieutenant colonel and then colonel of the regiment, which fought in West Virginia. Late in May 1862 he had a severe attack of jaundice. He was hospitalized in Nashville, Tennessee, and a change of climate was stated to be essential for his recovery. On June 5 he went home on sick leave and returned to his regiment on the twenty-seventh, although still not well. Promoted to brigadier general of volunteers in November

1862, he resigned from the army in January 1864.[1] He had served at Perryville, Stones River, Tullahoma, Chickamauga, Chattanooga, and in the relief of Knoxville. After the war, Beatty was a banker, a member of Congress from Ohio, and a writer. He died December 21, 1914, in Columbus, Ohio, and was buried in Oakland Cemetery, Sandusky. Internment card: Cause of death, heart disease.

1. CSR; John Beatty, *The Citizen Soldier*, 145–48.

SAMUEL BEATTY • *Born December 16, 1820,* in Mifflin County, Pennsylvania. Served in the Mexican War. His early life was spent in Stark County, Ohio, where he was county sheriff at the start of the Civil War. In April 1861 he was elected a company captain in the 19th Ohio Infantry and colonel of the regiment in May of that year. In November 1862 he was promoted to brigadier general of volunteers. During that year he had fought at Shiloh, Corinth, Perryville, and Stones River. He had a leave on surgeon's certificate in March 1863. During the Battle of Chickamauga on September 19, 1863, his horse fell while trying to leap over a ledge of rock. It fell over backwards and on top of Beatty. His left shoulder was dislocated when he hit the side of the bank; in addition, there was a small penetrating wound near the posterior border of the coracoid process of the scapula. After the injury was treated, he returned to his command and service at Chattanooga. For some months after the injury, there was an albuminous-looking discharge from the wound. A leave on surgeon's certificate was given to him on March 6, 1864. He was sick on May 23, and in June he received another leave on surgeon's certificate but did not leave the department. Transported in an ambulance, he continued in command during the Atlanta campaign and at Franklin and Nashville. In March 1865, while on a train near Stevenson, Alabama, he jumped from the stopped train and fell across a road tie. His left hip was severely injured, and the fall produced a right-sided inguinal hernia. Beatty, along with his surgeon, went to Knoxville for the fitting of a truss before he returned to duty. He was brevetted major general of volunteers in March 1865 and was discharged in January 1866. In January 1871, his left arm and shoulder were still almost useless. In 1877 the hernia was reduced easily by hand, but it was poorly retained by the truss. The shoulder was painful, and he usually carried the arm in a sling. Pain in his hip made him lame.[1] He died May 26, 1885, on his farm in Stark County, Ohio, and was buried in the Massillon City Cemetery.

1. *OR*, vol. 38, pt. 1:445; U.S. Army, CWS, roll 8, vol. 13, report 4, pp. 245–307; RVA, Pension SC 139, 566.

WILLIAM WORTH BELKNAP • *Born September 22, 1829,* in Newburgh, New York. After being admitted to the bar, he practiced in Keokuk, Iowa, and for two years was a member of the Iowa legislature. He was commissioned major of the 15th Iowa in December 1861. At Shiloh, on April 6, 1862, his horse was shot from under him and he was wounded but not disabled. He remained on the field and

moved along on foot. In the summer of 1862, he had chronic diarrhea and ulceration of his bowels, which was complicated by malarial fever. He was promoted to lieutenant colonel in August 1862 and colonel the following June. At
Vicksburg in June 1863 he had an attack of gout. He was made a brigadier general of volunteers in July 1864 and led a division in the Atlanta campaign, the
March to the Sea, and in the Carolinas. From January through March 1865 his
feet were so swollen that he had trouble wearing boots, and he complained of
pain in his knees and shoulders and soreness of the muscles of his lower limbs.
He was brevetted major general in March 1865. Belknap returned to Iowa after
the war and was appointed collector of internal revenue. In 1869 he became
secretary of war. A part of the period's corruption, he was impeached in 1876
and resigned before he could be convicted. He took up the practice of law in
Washington, D.C. Although he had diarrhea the rest of his life, it was not his
biggest health problem. During April and May 1886 he was treated for severe
gout of both feet. His feet were so greatly swollen that the upper parts of his
shoes had to be cut from the top to the toe. In June 1888, he had an attack of
gout and treated himself by immersing his feet and legs in cold water. His physician urged that instead he should use baths with liniment and cover his extremities in flannel. He also recommended, in addition to a raw diet, twelve
grams each of calomel, extract of colchicine acetate, extract aloes, and ipecacs,
divided into twelve pills, one of which was to be taken each hour. The medicine
apparently produced some improvement, and roller bandages were applied.
However, his shoes continued to be cut to the toes. His doctor in Keokuk decided it was an attack of acute articular rheumatism, possibly associated with
gout, for he had that diathesis. A particularly severe attack of arthritis occurred
from February through August 1890, involving both his feet, ankles, knees, el-
bows, wrists and the right hand. Belknap never fully recovered from the involvement of his right hand. During the 1890 attack, he developed a mitral
regurgitant murmur and there was albumin in his urine.[1] He died October 12,
1890, in Washington, D.C., and was buried in the Arlington National Cemetery.
DEATH CERTIFICATE: Cause of death, fatty degeneration of the heart. Duration
of last sickness, suddenly.

1. *OR*, vol. 10, pt. 1:289; RVA, Pension WC 284,336.

HENRY WASHINGTON BENHAM • *Born April 17, 1813,* in Connecticut. Graduated
from the USMA in 1837. At West Point he was seen one time each for a cold, a
headache, a sore throat, a toothache, and tonsillitis. During the Mexican War
he was wounded on February 23, 1847, while at Buena Vista. He had engineering duties prior to the Civil War and was commissioned brigadier general of
volunteers in 1861. On November 26, 1861, after service in West Virginia, he
applied for leave on a medical certificate and went to New York City. He was

arrested by order of Gen. William S. Rosecrans, who had not approved the leave. He was sick in camp at Falmouth as the result of exposure in March 1863. On April 29, while getting ready to lay the pontoon bridge over the river at Fredericksburg, he fell in a deep gully and injured his left temple, which produced considerable bleeding. In a later attack on his conduct, he was accused of being drunk when this happened, which was apparently not true. In May he was constantly exposed to the elements and had two or three very severe chills followed by malarial fever and rheumatism. At Gettysburg in July, Benham was present and under fire, but illness made him unfit for duty. Later in the fall and winter of 1863 he was often sick with the same symptoms he experienced in May. From the spring of 1864 until the end of the war he was in command of the engineer brigade of the Army of the Potomac. While at Fortress Monroe and City Point, Virginia, in May 1864, he had intermittent attacks of malaria and rheumatism. He received brevets of major general in the Regular and Volunteer Army. In March 1867 he was made colonel, Corps of Engineers. He continued having rheumatism for the rest of his life. One physician stated that it was a form of malaria probably contracted from exposure during the war. Between 1872 and 1877 he had repeated attacks of rheumatism and gout, and, during one severe episode, his weight was reduced by more than fifty pounds. However, in March 1875 he reported his health was good enough that he did not want to retire. For the last four years of his life he had frequent outbreaks of malaria and acute and chronic exacerbations of rheumatism and gout. Benham retired from active service in 1882. His heart had become weak due to degeneration of its walls and his condition was complicated by chronic interstitial nephritis and hypertrophy. His death on June 1, 1884, in New York City was due to a "complication of disorders."[1]

DEATH CERTIFICATE: Chief cause of death, fatty degeneration of the heart; contributing, asphyxia.

1. *OR*, vol. 5:669; LR, CB, roll 71, B447, 1864; WPCHR, vol. 603; Heitman, *Historical Register and Dictionary* 2:15; Gen. H. W. Benham's Narrative, pt. 1 of Narrative of Service with Army of Potomac from March 1863 to March 1864, Henry W. Benham Papers, USAMHI.

WILLIAM PLUMMER BENTON • *He was born December 25, 1828,* in New Market, Maryland. After his return from the Mexican War he completed his studies and was admitted to the bar in Indiana. He was made captain of the 8th Infantry, a three-month regiment, in April 1861 and regimental colonel in September upon the unit's reenlistment for three years. In April 1862 he was made brigadier general of volunteers and served in the Vicksburg campaign and at Mobile. He was given a sick leave from the end of May 1863 and was back by at least July. Brevetted major general in March 1865, he was mustered out in July. He returned to his law practice in Richmond, Indiana, but in 1866 went to New Orleans as an agent of the government. His death certificate does not provide a cause of death, and newspaper reports state only that he was seized with a congestive chill two weeks before he died. However, other sources have attributed his death on March 14, 1867, in New Orleans, to yellow fever.[1] He was buried in the Greenwood Cemetery in that city, but there is some question as to the possibility of his remains later being moved.

1. CSR; Death certificate; *New Orleans Times*, Mar. 15, 1867; *New Orleans Daily Picayune*, Mar. 15, 1867.

HIRAM GREGORY BERRY • *Born August 27, 1824,* in Rockland, Maine. Before the war he held a number of positions, including contractor, bank president, mayor of Rockland, and captain of the local militia company. In June 1861 he was made colonel of the 4th Maine Volunteers in time for First Bull Run. In poor health during the first week of January 1862, he was off duty for approximately five days and spent the time mostly away from his camp. Because of an injured thumb in February he had difficulty writing. During the Battle of Williamsburg on May 5, he did not have an overcoat and became drenched. Wet for thirty-six hours, he caught a bad cold. On the retreat to Malvern Hill on July 1 he was slightly wounded by a ball that severed his sword belt. A few days later he was wounded in the arm by a piece of shell and was also bruised by his horse falling on him when it was shot. Although already sick with malaria and injured, he continued on the field. By the middle of the month he was confined to his bed and did not return to duty until July 28. During this period he had a marked loss of weight, and the hair on his head and face started falling out. On August 4 he went home on sick leave; when he returned to duty in September, he was still weak and unable to undergo much exertion. Berry rapidly passed through ranks and was promoted to major general of volunteers in November 1862. That same month he reported that his health was better, but he could scarcely walk and his right arm was almost useless. The cold weather, he thought, would end his attacks of intermittent fever, but he would continue to take medicine daily to prevent a recurrence. In late December he was confined to his tent. By then all of his hair had fallen out, so he had his head shaved, and his scalp was washed daily according to his physician's instructions. He led a brigade at Fredericksburg but during February 1863 suffered severely from ague with chills and fever. He was mortally wounded on May 3, 1863, at Chancellorsville. After having a discussion with Gen. Gershom Mott, he was coming back across the road when a minié ball struck him in the arm close to the shoulder, passed downward, and lodged in his body. He died shortly afterward.[1] He was buried in Achorn Cemetery, Rockland, Maine.

1. *OR*, vol. 25, pt. 1:391, 447, 450, pt. 2:377, 569; RAGO, entry 623, "File D"; U.S. Army, CWS, report of O. M. Poe, roll 3, vol. 4, report 10, pp. 217–54; ibid., report of De Trobriand, roll 4, vol. 6, report 4, pp. 201–13; Edward K. Gould, *Major-General Hiram G. Berry*, 92, 101–2, 146, 183, 190, 192–93, 195–97, 205–6, 209, 211–12, 226–27, 235, 243–44.

DANIEL DAVIDSON BIDWELL • *Born August 12, 1819,* in Black Rock, New York. He resigned his position as police justice and enlisted as a private in the 65th New York Volunteers at the start of the war. After serving a short time with the 74th New York, he was appointed colonel of 49th New York in October 1861. He was in the Seven Days battles and at Fredericksburg, Chancellorsville, Gettysburg, and the Overland campaign. In March 1862 he was sick in Washington. From July through September 1862 he was on leave because of chronic diarrhea. During September and October of 1863 he had a continued low-grade fever with a strong tendency to the typhoid type, accompanied by extreme prostration and debility. His surgeon recommended that he have a change of climate. In August 1864 he was appointed brigadier general. On October 19, 1864, at Cedar Creek, he was knocked from his horse by a shell and was carried to an ambulance. He was admitted to the division hospital and died in a few hours.[1] He was buried in Forest Lawn Cemetery, Buffalo, New York.

1. CSR; *OR,* vol. 43, pt. 1:32, 54, 132, 196, 211, 215; RAGO, entry 534; Stevens, *Sixth Corps,* 420.

HENRY WARNER BIRGE • *Born on August 25, 1825,* in Hartford, Connecticut. A merchant in Norwich, Connecticut, when the war started, he was appointed major of the 4th Connecticut Volunteers. He resigned from this position so he could recruit the 13th Connecticut and was made its colonel in February 1862. He was at New Orleans, Port Hudson, the Red River campaign, and in the Carolinas. In September 1863 he was commissioned brigadier general of volunteers and was brevetted major general in February 1865. Birge resigned in October and engaged in cotton planting and the lumber business in Georgia. After being involved in a number of business enterprises in the West he took up residence in New York City, where he died. He had a stroke on May 30, 1888, and died June 1. He was buried in Yantic Cemetery, Norwich, Connecticut.
DEATH CERTIFICATE: Chief cause, cerebral apoplexy; contributing cause, rheumatic gout.

DAVID BELL BIRNEY • *Born May 29, 1825,* at Huntsville, Alabama. As a young man he went to live at Upper Saginaw, Michigan, which was a trading station with the Indians. However, the weather did not suit his health, and he returned to the East in the late 1840s. He was practicing law in Philadelphia when the Civil War started and was made colonel of the 23rd Pennsylvania when it became a three-year regiment. He was appointed brigadier general of volunteers in February 1862 and major general to rank from May 1863. Birney served on the Peninsula, at Fredericksburg, and at Chancellorsville. On July 2, 1863, two bullets struck him at Gettysburg but did not draw blood or cause him injury. However, he was given sick leave from July 9–29. He again had a sick leave from December 5–25. Birney received a contusion from a piece of shell at Spotsylvania on

May 12, 1864, but did not leave the field. He was under treatment for mild diarrhea from July to October but was able to function. He believed the causes for his illness were an improper diet and constant service in the saddle. Besides the diarrhea, he had symptoms of ague in September and considered asking for a leave, but duties prevented him from leaving. On October 4, 1864, his condition became worse and he remained in his tent for three days under the care of the medical director of the corps. He took to the saddle on October 7 when his presence was needed on the field; however, by that afternoon his poor condition required him to travel by ambulance. On October 9 his dysentery was so bad that the medical director felt he must be sent home. The working diagnosis was typhomalarious fever and severe dysentery. Birney reached Baltimore by boat on the tenth and Philadelphia the next day in a special railroad car. He was confused and could not remember his home address. After appearing to improve on October 18, he had severe intestinal hemorrhage that could not be stopped, and he died. His death has been attributed to a number of diseases, including malaria, but the most likely cause for at least the final sequence of events was typhoid fever. He was buried in Woodlands Cemetery in Philadelphia.[1]

DEATH CERTIFICATE: Cause of death, dysentery (contracted in camp).

1. CSR; *OR*, vol. 36, pt. 1:68, pt. 3:533; vol. 42, pt. 2:650, pt. 3:157, 275–76, 298; vol. 43, pt. 2:420; U.S. Army, CWS, roll 1, vol. 1, report 8, pp. 139–53; D. B. Birney to Gross, July 21 and Sept. 6, 1864, David Bell Birney Papers, USAMHI; Paul Steiner, "Medical-Military Studies on the Civil War. No. 3. Major General David Bell Birney, U.S.A.," *Military Medicine* 130 (1965): 606–15; Oliver Wilson Davis, *Life of David Bell Birney: Major-General United States Volunteers*, 7, 188, 220, 270, 275–78.

WILLIAM BIRNEY • *Born May 28, 1819,* on his father's plantation in Madison County, Alabama. Before the war he was a lawyer and lived in Cincinnati, Europe, and England before settling in Philadelphia. He joined the Federal Army as a captain of the 1st New Jersey and was made major of the 4th New Jersey in September 1861. Starting early in the spring of 1862, Birney was physically reduced from repeated attacks of intermittent fever and was confined to his bed the greater part of each day. However, his leave on surgeon's certificate in May was not allowed. On the Peninsula he was excused from duty for one day because of remittent fever. During the battle at Fredericksburg on September 13, 1862, he was hit twice but stayed on the field; a spent ball near his hip joint caused a severe contusion but no permanent injury. The other hit, from a shell fragment, struck him on the inside of the left foot, forward of the ankle joint. His foot was knocked out of the stirrup and he lost all muscular control over it for several days. He was treated in the field by the regimental surgeon. On December 30 he was ordered to report to Alexandria to take charge of the convalescents and stragglers. He was promoted to colonel of the 4th New Jersey in January 1863. In May he was given a surgeon's certificate because he required five days to have dental surgery. That same month he was appointed colonel of the

22nd U.S. Colored Infantry and brigadier general of volunteers. On September 1, 1864, he was admitted to a general hospital at Fort Monroe, Virginia, with chronic diarrhea and debility and given leave within a few days. He was brevetted major general in March 1865 and mustered out in August of that year. After the war, he practiced the law and was a prolific writer. Over the years his left ankle continued to be weak and painful. It particularly bothered him at night and deprived him of sleep. He was compelled to lie on his right side.[1] Birney died August 14, 1907, at Forest Glen, Maryland, and was buried in Oak Hill Cemetery, Georgetown, D.C. Burial record: Cause of death, old age.

1. CSR; U.S. Army, CWS, roll 1, vol. 2, report 2, pp. 217–20; RVA, Pension XC 2,678,874.

FRANCIS PRESTON BLAIR, JR. • *Born on February 19, 1821,* at Lexington, Kentucky. A lawyer before the war, he was also active in politics for the Union cause in Missouri and the nation. In 1860 he was elected to Congress, and in 1862 he enlisted seven regiments of troops. He was appointed a brigadier general of volunteers in August and major general in November. During the campaigns around Vicksburg in 1863, Blair received an injury to his leg from the kick of an artillery horse and also suffered from malarial poison. Initially he was confined to his tent, but since he could not receive adequate attention, he was transferred to the U.S. Van Buren Hospital located at Milliken's Bend, Louisiana. Blair commanded the 17th Corps during the Atlanta campaign, the March to the Sea, and in the Carolinas. In early 1865 he was in St. Louis, suffering great pain and nervous depression from an injury of his hand, which he received in front of Atlanta. He left the army in November 1865, practically destitute because he had spent all of his own funds for the Union. After failing as a cotton planter he returned to Missouri politics. In 1868 he was a Democratic candidate for vice president of the United States. From 1871 until 1873, when poor health forced him to retire, he was United States senator from his state. Blair died on July 9, 1875, in St. Louis and was buried there in Bellefontaine Cemetery. According to his attending physician, the cause of death was paralysis.[1]

1. RVA, Pension WC 177,303.

LOUIS (LUDWIG) BLENKER • *Born on May 12, 1812,* in Worms, Germany. In Europe he was a jeweler's apprentice, medical student, and revolutionary prior to his coming to the United States in 1849. Initially he farmed in Rockland County, New York, but at the start of the Civil War he was in business in New York City. He recruited a regiment that became the 8th New York Volunteers and was made its colonel. In August 1861 he was appointed a brigadier general of volunteers. He commanded a brigade at First Bull Run and at Cross Keys. Outside of Warrenton, Virginia, on April 6, 1862, his horse fell. Blenker was violently thrown to the ground with the horse's full weight on his side. According to his surgeon, he injured his thoracic and pelvic viscera. In spite of this, he continued on horseback to lead the division and attend to his duties. Over the next two months his surgeon advised Blenker to retire from active service, convinced that an organic injury had taken place as indicated from the almost-unremitting suffering and growing disturbance of Blenker's hepatic system.[1] Blenker was honorably discharged from the army in March 1863 and died October 31, 1863, on his farm in Rockland County. His remains were buried in Rockland Cemetery, Sparkill, New York.

1. *OR*, vol. 12, pt. 3:70–71; vol. 51, pt. 1:572; RVA, Pension Min. C 721,699.

JAMES GILLPATRICK BLUNT • *Born July 21, 1826,* in Trenton, Maine. As a boy he went to sea for five years; on his return he entered medical school. He practiced medicine in Ohio for a period and in 1856 moved to Greeley, Kansas. When the war started he commanded an irregular group, part of the "Kansas Brigade." He was appointed a brigadier general of volunteers in April 1862. His major service was at Cane Hill, Prairie Grove, Honey Springs, and in Missouri. Blunt was made a major general of volunteers in March 1863, to rank from the previous November. In late July he was sick after being in the saddle for forty-eight hours and was prostrate on the twenty-second. In August and September he had a fever that confined him to his bed for ten days in September and kept him from the saddle for even longer. He was taken to Fort Smith, Arkansas, in an ambulance and lay there in a private house for weeks. The illness affected him both physically and mentally, and he had periods of delirium and unconsciousness. Following this illness he was left with residual decreased memory, pain in his head, and insomnia. One of the physicians who treated him during this period stated that his problem was the result of a sunstroke with softening of the brain. In 1864 it was noted that Blunt confided in mere acquaintances instead of close associates and had no interest in his person or prosperity. He was discharged in July 1865. After the war he practiced medicine in Kansas, then moved to Washington, D.C. By the time he moved to Washington in 1869 he displayed impaired judgment and memory. He fell asleep during conversations and made sudden irrelevant remarks. These abnormalities were recognized by the surgeon general and others, and he was committed to St. Elizabeth's Hospital for the Insane in Washington, D.C. Here his symptoms progressed until he died July 25, 1881, and was buried at Leavenworth, Kansas.[1]

DEATH CERTIFICATE: Cause of death, primary, paresis, three years' duration; immediate, paresis with convulsions.

1. *OR*, vol. 22, pt. 2:392, 397, 472, 535, 586, 596, 666, 736; RVA, Pension WC 248,313; Paul E. Steiner, *Physician-Generals in the Civil War,* 17–21.

HENRY BOHLEN · *Born on October 22, 1810,* in Bremen, Germany. Served in the Mexican War. He was brought to the United States as a youngster and became financially successful as a liquor dealer. He helped recruit the 75th Pennsylvania Volunteers and was made its colonel in September 1861. In April 1862 he was promoted to brigadier general of volunteers. Bohlen was killed on August 22, 1862, near Freeman's Ford on the Rappahannock. Confederate troops found his body on the field still wearing the badge of a colonel, as he had not changed the insignia of rank.[1] He was buried in Laurel Hill Cemetery, Philadelphia.

1. *OR,* vol. 12, pt. 2:64, 251, 294; vol. 19, pt. 2:236.

JAMES BOWEN · *Born on February 25, 1808,* in New York City. Before the war, he was wealthy because of family money, was a railroad president, and took an active role in politics. After helping recruit a number of regiments he was made a brigadier general of volunteers in October 1862. Too old for field duty, he was made provost marshal general of the Department of the Gulf. In July 1864 he resigned and returned to New York where he took part in civic affairs. He died September 29, 1886, at Dobbs Ferry, New York, and was buried there in the Presbyterian Cemetery.

JEREMIAH TILFORD BOYLE · *Born May 22, 1818,* in what is now Boyle County, Kentucky. Before the Civil War he practiced law in Danville, Kentucky, and in November 1861 was made a brigadier general of volunteers. He was very sick on December 17, 1861. In May 1862 he took command of Federal forces in Kentucky and served with distinction at Shiloh. On March 28, 1863, he was confined to his house, too ill to see visitors. He was summarily relieved because of poor performance, and in July 1864 he resigned.[1] Returning to civilian life in Kentucky, he engaged in land speculation and the railroad business. He died July 28, 1871, in Louisville, Kentucky, and was buried at Danville.

1. *OR,* vol. 7:502; vol. 23, pt. 2:187, 190.

LUTHER PRENTICE BRADLEY · *Born December 8, 1822,* in New Haven, Connecticut. Prior to moving to Chicago in 1855, he held various commands in the Connecticut militia. He engaged in business in Chicago and served as a captain and as a lieutenant colonel of local militia. In November 1861 he was mustered into Federal service as lieutenant colonel of the 51st Illinois Volunteers and was made colonel in October 1862. During the Battle of Stones River in December he hurt his foot and "took a cold in it." He was still not able to get a boot or shoe on the foot by the first of February 1863 and had to wear an old moccasin. However, the foot was improving and he was able to ride a horse. Bradley was severely wounded in the right hip and right arm at the Battle of Chickamauga, September 19, 1863. He was absent on leave from September 25 to December 8 and joined Philip Sheridan in East Tennessee on January 1. His promotion as brigadier general of volunteers ranked from July. He was severely wounded in the left shoulder at Spring Hill, Tennessee, on November 29, 1864. His arm caused him pain day and night in late December, and even under the influence of morphine he slept poorly. He was unfit for travel, and his surgeon told him not to expect a rapid recovery. After Bradley reported for duty in March, he was ordered to serve as president of a court-martial from April 1 to May 5. He had a fall and severely injured his arm, which was quite useless and painful by May 8. The surgeons doubted that he would ever have the nervous action of the limb fully restored. Bradley remained in the army following the war and was made lieutenant colonel in July 1866 and colonel in 1879. He retired in November 1886.[1] He died in Tacoma, Washington, on March 13, 1910, and was buried in Arlington National Cemetery.

DEATH CERTIFICATE: Cause of death, cerebral hemorrhage of five days' duration, with senility; contributory, exhaustion.

1. *OR*, vol. 30, pt. 1:579, 581; vol. 45, pt. 1:114, 123, 269; RVA, Pension WC 706,626; U.S. Army, CWS, roll 4, vol. 7, report 49, pp. 837–45; Bradley to Buel, Feb. 1, 1863, Dec. 20, 1864; Bradley to mother, May 8, 1865, Bradley Family Letters, Luther P. Bradley Papers, USAMHI.

EDWARD STUYVESANT BRAGG • *Born February 20, 1827,* in Unadilla, New York. After obtaining an education in the legal field, he moved to Wisconsin where he practiced law and engaged in politics. When the Civil War started he was elected captain of a company that was made part of the 6th Wisconsin Volunteers. During the summer of 1862 he had an episode of erysipelas. Bragg was wounded in the left arm at Antietam on September 17, 1862. Two men bundled him into a shelter tent and hurried him to the rear. Although unfit for duty, he came back on the field about noon. In March 1863 he was appointed colonel. On May 29, 1863, near White Oak Church, he was kicked on the foot by a horse. He remained in his tent but by the first week of June had to go to Washington because his foot had become much worse. On the evening of July 8 he returned to duty but at the end of the month he had to go home because he could not endure the hot sun. He returned to camp on August 28. His promotion to brigadier general of volunteers ranked from June 1864. Following the war he returned to Wisconsin and politics. He served in Congress, as minister to Mexico, and as consul general at Hong Kong. A few months before he died, he was visited by a former soldier, who found him shrunken and sick in bed. On June 19, 1912, he suffered a paralytic stroke from which he never regained consciousness.[1] Died June 20, 1912, at Fond du Lac, Wisconsin, where he was also buried.

1. *OR*, vol. 19, pt. 1:248–49, 255; RVA, Pension WC 747,465; *MOLLUS* 3:256; Rufus R. Dawes, *Service with the Sixth Wisconsin Volunteers,* 89, 93, 146, 149, 185, 193, 201; *Fond du Lac Daily Reporter,* June 20, 1912.

JOHN MILTON BRANNAN • *Born July 1, 1819,* in Washington, D.C. Graduated from the USMA in 1841. He was treated at the Cadet Hospital twice each for headache and nausea and once each for sore feet, pain in groin, an inflamed eye, and back pain. Brannan was severely wounded during the fighting at Chapultepec on September 13, 1847. He was appointed brigadier general of volunteers in September 1861. During the war he commanded infantry and artillery troops in the Tullahoma campaign, at Chickamauga, at Chattanooga, and in the Atlanta campaign. At the end of the war he was brevetted major general in the regular and volunteer service and returned to the rank of major of the First Artillery. From March to May 1880 he was on leave, suffering from a malarial attack. According to his surgeon, he had malarial intercostal neuralgia, which had started in February. He had a similar attack with rheumatism from December 1880 through September 1881. Brannan was on court-martial duty and under treatment in New York City until June 1881 and on sick leave until he retired as a colonel in 1882. He died on December 16, 1892, in New York. According to his surgeon, his death was due to a condition from which Brannan had suffered for the past fourteen years. Brannan had gone out for a short walk and appeared well on his return. He went to his bedroom and a few minutes later was found by his servant lying dead across his bed. According to the attending surgeon, the cause of death was neuralgia of the heart.[1]

1. WPCHR, vol. 604; RVA, Pension WC 405,762; LR, ACP, 218, 1881, fiche: 000035; Heitman, *Historical Register and Dictionary* 2:16.

MASON BRAYMAN • *Born May 23, 1813,* in Buffalo, New York. After being an editor of various newspapers at a relatively young age, he became a lawyer and practiced in Michigan and Illinois. He enlisted at the start of the Civil War and in August 1861 was commissioned major of the 19th Illinois Volunteers. He fought at Belmont, Fort Donelson, and Shiloh. During the summer of 1862 he had a sunstroke. His appointment as brigadier general of volunteers ranked from September 1862. He suffered a similar sunstroke the last day of May 1863. That night, although unable to sit up, he followed his command. The next day, unable to proceed, he received a leave on surgeon's certificate. As soon as he was able, he went to his home in Illinois. In July 1863 he was assigned the command of the depot for drafted men at Camp Dennison, Ohio.[1] Brevetted major general at the end of the war, he moved extensively over the remaining years of his life. He lived in Missouri, Arkansas, the Idaho Territory, and Wisconsin. Brayman died February 27, 1895, at Kansas City and was buried at Ripon, Wisconsin.

1. *OR*, vol. 39, pt. 2:169; U.S. Army, CWS, roll 1, vol. 1, report 15, pp. 217–49.

HENRY SHAW BRIGGS • *Born on August 1, 1824,* in Lanesboro, Massachusetts. Prior to the war, he was a lawyer and politician. He was the captain of a local militia company and served in a three-month regiment before he was mustered in as colonel of the 10th Massachusetts in June 1861. A hypochondriac, Briggs was also a compulsive letter writer to his wife, and his letters to her throughout his period of service are filled with details of his health, diet, and treatment. During the summer of 1861 he had fatigue, diarrhea, and a recurring sore throat for which he wore a flannel wrap. Riding into camp on July 29, 1861, he was injured when a sharp stump hit his knee, which he bound with bandages he was carrying. Briggs received a flesh wound in both thighs at Seven Pines on May 31, 1862. Two musket balls had struck him simultaneously; one passed through the under part of the left leg and one lodged in the right thigh. Disabled, he had to be carried to the rear. He was taken by sea to Boston and then to his home. Briggs was appointed a brigadier general of volunteers to rank from July 1862. On January 19, 1863, he was ordered to report to duty at Baltimore as soon as his health would permit. It is of interest that after he returned he continued to write about his poor health but made no reference to any difficulties stemming from his wounds. During April 1863, while in Baltimore, a pain in his side caused him to worry about his liver, and he treated a persistent headache with medicine he had on hand after consulting his medical book. More medicine was sent to him from his family doctor, and he expressed concern that he did not think he could endure an active campaign. In August 1863 he was assigned to division command. In February 1864, while in Alexandria, Virginia, Briggs had severe spasms in his side. He put a hot-water bag to his feet and drank a pint or so of hot water. Also, he took a cup or two of graham crackers in the morning before getting up, then partook of beef tea and another cup of tea and crackers. After taking some saccharum and gelseminum that his doctor had sent, he also took some medicine that he had obtained in Boston and had carried in his bag for the last two and a half years. Starting in October 1864, most of his remaining service was spent on general court-martial duty in Washington, D.C. He had continued pains in the left and upper part of his stomach in October and November 1864, which he thought were like "wind pains." Pulvis china (cinchonae), something he had taken the previous winter, was prescribed. He was quite sick the first part of December with the pain and his bowels which were quite torpid. Magnesiae carbonas worked well as a mild cathartic. He continued to take his syrup regularly along with occasional cathartics, and he also fixed a cold compress on the sore spot as recommended by his doctor. He covered a folded napkin with a piece of a patent poultice preparation and an old piece of silk and then covered it all with his flannel band. The last of December and throughout January 1865 Briggs again had a sore throat and developed a severe cold. He thought he may have to stop his syrup because he was having too many bowel movements. The surgeon recommended he take ipecac and belladonna, to use cold compresses on his throat and chest at night, and to bathe the areas with cold water in the mornings. For his cold, he took a medication he obtained from his druggist in addition to powders, ale, and his old regular, the syrup. In March 1865 one of his syrup bottles exploded, so he took salt and whiskey before breakfast, unable to obtain good brandy. In late April his doctor thought he had damaged his stomach by eating so much shad and recommended he eat principally meat, bread, and no vegetables. Throughout the summer he had fewer symptoms. Another bottle of the syrup popped and fizzed in September, and by October he was considering stopping the syrup, since he had taken at least a gallon of it. He also wrote that although he had not commented on his stomach much in recent letters, the condition was on his mind almost all of the time. Displaying more insight into his problem, Briggs wrote that he believed his worst affliction was "stomach on the brain" and said, "I am ashamed of it now that I have spent so much time and ink on the subject but bottles (of tea) (and syrup) led me into it."[1] He was mustered out of service in December 1865 and returned to Massachusetts. For the last years of his life he was an appraiser at the Boston Custom House. Briggs died at Pittsfield, Massachusetts, on September 23, 1887, and was buried in that city.

DEATH CERTIFICATE: Immediate cause of death, heart disease.

1. CSR; *OR*, vol. 11, pt. 1:881, 906, 910, 912; vol. 21:981; vol. 51, pt. 1:1084; H. S. Briggs to Molly, May 1, 1861 (Letter Book of personal letters to his wife); July 31, Aug. 1, 1861, Apr. 11, 17, 30, 1863 (Personal letters written while Col. 10th Mass. Inf. Regt.); Feb. 2, 12, 1864 (Personal letters written while a General, Aug. 23, 1863–Feb. 12, 1864); Oct. 8, Nov. 29, Dec. 3, 7, 8, 10, 11, 17, 21, 25, 1864 (Personal letters written while on General Court-Martial Duty in Washington, D.C., Oct. 3–Dec. 31, 1864); Jan. 12, 15, Feb. 27, Mar. 6, 17, 1865 (Personal letters written while on General Court-Martial Duty Jan. 1–Mar. 31, 1865); Apr. 27, May 2, 12, 1865 (Personal letters written while on General Court-Martial Duty, Apr. 2–July 29, 1865); Sept. 9, 29, Oct. 2, 1865 (Personal letters written while on General Court-Martial Duty, Aug. 1–Nov. 4, 1865), all in Henry S. Briggs Papers, USAMHI.

JAMES SANKS BRISBIN • *Born on May 23, 1837*, in Boalsburg, Pennsylvania. A teacher at the start of the Civil War, he enlisted as a private. In April 1861 he was made a second lieutenant in the 1st U.S. Cavalry. At the Battle of Bull Run, July 21, 1861, he was struck in the side by a shell fragment and was so severely wounded that his men had to carry him off the field. He was taken back to nearby Centreville, but when he heard that the army was being defeated, he led his cavalry to fight. However, he was soon shot through the arm. In the retreat towards Centreville, he formed a line across the road at the side of old Germantown to try to stop the fleeing Federal troops. A fight ensued when a Federal lieutenant colonel attempted to force the line. Brisbin was knocked down and severely cut in the shoulder by a saber. On arrival at Arlington, he turned over command of his troops because of his wounds and went to Washington. Unable to get a pass to leave the city, he was taken care of at the home of Gen. Montgomery C. Meigs by the family physician. Brisbin finally went home to

Harrisburg where he was confined to bed for many weeks. Following recovery, he reported to his regiment in October 1861 and was sent to Ohio on recruiting duty. While leading a charge at Beverly Ford on June 9, 1862, he was thrown from his horse and temporarily disabled. From September 19 to November 10 and from June 23 to July 1,1863, he was absent on sick leave. While engaged in a skirmish at Greenbrier, Virginia, on July 26, 1863, he was shot through the calf of the leg. Because of the wound he had a disability leave from July 29 to November. At Sabine Cross Roads, Louisiana, on April 8, 1864, a shell took off his horse's head, and its body fell on Brisbin's right foot, crushing it. Following his promotion through grades he was made a brigadier in May 1865. After the war he remained in the army and was promoted to major in 1868, but his career seemed to consist of one illness after another. The foot injury from Sabine Cross Roads remained painful in February 1866. From December 1, 1868, to May 5, 1869, he was treated for rheumatism. In May 1871 he took a leave on certificate of disability and returned to his post in September. He was treated for an abscess from March 14–18, 1872. Epidemic catarrhal fever prompted hospital admission at Station Custer from January 20–22, 1874, and from January 24 to February 1875. Later in February he was admitted again for five days, and then beginning in September he began a 108-day admission for bronchitis and indigestion. While commanding in the field in Montana during April 1877 he was ordered to return to the post for health reasons and was not back in the field until July. He was under treatment for erysipelas from May 1–23, 1882. Brisbin was sick at Fort Robinson, Nebraska, from July 21 to October 1, 1888, with cerebral congestion. This produced paralysis of the left side of his face and tongue and the right side of his body, including his leg and arm. There was paralysis of motion only, and within a short time he improved and returned to duty. From November 12–27, 1888, he was treated for inflammation of the bladder and of the right testicle. In 1889 he was promoted to colonel of the 1st Cavalry. Late in January 1890, he had epidemic catarrh that relapsed. The relapse was complicated by chronic bronchitis and prompted a ninety-one day hospital admission. He returned to duty February 7, 1890, improved, but the bronchitis was still troublesome. He again had sick leave from September 29, 1890, to April 1, 1891, because of chronic bronchitis and indigestion. Although sick, in January he requested to go to Philadelphia to have a wart taken off his face. Soon after his return he left again and was gone from May 31 to June 30, 1891, because of chronic bronchitis. He spent most of the night of January 7, 1892, in transit on a railroad car and awoke about two o'clock A.M. with severe vomiting and a chill. Brisbin arrived at the Lafayette Hotel in Philadelphia and was treated by a physician, who made a diagnosis of grippe with severe and general acute bronchitis. Brisbin's temperature was 104°. After treatment his dry cough and fever improved. However, he developed jaundice, which persisted to the end of his life, and erysipelas of the nose, which spread over his face, head, ears, and sublingual glands.[1] He died January 14, 1892, and was buried at Red Wing, Minnesota.

DEATH CERTIFICATE: Cause of death, erysipelas.

1. RVA, Pension Min. C 405,387; U.S. Army, CWS, roll 4, vol. 6, report 5, pp. 215–55; LR, ACP, 2127, 1875, fiche: 000023.

JOHN RUTTER BROOKE • *Born on July 21, 1838,* in Montgomery County, Pennsylvania. Brooke entered the Civil War as captain of a three-month regiment and in November 1861 was made colonel of the 53rd Pennsylvania. The end of his right index finger was shot off at Fair Oaks, Virginia, on June 1, 1862. Brooke commanded a brigade at Antietam, Fredericksburg, and Chencellorsville. At Gettysburg on July 2, 1863, he was bruised on the left ankle and had great difficulty monitoring the enemies' activities. During September he had thirty days leave on certificate of disability. The following winter he commanded a convalescent camp at Harrisburg and was appointed brigadier general of volunteers to rank from May 1864. He was severely wounded during the assault at Cold Harbor on June 3, 1864, and was carried from the field insensible. He served on a general court-martial and in November was to report for assignment to light duty in December. In March 1865 he was assigned to take command of troops in the Shenandoah Valley.[1] He remained in the army and was appointed a lieutenant colonel in July 1866. After passing through ranks he was commissioned major general in 1897. He took part in the Puerto Rican campaign under Gen. Nelson A. Miles and was military governor, first of Puerto Rico and then of Cuba. He retired in July 1902. Brooke died in Philadelphia on September 5, 1926, and was buried in Arlington National Cemetery.

1. *OR,* vol. 27, pt. 1:369, 401; vol. 36, pt. 1:88, 167, 345, 414, 417; vol. 42, pt. 3:616; vol. 46, pt. 2:933; vol. 51, pt. 1:1192; U.S. Army, CWS, roll 6, vol. 10, report 37, pp. 299–313.

WILLIAM THOMAS HARBAUGH BROOKS • *Born January 28, 1821,* in Lisbon, Ohio. Graduated from the USMA in 1841. He served in the Florida and Mexican wars. Brooks developed a urethral stricture while in Mexico and, as a result, was in poor health on his return to the East in 1848. In 1855, following continued symptoms, he was advised to have surgery for a "radical cure." He returned to duty in 1856, but his urinary tract problem was not corrected. In March 1857 he was examined by a medical faculty member from Philadelphia and his prescriptions were administered by one of Brooks's army doctor friends in New York. It was a slow and tedious process, and the remedies themselves caused one or two severe attacks with chills and fevers. In order to be near his doctor he moved into his hotel. He arrived in Indianapolis on May 5, 1857, improved and full of hope. He was trying homeopathy in connection with allopathy surgery (when diseases are treated by producing a condition incompatible with or antagonistic to the condition to be cured or alleviated). On September 3, 1858, he wrote from Fort Defiance that he had not been able to go out on campaign. For the previous three weeks he had been troubled with his old complaints, which caused chills and fevers, sometimes twice a day. He went on an extended sick leave from 1858 to 1860. In May 1861, he had to leave his regiment for another operation and was absent for four months. He was appointed brigadier general of volunteers in September 1861. At Savage's Station on the night of June 29, 1862, he was wounded in the leg but continued with his duties. The ball had hit him on the underside of the thigh just above the knee, causing enough injury for it to be called a wound. A musket ball slightly wounded him in the face on September 17, 1862, during the battle of Antietam. He was a division commander at Fredericksburg, Chancellorsville, and Petersburg. He resigned in July 1864 because of continued poor health. After leaving the service, he resided on a farm near Huntsville, Alabama. Brooks continued having difficulties with his urethral stricture; there was an uncontrollable discharge of pus and the development of secondary kidney and bladder problems. Between the time he arrived in Alabama and August 1867 he had lost thirty pounds, so his weight was about 162 pounds, less than he had weighed when he left West Point. He died July 19, 1870, on the farm near Huntsville the result of a urinary tract infection secondary to the stricture, according to his wife.[1] Brooks was buried in Maple Hill Cemetery at Huntsville.

1. *OR*, vol. 11, pt. 2:50, 431, 464; vol. 19, pt. 1:377, 403, pt. 2:446; vol. 37, pt. 2:192; vol. 40, pt. 1:211, pt. 3:144, 177, 272; U.S. Army, CWS, roll 1, vol. 1, report 12, pp.179–84; RVA, Pension Old War file 27,687; W. T. H. Brooks to ———, Mar. 29, May 6, 1857, W. T. H. Brooks to father, Sept. 3, 1858 (New Mexico and Indianapolis letters), W. T. H. Brooks to father, July 8, 1862, Aug. 26, 1867 (Civil War letters), William H. T. Brooks Papers, USAMHI; Paul E. Steiner, "Medical-Military Studies on the Civil War. No. 1. Lieutenant General Ambrose Powell Hill, C.S.A.," *Military Medicine* 130 (1965): 225–28.

EGBERT BENSON BROWN • *Born October 4, 1816,* in Brownsville, New York. Brown sailed halfway around the world on a whaler as a young man before settling down in Toledo, Ohio, and becoming a grain dealer. After moving to St. Louis in 1852, he took up the railroad business. Initially a lieutenant colonel in the 7th Missouri Volunteers and a brigadier general of militia troops, he was appointed a brigadier general of volunteers to rank from November 1862. He was severely wounded near his left shoulder at Springfield, Missouri, on January 8, 1863, and the arm was totally disabled. Brown had been shot from a nearby residence while leading a charge of his bodyguard. He fell from his horse and, although able to remount, was unable to remain in the saddle and had to be carried off. The ball had entered the left arm four inches below the apex of the shoulder and struck the surgical neck of the humerus. The long head of the biceps was severed and the ball passed upwards and backwards, splintering the shaft and fracturing the head of the humerus. The projectile then struck the lower edge of the glenoid cavity of the scapula, which it also fractured, and finally lodged just back of the neck of the scapula. Forty-eight hours after the injury an excision was performed. The initial incision was V-shaped, and the head of the humerus and shaft of the bone, measuring five inches in all, and a small portion of the anterior surface of the scapula were removed. The wound had healed by granulation by the last of January and was closed except for a small opening that discharged moderate amounts of pus. The injured limb gradually shortened, eventually measuring two inches less than the other. Five weeks after the battle, he journeyed from Springfield to Sedalia, Missouri, on horseback, holding the reins in his good hand. Relieved of his command, he was on disability leave from February 2 until June 10, 1863, when he assumed command of the district of Central Missouri. Continued difficulties with his wound required another sixty days' leave on surgeon's certificate on July 20. Another person was temporarily assigned to the command of the Central District of Missouri in November because Brown was ill. Brown arrived at Warrensburg, Missouri, on May 29, 1864. During the fall of 1864 he was continuously in the saddle and in command of his brigade. Because of his disability, he was relieved from duty in April 1865 and ordered to report for assignment to such duty as the state of his health would permit. He resigned his commission in 1865. Following the war he was pension agent at St. Louis, a farmer in Illinois, and a member of the state board of equalization. In January 1866 his arm was useless. By November 1870, however, he had regained the functional use of the arm and was able to chop wood, play billiards, and use his fowling piece. However, a pension examination by two physicians in September 1873 reported that because of the deformity of the arm and the loss of power, he was totally disabled for manual work.[1] He died February 11, 1902, at West Plains, Missouri, and was buried in Cuba, Missouri.

1. *OR*, vol. 22, pt. 1:181, 185–86, pt. 2:716; vol. 34, pt. 4:113; vol. 41, pt. 2:571; vol. 49, pt. 2:384; *MSHW*, vol. 2, pt. 2:522, case 1495; U.S. Army, CWS, roll 2, vol. 3, report 18, pp. 517–83; RVA, Pension SC 65,018.

ROBERT CHRISTIE BUCHANAN • *Born March 1, 1811,* in Baltimore, Maryland. Graduated from the USMA in 1830. Served in the Black Hawk War of 1831–32 and the Florida and Mexican wars. Prior to the Civil War he had earned the brevet of lieutenant colonel and served on garrison and recruiting duty. His regiment defended Washington, D.C., until the spring of 1862, and he was appointed brigadier general of volunteers to rank from November of that year. He served on the Peninsula, at Antietam, and at Fredericksburg. While appearing in Washington as a witness in January 1863, he developed severe rheumatism under his right kneecap. In March he received permission to remain an additional fifteen days in Washington under treatment. His appointment as general expired in March without congressional confirmation, and he assumed command of the defenses of Fort Delaware. He became a colonel in 1864 and at the end of hostilities was brevetted brigadier and major general. Buchanan remained in the army after the war. He had sick leave from August 25 to December 1, 1865. When he retired from the army on December 31, 1870, he bore all the external traces of his declining years and as one who "has had organic changes in every tissue of his body." He died November 29, 1878, in Washington, D.C., and was buried in Rock Creek Cemetery. The attending surgeon listed the cause of his death as serous apoplexy, which he defined as an effusion of serum in the ventricles of the brain and at the base of the brain.[1]

1. U.S. Army, CWS, roll 1, vol. 2, report 9, pp. 93–98; RVA, Pension WC 191,614.

CATHARINUS PUTNAM BUCKINGHAM • *Born March 14, 1808,* in what is now Zanesville, Ohio. Graduated from the USMA in 1829. He resigned from the army in 1831 and, after teaching for a few years, became the proprietor of an ironworks in Ohio. Early in the Civil War, he held various state military posts in Ohio until his appointment as brigadier general of volunteers in July 1862. He resigned in February 1863 and returned to private business. Buckingham was involved in the grain business in New York and Chicago. He died August 30, 1888, at his home in Chicago, Illinois, and was buried in Woodlawn Cemetery at Zanesville.

RALPH POMEROY BUCKLAND • *Born January 20, 1812,* but it is uncertain as to whether he was born in Leyden, Massachusetts, or in Ravenna, Ohio. Buckland had a varied career before the war as a lawyer and politician and joined the Federal cause as colonel of the 72nd Ohio Volunteers in January 1862. He commanded a brigade at Shiloh and was appointed brigadier general of volunteers in July 1862. On July 1863, while at Vicksburg, he received a leave for twenty days because of a severe attack of fever. On September 25 his horse became frightened, reared, and fell backward. Buckland sustained a fracture of his right forearm, and his right hip and side were badly bruised. The fracture involved the wrist joint and was associated with marked displacement of the bone fragments. He had also sustained a severe shock, and there was extensive ecchymosis of his body. It was impossible to determine if any internal organs were injured. The injury to his arm was further complicated by severe and protracted inflammation, and the extremity was useless and the source of severe pain for a long time. His recovery was very slow, and on January 25, 1864, he was ordered to assume command of the district of Memphis. In January 1865 he resigned his commission and accepted a seat in Congress. After the war he often consulted his family doctor in regard to his right side and hip. His suffering was so continuous and severe that several other physicians were consulted. Following an examination it was proposed that his problem was due to a traumatic aneurysm from his abdominal injury. Buckland never had full use of his right hand again.[1] He died May 27, 1892, at Fremont, Ohio, and was buried there in the Oakwood Cemetery.

DEATH CERTIFICATE: Cause of death, aneurysm.

1. U.S. Army, CWS, roll 5, vol. 8, report 17, pp. 677–717; RVA, Pension SC 404,669.

DON CARLOS BUELL • *Born on March 23, 1818,* in what is the present-day city of Lowell, Ohio. Graduated from the USMA in 1841. Only two visits to the Cadet Hospital were recorded for him: one for bile and one for headache. Served in the Florida and Mexican wars. During the Mexican War on August 20, 1847, at Churubusco, Buell climbed to the top of an adobe house to get a better view, was shot in the shoulder, and fell from his perch. Everyone gave him up for dead. Since the bullet had not hit anything vital and Buell was in good physical condition, he recovered well and was back on duty at the end of six weeks. In 1855 he was on the river steamboat *Kate Kearney* when the boiler blew up. He helped save a number of passengers and was badly burned. Buell was commissioned brigadier general of volunteers in May 1861 and promoted to major general in March 1862. Buell was at Perryville on October 7, 1862, trying to get some men to rejoin their regiments. One of them seized his horse's bridle, causing the horse to rear up and fall over backwards. Severely bruised and unable to sit up or ride, Buell had to supervise his troops from a hospital wagon the next day. He was relieved of command on October 24, mustered out of volunteer service in May 1864, and resigned his regular commission in June.[1] After returning to civilian life he operated an ironworks and coal mine in Kentucky. He died November 19, 1898, near Paradise, Kentucky, and was buried in Bellefontaine Cemetery, St. Louis.

1. WPCHR, vol. 604; James Robert Chumney, Jr., "Don Carlos Buell, Gentleman General" (diss.), 4, 168–69; Glenn Tucker, *Hancock the Superb,* 48–49; Heitman, *Historical Register and Dictionary* 2:16; Daniel Marsh Frost, "Memoirs of Gen. D. M. Frost," typescript, Missouri Historical Society.

JOHN BUFORD • *Born March 4, 1826,* in Woodford County, Kentucky. Graduated from the USMA in 1848. He was treated twice for colica and once each for symptoms of ague, odontalgia, catarrhus, diarrhea, rash, and fever intermittent at West Point. After active service on the frontier, he had duty in various positions following the start of the Civil War and was commissioned a brigadier general to rank from July 1862. At Second Bull Run in August 1862, a spent ball struck his knee. He was a staff officer at Antietam and Fredericksburg and commanded a division of cavalry at Gettysburg. On August 2, 1863, he felt worthless. On November 18 he had a touch of rheumatism. For days he could not mount his horse without help, but once mounted was able to remain in the saddle all day. He contracted typhoid fever during the Rappahannock campaign in the autumn of 1863. He died from the disease on December 16, 1863, in Washington, D.C., and received his commission as major general of volunteers on his deathbed.[1]

1. *OR*, vol. 27, pt. 3:827; WPCHR, vols. 605, 606; Theodore Lymon, *Meade's Headquarters, 1863–1865*, 50; RVA, Pension C 27,614; "John Buford Memoir," John Gibbon Papers, Historical Society of Pa., Philadelphia, Pa.; Myles W. Keogh, "Etat de Service of Major Gen. Jno. Buford from his promotion from Brig. Gen'l to his death," Cullum Files, Special Collections, U.S. Military Academy Library, West Point, N.Y.

NAPOLEON BONAPARTE BUFORD • *Born on January 13, 1807,* in Woodford County, Kentucky. Graduated from the USMA in 1827. He resigned his commission in 1835 and became a civil engineer. In 1843 he moved to Rock Island, Illinois, and was a merchant and railroad president. He recruited the 27th Illinois at the start of the Civil War and was appointed colonel of the unit. Buford served at Belmont, Island No. 10, Corinth, and Vicksburg. He was made a brigadier general of volunteers in April 1862. On September 3 he applied for a sick leave. Early the next month his health was still poor from the climate and on the twelfth he obtained a twenty-day leave of absence. When he returned he reported to Washington for court-martial duty. In July 1864 he had diarrhea and headaches, which his surgeon attributed to deranged action of his liver and innervation. Early the next month he obtained a sick leave. Restored to health, he returned to duty by the end of September. On February 15, 1865, he reported that he had been in the South for the previous four summers and at Helena, Arkansas, considered an unhealthy post, for the last seventeen months, both of which seriously affected his health. He asked to be moved to a better climate and in March was given leave to go home. On the seventeenth he was delayed at St. Louis for treatment of his general condition and an acute inflammation of his eyes.[1] Mustered out of the military in August 1865, he held a number of Federal appointments as a civilian. Buford died March 28, 1883, in Chicago and was buried at Rock Island, Illinois.

1. CSR; *OR*, vol. 17, pt. 2:575; vol. 41, pt. 1:190, pt. 2:635, pt. 3:502; vol. 48, pt. 1:856, 1067; U.S. Army, CWS, roll 1, vol. 2, report 21, pp. 243–61; LR, CB, B45, 1863.

STEPHEN GANO BURBRIDGE • *Born August 19, 1831,* in Scott County, Kentucky. After practicing the law and being a farmer he was made colonel of the 26th Kentucky (Union) Infantry in August 1861. He served at Shiloh, Arkansas Post, and Vicksburg. Because his health had been exceedingly bad for the previous three months and he was unable to do his duty, he tendered his resignation to take effect May 1, 1862. Although he had returned home during this time to recuperate, he was still so debilitated that he was unable to assume command of his regiment. His surgeon certified that Burbridge had been afflicted with dyspepsia and a chronic sore throat for six weeks and was growing worse daily.

He felt a transfer to a better climate would help. His promotion as brigadier general of volunteers ranked from June 1862. Following a sick leave from July 4 to September 17, 1863, he assumed division command on September 20. In May and September 1864 he suffered with rheumatism and numbness of his feet and legs after several days of being exposed to a drenching rain. He resigned his commission in December 1865.[1] His administration of Kentucky during the war made him a postwar outcast in his state. Over the years he continued to suffer from rheumatism. He died on November 30, 1894, in Brooklyn, New York, and was buried in Arlington National Cemetery.

DEATH CERTIFICATE: Cause of death, cardiac valvular disease, cardiac syncope.

1. CSR; *OR*, vol. 26, pt. 1:319, 710; RVA, Pension WC 418,263.

HIRAM BURNHAM • *Born in Narraguagus (now Cherryfield)*, Maine, but the exact date is not known. Prior to the war he held a number of positions, including coroner. He was mustered into Federal service as colonel of the 6th Maine. Burnham was on the Peninsula and at Antietam, Fredericksburg, and Petersburg. He was absent on sick leave twice, in July and August 1862 and in January and February 1863. The last leave was due to chronic diarrhea. His commission as brigadier general of volunteers ranked from April 1864, at which time he was ordered to report at Yorktown. On September 29, 1864, during the assault on Fort Harrison, Burnham was wounded in the abdomen by a musket ball and survived for only a few moments.[1]

1. CSR; *OR*, vol. 33:939; vol. 42, pt. 1:799.

WILLIAM WALLACE BURNS • *Born on September 3, 1825*, in Coshocton, Ohio. Graduated from the USMA in 1847. He was treated three times for cephalalgia and once each for contusio and diarrhea at West Point. During the Mexican War he was on recruiting service. He had garrison duty until the beginning of the Civil War and was commissioned brigadier general of volunteers in September 1861. During the Seven Days battles he suffered from rheumatism in the back of his neck and shoulders. He always had a silk handkerchief around his neck to protect him from the elements, yet with every change in the weather complained of pain. Although wounded in the right cheek by a minié ball at Savage's Station, Virginia, on June 29, 1862, he continued in the field with his face bound in a handkerchief. The next day, during the Battle of Glendale, he was thrown from his horse as it jumped a concealed ditch, and his neck and back were injured. The facial wound would not heal, so he was sent to Philadelphia for treatment. The injury was cauterized every other day and then twice a week. The following month he was confined to the bed with his wound, malaria, and the effects of the constant strain. He joined his command on October 8 at Harpers

Ferry and commanded a division at Fredericksburg. In March 1863 he resigned his volunteer commission and reverted to his staff rank of major. After the Civil War he remained in the army and served in the commissary service until his retirement in September 1889. In January 1869, while on duty in New York, he had several severe attacks of rheumatism and had a civilian doctor take care of him. Although confined to his home, he remained on duty and had papers brought daily to his bedside for his signature. Several years prior to his retirement, he developed shortness of breath when ascending stairs. In the spring of 1871 he had another attack of rheumatism and was confined to his room for three months. The last ten years of his life he suffered from a cold feeling and pain at the base of his skull and along his spine. He would clasp his hands together at the back of his neck and say, "It's too cold," and the warmth of his hands lessened the pain. On the day of his death, April 18, 1892, at Beaufort, South Carolina, he complained of rheumatism in the back of his neck, and his daughter draped her fur cape around him when they returned from a walk. About midnight he was found lying on the floor in his bedroom. He was lifted onto a nearby bed, and mustard leaves were placed on his wrists and on the pit of his stomach. When the doctor arrived he was dead. A coroner's inquest was held and the cause of death was ruled to be apoplexy.[1] He was buried in Arlington National Cemetery.

1. *OR*, vol. 11, pt. 2:82, 90–93; RVA, Pension WC 379,914; U.S. Army, CWS, roll 1, vol. 2, report 27, pp. 425–32; *Battles and Leaders* 2:374; Coroners' Inquisitions Book, 1888–93, pp. 323–25, Beaufort, S.C.

AMBROSE EVERETT BURNSIDE • *Born May 23, 1824,* at Liberty, Indiana. Graduated from the USMA in 1847. While at West Point, he was treated for contusio four times, diarrhea three times, colica twice, and once each for nausea, morbi. varii., and vertigo. During the Mexican War, he served mainly on garrison duty in Mexico City. He was slightly wounded in the neck by an arrow in a skirmish with Apaches on August 23, 1849, at Las Vegas, New Mexico. During the winter of 1850, he had some type of gastrointestinal disease; granted a home leave, he did not return until May 1851. Burnside resigned his commission in 1853 and engaged in the manufacture of a breech-loading rifle that he had invented. At the start of the Civil War he organized a three-month regiment and was in command of a brigade at First Bull Run. He was commissioned brigadier general of volunteers in August 1861 and was promoted to major general to rank from March 1862. During May 1862, Burnside and many of his men had fever and diarrhea. The following August he had erysipelas of his foot and leg and was unable to wear his boot. Also, his weak ankle, which he had injured the previous winter and again during the summer, caused him to use a crutch. He was sick twice over the period of June and July 1863 and lost twenty pounds. In October he was very ill with an intestinal problem and felt he might be forced to ask to be relieved of the department command. From December 7–9, 1863, he was ill and confined to his room. He resigned from the service in April 1865. He had served in major campaigns from Roanoke Island to Petersburg without notable success. After the war, Burnside was engaged in the directorship of various railroads, was three times governor of Rhode Island, and was a United States senator. He died September 13, 1881, at Bristol, Rhode Island. The night before he had complained of chest pain and walked around the house for some time. The continued distress prompted a call to the doctor the next morning. Burnside asked for morphine and died.[1] He was buried in Swan Point Cemetery at Providence, Rhode Island.

DEATH CERTIFICATE: Cause of death, enlargement of heart.

1. *OR*, vol. 31, pt. 1:272, 278; WPCHR, vol. 605; William Marvel, *Burnside*, 10, 89–90, 102, 105, 258, 424; Heitman, *Historical Register and Dictionary* 2:16.

CYRUS BUSSEY • *Born October 5, 1833,* at Hubbard, Ohio. An Iowa businessman and politician, he was made an officer in the state militia at the start of the war. He entered Federal service as colonel of the 3rd Iowa Cavalry in August 1861. In February 1862, when the temperature was near zero and he was without a tent or camp equipment, he developed severe neuralgia and rheumatism in his head, neck, and back. On the subsequent march through Arkansas he was sick with malaria and was compelled to ride in an ambulance. In July he was still suffering from rheumatism in his back and neck and was granted a leave to go home on a surgeon's certificate. He left St. Louis on July 29 for Memphis against the advice of his physician. At the time, he was improving in health and thought he would soon be well. On the way he was violently attacked with fever and continued to get worse. He took the advice of several surgeons and returned to St. Louis. Bussey spent late August at his home in Keokuk, Iowa, on sick leave and returned to duty the next month. In November 1862 he was caught in a storm and was compelled to spend the whole night in a swamp standing in water. This rendered him unfit for duty for some time, supposedly due to malaria. In July 1863, after the surrender of Vicksburg, he was prostrated with malaria and was ordered to his home in Keokuk. Bussey was commissioned brigadier general of volunteers in January 1864 and reported to the headquarters at Little Rock, Arkansas, on May 17. He had malaria and jaundice in August and had a leave from September 8 to December 1, 1864. In March 1865 he was sick with erysipelas. On February 6 he was appointed to division command and was mustered out in September 1865. About the first of September 1866 he moved to New Orleans; ill with malaria on his arrival, he was confined to his bed for a month. In the summer of 1870 he spent some time in New York for treatment of his malaria and rheumatism. He lived in New Orleans until 1882, during which time he was under medical treatment for rheumatism, neuralgia, and malaria. In April, in an attempt to relieve his suffering, he spent several weeks at

Hot Springs, Arkansas. He moved back to New York in the fall of 1882, still under treatment for chronic rheumatism and malaria. During the summer of 1883, he spent several weeks at Saratoga in bad health, suffering from the same conditions. He sustained an injury to his left arm, nervous system, and heart from being run over by a runaway horse on February 11, 1895. The next December he was totally unfit by reason of rheumatism, lumbago, catarrh of his head and lungs, and a varicocele. By May 1897 his disabilities had greatly increased. For several years Bussey had not been able to attend to the business of his office and had to employ others to take charge. He had been confined to his room much of the time and had many attacks of pain in his back and side from rheumatism, some lasting two or three months. Daily he suffered agonizing pain in his heart. Confined to his bed or couch most of the time, he required the aid and attendance of other persons and hypodermic injections of morphine. After 1906 he was a semi-invalid with severe chest pain that required medication.[1] He died March 2, 1915, in Washington, D.C., and was buried in Arlington National Cemetery.

DEATH CERTIFICATE: Cause of death, primary, influenza and bronchial pneumonia, fifteen days' duration; immediate, cardiac insufficiency, gradual.

1. CSR; *OR*, vol. 34, pt. 3:637; vol. 48, pt. 1:1216; RVA, Pension SC 905,063; Steiner, *Physician-Generals*, 26.

RICHARD BUSTEED • *Born February 16, 1822,* in Cavan, Ireland. Before the Civil War he was admitted to the bar and for three years was corporation counsel of New York City. He was made captain of an artillery battery in October 1861 but resigned in a few weeks. The following August he was appointed a brigadier general of volunteers, but his name was not sent to the Senate for confirmation. After serving with the Federal occupation forces, he was appointed judge of the United States District Court for Alabama in 1863 and assumed the judgeship in Mobile in 1865. On the morning of December 28, 1867, Richard Busteed walked out of his room in the Battle House, crossed the street, and headed to his office in the United States Customs House. As he stepped onto the curbstone in front of his office, United States District Attorney Lucien Van Buren Martin walked up to Busteed with a Colt revolver and shot him. The trouble between Busteed and Martin had started as a personal matter and had become political. There was a debate as to whether they had words before Martin fired. The ball struck Busteed below the breastbone and knocked him into the gutter. Martin then walked up, adjusted his eyeglasses, and fired two more shots into Busteed's right leg. Busteed was helped up and assisted to a nearby physician's office where he was examined. One ball was cut out of his right thigh. He was moved by carriage to his room at the Battle House. By December 31 his recovery was announced as certain and he was well enough to hold court early in February

1868. Martin was released on bond and left the country; since Busteed was disinclined to appear in court, the case was dropped. He left Alabama in 1874, rather than face impeachment, and returned to New York City where he resumed his law practice. On September 27, 1888, he had a cerebral hemorrhage that resulted in a left-sided hemiplegia. The examining doctor on October 14, 1891, reported the following findings: There was a scar from an old gunshot wound of the abdomen located just below the ensiform cartilage. It was irregular in form and was one by two inches. There were two scars from gunshot wounds of the right leg and one surgical scar. One point of entrance was located on the anterior aspect of the leg over crest of the tibia. The point of extraction was situated on the inner aspect of the thigh, four inches above the knee joint, and was ¾ by ½ inches in area. The other point of entrance was five inches above the ankle joint, was circular in form, and a half inch in diameter. None of the scars was depressed, tender, or adherent, and none produced notable disability. As a result of his cerebral hemorrhage, his left arm was entirely useless, and he could only stand or walk with difficulty and had to be aided by an assistant.[1] He died September 14, 1898, in New York City and was buried there in Woodlawn Cemetery.

DEATH CERTIFICATE: Direct cause, apoplexy, duration of ten minutes; contributing, hemiplegia.

1. RVA, Pension SC 704,868; Sarah Woolfolk Wiggins, "Press Reaction in Alabama to the Attempted Assassination of Judge Richard Busteed," *Alabama Review* (July 1968): 211–19.

BENJAMIN FRANKLIN BUTLER • *Born November 5, 1818,* at Deerfield, New Hampshire. He was crosseyed and had the nickname of "Cockeye." In May 1838 he went swimming in the Kennebec River and sat on a cake of ice. He caught a severe cold, and his weight decreased to ninety-seven pounds. To help recover his health he sailed on a codfishing ship. He consumed large quantities of raw cod-liver oil; by the time he returned home he had regained twenty-five pounds. Before the Civil War he had a large legal practice and was elected to the Massachusetts House of Representatives and the state senate. He was a brigadier general of the Massachusetts militia and was appointed the first volunteer major general at the start of the war. His military service was varied and controversial. He was military governor of New Orleans and had command of the Army of the James. During the summer and again in September 1862 his health was not strong. He was relieved of his command in January 1865 after a particularly inept performance at Bermuda Hundred. After the war he served in Congress from 1866 until 1875. He was occasionally bothered by gallbladder symptoms. In January 1883 Butler had trouble signing the oath as governor of Massachusetts because he was so nearsighted. On February 14, 1890, he had a surgical procedure to remove a section from his eyelid because his left eye had almost closed. A half inch of the lid was cut out and the lower part sewn up to it, making the eye "wide open tight" to let in more light. The operation was performed by two surgeons at his home in Lowell. Butler refused an anesthetic and, following the procedure, entertained the doctors at dinner. In November 1891 he had an abscess in his ear. On January 10, 1893, one day after arguing a case before the Supreme Court in Washington, D.C., he developed a cold. Soon after midnight on the eleventh, his coughing and heavy breathing awakened his valet, who noted that his expectorant was blood-stained. A physician was called who thought nothing could be done, and soon Butler died. Supposedly his last hours were complicated by the bursting of a small blood vessel secondary to the violent coughing.[1] He was buried in his wife's family cemetery in Lowell, Massachusetts.

DEATH CERTIFICATE: Cause of death, primary, pulmonary congestion. Immediate, heart failure.

1. *OR*, vol. 15:558, vol. 46, pt. 2:70; Howard P. Nash, Jr., *Stormy Petrel: The Life and Times of General Benjamin F. Butler, 1818–1893*, 28, 171, 264–65; Richard S. West, Jr., *Lincoln's Scapegoat General; A Life of Benjamin F. Butler, 1818–1893*, 354, 373, 417; Robert Stuart Holzman, "Benjamin F. Butler: His Public Career" (diss.), 2:363–64; Ames, *Chronicles from the Nineteenth Century* 1:427, 678; 2:583, 593.

DANIEL BUTTERFIELD • *Born October 31, 1831,* in Utica, New York. Prior to the Civil War, he studied law and was superintendent of the eastern division of the American Express Company. He entered the Federal service as a sergeant in April 1861 and the following month was commissioned colonel of the 12th New York Militia. His appointment as brigadier general of volunteers ranked from September. Ill, he gave up command of the brigade in May 1862. Back on the field on June 27 at Gaines' Mill, he was enfeebled by the extreme heat. On July 2 he had a return of the weakness and illness from which he had been suffering for some time and was admonished to rest and remain quiet. At Harrison's Landing that month he received a furlough in consequence of a diagnosis of typhoid fever but returned before expiration of his leave. It was at Harrison's Landing that he composed "Taps." In September 1862, near Alexandria, he was again afflicted with fever. During this illness he was unable to leave the house and could not take command. About September 6 he received sick leave and did not report back to the army until late October. He commanded the Fifth Corps at Fredericksburg and was chief of staff for both Hooker and Meade. On December 30 he had another sick leave and returned after the first of the year. Wounded at Gettysburg on July 3, 1863, he left the army on July 6 and in October accompanied Hooker to the west. He was sick in his quarters on November 13 and by the fifteenth had moved to Hooker's headquarters, where he was seen by the surgeon every day. On December 15, 1863, he was given another leave of absence for twenty days on surgeon's certificate. He was lying down and was unable to sign his communications due to diarrhea on June 21, 1864. On June

24 he was obliged to leave the command on account of his health. In July he was home on sick leave. He was brevetted brigadier and major general, U.S. Army, in 1865.[1] In 1870 he resigned from service. Until his death he held a number of business and civic positions. He died July 17, 1901, at Cold Springs, New York, and was buried at West Point.

DEATH CERTIFICATE: Cause of death, chief cause, softening of brain; contributing cause, apoplexy. Duration, several weeks.

1. *OR*, vol. 11, pt. 1:727, pt. 2:315–21; vol. 19, pt. 2:514; vol. 27, pt. 1:1041; vol. 38, pt. 2:203, 337, pt. 4:549, 563; U.S. Army, CWS, roll 3, vol. 4, report 4, pp. 69–123; Hubbard to Nellie, Nov. 13, 15, 1863 (bound book of typed copies), Robert Hubbard Letters, USAMHI.

C

GEORGE CADWALADER • *Born May 16, 1806,* in Philadelphia. Prior to the Civil War he was brevetted a major general of volunteers for his gallantry in the Mexican War and was major general of Pennsylvania troops. In April 1862 he was commissioned a major general of volunteers, and early in the war he served in various staff and advisory positions. On September 1, 1862, he was treated for a contusion of his knee and on November 19 was under care in Washington, D.C., for synovitis.[1] He was made commander of the post at Philadelphia in August 1863 and held this position until he resigned in July 1865. After the war he returned to his private interests. Cadwalader died February 3, 1879, in Philadelphia and was buried there in the cemetery of Christ Church.

DEATH CERTIFICATE: Cause of death, apoplexy, cerebral.

1. RAGO, entry 534.

JOHN CURTIS CALDWELL • *Born on April 17, 1833,* in Lowell, Vermont. A prewar teacher, he entered Federal service as colonel of the 11th Maine in November 1861. His promotion to brigadier general ranked from April 1862. He was wounded at Fredericksburg on December 13, 1862. He was near a brick building in the town when he was struck by a musket ball in the left side. He did not leave the field and was struck a second time in the left shoulder. Caldwell then passed down the road to direct one of the regiments. Afterward he went to a nearby hospital to have his wounds dressed and did not return to the field. In February he was back in command. He was at Chancellorsville and Gettysburg, and in the fall of 1863 he commanded the Second Corps during the Mine Run campaign. He was mustered out of service in January 1866.[1] Following the war he was admitted to the Maine bar and held a number of state and Federal appointments. He died August 30, 1912, in Calais, Maine, and was buried in East Machias, Maine.

DEATH CERTIFICATE: Cause of death, senile decay.

1. CSR; *OR*, vol. 21:233–34.

ROBERT ALEXANDER CAMERON • *Born February 22, 1828,* in Brooklyn, New York. Although he graduated from medical school, he seemed to have little interest in the profession and published a newspaper in Indiana before the war. He joined the Federal Army as a captain, rose through ranks, and became a brigadier general of volunteers from August 1863. He had seen service at Island No. 10, New Madrid, and Memphis. At the Battle of Port Gibson on May 1, 1863, he sustained an injury to his eyes from foreign material, which produced an acute conjunctivitis. He was unable to take part in the Battle of Champion's Hill on May 16 and had to be transported at times in an ambulance. Because of partial blindness due to acute purulent ophthalmia, he was sent home. After returning to the field at Vicksburg he developed diarrhea, which stayed with him to his grave. He was never in the hospital for the illness but was treated by regimental surgeons. In August 1863 he suffered from chronic inflammation of the stomach and bowels along with his chronic diarrhea and was given a sick leave. He later claimed that the diarrhea caused hemorrhoids and an umbilical hernia. Cameron commanded a division in the Red River campaign. He was brevetted major general as of March 1865 and soon resigned his commission. For the first one to two years after his discharge he continued to have trouble with his eyes. Not able to do anything, he had to stay in a dark room. Later, Cameron spent much of his time trying to establish farm colonies in Colorado. During 1883 he was working as a physician and a post office inspector. Starting in 1892 he required narcotics for the severe attacks of abdominal pain superimposed on his chronic diarrhea. He was reduced to a low residue, soft diet. He died March 15, 1894, near Canon City, Colorado, and was buried in that city. His attending physician found at necropsy four areas of contractions and induration, each about six inches long: one in the jejunum and three in the ileum. Only fluids could pass through these strictures. They were attributed to the healing of ulcers, and the cause of death was diagnosed as chronic enteritis. Paul E. Steiner, M.D., speculated that it might have been regional enteritis.[1]

1. CSR; *OR*, vol. 24, pt. 2:51; vol. 48, pt. 2:363; RVA, Pension WC 401,575; Steiner, *Physician-Generals*, 28.

CHARLES THOMAS CAMPBELL • *Born on August 10, 1823,* in Franklin County, Pennsylvania. He was wounded during the Mexican War. Before the Civil War, he served in the lower house of the Pennsylvania legislature. He was first a captain and then colonel of artillery until February 1862, when he was made colonel of the 57th Pennsylvania. He was severely wounded at Fair Oaks on the evening of May 31, 1862. Not conscious of what was happening, he was carried with difficulty from the field to the rear. He had received one wound through the right wrist, one through the groin and pelvic bone, and a slight wound in the left leg. Campbell was sent to a hospital in Philadelphia where he had a rapid recovery. He obtained a leave of absence starting late in June. Still lame in August, he was back in command about the middle of September. With his arm still in a sling, he was severely wounded December 13, 1862, at the Battle of Fredericksburg. He received three wounds, one through the body and two through the right arm. The right elbow joint was fractured. The same day he had a primary resection of his elbow joint and four inches of the ulna and radius. He was sent to Washington, where his recovery was rapid following several nonspecified surgical procedures. His final appointment as brigadier general ranked from March 1863. From March 13 to May 12 he was on leave. On his return he was placed on inspection and court-martial duty. He was ordered to St. Paul, Minnesota, on July 30, 1863, to await orders. From the following summer until the end of the war he had district command in Wisconsin. After the war he went to the Dakota Territory, where he was an inspector of Indian agencies and an operator of a stage line. He later helped establish the town of Scotland, South Dakota, and operated a hotel there. In the 1880s his right hand was almost worthless and there was ancholosis of the right elbow. He required the attendance of another person in putting on and taking off his clothing, in washing his person, and in getting in and out of any conveyance. By 1889 he needed extra-large clothing so he could, with assistance, get his crooked arm into the sleeve of his coat. His condition was further complicated by a lame back and rheumatism in his left arm and shoulder. The back pain was particularly bad in the area where the bullet had exited. On April 9, 1895, he fell down the steps of his hotel, the Campbell House. He broke an arm and two ribs and injured himself internally. He died in the hotel on April 15 as a result of the fall. His body was taken to Yankton and buried in the Yankton Cemetery.[1]

1. CSR; *OR*, vol. 11, pt. 1:846–47; vol. 21:364, 369; *MSHW*, vol. 2, pt. 2:852, case 33; RVA, Pension WC 428,037; U.S. Army, CWS, roll 1, vol. 1, report 49, pp. 921–30; *Scotland (South Dakota) Journal*, Apr. 20, 1895; South Dakota Grave Registration Project, Field Data, Yankton Cemetery.

WILLIAM BOWEN CAMPBELL • Born February 1, 1807, in Sumner County, Tennessee. Served in the Florida and Mexican wars. Prior to the Mexican War he practiced law and served in Congress for three terms. A one-time governor of Tennessee, he was appointed a brigadier general of volunteers in June 1862. He resigned from this position in January 1863. For his few remaining years after the war he worked for reconstruction in Tennessee. Campbell died August 19, 1867, in Lebanon, Tennessee, and was buried there in Cedar Grove Cemetery.

EDWARD RICHARD SPRIGG CANBY • *Born November 9, 1817,* at Piatt's Landing, Kentucky. Graduated from the USMA in 1839. As a cadet, he was treated for a headache seven times, a cold four times, nausea twice, and once each for toothache, bruise, sore throat, sore foot, cough, and wound. He fought in the Florida and Mexican wars and served on frontier and garrison duty. On January 25, 1841, he was granted a three-month leave of absence because of poor health and went home to recuperate. He had a severe attack of fever while in Indianapolis in October 1848 and did not return to duty until the next month. On New Year's Eve 1854 he was detained in Louisville with rheumatism and remained there for almost a month. He was promoted to colonel in May 1861 and was put in command of the Department of New Mexico. Canby was appointed brigadier general of volunteers in May 1862 and ordered east. In March 1864 he was sick and nearly broken down, supposedly from his duties in the War Department. He performed staff duties until the next month when he was appointed major general of volunteers and was placed in command of the Military Division of West Mississippi. He helped plan the expedition against Mobile. On November 8, 1864, while travelling on the gunboat *Cricket* upon the White River near Prairie Landing, Canby was wounded in the upper part of the thigh by a single shot from guerrillas. The ball passed below his hip, went through the scrotum, and hit his penis. He returned to New Orleans on November 10 and was cared for by his wife. He had a severe episode with "unnatural excitement" on November 12–13 associated with great pain and fever. By November 30 he was rapidly improving. The wound was discharging freely and his appetite was good. He accepted the surrender of Confederate generals Richard Taylor and Edmund Kirby Smith and their troops in May 1865. In 1866 he was promoted to brigadier general, U.S. Army. During May of that year he requested to be relieved from duty in the Department of Louisiana, mainly for health reasons. After assuming command of the Department of the Columbia in August 1870 he had occasional attacks of neuralgia and rheumatism due to the damp climate. He and the peace commissioner were killed by Modoc Indians at Van Bremmer's Ranch, Siskiyou County, California, on April 11, 1873. Captain Jack, chief of the Modocs, drew a pistol and shot Canby, the ball striking him in the face. Canby did not fall until he had run forty or fifty yards and was struck in the back of the head by another shot. His assailants came upon him, shot him again, stripped him of his clothing, turned his face downward, and left him.[1] He was buried in Crown Hill Cemetery at Indianapolis, Indiana.

1. CSR; *OR*, vol. 36, pt. 2:329; vol. 41, pt. 4:450–51, 484–85, 500, 504, 529, 532, 568, 602, 653, 717, 1075; vol. 52,pt. 1:653; Max L. Heyman, Jr., *Prudent Soldier: A Biography of Major General E. R. S. Canby, 1817–1873*, 42, 70, 87–89, 219–23, 293, 349.

JAMES HENRY CARLETON • *Born December 27, 1814,* in Lubec, Maine. He was appointed a second lieutenant of the 1st U.S. Dragoons in October 1839 and participated in Kearny's Rocky Mountain expedition. Served in the Mexican War. He suffered from fatigue and exposure to cold after four days of constantly being in the saddle, from February 20, 1847, to noon on February 24. This resulted in severe rheumatic and neuralgic affections of his head and great prostration of his health. However, he remained on duty except for intervals of only a few days. Because of his illness, he was ordered to Washington, D.C., on a surgeon's certificate of disability. He arrived in New Orleans on October 28, 1847, and was under a doctor's care in that city. In December he went to Washington. During February through April 1848, he was in Bangor, Maine, in poor health and with an obstinate cough. In June he placed himself under the care of a Boston physician. He continued having a most painful and lingering neuralgia of his head, which made him unfit for exposure to the sun. The physician attributed Carleton's illness to previous attacks of fever and ague and to his exposure and fatigue during service in Mexico. By September he improved so he could perform light duty if he was not exposed to the sun. In October 1848 he took command of a company of dragoons at Carlisle, Pennsylvania. In March 1858 he was made recruiting officer in Lexington, Virginia, and over the next three months had three severe episodes of congestion of his liver and stomach. Each episode prostrated him for days. During the May attack he had chills and fever and was confined to his room. He was commissioned brigadier general of volunteers to rank from April 1862 and was made commander of the Department of New Mexico. Carleton was brevetted through grades to that of a major general of the Regular Army and the volunteer service. In July 1866 he was commissioned lieutenant colonel of the Fourth Cavalry. While stationed at San Antonio in April 1872, he suffered from chronic eczema rubrum of both legs. The summer heat made the affected parts swell to such an extent that walking was impossible and riding extremely painful. On May 6 he left on sick leave for Hot Springs, Arkansas, on the advice of his surgeon. In October one physician reported that the chronic eczema of both legs was the result of edema, which was probably due to impropriety of the blood resulting from a scorbutic condition of his system. The following month, another surgeon stated that it was the result of feeble capillary circulation and impaired nerve force. In December, while in New Orleans, he had a severe attack of catarrh and acute catarrhal bronchitis that developed into pneumonia of the right lung. He died on January 7, 1873, in San Antonio.[1] The death certificate has January 8 as the date of his death but most sources report the seventh.

DEATH CERTIFICATE: Cause of death, pneumonia, eight days' duration.

1. U.S. Army, CWS, roll 2, vol. 3, report 35, pp. 1035–111; LR, ACP, 5058, 1872, fiche: 000010.

WILLIAM PASSMORE CARLIN • *Born November 24, 1829,* near Carrollton, Illinois. Graduated from the USMA in 1850. As a cadet he was seen for diarrhea twice and once each for catarrhus, cephalalgia, contusio, cynanche tonsillitis, febris intermittent, febris ephemeral, febris remittent, tonsillitis, pyrosis, subluxatio, vulnus laceratum, and vulnus punctum. In May 1855, during a march from Fort Leavenworth to Fort Laramie, he, along with many of the troops, had cholera, and he was sick for many weeks. After his recovery, he marched over three hundred miles from Fort Laramie to Fort Pierre, South Dakota. During the Indian campaign of August 1857, about forty miles north of old Fort

Atkinson, he injured his left ankle and was compelled to ride on a captured Indian pony. Carlin was a captain in the Regular Army at the start of the Civil War and was commissioned colonel of the 38th Illinois Volunteers in August 1861. He was sick in bed October 21, 1861, the beginning of the battle of Frederickstown, Missouri. Although he was on the field in the afternoon, he had to turn over a portion of his command the next day. He served with distinction at Perryville and in November 1862 was promoted to brigadier general of volunteers. He was sick in January 1863 due to exposure and fatigue at Stones River and went home for about twenty days. At Chickamauga, on September 19, 1863, Carlin's horse was shot; he was slightly wounded but remained on the field. He went north on sick leave on December 2 and returned to duty January 19, 1864. Carlin commmanded a division in the Atlanta campaign and in the Carolinas. On March 23, 1865, the troops arrived at Goldsborough, North Carolina, where Carlin became sick from exhaustion, fatigue, and the hardships of the long march. He was admitted March 30 to the USA hospital steamer, *Cosmopolitan*, with a diagnosis of chronic dysentery. He did not report back until late in May.[1] After being brevetted through ranks to major general in both the volunteer and regular service, he assumed his regular rank of major of infantry following the war. Carlin served in garrison command in the South before returning to frontier duty. In May 1893 he was appointed brigadier general and retired that year. He died near Whitehall, Montana, on board a Northern Pacific train on October 4, 1903. He was buried in Carrollton, Illinois.

1. *OR*, vol. 3:216, 220; vol. 47, pt. 1:107; vol. 51, pt. 1:1216; *OR Suppl.*, vol. 1, pt. 1:257; WPCHR, vols. 605, 606, 607; RAGO, entry 534; U.S. Army, CWS, roll 1, vol. 1, report 58, pp. 1029–51; ibid., roll 3, vol. 5, report 1, pp. 1–233.

EUGENE ASA CARR • *Born March 20, 1830,* in Erie County, New York. Graduated from the USMA in 1850. Carr was seen at the Cadet Hospital for catarrhus five times, cephalalgia, clavus, and contusio each three times, diarrhea, vulnus incisum, vulnus incip., and odontalgia each twice, and once each for vulnus laceratum, morbii. cutis, pleurodynia, and subluxatio. On October 10, 1854, at Fort Davis on the Texas frontier, he was hit in the side by an Indian arrow. Although some sources report he was wounded on the third, the tenth appears to be correct. Two weeks later he was still barely able to travel. In May 1859 he was ill with what was diagnosed as cerebritis. A captain at the start of the Civil War, he was promoted to colonel in August 1861 and brigadier general of volunteers in March 1862. At the Battle of Pea Ridge on March 7, 1862, Carr was wounded three times. A grapeshot glanced off his wrist a little above the joint, passed in and out of the coat sleeve, and caused an injury similar to a sprain. Another ball struck him on the neck, partially paralyzing him for a moment but causing no further problems except for a flesh wound. He was in severe pain after having been hit on the left ankle, but the pain lasted only about half an hour. The arm wound was probably worse than he reported, and after his arm was bandaged, he returned to the field and stayed with the army. In October 1862, while at Helena, Arkansas, he was given a sick leave because of malarial fever. On his return, he was stopped at St. Louis where he was made district commander. In April 1863, he had a "tendency" to intermittent fever and diarrhea associated with inflammation and irritation of the neck of the bladder and the prostate. He had a recurrence of malaria in June and had to take palliative medicine just so he could perform his duties. The urinary tract symptoms continued and the disease, along with the medicines he required, produced diarrhea. At the time of the surrender of Vicksburg in July, Carr was suffering severely and was hardly able to walk. He obtained a sick leave and did not return until September. He served in the Camden campaign and in the campaign against Mobile in 1865. Following the Civil War he had occasional headaches, stated to be secondary to malaria. Carr was brevetted major general in both the volunteer and regular services and reverted to his rank of major. On May 22, 1865, he bruised his hand and had to wrap it in a wet handkerchief. In July he was not feeling well and had a severe fever for a day. He participated in a number of campaigns in the West and was promoted through ranks to brigadier general in 1892. In February 1871 he was treated for a contusion. The next month he was sick with a headache, and by April his condition had become worse. Although appointed to court-martial duty, he was unable to attend its sessions. In June he received a two-month sick leave. During the summer of 1873 he continued to have malarial headaches. In March 1874 his surgeon's certificate stated that for the previous few months he had suffered from dyspepsia accompanied by torpidity of the liver, obstinate constipation, a severe and almost constant headache, and general debility that had been complicated by malarial fever. During May the headaches and fevers became a daily occurrence, increasing in severity. His physician reported that he needed a year's leave to recover, so he obtained a sick leave from June 1874 to June 1875 and spent part of the time in Europe and England. During September 1876 he was on the field in the West and was almost out of quinine, which he used to prevent headaches. From August 31 to September 3, 1887, he was excused from musters and inspections but not his other duties because of a bilious headache. In November and December of that year he had acute bronchitis and a boil on the posterior aspect of his neck. Carr was hospitalized at Fort Wingate, New Mexico, from December 31, 1889, to April 3, 1890, with acute bronchitis complicated by catarrh. In March he was unable to do his duties as post commander because he was sick with influenza. He retired from the army in 1893. He died December 2, 1910, at his home in Washington, D.C. According to his attending surgeon, the cause of death was asthenia due to chronic cholecystitis.[1] Carr was buried at West Point.

1. CSR; *OR*, vol. 8:200; vol. 13:781; vol. 53:542; U.S. Army, CWS, roll 2, vol. 3, report 24, pp. 661–74; LR, ACP, 467, 1873, fiche: 000011; RVA, Pension C 721,025; Eugene A. Carr Biographies; E. A. Carr to father, Mar. 15, Nov. 1, 1862, E. A. Carr to ———, May 22, July 24, 1865, Son to father, Mar. 20, Nov. 29, 1874, E. A. Carr to wife, May 7, 14, 1874, Eugene A. Carr Papers, USAMHI.

JOSEPH BRADFORD CARR • *Born August 16, 1828,* in Albany, New York. He was engaged in the tobacco business at the start of the Civil War and was colonel of a New York militia. Carr entered Federal service as colonel of the 2nd New York Volunteers in May 1861 and was appointed brigadier general of volunteers in September 1862. He saw service on the Peninsula and at Second Bull Run, Fredericksburg, and Chancellorsville. His nomination was not acted on by the Senate and he was reappointed in March 1863. At Gettysburg in July 1863, his horse was killed under him; though injured, he continued to direct his brigade. About December 1864 he contracted an inflammatory eye disease. His surgeon reported that the problem was due to exposure to cold and the peculiarities of the atmosphere at Fort Pocahontas, Virginia. He was treated for several weeks in his quarters. When the war ended he was brevetted major general of volunteers and was discharged in August 1865. He entered business in Troy, New York, and was New York secretary of state for five years. By 1879 he had lost the sight of his left eye, and the vision of the other eye was seriously impaired. In 1889 a cancerous growth developed on the inner surface of his jaw. Although he underwent repeated operations for its removal, it proved incurable. On February 24, 1895, he died in Troy and was buried in that city at Oakwood Cemetery.[1]
DEATH CERTIFICATE: Cause of death, carcinoma of the neck.

1. U.S. Army, CWS, roll 1, vol. 2, report 17, pp. 199–215; RVA, Pension WC 440,865; New York Monuments Commission for the Battlefields of Gettysburg and Chattanooga, *Final Report on the Battlefield of Gettysburg* 3:1351–53.

HENRY BEEBEE CARRINGTON • *Born on March 2, 1824,* in Wallingford, Connecticut. A lawyer and strong abolitionist, he helped reorganize the Ohio militia and was state adjutant general before the Civil War. In 1861 he was commissioned a colonel in the Regular Army and in 1862 was made brigadier general of volunteers. After service in West Virginia he recruited troops in Indiana and suppressed those with Southern leanings in Ohio and Indiana. In April 1865 he was too ill to travel because of hemoptysis. He was mustered out of volunteer service in 1865. Carrington participated in Indian affairs after the war and was a productive writer on historical matters. While en route from Fort Casper to Fort Laramie in February 1867, he accidently received a gunshot wound of the left thigh. In May he was at Fort McPherson, Nebraska, suffering with contractions and pain in his leg and also from localized consolidation of the superior lobe of the left lung. By the end of the year, use of the knee was insecure; at times it failed to support him.[1] He died October 26, 1912, in Boston and was buried in Fairview Cemetery, Hyde Park, Massachusetts.
DEATH CERTIFICATE: Cause of death: senility, one year plus.

1. U.S. Army, CWS, roll 3, vol. 4, report 20, pp. 679–703; LR, CB, C485, 1868.

SAMUEL SPRIGG CARROLL • *Born September 21, 1831,* in Takoma Park near Washington, D.C. Although many sources report the year of his birth as 1832, in a response to an inquiry when he was to retire in 1891 Carroll wrote that he had been born in 1831. He graduated from the USMA in 1856. During his period as a cadet he was treated for catarrhus six times, excoriatio and febris intermittent tertian each three times, vulnus incisum, subluxatio, colica, and clavus each twice, and odontalgia, neuralgia, contusio, intoxicatio, phlegmon, nausea, and cephalalgia each once. Following frontier service he was appointed colonel of the 8th Ohio Infantry in December 1861. While visiting the outpost on the Rapidan and beyond Cedar Mountain on August 14, 1862, he was wounded in the right breast. He returned to duty and took part in the battle at Fredericksburg in December. Starting January 12, 1863, he had sick leave because of his old wound and other complications. The surgeon's justifying certificate reported that he had also had remittent fever for the previous week and diarrhea for two months. The next month he was convalescing from remittent fever and had partial solidification of the upper lobe of the right lung accompanied by cough and some hemorrhage. In March he was still under treatment for disease of his lung consequent upon the wound of the right side. The following month, in addition to his continued cough, he had rheumatism of his left hip and knee. He was back in time to fight at Chancellorsville and Gettysburg. On July 23, 1863, he was unable to travel because of acute dysentery and remained in Washington, D.C., for treatment. On October 14 he was slightly wounded at Bristoe Station, Virginia. In May 1864, Carroll was wounded three times. The first was at the Wilderness on May 5, where he received a flesh wound of the right arm but was able to remain on the field. Later he went to the rear for medical attention and resumed command the following morning. On May 10 he was slightly wounded but continued on duty. On May 13, during a reconnaissance at Spotsylvania Court House, Carroll was suffering from his wounded right arm when his left elbow was shattered by a rifle bullet. He had to be carried to a field hospital where cold-water dressings were applied to his elbow. Before the examination of the injury was made under chloroform, Carroll insisted that an effort be made to save the arm. The ball had entered in the internal condyle of the left humerus of the outstretched arm and, ranging downwards and outwards, made its exit upon the radial aspect of the forearm. The internal condyle was fractured, and there was a comminuted fracture of the radius. The wound was enlarged with a scalpel; using a chainsaw, about four inches of the radius, including the head, were resected. Forceps were used to pick out the loose spicules of bone. Leaving the wounds patulous, the surgeon put the arm up in a hollow obtuse angle splint. Erysipelas soon developed and extended up the arm and over the shoulder. His recovery was further complicated by bedsores, great emaciation, and an irritative fever that lasted all summer. Carroll was confined to his bed at his mother's home in Washington, D.C., for almost three months. In October 1864 he developed eczema adjacent to the wound. By early November the wound was still uncicatraized and there was complete ankylosis of the joint. His appointment as brigadier general of volunteers ranked from May, and in December 1864 he was assigned to court-martial duty. For two years after he was wounded he still suffered with pain in the arm. Abscesses occasionally developed, and particles of necrosed bone were discharged. For six to eight months in 1866 he had hemorrhage from his lungs. He was given a sick leave from January 24 to February 22, 1868. In June 1869 Carroll was examined by a retirement board, who reported that he was having a great deal of trouble with his lungs due to the old wound received at Cedar Mountain. His left elbow was ankylosed and flexed at a right angle with loss of rotation of the forearm. There was also loss of the sensation and power of flexion of the left hand and fingers. He could not use the bridle with his left hand. On June 9, 1869, he was retired as a major general, U.S. Army, for disability resulting from wounds. In 1892 and 1893 he had nasopharyngolaryngeal catarrh. He had a considerable paroxysmal cough, which the physician felt could not be accounted for by these conditions alone. On examination of the chest there was a circumscribed area of chronic interstitial pneumonia in the right lung, corresponding to the area where he had received the gunshot wound. Although the elbow joint remained immobile, he regained the use of the wrist joint and of the hand and fingers. He could hold a fork firmly while carving and the arm was invaluable.[1] He died in Takoma Park, D.C., on January 28, 1893, and was buried in Oak Hill Cemetery at Georgetown.

DEATH CERTIFICATE: Cause of death, pneumonia. Duration, six days.

1. CSR; *OR*, vol. 25, pt. 2:134; vol. 36, pt. 1:69, 326, 430–31, 448, pt. 2:711; vol. 42, pt. 2:424; vol. 51, pt. 1:1193; WPCHR, vols. 608, 609; RVA, Pension WC 383,676; *MSHW*, vol. 2, pt. 2:848, case 1781; ibid., pt. 2:852, case 34; RAGO, entry 623, "File D"; U.S. Army, CWS, roll 4, vol. 6, report 6, pp. 257–60; LR, ACP, 1639, 1875, fiche: 000049.

SAMUEL POWHATAN CARTER • *Born August 6, 1819*, in Elizabethton, East Tennessee. He graduated from the United States Naval Academy in the class of 1846. Until the start of the Civil War he served in various capacities in the U.S. Navy and had risen to the rank of lieutenant. Extensive notes from the Bureau of Medicine and Surgery on his medical conditions while serving in the navy before and after the Civil War provide insight into the prescribing practices of the time.

Admitted January 16, 1847, with cough and dizziness of head. Rx. Iris fluid extract. Origin not stated. Discharged, January 18, 1847. Admitted April 9, 1847, with fever which was preceded by a chill. Had a bad cough for some weeks past, which has been aggravated by late exposure on shore. Rx. Carbonate and bitartrate potassium, zingiber pulvis powder, vinum ipecacuanhae, tincture oppii, Spr. ether. April 13. Oleum tiglium to chest. Discharged April 27, 1847, to Naval Hospital Pensacola with bronchitis. Hospital journals are not on file. Admitted May 7, 1854, was taken with a chill followed by fever and sweating. Has had intermittent fever before. Rx. Quinine sulfate, Calomel. May 8. Dover's powders. Origin not stated. Discharged

May 14, 1854, to duty. San Jacuita. Admitted March 14, 1856, with catarrh. Rx. Seidlitz powders. Origin not stated. Discharged March 15, 1856, to duty. Admitted June 15, 1856, with haemoptysis. Rx. Rest, low diet, cooling drinks. Improved. Origin not stated. Discharged June 29, 1856, to duty. Admitted Dec. 31, 1856, with eczema of some standing. Lymphatic glands in axilla, inflamed and swollen. Painful and stiff. Had cough and some diarrhea. Rx. Potassium iodide, poultice to axilla. Jan. 4, 1857. Goulards cerate. Origin not stated. Discharged Jan. 6, 1857, to duty. Admitted Jan. 11, 1857, with diarrhea, bloody stools. Jan. 17, debilitated. Jan. 20, disease of bowels complicated with intermittent (fever). Rx. Quinine sulfate, calomel and oppii. He went on shore January 28.

In July 1861 Carter was detailed from the navy to the War Department and in May 1862 was commissioned brigadier general of volunteers. Carter served in East Tennessee and in the Carolinas. He was brevetted major general of volunteers to rank from March 1865. The following January he was discharged from the army and took his naval rank of commander.

Admitted July 4, 1871, with dysentery. Rx. plumbi acetate, oppii, ipecac. July 9, bismuth carbonate. July 10, discharged. Admitted Naval Dispensary, Washington, Dec. 31, 1877, with erythema. Rx. Sodium bicarbonate, extract Columbae fluid. Discharged Jan. 9, 1878 to duty. Admitted Mar. 20, 1878, with tonsillitis. Rx. Nitrate of silver. Discharged April 2, 1878, to duty. Admitted April 8, 1878, with bronchitis. Rx. Counter irritant to chest. Muriate of ammonia. Discharged May 1, to duty. Admitted April 22, 1880, with ulcer-corneal. Not in line of duty. Discharged May 7, 1880, to duty. Well. Admitted Dec. 4, 1880, with catarrhus. Not line of duty. RX. Emp. caffeine. Discharged Dec. 7, 1880, to duty. Admitted April 2, 1881, with malarial cachexia. Rx. Quinine. Discharged April 1881, to duty. Admitted May 17, 1881, with malarial cachexia. Rx. Quinine. Discharged May 21, 1881. Admitted October 13, 1881, with rheumatic chorea. Rx. Sodium salicylate. Discharged October 20, 1881, to duty.

He retired from the navy in 1881 as a commodore and the following year was advanced to rear admiral on the retired list.

Admitted March 15, 1882, with catarrhus epidemic. Discharged March 30, 1882. Admitted March 4, 1883, with febris intermittent. Rx. Chloral hydrate, potassium citrate. March 6. Quinine sulfate. Discharged March 11, 1883. Admitted August 27, 1883, with rheumatism acutus. Pain in broad muscles of back and hips. Some febrile disturbances. Sodium salicylate.

Carter was admitted to the hospital in Washington, D.C., on May 24, 1891, with typhlitis. The surgeon was called and found him suffering with pain and tenderness in the right iliac fossa due to what he presumed was an ulcerative inflammation of the caecum. His suffering was controlled by opiates and the usual

remedies; however, he died on May 26, 1891. According to his attending surgeon, the cause of death was typhlitis.[1]

1. RVA, Pension Navy WC 10,528.

SILAS CASEY · *Born July 12, 1807,* at East Greenwich, Rhode Island. He graduated
from the USMA in 1826. Served in the Florida and Mexican wars. While in
Florida, he had medical leave from June 30 to December 31, 1841, because of
great debility and emaciation as the result of an attack of congestive fever. In
the assault on the works of Chapultepec on September 13, 1847, he was seriously
wounded. After duty, mainly on the Pacific Coast, he was appointed lieutenant
colonel in 1855. Casey was on sick leave from March 1 to November 10, 1857. In
August 1861 he was appointed a brigadier general of volunteers, and in May
1862 he was brevetted brigadier general in the Regular Army and commissioned
major general of volunteers. He served creditably on the Peninsula but was
ordered to Washington in July 1862 because his health and years did not fit him
for active command of troops in the field. Discharged from volunteer service in
July 1865, he resumed his regular rank of colonel. Casey retired from the army
in 1868. He died on January 22, 1882, in Brooklyn, New York, and was buried on
the Casey family farm at North Kingstown, Rhode Island. According to the
attending surgeon, he died as the result of "general destruction of the vital forces"
due to failure of his digestive system.[1]

1. *OR,* vol. 11, pt. 3:298; LR, ACP, 1001, 1882, fiche: 000067; Heitman, *Historical Register and Dictionary* 2:17.

ROBERT FRANCIS CATTERSON · *Born on March 22, 1835,* near Beech Grove, Indiana. A medical graduate, he had just started his practice at the beginning of the
Civil War. Catterson entered Federal service and passed through first sergeant,
second lieutenant, first lieutenant, captain, lieutenant colonel, and colonel of
the 97th Indiana by November 1862. He was wounded four times at Antietam
on September 17, 1862. One ball entered the right gluteus muscle just posterior
to the rim of the right acetabulum, passed backward, made its exit in the posterior portion of the lacerated sphincter ani, and then passed into part of the left
gluteus muscle. At the same time a musket ball struck across the base of the left
thumb, disabling it. Another musket ball entered the outer side of the left foot,
struck the bone, and passed backward, finally lodging under the skin beneath
the middle of the os calcis. It was later extracted from this location. In addition,
a piece of shell struck his right leg just above the kneecap. Taken first to the
division hospital, he was moved on the twenty-fourth to a general hospital at
Frederick. Catterson reported that his wounds were not dressed for eleven days
and no explanation was provided. About September 28, he was transported to

the Seminary Hospital, D.C., where he remained for thirty days until he went home on leave. During January and February 1864 he was sick in camp and was in the division hospital from June 25 to August 1. A surgeon's certificate on August 9 reported that he was suffering with chronic diarrhea and general debility. His promotion to brigadier general of volunteers ranked from May 1865. Following the war, he engaged in politics and a number of unsuccessful businesses. A pension board in 1900 found that his rectal wound had been three or four inches up and that in healing had formed a pouch that was still present. The pouch sometimes filled with a mass of coagulated blood that interfered with defecation.[1] Incapacitated by a stroke, he died in the veterans' hospital in San Antonio, Texas, on March 30, 1914, and was buried there in the National Cemetery.

DEATH CERTIFICATE: Cause of death, senility.

1. CSR; *OR*, vol. 38, pt. 1:106, pt. 3:283; RVA, Pension WC 779,170; Steiner, *Physician-Generals*, 35–37.

JOSHUA LAWRENCE CHAMBERLAIN • *Born on September 8, 1828*, in Brewer, Maine. On his twenty-first birthday, he had a fever and was delirious. After the family physician gave up on the case, his mother called in a homeopathic physician. The illness was protracted, and it was some months before he fully recovered. A professor at Bowdoin College at the start of the Civil War, he entered Federal service as a lieutenant colonel of the 20th Maine in August 1862. He received a deep scratch on his right ear and neck from a musket ball at Fredericksburg on December 13, 1862. During June 1863 he had a sunstroke and remained in a house at Gum Springs, Virginia, when his troops moved out. However, in a few days, although still not well, he rejoined his men. At Gettysburg on July 2, 1863, a rock splinter or piece of shell penetrated his right instep. He also received a contusion of his left leg when a minié ball smashed against his sword scabbard. On July 27 he requested medical leave because of a severe attack of nervous prostration and neuralgia. In August he contracted malaria and went home on sick leave for about two weeks. On November 7, 1863, he had recurrence of the malaria with chills, fever, and nausea. He slept in the snow on the night of November 10 and collapsed with malaria-like symptoms. Along with his orderly, he was taken in a freight train to Washington. He was placed in the officers' hospital at Georgetown Seminary where his sister came to help with his care. On November 28 he was confined to the hospital bed by what the physician reported was typhomalarial fever. He went home in December, and the next month, when he was able to do light duty, he was appointed to a general court-martial. He returned to his command six months later. On June 18, 1864, at Petersburg, Chamberlain was wounded again and received a field promotion to brigadier general. Unable to move, he leaned on his sword, ordered his troops forward, and then sank to the ground. He was carried a short way to the rear by his aides and then for three miles on a stretcher to the field hospital. The minié ball had entered his right hip, severed arteries, nicked his urinary bladder, fractured the left pelvic bones, and came out behind the left hip joint. Two surgeons worked on him in the field hospital tent and did the best repair they could. On June 19 he was sent on a stretcher the sixteen miles to City Point on the James River. Next he was taken aboard the hospital ship, *Connecticut,* and was brought to Annapolis where he was put in the naval academy hospital. Recovery was complicated by convulsive chills and fever. The use of an indwelling catheter produced pressure necrosis and a urethral fistula that caused him difficulties for the rest of his life. The catheter would become encrusted with a calculous deposit after being used for just five days. When he reported back to duty in November 1864, he was still unable to ride a horse or walk very far but resumed command of his brigade. Poor health prompted a hospitalization in Philadelphia in December 1864 and a sick leave. In the fight on the Quaker Road, March 29, 1865, he was wounded. A ball, after passing through his horse's neck, hit his arm and struck him just below his heart. The projectile, deflected by a leather case of field orders and a brass-backed pocket mirror, followed around two ribs and came out his back. Unconscious, he slumped onto his horse but soon regained consciousness and was able to rally his troops. He was assigned to brigade command on April 10, 1865, and when he went home in July he applied for leave to have surgery. His original discharge was revoked so he could have continued treatment of his wounds. Chamberlain was brevetted major general and discharged in January 1866. He served as governor of Maine from 1866 until 1870 when he became president of Bowdoin College. In February 1869 he was having bladder irritation, and the lower part of his abdomen was tender and sensitive. The large urinary fistula at the base of his penis in front of the scrotum was bothersome. Also, an area in the left breast was causing him pain. A pension examination in September 1873 provided more information on the initial wound and his subsequent course. It appeared that the ball had entered the right hip in front of and a little below the right trochanter major, passed diagonally backward, and had exited above and posteriorly to the left great trochanter. The bladder had been injured in some manner as demonstrated by the subsequent passage of urine from the track of the wound and its extravasation. Although he suffered severe pain, his chief disability resulted from the fistulous opening of the urethra. It was half an inch or more in length, just anterior to the scrotum, and frequently became inflamed. The greater part of his urine was voided through the fistula, which the examining physician speculated was secondary to the long use of a catheter. In early 1883 he submitted to some type of surgery and almost died. Because of his poor health, he resigned the presidency of Bowdoin College in the fall of 1883 and gave up his lectures in 1885. Chronic cystitis caused frequent attacks of epididymitis and orchitis that totally disabled him. In December 1890 he was sick for weeks with infection and was confined to his room. During February 1893 he was in New York City to obtain treatment. He had been suffering from an another attack of cystitis, epididymitis, and orchitis since the previous August. This had culminated in a severe abscess from which he still suffered in the last week of December. He continued having infections, and near the end of 1913 he was confined to his bed or to a bedside chair and required a trained nurse.[1] Chamberlain died February 24, 1914, in Portland, Maine, and was buried in Pine Grove Cemetery, Brunswick, Maine.

DEATH CERTIFICATE: Cause of death, chronic cystitis and chronic posterior urethritis caused originally by gunshot wound.

1. CSR; *OR*, vol. 27, pt. 1:614; vol. 40, pt. 1:223, pt. 2:182, 216, pt. 3:520; vol. 42, pt. 3:256, 662, 731; vol. 46, pt. 1:800, pt. 2:193, pt. 3:691, 731; RVA, Pension SC 96,956; LR, CB, roll 248, C411, 1866; Willard M. Wallace, *Soul of the Lion: A Biography of General Joshua L. Chamberlain*, 99–100, 115, 119–23, 131–38, 140, 246–47, 288, 294–96, 309–10; Joshua Lawrence Chamberlain, *The Passing of the Armies*, 45–46; Alice Rains Trulock, *In the Hands of Providence: Joshua L. Chamberlain and the American Civil War*, 42, 103, 120–21, 330, 466; Paul E. Steiner, "Medical-Military Studies on the Civil War. No 1. Lieutenant General Ambrose Powell Hill, C.S.A.," *Military Medicine* 130 (1965): 225–28.

ALEXANDER CHAMBERS • *Born August 23, 1832,* in Great Valley, New York. Graduated from the USMA in 1853. As a cadet, he was seen for excoriatio five times, diarrhea, catarrhus, and cephalalgia each four times, and febris intermittent and febris ephemeral each twice. Served in the Florida wars. Chambers had duties on the frontier and in garrison until the start of the Civil War. He was sick at Camp Floyd, Utah, from December 1859 through January 1860. Following recruiting duty in Iowa, he was appointed colonel of the 16th Iowa Infantry in March 1862. He was wounded twice at Shiloh on April 6, 1862. One wound was in his arm, and the other, from a spent ball that hit him on the hip joint, was very painful and made him lame. On April 29 he reported from St. Louis that he had been having chills and fever for several days. At the battle of Iuka, Mississippi, on September 19, 1862, Chambers was severely wounded by a musket ball and two buckshot in the right shoulder and neck. Taken prisoner, he was left by the Confederate troops in the hospital at Iuka and was recaptured by Federal forces on September 20th. He was on home leave in November and December and suffered from a severe contraction and rigidity of the muscles of the injured arm and shoulder. He rejoined his command in January 1863. He went on sick leave again in April and assumed brigade command when he returned in June for the Vicksburg campaign. His appointment as brigadier general of volunteers to rank from August 1863 was negated by the Senate in April 1864, supposedly because he was not a legal resident of Iowa. In October he was still disabled from his shoulder wound. He was finally brevetted brigadier general in the U.S. Army in March 1865. Following the war he was on garrison duty, frontier service, and had frequent sick leave. In August 1880 he went on sick leave to help eradicate from his system the malaria contracted while at the post of Fort Lapwai, Idaho. He returned on September 20. Chambers was present sick from April 30 to May 13, 1881. In March 1883 he was treated for catarrh and was on sick leave from July 26 to August 24, 1884. He was present sick from December 25, 1884, to January 1885, March 16–23, and from March 31 to April 13. His surgeon at Fort Bridge, Wyoming, reported on March 20, 1885, that Chambers had been disabled by severe neuralgia of his right arm and shoulder for the previous five months. Because of the constant pain, he suffered from loss of sleep, and a change of climate to a drier area was recommended. In October 1885 he applied for an extension of his sick leave based on a medical certificate that reported he was suffering from a pericardial effusion. He had frequent attacks of pain over his entire chest. As a result of his combined problems he had been unable to sleep for many days and nights, except when leaning forward on a table or other support, and was very weak and emaciated. By December his condition had not improved. He still had a pericardial effusion and consequent congestion of his lungs with a cough and occasional dropsical swelling of his feet. He was weak and had little appetite. In March 1886, although still weak, he appeared to have improved and was advanced to colonel that month. Though still confined to his room, he was able to sleep in a horizontal position, his appetite was better, and he no longer had swelling of his feet. He was back on duty in June; however, his health remained poor. In October his physician reported that Chambers had been suffering from chronic bronchitis with frequent acute attacks for at least the previous eighteen months. He was on almost constant sick leave from October 10, 1886, to the date of his death. He went to San Antonio, Texas, in hopes that the climate would be an improvement over the Wyoming Territory's winter. Chambers died in the Meager Hotel in San Antonio, Texas, on January 2, 1888. According to his attending surgeon he died of pleuropneumonia following chronic asthma produced by the old gunshot wound.[1] He was buried in Owatonna, Minnesota.

1. CSR; *OR*, vol. 10, pt. 1:287; vol. 17, pt. 1:95, 101; WPCHR, vols. 607, 608; LR, ACP, 5006, 1874, fiche: 000020; RAGO, entry 534; *San Antonio (Texas) Daily Express,* Jan. 4, 1888.

STEPHEN GARDNER CHAMPLIN • *Born July 1, 1827,* in Kingston, New York. He practiced law prior to entering Federal service as a major of the 3rd Michigan Infantry in June 1861. The following October he was promoted to colonel of the unit. At Fair Oaks on May 31, 1862, he was severely wounded and unable to take further part in the action. A musket ball had passed through the muscles of his hip. Initially placed in a field hospital, he was transferred to a hospital in Philadelphia on June 12. In July he was on leave in Michigan but was still confined to his bed most of the time. Although his wound was not healed, he led his regiment on August 29, 1862, at Groveton during the Second Bull Run campaign. Due to his overexertion the wound broke down, and he was completely prostrated. His promotion to brigadier general of volunteers ranked from November. During November through January 1863 he was absent with anemia, fever, and repeated attacks of diarrhea. He assumed command of the post at Grand Rapids, Michigan, on September 24, 1863. He died from the effects of his wound and complications on January 26, 1864. His surgeon reported that he had developed evidence of tubercular disease in December 1862, which was a factor in his death.[1] He was buried in Fulton Street Cemetery in Grand Rapids.

1. CSR; *OR*, vol. 11, pt. 1:838, 865, 869; vol. 12, pt. 2:435–36; RVA, Pension C 22,583; Heitman, *Historical Register and Dictionary* 1:294.

EDWARD PAYSON CHAPIN • *Born August 16, 1831,* in Waterloo, New York. A practicing lawyer, he was involved in local militia affairs prior to the Civil War. He entered service as a captain of a company that later became part of the 44th New York. Chapin was seriously wounded early on May 27, 1862, at Hanover Court House. As soon as his condition permitted he was sent north. Still recovering, he was sent to Buffalo to take charge of a recruiting office for the 44th New York regiment. In July, while on this duty, he was commissioned a colonel. He was instantly killed May 27, 1863, at Port Hudson by a bullet that struck him in the face and penetrated his brain. Posthumously, he was promoted to brigadier general of volunteers to rank from the day of his death.[1] He was buried at Waterloo, New York, in Maple Grove Cemetery.

1. *OR*, vol. 11, pt. 1:729, 732; vol. 26, pt. 1:67, 511; Nash, *Forty-Fourth New York*, 341.

GEORGE HENRY CHAPMAN • *Born November 22, 1832,* in Holland, Massachusetts. Chapman served three years in the navy as a midshipman; after his resignation, he published a newspaper and took up the law. In October 1861 he was made a major of the 3rd Indiana Cavalry. After passing through ranks he was promoted to brigadier general of volunteers in 1864. He was slightly wounded September 19, 1864, near Winchester but was only partially disabled for several hours. The wound did not prevent him from riding ninety miles on horseback over the next seven days. He was brevetted major general in 1865 and resigned in January 1866.[1] He had served at Second Bull Run, Antietam, Fredericksburg, Gettysburg, Petersburg, and in the Shenandoah. Following the war he served as a judge for five years and finally in 1880 was elected to the Indiana state senate. He died near Indianapolis on June 16, 1882, and was buried there in Crown Hill Cemetery.

DEATH CERTIFICATE: Immediate cause, aneurysm of aorta; contributing, aorta was found ruptured near the cardiac valves. The pericardium was full of blood.

1. *OR*, vol. 43, pt. 1:25, 55, 428, 518, pt. 2:110, 119, 183.

AUGUSTUS LOUIS CHETLAIN • *Born December 26, 1824,* in St. Louis, Missouri. A rich, self-made businessman, he was made captain of a volunteer company at the start of the war. By April 1862 he had risen to colonel of the 12th Illinois Volunteers. He was at Forts Henry and Donelson and rose from his sickbed to take command of his regiment for the Battle of Shiloh on April 6, 1862. During the action his horse was shot, he was thrown, and his face and breast were badly bruised. After the battle he returned to camp, sick and completely exhausted. He was put on the steamer *Laton* where he remained for two days, unable to leave his bed. In December 1863 he was promoted to brigadier general of volunteers. He was discharged in January 1866 after having been brevetted major general of volunteers the previous June. After the war he held Federal offices and became a prominent and successful banker. In October 1893, in his declaration for an original invalid pension, he reported that he had chronic diarrhea and severely impaired vision.[1] He died March 15, 1914, in Chicago and was buried in Greenwood Cemetery, Galena, Illinois.

DEATH CERTIFICATE: Cause of death, exhaustion and inanition (1 year); contributory, chronic organic heart (years).

1. *OR,* vol. 10, pt. 1:156–58; RVA, Pension WC 11,949.

MORGAN HENRY CHRYSLER • *Born September 30, 1822,* in Ghent, New York. Prior to the war he spent most of his time as a farmer and entered Federal service as a private. In June 1861 he was made captain of the 30th New York. He received a thirty-day sick leave on November 22, 1861, because of a sprained ankle. Chrysler was promoted to major in March 1862, lieutenant colonel in August 1863, and colonel in December. He served on the Peninsula, in the Second Bull Run campaign, at Antietam, and at Chancellorsville. In early 1864 he and his regiment were ordered to Louisiana. During a skirmish on the Morgan's Ferry Road near the Atchafalaya River, Louisiana, on July 28, 1864, he was severely wounded. A minié ball had entered at the interclavicular notch of the sternum, just at the point of the right clavicle, passed to the right, and emerged at the superior point of the shoulder. The trachea and the origin of the sternocleidomastoid muscle were injured. He was sent home and, after being treated for about two and a half months, returned to duty. He was appointed a brigadier general of volunteers in November 1865 and was discharged in 1866. Following the war he was unable to resume his farming because of his old wound. A certificate from the pension examining board in 1870 reported that Chrysler could scarcely extend his right arm above the horizontal plane of his shoulder joint. The cicatrix at the entrance of the minié ball extended across the clavicular origin of the sternocleidomastoid muscle. Pressure upon the scar caused a cough and spasmodic contraction of the laryngeal and pharyngealmuscles, which were visible on the surface. A similar spasm was produced when he spoke loudly or when he swallowed fragments of food of sufficient size to press upon the trachea in passing through the esophagus. He had attacks, usually nocturnal, of extreme dyspnea, with a sensation of complete constriction of the lower part of the trachea. These were transient but occurred often, sometimes without a recognizable cause, but frequently after fatigue or exposure. His physician suggested the hyperaesthetic condition of his inferior laryngeal nerves seemed to depend upon deep cicatricial contraction rather than upon a neuritis. In 1879 Chrysler reported that there was no improvement in his condition and he was not able to farm. His right shoulder had gradually dropped and his right eye was inclined to act independent of the left. There was also a tendency of his right side to become numb.[1] He died August 24, 1890, in Kinderhook, New York, and was buried at Valatie, New York.

DEATH CERTIFICATE: Cause of death, peritonitis superinduced by gastritis and injury of the pneumogastric nerve by gunshot wound received in the late war.

1. CSR; *OR*, vol. 41, pt. 1:179, pt. 2:450, 549; *MSHW*, vol. 2, pt. 1:407; RVA, Pension WC 276,603.

WILLIAM THOMAS CLARK • *Born June 29, 1831, in Norwalk,* Connecticut. Clark left his law practice in 1861 and became first lieutenant in the 13th Iowa Infantry, a unit he had helped recruit. During the war he held staff rank and was finally appointed brigadier general of volunteers in May 1865. He went to Texas after the war and became involved in Reconstruction politics. In his application for an invalid pension on November 27, 1897, he reported that he suffered from disease of his eyes, rheumatism, senility, and general debility. While staying at the Windsor Hotel at Seward, Nebraska, on January 27, 1898, he fell down a flight of wet stairs. Although pale, nauseated, and in pain, he apparently sustained no severe injury.[1] He died October 12, 1905, in St. Luke's Hospital in New York City and was buried in the Arlington National Cemetery.

DEATH CERTIFICATE: Cause of death, asthenia following operation for an epithelioma of the pharynx.

1. RVA, Pension WC 600,425.

CASSIUS MARCELLUS CLAY • *Born October 19, 1810,* in Madison County, Kentucky. Served in the Mexican War. In 1843 Clay was attacked by a paid assassin, Samuel M. Brown. Brown fired his pistol at Clay, who severely cut Brown's face with his bowie knife. The bullet was aimed at Clay's breast but a knife scabbard, strapped to his chest with a silver-lined point, was hit instead, and his chest was only bruised. About the middle of July 1845 Clay contracted typhoid. During the rest of the month and throughout August, others had to edit his newspaper for him. While he dictated from his sickbed, his hands and head had to be bathed in cold water to keep him from being delirious from fever. By October his health was back to normal. He volunteered for the war with Mexico and on January 23, 1847, he was captured by Mexican troops. In Mexico City he and the other men were put in the monastery of Saint Jago, which had been converted into a prison. Clay became sick apparently from the lead in the water pipes. He was attacked while making a political speech in Foxtown, Kentucky, on June 15, 1849. Following an argument, he was grabbed by members of the crowd, his knife taken away from him, and he was beaten in the area of his spine and pelvis with clubs. Next, he was stabbed in the right chest, and his sternum was severed. While getting his knife back, he cut two of his fingers to the bone. Using his knife, he killed one of the attackers. Luckily, when a member of the crowd placed a pistol against Clay's head it misfired. Faint from loss of blood, Clay was carried off and was not well until the spring of 1850. He was a major general of volunteers from April 1862 until he resigned in March 1863. From 1863 until 1869 he was United States minister in Russia. After divorcing his first wife, he married a fifteen-year-old girl in 1894. This marriage lasted for only two years, and in January 1900 he was attacked by a group of men who were possibly influenced by his first wife's new husband. Although wounded, he killed two of them. His wound was not serious but he never completely recovered his health, and he became more mentally unstable and suspicious. He believed that there was a conspiracy to kill him, which seems a reasonable assumption, and for some years he fortified his home, Whitehall, and led a life of seclusion. He felt it necessary to keep the premises guarded and himself and his servants heavily armed. Only those who were in his favor were allowed to pass through into his stronghold. Two weeks before his death, doctors from Lexington and Louisville were called in consultation. His family considered it necessary to take steps to have him legally pronounced of unsound mind, and this was done. A committee was appointed by the court to take charge of him and his effects. It was reported that he suffered from kidney disease and an enlarged prostate and cystitis. Due to his paranoid tendencies, even his doctors had trouble getting in to see him. However, during his last few days the weapons were removed and friends could come and go. It is doubtful that he recognized any of his children, whom he had not seen for years. On July 22, 1903, he died peacefully on his estate in Madison County, Kentucky, and was buried in nearby Richmond Cemetery.[1]

1. H. Edward Richardson, *Cassius Marcellus Clay*, 35–36, 48–54, 60, 64, 69, 71, 128, 133, 135; *Louisville (Ky.) Courier-Journal*, July 23, 1903.

POWELL CLAYTON • *Born August 7, 1833*, in Delaware County, Pennsylvania. Clayton was a civil engineer prior to the war and entered Federal service as a captain in May 1861. The following December he was appointed lieutenant colonel of the 5th Kansas Cavalry and in March was made its colonel. His major military service was in Missouri and Arkansas. From July through September 1862, he was absent sick in St. Louis with what was initially diagnosed by one physician as bilious remittent fever and later by another as dysentery and typhoid fever. His debility was severe and by the end of August he was nothing but a skeleton. He returned to duty in October. On June 24, 1863, he requested permission to visit Memphis for a dental operation. Because of sickness, he had to turn over his command October 27. He was promoted brigadier general of volunteers in August 1864. Through September and October he was sick in his quarters with bilious fever. After the war, he went to Arkansas where he was governor, senator, and a businessman. From 1897 until 1905 he was ambassador to Mexico. Clayton died August 25, 1914, in Washington, D.C.[1] He was buried in Arlington National Cemetery.

DEATH CERTIFICATE: Cause of death, primary, senile pneumonia, three days' duration. Immediate, (illegible) three days' duration.

1. CSR; *OR*, vol. 22, pt. 1:728; vol. 41, pt. 3:104, 213, 633; RVA, Pension WO 1,036,393.

GUSTAVE PAUL CLUSERET • *Born on June 13, 1823*, in Suresnes, France. Cluseret graduated from St. Cyr, France, and served in Algeria and in the Crimea. He commanded in the French Legion in Giuseppe Garibaldi's forces and was wounded at the siege of Capua. Cluseret came to the United States in January 1862 and was commissioned a colonel and aide-de-camp on the staff of Gen. George B. McClellan. He was promoted to brigadier general of volunteers in October and resigned in March 1863. For a time he edited a weekly newspaper in New York before returning to Europe in 1867. He died August 22, 1900, near Hyeres, France, and was buried in the Old Cemetery of the Commune in Suresnes.

JOHN COCHRANE • *Born on August 27, 1813*, in Palatine, New York. Before the Civil War he was a lawyer and politician. In June 1861 he joined the Federal service as colonel of the 65th New York Infantry and was promoted to brigadier general of volunteers in July 1862. He served at Fair Oaks, Antietam, and Fredericksburg. He had a sick leave in June and in October 1862. Cochrane resigned February 1863 because his chronic bronchitis had become worse. Also, his long-standing double inguinal hernia was increasing in size and was impossible to control by mechanical appliances.[1] After his discharge from the military, he spent most of his remaining years engaged in politics. Cochrane died February 7, 1898, in New York City at his residence and was buried in the Rural Cemetery at Albany, New York.

DEATH CERTIFICATE: Direct cause, interstitial nephritis. Indirect cause, slight edema.

1. *OR*, vol. 21:999; U.S. Army, CWS, roll 1, vol. 2, report 30, pp. 457–64; LR, CB, roll 11, C81, 1863.

PATRICK EDWARD CONNOR • *Born March 17, 1820,* in County Derry, Ireland. Served in the Florida and Mexican wars. At Buena Vista on February 23, 1847, he was wounded in his left hand by a musket ball but stayed with his troops. By that evening he had lost so much blood on the cold rainy battlefield that it was necessary to keep him warm. Two of his companions huddled close to him on both sides during the night. He recuperated, then left the army in May 1847 and was discharged while in camp at Monterrey. The reason given for his separation from service was rheumatism.[1] At the start of the Civil War he was engaged in mining in California. In September 1861 he was appointed colonel of the 3rd California Infantry and was assigned to command of the District of Utah. His successful handling of hostile Indians won him an appointment as brigadier general of volunteers to rank from March 1863 and a brevet of major general at the end of the war. In 1866 he was discharged from the military and took up publishing a newspaper and mining interests in Salt Lake City. He died December 17, 1891, at Salt Lake City and was buried there in Fort Douglas Cemetery. DEATH CERTIFICATE: Immediate cause of death, urethral fever and general debility. Remote, urethral stricture, chronic cystitis, four weeks' duration.

1. *MOLLUS* 25:95; James F. Varley, *Brigham and the Brigadier: General Patrick Connor and His California Volunteers in Utah and Along the Overland Trail,* 4–5.

SELDON CONNOR • *Born January 25, 1839,* in Fairfield, Maine. When he was seventeen years of age he had typhoid fever. Initially he entered Federal service as a private in a three-month regiment, the 1st Vermont Volunteers, in May 1861. While in camp he had a severe cold that developed into chronic catarrh, and he did not recover from it until the next winter. He was appointed lieutenant colonel of the 7th Maine in August 1861. When his regiment was returning from the Peninsula, he was compelled by sickness to remain in Alexandria. He had an attack of dumb ague and diarrhea, which he treated in part by wearing a flannel bandage around his waist. He rejoined his regiment in September 1862 and was at Antietam. Connor was slightly wounded at Fredericksburg on May 4, 1863, but was able to serve at Gettysburg. In January 1864 he was appointed colonel of the 19th Maine. On May 6, 1864, in the Wilderness, his left thigh was shattered by a musket shot. The bullet passed through the leg, from the inner aspect directly through the thigh to the outer aspect, under the quadriceps tendon. He had a compound and comminuted fracture of the left femur, eight inches below the hip. Unable to ride, he was carried by his men on a blanket to the rear. He weighed two hundred pounds, and the way was rough, so it was difficult taking him to the road. At the field hospital, a primary excision of three-and-one-half inches of his fractured femur was performed. He was first moved to the hospital at Fredericksburg where the limb was kept on a double-inclined plane, made on the field from bread boxes. Sores caused by abrasions under the knee and the wound itself became maggoty. When water transportation was open, he was transported to the Douglas Hospital in Washington, D.C. On arrival there, he was taken from the inclined plane to a bed and the wounded leg was put in a bran box. He had been in the hospital some four or six weeks when a secondary hemorrhage occurred. The surgeons were hastily summoned, and preparations for amputation were made. However, he had lost so much blood and was in such a weakened condition they decided such treatment would be fatal. The tourniquet was removed and the bleeding was stopped by digital compression. Day and night for the next few weeks someone was at his side to apply pressure if needed. The thigh became greatly distended, and at the end of four weeks, when the clots were allowed to dislodge, the discharge was pus rather than blood. After being in the hospital for several weeks, while lying on his back, he felt something pricking through the skin on the underside of his thigh. A surgeon extracted a flattened piece of lead equivalent to about a third of the ordinary elongated bullet. It was a split-off portion of the ball, which had made its own track. The rest of the ball had passed through the thigh. Connor's promotion to brigadier general of volunteers ranked from June 1864. While in the hospital, he wrote a friend on October 18, 1864, and reported that the dead bone had hindered healing. Within the previous month, the doctor had extracted a small handful of osseous structures. One piece was left but was not loose enough to be removed. He was still flat on his back and his leg was suspended by a surgical appliance. The injury and surgery would result in a leg that would be four to five inches shorter than the other. In later years there was ankylosis of the knee joint, and the leg was entirely useless. During the spring of 1865 the bones seemed to be uniting, and a Smith anterior splint was applied. Before long he had pain in the knee and the splint was taken off. The knee joint was inflamed but responded to the application of ice for four weeks. At one time, extension of the limb was maintained by a weight attached to a strip of adhesive plaster on each side of the limb. It produced a little sore at the ankle that soon became an inflamed ulcer, extending for some distance around the ankle. Healing occurred following the application of dry calomel. Connor was allowed to witness the Grand Review of the Army of the Potomac on May 23, 1865, from an ambulance with his leg in a plaster of paris bandage. In August he was taken by stretcher to his father's home. After a week or so he developed dysentery and dropped to one-half his normal weight. His stomach rejected everything, including water. A consultant recommended brandy and a change in diet. While in his weakened condition Connor's right leg drew up. However, on January 1, 1866, he stood up for the first time in almost two years with the aid of crutches. He was discharged from Federal service in April.[1] In the spring of 1866, he fell and fractured the femur again, and it was over a year before he could put weight on the limb. For the majority of the rest of his life he held state and Federal political positions. In spite of his stiff leg and having to use crutches, he was quite active and would walk down to his office, coming back up the hill in a carriage. In 1891 he had a sudden attack of abdominal distress and severe chills, and there was pus in his urine. His surgeon, Stephen H. Weed, saw him and thought the problem was in the pelvis of the right kidney. In June he was confined to bed and did not recover until August. During the spring of 1892 two large painless swellings appeared, one in his right groin and one in his right thigh a few inches below the groin. Weed applied lotions and finally ordered poultices. The lesions softened, and when they felt fluctuant, he opened them. For several weeks there was a slight discharge of pus. One morning while dressing the wound he found a calculi. Next day he placed Connor under ether, made a free incision into the swelling in the thigh, enlarged the opening in the groin, and removed from each a renal calculus as large as a cranberry bean. The sinus in the groin was kept open and washed out daily, sometimes with a bichloride of mercury solution, then with tincture of iodine or peroxide of hydrogen. There was no urine in the discharge. The lower sinus healed immediately after opening and removal of the calculus, being simply under the skin. Over the years the sinus in the groin continued to discharge about four or five tablespoonsful of laudable pus each day. A catheter would pass without interruption through the sinus into the pelvis of the kidney and was kept there to be withdrawn for the exit of pus and for injections. Connor required the daily aid of a trained nurse and was wholly confined to his bed. The sinus never closed after it was first opened except for one short month, and there was no pus in his urine once the sinus had healed open. Frequently Connor showed signs of septic and uremic poisoning. Weed operated on Connor on February 13, 1895, and made a flank incision as if to remove the kidney. When he reached the area there was a large cavity behind the pelvis of the kidney. The cavity was filled with pus and considerable sand of uric acid formation and contained a calculus of uric acid, larger than those that had been removed from the groin. The cavity communicated with the sinus and was discharging its pus into it. He speculated that this stone had escaped from the pelvis of the kidney at the same time as the others and had remained there during the three years the discharge had been present. The kidney problem was not considered to be related to his old wound.[2] He died July 9, 1917, in Augusta, Maine, and was buried there in Forest Grove Cemetery.

DEATH CERTIFICATE: Cause of death, nephritis of twenty-two years or more duration; contributing cause, abscess of kidney.

1. *OR*, vol. 36, pt. 1:441; U.S. Army, CWS, roll 4, vol. 6, report 27, pp. 521–33; RVA, Pension C 83,546; *MSHW*, vol. 2, pt. 3:203; Connor to Dr. Edward D. Sabine from Douglas Hospital, Washington, D.C., Oct. 18, 1864 (copy sent to author by David B. Sabine); *MOLLUS* 19:221, 225.

2. RVA, Pension C 83,546; *Lewiston (Me.) Journal, Illustrated Magazine Section*, n.d., Maine State Library, Augusta, Me.; *Biographical Encyclopaedia of Maine in the Nineteenth Century*, 147.

JOHN COOK • *Born June 12, 1825,* in Belleville, Illinois. He was a businessman and an elected official before the war. He was commissioned colonel of the 7th Illinois Infantry in April 1861 and brigadier general of volunteers the next March. In March 1862, after fighting at Fort Donelson, he went on sick leave and re-

turned to duty in April on the morning of the Battle of Shiloh. His health remained poor, and after the battle he was granted another leave of absence. A
surgeon's certificate in July 1862 reported that Cook was suffering with chronic
diarrhea; as a result his constitution was so impaired that exercise and exposure
to the sun produced syncope, pulselessness, and entire prostration. A different
surgeon's certificate of disability two weeks later stated that Cook had general
debility, a severe cough, and derangement of his alimentary canal. The next
month he was ordered to report for duty. On May 23, 1864, he reported that his
health was too impaired for active duty and he required a dry climate such as
that found in New Mexico. No specific diagnosis was given. In September he
was ordered to command the District of Illinois. During April through July
1865 he suffered from chronic diarrhea. In August he was brevetted major general of volunteers and discharged. He was elected to the lower house of the
Illinois legislature in 1868 and in 1879 was awarded the South Dakota Sioux
agency. In June 1901 he was knocked down by a horse and injured. He was weak
and had difficulty getting around. Supposedly he had an enlarged prostate dat-
ing back to his army days, but it did not cause him any disability until 1904. He
died October 12, 1910, in Ransom, Michigan, and was buried in Oak Ridge Cemetery, Springfield, Illinois.[1]

DEATH CERTIFICATE: Cause of death, prostate abscess; contributory, cystitis.

1. CSR; RVA, Pension XC 2,694,302; U.S. Army, CWS, roll 4, vol. 7, report 52, pp. 863–79; LR, CB,
roll 248, C401, 1866.

PHILIP ST. GEORGE COOKE • *Born on June 13, 1809,* in Leesburg, Virginia. Graduated from the USMA in 1827. Served in the Black Hawk War, the Mexican War,
and the Utah expedition of 1857–58. In the Kansas Territory on September 14,
1856, he was sick and had to turn the command of his troops over to another.
He was sick again during April and July 1857. Ill for months in 1858, he left Utah
in July. He was commissioned brigadier general in the Regular Army in November 1861. Supposedly on February 24, 1862, at a camp east of Washington,
D.C., he was somewhat injured when his carriage blew over onto the hard, frozen ground. He was sick for a short time in 1862 but led a division on the Peninsula. For the rest of the war he held no field command but had recruiting
duties, district command, and court-martial duties. He retired from the army
in 1873. In December 1887 he requested permission to go to Bermuda for a couple
of months for the benefit of his health. He died March 20, 1895, in Detroit,
Michigan, and was buried there in Elmwood Cemetery. Medical report: Cause
of death, senesctus.[1]

1. *OR,* vol. 11, pt. 1:1010; *OR Suppl.,* vol. 1, pt. 1:360; U.S. Army, CWS, roll 1, vol. 2, report 56, pp.
775–77; LR, ACP, 4270, 1873, fiche: 000016; Jerry Thompson, *Henry Hopkins Sibley: Confederate
General of the West,* 119, 134–35, 162, 168.

JAMES COOPER • *Born May 8, 1810,* in Frederick County, Maryland. Prior to the war, Cooper was a lawyer and a politician. His political views prompted his appointment as a brigadier general of volunteers to rank from May 1861. Cooper was at Front Royal, Virginia, on June 6, 1862, having had an accident that was thought would disable him for field service. However, the next month he was on the march with his troops. In September he was placed in charge of a paroled prisoner-of-war camp near Columbus, Ohio, and was soon made commandant of the nearby Camp Chase. He became very sick in late February and died at Columbus on March 28, 1863. He was buried in Mount Olivet Cemetery in Frederick, Maryland. According to the surgeon's certificate, he died from congestion of the lungs.[1]

1. *OR,* vol. 12, pt. 3:457–58; RVA, Pension WC 4,736; LR, CB, B180, 1863.

JOSEPH ALEXANDER COOPER • *Born November 25, 1823,* near Cumberland Falls, Kentucky. Served in the Mexican War. He engaged in farming prior to the Civil War and entered Federal service in 1861 as a captain. In March 1862 he was promoted to colonel of the 6th Tennessee. Cooper, although sick in January and February 1864, was present. His commission as brigadier general ranked from July 1864, and he was discharged in 1866 after being brevetted major general. He served at Mill Springs, Stones River, Chickamauga, Chattanooga, in the Atlanta campaign, and at Franklin and Nashville. Following the war he was a collector of internal revenue for ten years in Knoxville, Tennessee, and in 1880 returned to farming in Kansas. He received an injury on April 3, 1891, when hit by a railroad car at Larned, Kansas. Old age had resulted in the weakening of his eyesight and hearing, and he was within a few feet of a railroad crossing when his horses became unruly. The train sounded no whistle or alarm until Cooper's team was within fifteen feet of the track. Hearing the alarm, the team became more unmanageable. The train continued at full speed as the alarm was sounded again, further frightening the horses. The only way Cooper could go forward was to cross the track; in doing so his buggy was struck. He received a severe wound on his head and was so stunned that he was helpless. He was under the care of a physician and surgeon for several weeks, during which time he was confined to his bed. He had complained about a sore shoulder and ankle for ten years, and in January 1893 he was almost entirely disqualified from manual labor by a fractured shoulder and ankle. It is not clear how he had sustained these prior injuries. He also had a diseased stomach. In October 1909 he had to give up his position as honored moderator of the South Central Kansas Baptist Association because of failing health. He died May 20, 1910, in Stafford, Kansas, and was buried in the National Cemetery at Knoxville, Tennessee. Burial records: Cause of death, senility.[1]

1. *OR,* vol. 32, pt. 1:52; RVA, Pension WC 708,155; *St. John (Kans.) Weekly News,* May 26, 1910; District Court Case no. 2396. Appr. Docket no. F, p. 296, filed Apr. 18, 1892; Minnis Funeral Home Records (holder of M. S. Barber, undertaker records), St. John, Kans.

JOSEPH TARR COPELAND · *Born May 6, 1813,* at Newcastle, Maine. Prior to the war he was a lawyer and judge. Initially commissioned a lieutenant colonel of the 1st Michigan Cavalry in August 1861, he was made a colonel of the 5th Michigan Cavalry in August 1862 and was appointed brigadier general of volunteers to rank from September 1862. Although just recovering from a protracted illness, he took command of the troops in May 1862 against the advice of his surgeon. He only left his command when utterly unable to keep his saddle. On June 3, 1862, he left on sick leave for fifteen days. From July 1863 until the end of the war he had no active field duty. On February 28, 1865, he obtained a thirty-day leave on surgeon's certificate and resigned in November.[1] After the end of hostilities he operated a hotel near Pontiac, Michigan, until 1878, when he moved to Florida. He died May 6, 1893, in Orange Park, Florida, and was buried there in Magnolia Cemetery.

1. *OR,* vol. 12, pt. 1:579–80, 596; U.S. Army, CWS, roll 1, vol. 2, report 20, pp. 231–41; ibid., roll 4, vol. 7, report 21, pp. 325–31.

MICHAEL CORCORAN · *Born September 21, 1827,* in Carrowkeel, County Donegal, Ireland. After serving in the Revenue Police and being a member of the Ribbonmen, a society of rural guerrillas, he emigrated to the United States in 1849. He was active in Tammany Hall politics and enlisted as a private in the 69th New York Militia in 1851. In 1859 he was elected colonel of the unit; because of his refusal to parade his regiment in honor of the Prince of Wales he was court-martialed in 1860. He became very ill in February 1861 and was still very weak when the Civil War started. The charges against him were dismissed on April 20, 1861; ordered to resume command of his regiment, he accompanied his men in an ambulance. Corcoran was wounded in the leg and captured at the Battle of First Bull Run on July 21, 1861. He was moved from prison to prison and, at one point, while in solitary confinement, contracted typhoid fever. After being released in August 1862, he returned to New York. His promotion as brigadier general of volunteers was ranked from the date he was wounded. He was with his troops at Camp Scott, Staten Island, in October 1862 when he had a high fever. His recovery was slow. In October 1863 he returned to New York to see a specialist because he was unwell and in need of rest. The physician reported that the illness was due to the poor food and bad air he was subjected to during his imprisonment. He recommended rest and a diet of oatmeal and barley water to build up his strength. Corcoran returned to duty in November. While riding with Gen. Thomas Meagher on December 22, 1863, he rode ahead and out of sight of the group. He was later found on the ground having a violent convulsion, his face purple. Unconscious, he was taken by wagon to the camp where surgeons bled him and then pronounced him dead. His death has been variously attributed to a fracture of the base of the skull, fit, or apoplexy. Apparently, he had previously had one or two fainting fits. However, the surgeon of the 69th Regiment who saw him immediately after the injury said he died from a fracture of the base of the skull. Although not stated, if this was a depressed fracture, it should have been an obvious diagnosis.[1] He was buried in Calvary Cemetery, Long Island City, New York.

1. CSR; RVA, Pension C 50,379; Daly, *Diary of a Union Lady,* 166, 186, 196, 256, 270; D. P. Conyngham, *The Irish Brigade and Its Campaigns,* 20, 40–41, 540; Phyllis Lane, "Michael Corcoran: Notes Toward a Life," *The Recorder* 3, no. 3 (Summer 1990): 42–54.

JOHN MURRAY CORSE • *Born April 27, 1835,* in Pittsburgh, Pennsylvania. Corse was a student at USMA for two years and left there in 1855. Only one visit for cephalalgia was recorded for Corse while he was a cadet. A lawyer and politician, he was commissioned a major in the 6th Iowa in July 1861. He had a thirty-day sick leave starting December 14, 1861, and reported back for duty the next month. In the middle of January 1863 his surgeon reported that he was suffering from hepatitis and bilious fever along with pain and irritation of his kidneys. A change of climate was suggested for the benefit of his health. The last of May he was present sick in his quarters. After passing through grades and doing good service in the Vicksburg campaign, he was promoted to brigadier general of volunteers to rank from August 1863. During the assault on Tunnel Hill near Missionary Ridge on November 25, 1863, he received a contusion of his leg from a shell and was taken off the field. The next day he had to give up his command. He was sent home on sick leave to Burlington, Iowa, on December 4. He remained in bed until the middle of January when he was carried to Springfield, Illinois, to assume command of the draft rendezvous. However, he was relieved February 1 on a surgeon's certificate because his wound had not sufficiently healed for active service, and he returned to Iowa. He returned to duty in April. In the defense of Allatoona Pass, Georgia, on October 5, 1864, he was slightly wounded in the cheek. The ball struck the point of the left malar bone and passed externally to the ear. He was insensible for thirty to forty minutes but remained on the field and in command. Because of continued pain in his head over the next few days he was unable to make a detailed report. He was discharged in 1866 with the brevet of major general.[1] Corse returned to Chicago where he was appointed collector of internal revenue. Later he moved to Massachusetts and was made postmaster of Boston. He died April 28, 1893, at Winchester, Massachusetts, and was buried in Aspen Grove Cemetery, Burlington, Iowa.

DEATH CERTIFICATE: Immediate cause of death, cerebral hemorrhage.

1. CSR; OR, vol. 31, pt. 2:69, 87, 575, 636–37; vol. 32, pt. 2:137, pt. 3:486; vol. 39, pt. 1:731, 761, 765, pt. 3:92, 96–97, 108, 150; U.S. Army, CWS, roll 1, vol. 2, report 36, pp. 525–31; RAGO, entry 534.

DARIUS NASH COUCH • *Born on July 23, 1822,* in Putnam County, New York. Graduated from the USMA in 1846. During the Mexican War he contracted dysentery, which bothered him the rest of his life. Although he was ill, he remained with his regiment in 1846. He had sick leave on August 7, 1847, and went back to New York. After his recovery, he returned to his regiment in Mexico in January 1848. He received a sick leave again in July 1852 and went to Hot Springs, Virginia. On September 21, 1852, he was able to come back to duty. Couch resigned his commission in 1855 and entered business. He reentered Federal service as a colonel of the 7th Massachusetts Volunteers and was commissioned brigadier general of volunteers to rank from May 1861. He was sick April 25, 1862, and though still ill on May 5, he accompanied Gen. John James Peck in the field and advised him on troop disposition. Couch felt that the exposure and fatigue incident to a battle always seemed to aggravate his dysentery, and he frequently had to command his troops while lying on his back. Because of his continued poor health he submitted his resignation, which was refused. On July 22 he took leave from camp. On August 12 he returned to Harrison's Landing and the army. He was at Antietam and Fredericksburg, but because of a severe attack of dysentery, he left the field on December 24 on a twenty-day leave. On January 15, 1863, he returned to the army and resumed command. He never went to a hospital for any of his illnesses but was always cared for in camp or else returned home for rest and treatment. At Chancellorsville on May 3, 1863, he was wounded twice and his horse was killed. After a short leave, he returned on June 6 and assumed corps command. After Gettysburg he was in the West, at Nashville, and in the Carolinas campaign. In May 1865 he resigned. Following the war he continued to have frequent attacks of diarrhea and dysentery, which caused great pain and general prostration.[1] He died February 12, 1897, in Norwalk, Connecticut, and was buried in Taunton, Massachusetts.

1. *OR*, vol. 11, pt. 1:390, 520, 522; vol. 51, pt. 1:1045; U.S. Army, CWS, roll 5, vol. 9, report 6, pp. 39–115; RVA, Pension WC 549,269.

ROBERT COWDIN • *Born September 18, 1805,* in Jamaica, Vermont. When the Civil War started, he was involved in the lumber business and was colonel of a Massachusetts militia regiment. In May 1861 he entered Federal service as colonel of the 1st Massachusetts Infantry. While at Fair Oaks his health was impaired due to the unhealthy location of his camp, and on September 1, 1862, he had a violent cold. In spite of his illness he continued with his duties, and his promotion as brigadier general of volunteers ranked from that month. On September 16 his surgeon stated that he had suffered for two weeks from remittent fever and intestinal irritations caused by exposure to the cold rain. On October 10 he was ordered to report for assignment. His appointment as brigadier general was not confirmed by the Senate and in March 1863 he was relieved from duty and sent home.[1] After he returned to Boston he was involved in various public institutions. He died July 9, 1874, in Boston and was buried in Mount Auburn Cemetery, Cambridge, Massachusetts.

DEATH CERTIFICATE: Immediate cause of death, gastrosarcoma.

1. CSR; *OR*, vol. 51, pt. 1:879.

JACOB DOLSON COX • *Born October 27, 1828,* in Montreal, Canada. As a result of his position as a lawyer and politician, he was made a brigadier general of Ohio state troops in April 1861. He was appointed a brigadier general of volunteers to rank from May of that year. Cox served with distinction in West Virginia, at Antietam, in the Atlanta campaign, at Franklin and Nashville, and in North Carolina. When his appointment as major general expired he was reappointed and confirmed in December 1864. On December 16 he developed symptoms of malarial poisoning. He continued on duty until December 23, when he was forced to find quarters in a private home along the Duck River, Tennessee. His surgeon reported it was due to his drinking contaminated water during the time of the encampment at Nashville and prescribed medications. His request for a medical leave to go home was granted. He learned his unit was on the move and rejoined his division at Washington on January 29. However, he did not return to his full strength for a month. In 1866–67 he was governor of Ohio and served for a time as secretary of the interior under President U. S. Grant. For the rest of his life he held a number of positions, including president of a railroad company, dean of a law school, lawyer, and writer. Cox had heart disease, and his health deteriorated during the last part of the 1890s. After a full day of sailing on July 30, 1900, he went to bed and was later found unconscious. He died on August 4 from a massive heart attack near Gloucester, Massachusetts.[1] Cox was buried in Spring Grove Cemetery, Cincinnati, Ohio.

1. *OR,* vol. 45, pt. 1:361; Jerry Lee Bower, "The Civil War Career of Jacob Dolson Cox" (diss.), 184–85, 236, 241; Jacob Dolson Cox, *Military Reminiscences of the Civil War* 2:376–77, 385, 391.

JAMES CRAIG • *Born February 28, 1817,* in Washington County, Pennsylvania. Served in the Mexican War. Another lawyer and politician whom Abraham Lincoln appointed as a brigadier general of volunteers, Craig ranked from March 1862. In May 1863 he resigned his Federal commission and the following May was made a brigadier general in the Missouri state militia. He resigned this position in January 1865 and for the majority of the rest of his life was involved with railroads. He died of cancer at his home on October 21, 1888, in St. Joseph, Missouri, and was buried there in Mount Mora Cemetery.[1]

1. Sheridan A. Logan, *Old Saint Jo: Gateway to the West, 1799–1932.*

SAMUEL WYLIE CRAWFORD • *Born November 8, 1827,* in Franklin County, Pennsylvania. After three requests when he was considered for retirement, Crawford finally reported that he was born in 1827. Following graduation from medical school in 1850, he served as an army surgeon. He had a bad sore throat the last of 1860 and the first of 1861. In 1861 he was made major of the Thirteenth Infantry and his assignment as brigadier general of volunteers ranked from April 1862. He mentioned that he was wounded in February 1862, but further details are lacking. At Antietam on September 17, 1862, he received a gunshot wound on the lateral side of his right thigh. Judging from later developments, the bone must have been injured. He remained in command until he became weak through blood loss and had to be carried to the hospital. The next day he was taken by ambulance first to Hagerstown, Maryland, and then to Chambersburg, Pennsylvania, where he remained in his father's house. When Confederate cavalry approached the house in October, he had to leave by ambulance. From the end of October through January, he had an ecchymotic, erythematous, papular eruption on his right hip near his wound. One surgeon speculated that the skin changes were the result of an injury of the external cutaneous nerves, while another reported they were due to gastroenteric irritability, irregular nervous action, and an impoverished general system induced by nervous temperament, exposure in the field, and a deficient diet. The ball was removed at some point in his treatment but the exact date is not clear. Crawford was unable to do field duty for five months but was placed on an examining board and on court-martial duty. In May 1863 he was assigned to command of the Pennsylvania Reserve Corps and led them at Gettysburg in July. On August 26, 1863, he had the onset of dysentery, which continued through October; one physician suggested it was due to malaria. There was an extensive, diffuse inflammation of his right thigh and reopening of the wound in February 1864. The wound sloughed and there was discharge of foreign material, including pieces of clothing or India rubber cloth. That same month he was commissioned lieutenant colonel of the U.S. Second Infantry. In March he was in Philadelphia under medical care, and in April he was diagnosed as having intermittent fever. He gave up his command for a few hours at Spotsylvania on May 8, 1864, when injured by a tree limb that fell after being hit by a cannonball. During the fighting on the Weldon Railroad on August 18 he was slightly wounded in the breast. His thigh wound still required a constant change of bandages, and after the battles of early February 1865 he had to give up his command because he was unable to remain in the saddle. Crawford was brevetted through all grades to major general of both the regular and volunteer service. Discharged from volunteer service in 1866, he continued to serve with his regiment. He required frequent treatment of his leg wound over the next two years. Walking or exertion was painful, and horseback riding was so irritating that he could not ride. In 1869 he was promoted to colonel. In December 1870, he developed abscesses and a fistulous opening with discharge of bone fragments and tissue as a consequence of necrosis of the shaft of the right femur. These events were associated with considerable constitutional disturbances. There was no improvement in his condition between March and August 1871, and because of continued discharge of bone particles, he was almost entirely confined in his room for a few weeks. In December, while at Huntsville, Alabama, his condition worsened. The two large openings of his wound discharged freely and were accompanied by swelling of the leg. He left his post on December 21. His wound was unchanged during 1872 and he had severe constitutional symptoms. He retired from the army in 1873 because his wound had broken down again and was discharging pus. For some weeks he had suffered from a sensation of coldness in the wounded limb to such a degree that it interferred with his sleep. The cold sensation could only be overcome by friction of the surface or by using some method to maintain the temperature. One physician suggested that the cold sensation was due to nerve damage or to interference with the blood circulation resulting in pressure on the vessels by the muscles hardened from continuous inflammation. Offensive pus came from three openings on the outer side of the right thigh about six inches above the knee joint. Examining surgeons had no doubt that the bone was diseased and that surgery might be required to remove part of it. His condition continued to deteriorate, and by March 1892 he was so disabled that he could not get around much and required the attention of a physician almost daily. According to the attending physician, he suffered a stroke on the night of November 2–3, 1892, and died on the evening of the third in Philadelphia.[1] He was buried in Philadelphia's Laurel Hill Cemetery.

1. OR, vol. 19, pt. 1:484–86; U.S. Army, CWS, roll 8, vol. 13, report 1, pp. 3–209; LR, ACP, 74, 1873, fiche: 000088; RAGO, entry 534; Steiner, *Physician-Generals,* 41–44.

THOMAS LEONIDAS CRITTENDEN • *Born May 15, 1819,* in Russellville, Kentucky. Served in the Mexican War. A prewar lawyer, he was appointed brigadier general of volunteers in September 1861. Crittenden was sick at the time the division was encamped at Shiloh in late April 1862. He was confined to his room for eight to ten days and did not join his command until May 3. In July 1862 he was commissioned major general. After service in the Tullahoma campaign and Chickamauga, Crittenden, at his own request, was relieved of command on June 8, 1864, and his resignation took effect in December. After serving for a period as state treasurer of Kentucky he accepted a position as a colonel in the Regular Army. Unable to discharge his duties on the frontier because of his age, the exposure, and his rheumatism, he requested to be retired in 1881. His health poor in April 1888, he requested permission to go to Mexico City for a short visit. He died October 23, 1893, at Annadale, Staten Island, New York, and was buried in Frankfort, Kentucky. Cause of death, progressive paresis.[1]

1. OR, vol. 10, pt. 1:700, 703; vol. 36, pt. 1:147, 915; vol. 42, pt. 3:998; LR, ACP, 1862, 1881, fiche: 000037; Records of death, Town Clerk, Westfield, N.Y.

THOMAS TURPIN CRITTENDEN • *Born October 16, 1825,* in Huntsville, Alabama. Served in the Mexican War. He was practicing law when he was appointed captain of the 6th Indiana in April 1861. Crittenden was promoted to colonel a week later and in April 1862 was commissioned brigadier general of volunteers. He had fought in West Virginia and at Shiloh. He was captured in July 1862 under rather embarrassing circumstances and resigned in May 1863. For the rest of his life he mainly practiced the law. He died September 6, 1905, in the Hawthorne Inn at East Gloucester, Massachusetts, and was buried in Arlington National Cemetery.

DEATH CERTIFICATE: Cause of death, primary, heart disease; contributory, senility.

MARCELLUS MONROE CROCKER · *Born on February 6, 1830*, in Franklin, Indiana. He entered the USMA with the class of 1851 but left in February 1849 to study law. While at West Point he was treated twice each for phlegmon and cephalalgia and once each for diarrhea, dysentery, and catarrhus. Crocker was practicing law at the start of the Civil War. U. S. Grant stated that Crocker was already dying from tuberculosis at the time he volunteered for military service. He rapidly rose from captain of the 2nd Iowa Infantry to colonel of the 13th Iowa by December 1861. Crocker was present sick in June 1862. His promotion as brigadier general of volunteers ranked from November 1862. Another officer had to be temporarily assigned to take his command because he was ill on May 27, 1864. He had held field commands at Shiloh, Corinth, and Vicksburg. His resignation, submitted because of poor health, was not accepted in June, and he was sent to New Mexico to improve his physical condition in the drier climate. By December Crocker reported that he was well enough to return to duty and went back east. He died August 26, 1865, in Washington, D.C., and was buried in Woodland Cemetery, Des Moines, Iowa.[1]

1. *OR*, vol. 34, pt. 4:504; vol. 38, pt. 3:578; vol. 40, pt. 2:303; vol. 45, pt. 2:388; vol. 48, pt. 1:829, 1157; vol. 49, pt. 1:860; WPCHR, vol. 606; RVA, Pension C 74,057; *Battles and Leaders* 3:503.

GEORGE CROOK · *Born September 8, 1829*, near Dayton, Ohio. On a form he sent to the adjutant general on August 24, 1881, he reported that he was born in 1829. Graduated from the USMA in 1852. At West Point he was treated for morbi. varii., cephalalgia, catarrhus, subluxatio, and colica once each. Crook was scheduled to leave Benicia Barracks, California, with his company in January 1853 when he developed erysipelas of both ankles. Two doctors treated him. The first painted the area with creosote and iodine, which only made the lesions worse. The following day the next doctor gave him calomel and jalap. Crook thought he had improved enough to go with his men. In January 1854, while pursuing Indians in the cold weather, he was trying to extinguish some burning blankets when molten rubber got on his hands, burning them. In early 1856 he had sudden onset of acute rheumatism of his left shoulder associated with erysipelas of the left arm. A contract doctor who was frequently drunk took care of him, but with minimal success, and the arm shrunk in size and was useless. A large abscess extending from the elbow to the shoulder developed and had to be lanced. Medical books available to Crook suggested that brandy was good for erysipelas but was not good for rheumatism. One out of two did not seem bad, so he took the brandy. An Indian woman came into his room and asked who he was leaving his things to when he died, so he decided to take his case in hand. He again medicated himself with calomel and jalap until he started to improve. Then each day he poured cold water over the arm. For nearly a year afterward the arm was so weak that he could hardly raise it. In addition, he had taken so much morphine that he had difficulty going to sleep without it. On June 10, 1857, during a skirmish with Indians at Pit River Canyon, California, he was hit in the right hip by an arrow. Although he pulled out the shaft, the arrowhead remained in his leg. It was necessary for him to make the painful trip back to camp on horseback. When he arrived his groin was discolored by blood. He remained in camp a few days, but his leg became worse, and he requested that a doctor come and remove the arrowhead. The surgeon arrived and stated that it was best to leave the arrowhead alone, so it remained with Crook until he died. Seventeen days after he was wounded, he participated in another expedition after raiding Indians. While on a stagecoach in the fall of 1859 he had severe pain in his stomach, which seemed like a ball of fire. He ate little, and the doctor reported it was due to his liver and prescribed some form of medicine. Apparently the pain went away without any residual. In the fall of the next year, while on another stagecoach going to the East, he experienced an attack of malaria while in Sherman, Texas. In September 1861 he was appointed colonel of the 36th Ohio. A spent musket ball struck him on the foot during the battle of Lewisburg, Virginia, on May 23, 1862. At first he had little distress, but by nightfall he was in severe pain. He did not rest the foot and improvement was slow. In August 1862 he was promoted brigadier general. He had what was termed "serious liver trouble" in January 1863; however, there are no further details of this episode. At the end of the war he was brevetted major general in the Regular Army. Crook remained in the military and in 1866 was made lieutenant colonel of the 23rd Infantry. His remaining years were spent mainly on the western frontier, and he rose to the rank of major general. In the summer of 1887 he had difficulty sleeping, felt unwell during the day, and took frequent doses of a quinine solution for attacks of malaria. At one point he took up to eighteen grains at a time. He had some type of recording of his pulse in Chicago the next year that demonstrated an irregularity. For a number of years he had episodes of bleeding from his lungs and in October 1888 had another bad attack. The consulting doctor told him that his lungs were distended and pressed on his heart. Apparently he thought the diagnosis was emphysema. The physician who took care of him for the last few years of his life did not think he had emphysema but rather chronic gastric catarrh. He stated, "When his stomach was distended by gases it produced active sympathetic action of the heart, characterized by rapid irregular and intermittent beats. The episodes were easily treated. The general had not contributed to his condition since he was absolutely temperate and did not drink or smoke." Crook arose early on March 21, 1890, and started his exercises with a dumbbell in his parlor at the Grand Pacific Hotel in Chicago. He experienced chest pain and difficulty breathing and called his wife. Shortly afterward he died from what was diagnosed as heart failure by the hotel physician but what from the description sounds more like a myocardial infarction. Dr. McClellan, the U.S. Army surgeon who took care of him over the previous few years, stated in a report that Crook died with gastric catarrh and heart failure.[1] He was buried in Arlington National Cemetery.

1. WPCHR, vol. 606; LR, ACP, 2229, 1882, fiche: 000017; autobiography of Major Gen. George Crook, 1885–1890 (handwritten), Crook-Kennon Papers; Crook's diaries, Aug. 13, 1885–Mar. 13, 1890, pp. 137, 148–49, 156–58, USAMHI; RVA, Pension C 276,308; U.S. Army, CWS, roll 1, vol. 2, report 22, pp. 263–89; Heitman, *Historical Register and Dictionary* 2:19; George Crook, *General George Crook: His Autobiography*, 90–91, 102, 281; *Maury (Tenn.) Democrat*, Mar. 27, 1890.

JOHN THOMAS CROXTON • *Born on November 20, 1836*, in Bourbon County, Kentucky. Croxton left his law practice and entered Federal service as lieutenant colonel of the 4th Kentucky Mounted Infantry in October 1861. The following May he was promoted to colonel. Croxton served at Mill Springs, Perryville, and in the Tullahoma campaign. He was confined to his bed with typhoid fever from March 28 until April 20, 1863, and did not rejoin his command until April 30. During May and June he was absent sick in Paris, Kentucky. On September 20, 1863, at Chickamauga, he was wounded in the left thigh and exited the field when he became so exhausted that he was unable to sit up. He was sent to the officers' hospital in Nashville, Tennessee, for treatment. Croxton returned to duty before he was fully recovered from the effects of the wound. During the Battle of Missionary Ridge on November 25, 1863, his previously wounded leg was severely bruised by the explosion of a shell. In July 1864 he was appointed brigadier general of volunteers. After the Atlanta campaign and the Battle of Nashville he resigned from Federal service in December 1865 and returned to his law practice. In 1874 he accepted the office of U.S. minister to Bolivia and died there on April 16, 1874. A few weeks prior to his death, a cavity in his left lung had increased in size and the material it contained could not be discharged by coughing because he was so weak. He was debilitated and feverish. After his death, an examination of his abdominal organs was made prior to embalming the body. The stomach, intestines, liver, and kidneys were normal while the mesenteric lymph nodes showed evidence of prior tuberculous involvement. His wife reported that he died from consumption.[1]

1. CSR; *OR*, vol. 30, pt. 1:172, 417, 423; vol. 31, pt. 3:202; LR, ACP, 2245, 1878, fiche: 000089; RVA, Pension Min. C 224,681.

CHARLES CRUFT • *Born on January 12, 1826*, in Terre Haute, Indiana. Before entering Federal service as a colonel of the 31st Indiana Infantry in September 1861, he had spent a varied life as teacher, clerk, lawyer, and president of a railroad. Cruft was listed as wounded at Fort Donelson on February 15, 1862, but he does not mention such an event. At Shiloh on April 6, 1862, he was wounded in the head, shoulder, and left thigh. He was confined on the steamer *New Uncle Sam* at Pittsburg Landing for some time because of his wounds. His promotion as brigadier general of volunteers ranked from July, and he was back in command in August. He was wounded at Richmond, Kentucky, on August 30, 1862. He was at Stones River, Chickamauga, and Chattanooga. On June 10, 1864, he was ordered to Chattanooga on account of a severe fever, and in the middle of July he was recovering in the hospital. In November he was in command of a detachment at Chattanooga, but his health was still not good. However, he led a division at Nashville. Having been brevetted major general, he was discharged in August 1865.[1] Cruft returned home and resumed his law practice. He died March 23, 1883, in Terre Haute and was buried there in Woodlawn Cemetery.

DEATH CERTIFICATE: Immediate cause of death, hemoptysis, three days.

1. CSR; *OR*, vol. 10, pt. 1:234, 236; vol. 16, pt. 2:466; vol. 38, pt. 1:90, 231; vol. 52. pt. 1:275; U.S. Army, CWS, roll 2, vol. 3, report 19, pp. 585–97; Alfred Lacey Hough, *Soldier in the West: The Civil War Letters of Alfred Lacey Hough,* 204, 229.

GEORGE WASHINGTON CULLUM • *Born on February 25, 1809,* in New York City. Graduated from the USMA in 1833. At West Point he was treated for a cold twice and a boil once. As an instructor at the academy in 1850 he was treated for catarrhus. After serving as an engineer during the years before the Civil War, he was made a brigadier general of volunteers to rank from November 1861 and served on Gen. Henry W. Halleck's staff. Although sick, he was in his office in Cairo, Illinois, on March 3, 1862. The next day he rose from his sickbed to go on the expedition and examine the works at Columbus, Kentucky. After the war he remained an engineer in the army until 1874. Cullum's most outstanding contribution was the compilation of the *Biographical Register of the Officers and Graduates of the United States Military Academy* and the provisions for its supplementation in his will. He died February 28, 1892, at his residence in New York City. He was buried in Green-Wood Cemetery, Brooklyn. According to the attending physician, he died of pneumonia.[1]

1. *OR*, vol. 7:435, 437; LR, ACP, 692, 1873, fiche: 000090.

NEWTON MARTIN CURTIS • *Born May 21, 1835,* in De Peyster, New York. After serving as a teacher, postmaster, and farm manager, he entered the U.S. Army as a company captain in the 16th New York. At West Point, Virginia, on May 7, 1862, a musket ball entered his left axilla and came out at the lower angle of his scapula, injuring the nerves. The wound impaired the use of his arm. In December 1862 he had chronic diarrhea and developed a fistula in ano. Curtis left on sick leave in March and rejoined his regiment the following month. He requested permission in August 1863 to be sent to Alexandria to receive medical treatment from his private physician, who was in charge of Fairfax Hospital. From January through April 1864 he was present sick. He was seriously wounded during the fighting at Fort Fisher, North Carolina, on January 15, 1865. A shell fragment struck him over the left eye and destroyed its sight. For many weeks he was at the officers' hospital at Hampton. In March he was on sick leave and improving in health except for a few days when he had a slight fever and dizziness due to his head wound. Curtis reported back for assignment to light duty in April 1865 and was temporarily attached to the department staff. He was made brigadier general primarily for his actions at Fort Fisher and was brevetted major general. He was mustered out in 1866.[1] Following hostilities he served in a number of capacities for the state of New York. In April 1867 he continued to have chronic diarrhea and developed three large sinuses associated with his fistula in ano. By September 1873 he had been operated on three times for his fistula in ano; it had healed, but fissures were still present. When examined in September 1875 and in September 1877 he was having severe neuralgic pains from his left shoulder to his hand, and the hand was weak. The head wound had not only destroyed the use of the left eye, but he had severe pain in the eye socket and the left side of his head. He also still had several fistula in ano but they had improved.[1] He died at New York City on January 8, 1910, and was buried in Ogdensburg, New York.

DEATH CERTIFICATE: Cause of death, cerebral apoplexy.

1. CSR; *OR*, vol. 46, pt. 1:400, 416, pt. 3:763; RVA, Pension SC 84,564; *MOLLUS* 17:49; John Weslely Turner Papers (Official Correspondence, Jan.–Mar. 1863), USAMHI.

SAMUEL RYAN CURTIS • *Born on February 3, 1805,* in Clinton County, New York. Graduated from the USMA in 1831 and resigned his commission the next year. Served in the Mexican War. Curtis had engaged in the practice of the law, engineering, and politics and was a member of Congress at the start of the Civil War. He entered the Federal service as a colonel of the 2nd Iowa but was soon appointed brigadier general of volunteers to rank from May 1861. His major service was at Pea Ridge. In February 1862, dysentery had broken out among the troops; Curtis fell sick on the seventh. He was appointed major general in March 1862. He was ill again in August and obtained leave the next month to return to Iowa. On September 22 his leave was revoked and he was ordered to immediately assume command of the Department of Missouri in St. Louis. In early October 1864 he was sick. He had to be carried in an ambulance from which he directed the movement of his troops. According to his son, after the war he suffered from a nervous affection of his back to such an extent that he was unable to sit up. In July 1865 he was in Milwaukee, Wisconsin, recovering from having injured his arms in a fall. It hurt him even to write. In August 1865

he was assigned to negotiate with the Plains Indians and in November was ordered to report on the construction of the Union Pacific Railroad. He was mustered out of service in April 1866 and died December 26, 1866, at Council Bluffs,
Iowa. He was buried in Oakland Cemetery, Keokuk, Iowa. Two physicians speculated that his death was caused by the strain and his exposure to the elements,
particularly during the Sioux campaign of 1864. His wife reported that he died
from heart disease.[1]

1. *OR*, vol. 8:547; vol. 13:553, 556, 609, 656; vol. 41, pt. 1:512; vol. 48, pt. 2:1074; RVA, Pension Min.
C 252,668.

GEORGE ARMSTRONG CUSTER • *Born December 5, 1839,* in New Rumley, Ohio.
Graduated from the USMA in 1861. While at West Point, he was treated for
contusio and catarrhus seven times each, diarrhea, excoriatio, and subluxiatio
each three times, cephalalgia twice, and once each for nausea, odontalgia, clavus, erysipelas, and gonorrhea. Custer entered the Civil War as a lieutenant and
did staff duty until he was appointed brigadier general of volunteers in June
1863. He had sick leave from October 3 to December 2, 1861. While trying to put
out a fire on the Skiff Creek before Williamsburg, Virginia, on May 4, 1862, he
burned his hands. During a charge to capture enemy guns near Raccoon Ford
on September 13, 1863, he received a gunshot in the area of the tibia, which tore
his boot. The soft structures were injured along with the periostium of the
bone. He returned to duty in October. Custer was thrown from a carriage on
March 14, 1864, and suffered a concussion of the brain. He received a leave and
was back in April. In July he had remittent fever and diarrhea. He was given the
full rank of major general of volunteers in April 1865 and was appointed lieutenant colonel of the Seventh Cavalry in 1866. During October 1867, while on
court-martial duty, he had a boil on his right thigh. Custer died at Little Big
Horn, Wyoming, on June 25, 1876. The confusion concerning the details of
Custer's death at Little Big Horn are reflected in the number of articles and
books dealing with the subject. Reports by the only survivors of the battle, the
Indians, say he was killed midstream of the Medicine Tail Coulee and then
carried to the spot where he was found. Others report he was killed where he
was found.[1]

1. *OR*, vol. 11, pt. 1:526, pt. 3:140; vol. 29, pt. 1:112; RG 94, Records of the AGO, 1783–1917, Military
Service Records of George A. Custer, 1856–79, microfilm; Lymon, *Meade's Headquarters,* 17; Robert
M. Utley, *Cavalier in Buckskin,* 193; David Humphreys Miller, *Custer's Fall: The Indian Side of the
Story,* 128, 245.

LYSANDER CUTLER • *Born on February 16, 1807,* in Worcester County, Massachusetts. Essentially a self-educated man, he was among other things a teacher,
businessman, and grain broker before the war. He entered Federal service as
colonel of the 6th Wisconsin. During the Second Bull Run campaign, on Au-

gust 28, 1862, he was wounded in the right thigh and received treatment both in the hospital and at home. In late October, his wound partially healed, he developed sciatica. Although still suffering from the wound, he reported back to duty November 4. However, another had to command the regiment initially. Cutler's commission as brigadier general of volunteers ranked from that month. Because of the lameness and stiffness of his leg, he had to be assisted on and off his horse. At Fredericksburg on December 13, 1862, he turned over his command in the evening because of the effects of his previous wound, the sciatica, and a contusion to the other leg from being kicked by a horse. He went on leave in January and reported back for duty on March 25, 1863, in time for Chancellorsville and Gettysburg. At City Point, Virginia, on August 21, 1864, he was wounded in the face by a piece of shell, which caused great disfigurement. Relieved from duty at his own request in September, he spent the rest of the war directing the draft rendezvous at Jackson, Michigan. He resigned in June 1865. Cutler returned home an invalid and had to be under care most of the time up to his death. The gunshot wound of his thigh caused wasting of his flesh and strength. His health continued to decline, and on July 19, 1866, he had a slight stroke that further paralyzed the wounded right leg. On the twenty-fifth he had a more severe stroke, which resulted in hemiplegia of his entire right side and, according to his attending physician, his death on the thirtieth.[1] Died in Milwaukee and was buried there in Forest Home Cemetery.

1. CSR; *OR*, vol. 12, pt. 2:337, 378, 382; vol. 21:477; vol. 42, pt. 1:19, 31, pt. 2:356; vol. 51, pt. 1:995; RVA, Pension WC 184,226; U.S. Army, CWS, roll 1, vol. 2, report 6, pp. 71–79; Dawes, *Sixth Wisconsin*, 104–5, 109–10.

D

NAPOLEON JACKSON TECUMSEH DANA • *Born April 15, 1822,* at Fort Sullivan, Eastport, Maine. Graduated from the USMA in 1842. Dana was seriously wounded in the hip at the battle of Cerro Gordo on April 18, 1847. He lay on the field for over a day before he was brought in by a burial detail. He was absent on sick leave because of his wound and on recruiting service until March 1849. In 1855 he resigned from the U.S. Army and took up banking in Minnesota, where he became a brigadier general of militia. He was appointed colonel of the 1st Minnesota in October 1861 and became a brigadier general of volunteers the next year. After arriving at Harrison's Landing, he was very ill with a fever and rheumatism and was confined to his bed on July 5, 1862. He was sent to Philadelphia on the tenth and remained there for six weeks in such bad condition that there was concern for his life. In August a surgeon in Philadelphia reported that he had remittent fever. Dana was back in command of his brigade on September 2. At Antietam, September 17, 1862, he was carried from the battlefield seriously wounded. The ball entered the lateral side of the lower third of the left leg and passed forward. After spending two days in a field hospital at Readysville, Maryland, he was sent to private residences in Washington and Philadelphia. He remained in bed for two months and at some point the ball was removed from the anterior surface of the leg, two and one-half inches from the entrance. His promotion as major general ranked from November 1862. An examination on November 11 revealed an irritable ulcer at the point of entrance of the ball over the fibula and the development of enlarged veins of the leg. In late November he stated he could do any sedentary duty. He left Philadelphia and sat on a military commission until May 1863. In November 1864 he was confined to his room for several days because of sickness. He was relieved of his command May 1, 1865, and ordered to report by letter from his home. After the war Dana entered business and served as deputy commissioner of pensions for the United States government from 1895 until 1897. By April 1881 his wounded leg had medium-sized varicose veins that were particularly prominent just at the lower border of the patella. The cicatrix of the exit of the ball was depressed and somewhat adherent. According to the local commanding officer, he died of apoplexy on July 15, 1905, in Portsmouth, New Hampshire, and was buried there.[1]

1. *OR*, vol. 11, pt. 2:95; vol. 19, pt. 1:57, 173, 276, 307, 319–20; vol. 41, pt. 4:585; vol. 48, pt. 2:280; RVA, Pension SC 216,143; U.S. Army, CWS, roll 1, vol. 2, report 4, pp. 51–57; LR, ACP, 137, 1874, fiche: 000048; RAGO, entry 534; Huger journal from Mexico, B. Huger Papers, University of Virginia Library, Manuscript Division, Special Collections Department, Charlottesville, Va.; Cadmus M. Wilcox, *History of the Mexican War*, 297.

JOHN WYNN DAVIDSON • *Born August 18, 1824*, in Fairfax County, Virginia. Graduated from the USMA in 1845. During the Mexican War he served mainly in California. Late in September 1852 he developed a severe cold and was on the sick list. He did not improve and remained on sick leave until May 12, 1853, when he was ordered to join his company. In August 1853 he arrived in New Mexico. Davidson was wounded by Indians at Cienequilla, New Mexico, on March 30, 1854, but was back on duty the next month. His appointment as brigadier general of volunteers ranked from February 1862. During the siege of Yorktown he was disabled by a strain on April 27, 1862, and was given a leave of fifteen days. On June 29, in the Battle of Savage Station, he had a sunstroke. He remained insensible for some time, lying on the ground and appearing dead. He was carried in a litter by men of his brigade during the retreat. The next day, although weak, he was back in the saddle. On July 24 at Harrison's Landing he received a leave of absence on a surgeon's certificate, reporting that he suffered from nervous prostration consequent to the sunstroke. Davidson assumed temporary command of the St. Louis Division of Missouri on August 6, 1862. For the next year and a half, whenever he was exposed to the sun, he had mild symptoms similar to his sunstroke. When in malarial districts he also suffered from fevers and general biliary derangements. During the middle of December

1864 he arrived in New Orleans and had a high fever, which may have been malaria. He remained in the army after the war and served in the inspector general's department, taught at Kansas Agricultural College, and held various commands on the frontier. While on an inspection tour of the Southern District of Mississippi in late June 1865 he became violently ill when exposed to the hot weather. The surgeon stated that the symptoms were those of one who had previously suffered a sunstroke. In August a surgeon at Natchez, Mississippi, reported that Davidson was suffering from debility resulting from the malarious influences he had been exposed to over the last three years. In October a different surgeon stated that he had chronic congestion of the liver, dyspepsia, and remittent fever that had been aggravated by a recent attack of severe dengue. He was sent on a leave of absence the next month and in January 1866 was offered the command of the Second Cavalry Regiment at Fort Riley, Kansas. During February 1867 a surgeon at Fort Leavenworth, Kansas, attempted to put all of his medical problems together and reported Davidson suffered from the effects of sunstroke, remittent fever, and dengue. He recommended that Davidson reside in the high regions in the West away from the malarious areas. In June 1867, after they started out on an inspection of Fort Arbuckle, Cherokee Nation, Davidson became sick from the heat. He had to go back and was placed on court-martial duty. After two bouts of his old malaria, he requested retirement in August 1869 because of his poor health and continued sensitivity to sun exposure. However, the next year it was refused because the retirement list was full and the reviewing surgeon did not think an individual who had previously suffered sunstroke was more sensitive to a second attack. While at Fort Sill in 1874 he had a few slight attacks of malaria that forced him to go to bed. Following his arrival at Fort Griffin, Texas, in March 1875, he had recurrent attacks of malaria. Because of the severity of his illness, Davidson obtained a four-month leave and went with his family to their home in Manhattan, Kansas. They arrived there in August, and he was cared for by a private physician. In November Davidson wrote that he was still suffering from chronic diarrhea with derangement of the stomach and liver caused by the malarial poisoning. His kidneys were badly affected and there were symptoms of diabetes. In December 1875 he had similar symptoms but also had developed rheumatism. He kept obtaining leaves, and in May 1876, after his strength had improved, he was ordered to report for duty as recruiting officer at Louisville, Kentucky. Soon after his arrival there, he had a recurrence of diarrhea and malarial fever, and in June 1876 he returned home on leave. When his health had improved, he returned to duty in Texas on December 20, 1876. From June to October 1878 he had repeated attacks of malarial fever. In November his surgeon stated that he was suffering from the chronic results of the malaria, which consisted of a deranged function of his liver, spleen, and stomach. On the morning of February 7, 1881, at Fort Custer, Montana, an officer reported that the beef cattle were

being fed on refuse forage from the stables. When Davidson rode down to inspect the forage, his horse slipped on the ice and fell down a twenty-foot embankment. His saddle struck him in the side and stomach and broke two of his
ribs. The pain continued over the months, making him unfit for duty. In May
1881 he obtained a one-year leave on surgeon's certificate, reporting he had subacute gastritis and general nervous debility. He went as far as St. Paul, Minnesota, where he died June 26, 1881, with an enlarged liver, which attending surgeons variously diagnosed as due to inflammation or cancer.[1]

1. OR, vol. 11, pt. 1:390, 511, 513, pt. 2:464, 481; vol. 51, pt. 1:585; U.S. Army, CWS, roll 3, vol. 4,
report 13, pp. 283–459; LR, ACP, 4376, 1875, fiche: 000060; RVA, Pension C 195,176; Homer K. Davidson,
Black Jack Davidson: A Cavalry Commander on the Western Frontier, 67, 72, 75, 130, 133, 145, 150–53;
Heitman, *Historical Register and Dictionary* 2:19.

HENRY EUGENE DAVIES • *Born on July 2, 1836,* in New York City. He left his law
practice at the start of the war and was made a captain of the 5th New York
Infantry. Davies was appointed major in August 1861, lieutenant colonel in December 1862, colonel in June 1863, and brigadier general in September 1863. He
served on the Peninsula, in the Second Bull Run campaign, and in the
Shenandoah. In April 1862 he suffered from irritative fever and urticarial eczema. He received a sick leave the middle of June 1863 because of chronic diarrhea and general debility; when restored to health he returned to duty on August 10. On July 29, 1864, he went to the Cavalry Corps' hospital at City Point
because of an attack of malaria and after a few days was sent north to recuperate. He returned in September to command his brigade. At the Battle of Hatcher's
Run, February 6, 1865, Davies received a contusion of the right breast from a
bullet and was carried to the rear. After having a sick leave, he returned and
assumed temporary division command on the twenty-third. He was promoted
to major general and resigned in January 1866. Following his return to New
York, he resumed his law practice. According to the death certificate he died
September 7, 1893, in Middleboro, Massachusetts, and was buried in the yard of
St. Luke's Church at Beacon, New York. His gravestone records his death as on
September 6, 1894.[1]

DEATH CERTIFICATE: Cause of death, hemorrhage of lungs.

1. CSR; OR, vol. 40, pt. 1:615, 618–19; vol. 42, pt. 1:80, 82, pt. 2:449; vol. 46, pt. 1:68, 366, 622, pt.
2:449; RVA, Pension WC 679,218; U.S. Army, CWS, roll 2, vol. 3, report 4, pp. 109–22; ibid., roll 7, vol.
11, report 9, pp. 637–815; RAGO, entry 534; Fishkill Historical Society, N.Y.

THOMAS ALFRED DAVIES • *Born on December 3, 1809,* in St. Lawrence County,
New York. Graduated from the USMA in 1829. Davies resigned his commission
in 1831 and was first a civil engineer and then a merchant. He reentered Federal
service as colonel of the 16th New York at the start of the Civil War. His major
service was at First Bull Run and Corinth. On September 6, 1861, he had a

surgeon's certificate that stated he was suffering from chronic bronchitis with a severe cough. In addition, he had symptoms of typhoid fever, which was epidemic at the time. Davis was made brigadier general of volunteers in March 1862. Early in June he went north on sick leave and returned to field duty by the end of the year. For the rest of the war Davies had mainly district commands. He was discharged with the brevet of major general in August 1865.[1] After his return to New York he became a writer. He died August 19, 1899, near Ogdensburg, New York, and was buried in the family cemetery at Oswegatchie, New York.

DEATH CERTIFICATE: Cause of death, bronchopneumonia.

1. CSR; Steiner, *Disease*, 177–79.

EDMUND JACKSON DAVIS • *Born October 2, 1827,* at St. Augustine, Florida. Prior to the war he was a lawyer, judge, and district attorney. Davis raised the 1st Texas Cavalry and was made a colonel of volunteers in October 1862. In November 1864 he was promoted to brigadier general of volunteers. Following the war he became a politician and practiced the law. He died February 7, 1883, in Austin, Texas, and was buried there in the State Cemetery.

JEFFERSON COLUMBUS DAVIS • *Born March 2, 1828,* in Clark County, Indiana. Served in the Mexican War. In June 1848 he was commissioned directly into the Regular Army as a second lieutenant. While at Fort Myers, Florida, he had sick leave from May to December 1853. A captain at the start of the Civil War, Davis was appointed colonel of the 22nd Indiana in August 1861. On October 29 he was sick all night, due in part to the medicine he had taken, but was better the next day. Davis was promoted brigadier general of volunteers in December 1861. He commanded a division at Pea Ridge and Corinth. In July 1862 he returned home on sick leave. Although advised to rest, he wanted to return and was ordered to report to Louisville. During a quarrel on September 29, 1862, he shot and killed Gen. William Nelson. Davis was restored to duty and served with distinction at Stones River, Chickamauga, in the Atlanta campaign, and in the March to the Sea and Carolinas campaign. He was ill on July 28, 1864, and turned over command a of his troops until August 23. In 1866 he was breveted major general and was made a colonel in the regular service. For many years after the war Davis was afflicted with ill health. His disease manifested itself by chronic jaundice and anemia. He had sick leaves from August 1–19, 1876, November 5 to December 9, 1876, December 19–29, 1876, February 3 to May 16, 1878, and July 31 to September 1879. Although no specific diagnosis is available for these leaves, it was stated that his disease had the appearance of chronic jaundice. He was a member of a military board at Chicago, Illinois, when he died there on November 30, 1879. His attending physician reported the cause of death as pneumonia complicated by jaundice and anemia, which had existed for several years.[1] He was buried in Crown Hill Cemetery, Indianapolis.

1. CSR; *OR,* vol. 38, pt. 1:78, 95, 635–36, 650–51; RVA, Pension WC 191,233; Joseph P. Fried, "How One Union General Murdered Another," *CWTI* 1 (June 1962): 14–16.

GEORGE WASHINGTON DEITZLER • *Born November 30, 1826,* in Pine Grove, Pennsylvania. He was a farmer and antislavery politician at the start of the war and was made colonel of the 1st Kansas Volunteer Infantry. At Wilson's Creek, Missouri, on August 10, 1861, he was shot in the front of his right leg, just above the knee. The bullet struck the bone, glanced to the right, and lodged in the muscles near the bone, causing great pain and blood loss. Deitzler was carried from the battlefield to Springfield, Missouri, and then with the retreating army to Rolla. He was not treated in the hospital but was cared for by the regimental surgeon. The bullet was removed approximately eight months after he was wounded. The ball was flattened like a wafer with serrated edges. The wound healed, leaving a weak and painful joint. Unfit for field duty for about ten months, he performed mostly post duties in Missouri and Kansas. His promotion as brigadier general ranked from November 29, 1862. Deitzler was off duty from April 1863 until he resigned. He was treated for diarrhea and jaundice in Memphis, Tennessee, in May 1863, and a change in climate was recommended. He had sick leave the next month, and when the diarrhea became chronic it prompted his August resignation from Federal service. In 1864 he was a major general of the Kansas militia. After the war he was mainly a mining and railroad official. He returned to Kansas, but since his disease failed to respond to medical treatment it was suggested, again, that a change in climate might be helpful. Despite a move to California in July 1872, Deitzler continued to require treatment for his chronic diarrhea and jaundice. It was stated that his bloody, mucus discharges in conjunction with emaciation and great muscular debility indicated ulceration of the colon. On the morning of April 11, 1884, Deitzler and a passenger went out to the foot of Santa Catalina mountain in a buggy to examine some water rights for irrigation. Instead of coming directly back to Tucson, Arizona, they skirted along the foothills of the mountain. After about a mile, one of the lugs on the buggy became loose. Deitzler tried to quiet the terrified horses but the neck-yoke slipped from the poles, further frightening them and causing them to overturn the buggy. Deitzler was thrown onto the road about thirty yards to the rear. He took several breaths, uttered a faint groan, and died. A slight cut on his forehead and another on the left side of his nose were the only visible marks of injury. Close examination revealed his neck had been broken close to the shoulders. He was buried in Oak Hill Cemetery, at Lawrence, Kansas.[1]

1. CSR; RVA, Pension WC 400,802; *OR,* vol. 3:70, 83; vol. 22, pt. 2:472; *(Tucson) Arizona Daily Star,* Apr. 11, 1884.

RICHARD DELAFIELD · *Born September 1, 1798,* in New York City. Graduated from USMA in 1818. Delafield served as an engineer and in other positions during his forty-three-year military career prior to the Civil War. In May 1864 he was promoted to brigadier general. In 1866 he was retired from the army and spent the rest of his life engaged in engineer-related activities. He died November 5, 1873, in Washington, D.C., and was buried in the family plot in Green-Wood Cemetery, Brooklyn, New York. According to his attending physician, he died of softening of the brain.[1]

1. LR, ACP, 4354, 1873, fiche: 000092.

ELIAS SMITH DENNIS · *Born December 4, 1812,* in Newburgh, New York. Dennis was an Illinois politician and a U.S. marshal in the Kansas Territory before the Civil War. In August 1861 he was mustered into Federal service as lieutenant colonel of the 30th Illinois Volunteers. He served at Fort Donelson, Vicksburg, and Mobile. He developed a rupture in November 1862 but remained on duty. His promotion as brigadier general of volunteers ranked from that month. He was present sick in December 1862 and January 1863. He was brevetted major general at the end of the war and discharged in August 1865.[1] Dennis died December 17, 1894, at Carlyle, Illinois, and was buried in the City Cemetery. DEATH CERTIFICATE: Cause of death, pneumonia. Duration of disease, about ten days.

1. RVA, Pension SC 415,566.

FREDERICK TRACY DENT · *Born December 17, 1820,* near St. Louis, Missouri. Graduated from the USMA in 1843 with Ulysses S. Grant, his future brother-in-law. During his period at the academy he was treated for a toothache twice and sore feet once. Served in the Mexican War. He was wounded at Molino del Rey on September 8, 1847.[1] At the start of the Civil War he was a captain posted in San Francisco. Promoted to major in March 1863, he went to New York City and served on a military commission. In the spring of 1864 he was appointed aide-de-camp to Grant and a lieutenant colonel. He was made a brigadier general of volunteers to rank from April 1865. Dent remained in the army. Following a stroke, he had a left hemiplegia and in January 1881 took an extended leave. By the following year he was compelled to lie down if he walked more than a hundred yards, and he retired as a colonel in December 1883. He died December 23, 1892, at Denver, Colorado, and was buried in Arlington National Cemetery.

1. LR, ACP, 689, 1881, fiche: 000093; Heitman, *Historical Register and Dictionary* 2:20.

JAMES WILLIAM DENVER · *Born October 23, 1817,* near Winchester, Virginia. During the Mexican War he was sick in August and September of 1847.[1] A California politician, he killed an editor who had criticized his actions during a duel in

1852. He was commissioner of Indian Affairs in 1857 and the next year was governor of the Kansas Territory. While in this capacity he helped establish the city of Denver, Colorado, which was named in his honor. After he returned to Ohio, he was appointed brigadier general of volunteers in August 1861 by President Lincoln. He led a division at Corinth. Denver resigned his commission in March 1863 and spent the rest of his life in politics. He died August 9, 1892, in his residence at Washington, D.C., and was buried in Wilmington, Ohio.

DEATH CERTIFICATE: Cause of death, primary, nephritis; immediate, uremia, coma. Duration last sickness, three days.

1. "Official List of Officers who Marched with the Army under Command of Major General Winfield Scott," Circular, Adjutant General's Office, Mexico, Feb. 7, 1848. American Star Print, Mexico, 1848, USAMHI.

GUSTAVUS ADOLPHUS DE RUSSY • *Born on November 3, 1818,* in Brooklyn, New York. He entered the USMA but resigned in 1838 after three years. Served in the Mexican War. In 1847 he was commissioned directly into the army as a second lieutenant. From May 12–13, 1855, he was in the post hospital, Fort Hamilton, New York Harbor, with diarrhea. At the start of the Civil War he was a captain. De Russy was sent home on sick leave from August 4, 1862, until September, when he was placed on mustering duty in New York City. In November he returned to the army and in March 1863 entered volunteer service as colonel of the 4th New York Artillery. His major field service was at Malvern Hill and Fredericksburg. His commission as brigadier general of volunteers ranked from May 1863. Following the war, he remained in the Regular Army as a major but was frequently in and out of post hospitals. He was sick in the post hospital, Fort Independence, Boston Harbor, Massachusetts, from January 23 to February 7, 1868, with rheumatic gout. From August 23–29, 1870, he was in the post hospital, Oglethorpe Barracks, Savannah, Georgia, with rheumatism. He was in the post hospital, Fort Monroe, Virginia, because of gout or rheumatic gout on the following dates: August 30 to September 6, 1871; December 13–19, 1871; December 31, 1871, to January 4, 1872; April 8–26, 1872; August 16 to September 14, 1872; June 5–10, 1873; June 18–26, 1873; and October 16 to November 17, 1873. He was in the post hospital, Fort Niagara, Youngstown, New York, with acute or chronic rheumatism on the following dates: February 8–23, 1877; February 28 to March 5, 1877; December 10–16, 1878; and December 28, 1878, to January 7, 1879. De Russy was in the post hospital, Fort Hamilton, New York Harbor, for acute or chronic rheumatism as follows: August 14–27, 1880; October 22 to November 5, 1880; December 31, 1880, to January 5, 1881. He was in the post hospital, St. Augustine, Fort Marion, Florida, for gout on the following dates: June 29 to July 1, 1882, July 14–16, 1882. In 1882 he retired from military service as a colonel. The physician who took care of him from 1883 to 1891 reported that he had first treated De Russy for muscular and articular rheumatism in 1883 and subsequently for repeated attacks over the years. During a period of such illness in

1886 or 1887 he observed evidence of pericarditis and nephritis in consequence of the rheumatism. He deduced this from the condition of some of De Russy's joints (wrist and fingers) at the time he had first seen him, and that he had probably had attacks of rheumatism rather than gout. De Russy was treated on January 8, 1891, for dyspnea, gastric disturbances, and for chronic Bright's disease. The physician stated that an analysis of his urine revealed the presence of the form of Bright's disease termed chronic interstitial nephrotic (contrasted to gouty kidneys). It was not possible for him to state the probable duration of the illness. However, he reported that a careful investigation into De Russy's past history suggested that it must have existed for a year or more, and that it was a complication of chronic rheumatism. He died in uremic coma on May 29, 1891, at Detroit, Michigan, and was buried there in Elmwood Cemetery.[1]
DEATH CERTIFICATE: Cause of death, Bright's disease. Duration about one year.

1. RVA, Pension WC 367,066; U.S. Army, CWS, roll 3, vol. 4, report 21, pp. 705–7.

PHILIPPE RÉGIS DÉNIS DE KEREDERN DE TROBRIAND • *Born June 4, 1816*, near Tours, France. He followed a number of occupations prior to the war and in August 1861 entered Federal service as colonel of the 55th New York. He held major commands on the Peninsula and at Fredericksburg, Chancellorsville, Gettysburg, and Appomattox. On May 21, 1862, he was left behind in a shanty with remittent bilious or swamp fever of a dangerous character. He was ordered north to New York City on sick leave on a surgeon's certificate on June 9. On June 21 a New York City physician stated he was recovering from remittent congestive fever and that he was still too ill to go back to duty. He returned to Harrison's Landing on July 10, 1862, and resumed regimental command. He was commissioned as a brigadier general of volunteers to rank from January 1864 and as a major general by brevet from April 1865.[1] He remained in the army after the war and retired in March 1879. Died July 15, 1897, at Bayport, New York, and was buried in St. Anne's Cemetery in Sayville, New York.
DEATH CERTIFICATE: Cause of death, congestion of lungs; contributing cause, cystitis.

1. CSR; *OR*, vol. 11, pt. 1:874, 888; U.S. Army, CWS, roll 4, vol. 6, report 4, pp. 201–13.

CHARLES DEVENS, JR. • *Born on April 4, 1820*, in Charlestown, Massachusetts. Before the Civil War, he was a lawyer, politician, and militia brigadier general. He was commissioned colonel of the 15th Massachusetts in the early days of the war. He was appointed brigadier general of volunteers in April 1862. On May 31, during the Battle of Fair Oaks, he received a bullet wound in the leg but only left the field when the fighting was over. Disabled, he did not resume command for about two weeks. He led a brigade at Fredericksburg and a division at Chancellorsville. At Chancellorsville, May 2, 1863, his right foot was struck by a musket ball. He tried to keep his troops together but had to be carried off of the field. Still disabled in July, he was ordered to take command of the rendezvous for the disabled. The bullet in his leg had not been extracted by April 1864. On May 12, 1864, he was hospitalized for ten days with a diagnosis of tonsillitis. The next month an attack of acute rheumatism caused Devens to be carried about on a stretcher and prompted him to be relieved on the fourth. He was admitted to the USA hospital steamer *Atlantic* on July 11 and was transferred to a general hospital within a few days. He returned to duty in the middle of October. When recommended for a brevet in April 1865 it was reported that he was always with his command in the field, even when his condition rendered him unable to walk or ride on horseback.[1] Following the war he was a judge of the superior court, justice of the Massachusetts supreme court, and was appointed attorney general of the United States by President Rutherford B. Hayes. He died January 7, 1891, in Boston and was buried in Mount Auburn Cemetery, Cambridge, Massachusetts.

DEATH CERTIFICATE: Immediate cause of death, cardiac failure, due to fatty degeneration of the heart.

1. *OR*, vol. 11, pt. 1:761, 876, 881, 905–7; vol. 25, pt. 1:632–35; vol. 36, pt. 1:179, 1005; vol. 46, pt. 3:1015; U.S. Army, CWS, roll 2, vol. 3, report 34, pp. 1023–33; RAGO, entry 534.

THOMAS CASIMER DEVIN • *Born December 10, 1822,* in New York City. A house painter, he was a lieutenant colonel of a militia regiment when the Civil War started and in November 1861 was made colonel of the 6th New York Cavalry. He was at Antietam, Fredericksburg, Chancellorsville, Gettysburg, the Shenandoah, and Appomattox. In the action near Front Royal, Virginia, on August 16, 1864, his foot was hit by a minié ball. He left his command on August 19 and returned on September 1. His promotion as brigadier general of volunteers ranked from October 1864. He was brevetted major general of volunteers in 1865 and discharged in January 1866. After the war Devin remained in the army and in 1866 was appointed lieutenant colonel. His health was poor in later years, and he was on sick leave from June 1873 to May 1874. During the summer of 1873, he had a polyp removed from his left middle ear by a specialist in Paris. A physical examination on December 22, 1873, revealed that he had a perforation of the left eardrum, which had been destroyed by the polyp. Chronic inflammation of both eustachian tubes rendered them almost impervious to treatment, and there was an associated chronic pharyngitis. His hearing was very impaired and no permanent improvement could be expected. Although he had almost no pain by April 1874 and the perforation was smaller, there was no other improvement in his condition. In August 1877 he was on sick leave at White Sulphur Springs under medical treatment for a malarial rheumatic affliction of his back and lower lumbar area. In addition, he was considering going "beyond the sea" for medical treatment if the condition of his throat did not improve. Devin was on sick leave from February 18 until his death in New

York City on April 4, 1878.[1] He was buried in Calvary Cemetery, Long Island City, New York.

DEATH CERTIFICATE: Primary, inflammation of the stomach, angina pharynges (pharyngitis); immediate, apoplexy, [illegible word] of high degree of inflammation of the above named parts. Duration, the attack of inflammation began on March 31, 1878, and continued until the end.

    1. *OR,* vol. 43, pt. 1:439, 474–75; RVA, Pension WC 184,875.

JOEL ALLEN DEWEY • *Born on September 20, 1840,* in Georgia, Vermont. Dewey left college in 1861 and entered Federal service as a second lieutenant of the 58th Ohio. After being promoted through ranks, he was appointed brigadier general of volunteers in November 1865. He had served at Iuka, Corinth, and in the Atlanta campaign. Dewey studied the law after the war and became a lawyer and a politician. He was summoned to Knoxville, Tennessee, and testified in the Circuit Court on June 16, 1873. Although he woke up that night at 1:00 A.M. and 3:00 A.M., planning to take the early morning train, he was persuaded to take the noon train instead. However, he took no train. He went back to the court the next day; soon afterward his head fell on his chest and he slumped to the floor. He was gasping and struggling for breath, and those nearby picked him up and carried him to the door. In a few minutes he died assumably of heart disease. He was buried at Dandridge, Tennessee.[1]

    1. RVA, Pension WC 841,211; *Knoxville Daily Press and Herald,* June 18, 1873; *Knoxville (Tenn.) Chronicle Daily,* June 18, 1873.

JOHN ADAMS DIX • *Born July 24, 1798,* in Boscawen, New Hampshire. Dix practiced the law and was a New York state official and politician. At the start of the Civil War he was U.S. secretary of the Treasury. President Lincoln appointed him one of the first major general of volunteers to rank from May 1861. Too old for field service, he performed department and garrison duties during the war. He died April 21, 1879, at New York City and was buried there in Trinity Cemetery.

DEATH CERTIFICATE: Primary cause, chronic cystitis and pyelonephritis, several years' duration; immediate, uremia.

CHARLES CLEVELAND DODGE • *Born September 16, 1841,* at Plainfield, New Jersey. In December 1861 he entered Federal service as a captain of the 7th New York Cavalry. By the following August he had been appointed colonel of the unit, and his appointment as brigadier general of volunteers ranked from November 1862. Because of command differences, he resigned his commission in June 1863 and went into business. He died November 4, 1910, in a private hospital in New York City and was buried in Woodlawn Cemetery.

DEATH CERTIFICATE: Cause of death, hypostatic pneumonia, gastroduodenitis.

GRENVILLE MELLEN DODGE • *Born April 12, 1831,* at Danvers, Massachusetts. As a young man he was engaged in civil and railroad engineering. During a survey trip in March 1857, Dodge and his crew all developed snow blindness. They were taken back to Iowa City in a wagon, and it was recommended they stay in a dark room for a month. He organized a militia company in Iowa, and in July 1861 he entered Federal service as colonel of the 4th Iowa Infantry. Ill with typhoid fever during August 1861, he visited St. Louis in September for the benefit of his health. On the night of December 27, 1861, near Rolla, Missouri, his horse fell and a small pistol that was in his coat pocket discharged and wounded him in the left leg. The wound was nearly through the fleshy part of the thigh above the knee and ranged downwards. He was treated by the regimental surgeon and an incision was later required to remove the ball. Dodge was confined to his quarters for a few weeks, but it took a much longer period for the wound to heal. He was assigned to brigade command in late January 1862 and his promotion to brigadier general ranked from March. On March 1, he contracted a cold and severe bronchitis. Still pale and suffering with his recent illness, he was injured at Pea Ridge on March 7, 1862. The records and reports are somewhat confusing as to what exactly happened. Three horses were shot from under him, one of them being struck with twenty balls. Dodge apparently had two knuckles knocked out of joint in his left hand by the glancing blow of a grapeshot and he was also knocked off his horse by a falling tree limb. Other records report he was hit in the side by a grapeshot. He was sent to St. Louis under the charge of the surgeon of the 3rd Iowa. His condition was complicated by chronic diarrhea during the last of April. He returned to duty in June 1862, but in July the strain brought about by his duties did little to improve his health. On August 17, 1863, he had sick leave and went north. He returned for duty at Corinth on October 15. He was quite sick March 23, 1864. In June he was commissioned major general and was placed in command of the Sixteenth Corps in the Atlanta campaign. During an argument on July 25, Dodge slapped Maj. Gen. Thomas W. Sweeny. Sweeny hit him on the nose with his fist and Dodge's face was covered with blood. The affair led to Sweeny's court-martial, but he was later reinstated. While superintending preparations outside of Atlanta, Georgia, on August 19, 1864, Dodge was wounded in the head by a sharpshooter. The ball hit near the center of his frontal bone, glanced upward, and fractured the external table of the bone. Knocked unconscious, he had to be carried to the rear on a blanket. There was a severe concussion of the brain. He remained in his tent and on August 24 received sick leave. On the basis of the symptoms, which he did not describe, the surgeon reported there was derangement of his brain and nervous system. Dodge's wife and the regimental surgeon took him to Greenfield, Indiana, to stay with relatives. Some sort of surgical treatment was performed. By September the scalp wound was only partially healed. Dodge took command of the Department of Missouri, located at St. Louis, on December 9. The surgeon who had originally treated him for his head wound examined him again in December. He found that there was necrosis of the frontal bone and Dodge still had pain and derangement of the nervous system. Dodge resigned from the army in May 1866 and spent the rest of his life associated with railroads. In 1867 he had trouble with his side for five months and had some type of unspecified surgery. In January 1872 he required crutches because of rheumatism. He spent a portion of each year from 1874 to 1879 in Europe for his health. During 1889 and 1890 he suffered with gout. He spent the winter of 1893–94 at Hot Springs for the benefit of his health. In December 1914 he was in bed with cancer and by the next spring had lost fifty pounds. He went to New York in August for radium treatment and underwent an exploratory operation, which for some reason was done without benefit of an anesthetic.[1] He died January 3, 1916, at Council Bluffs, Iowa, and was buried there in the Walnut Hill Cemetery.

DEATH CERTIFICATE: Cause of death, cancer of rectum and bladder.

1. CSR; *OR*, vol. 8:261; vol. 17, pt. 1:27, pt. 2:310; vol. 30, pt. 4:378; vol. 32, pt. 3:123; vol. 38, pt. 3:375, 387, pt. 5:662; vol. 39, pt. 3:702; vol. 41, pt. 4:673; U.S. Army, CWS, roll 5, vol. 8, report 6, pp. 199–500; RVA, Pension SC 127-386; G. M. Dodge to Gen. John C. Black, Jan. 16, 1915, Grenville M. Dodge Papers, State Historical Society of Iowa, Des Moines, Iowa; Stanley P. Hirshson, *Grenville M. Dodge: Soldier, Politician, and Railroad Pioneer*, 26, 53, 57–58, 103, 152, 181, 223–24, 227, 259–61.

CHARLES CAMP DOOLITTLE · *Born March 16, 1832,* in Burlington, Vermont. In June 1861 he was appointed a first lieutenant of the 4th Michigan Infantry. He was promoted to captain in August and to colonel in August 1862 after service on the Peninsula. In April 1864, while on duty at Nashville, Tennessee, he was disabled by acute inflammatory rheumatism. He commanded a brigade at the Battle of Nashville. His promotion to brigadier general ranked from January 1865, and he was discharged the following November. After the war he was a bank employee. The rheumatism continued the rest of his life and it was stated that his prior acute rheumatism resulted in his heart disease. He died February 20, 1903, at the "Hattersley" in Toledo, Ohio, and was buried in Woodlawn Cemetery in that city.[1]

DEATH CERTIFICATE: Cause of death, chief, prostration; contributing, chronic heart disease and rheumatism.

1. CSR; RVA, Pension WC 555,341.

ABNER DOUBLEDAY · *Born June 26, 1819,* at Ballston Spa, New York. Graduated from the USMA in 1842. During his time as a cadet he was treated for pain in the side four times, a cold three times, nausea and cough each two times, and a sprain, sore hand, ulcer, toothache, and sore throat each once. Served in the Mexican War. Following routine garrison duty and minor service at the start of the Civil War, he was commissioned brigadier general of volunteers in 1862. He was actively engaged at Second Bull Run, Antietam, and Fredericksburg. While riding out on reconnaissance on July 27, 1861, Major Doubleday had a serious injury to his left leg from hitting a six-mule team that blocked his path as his horse was passing through at full speed. A shell exploded under his horse's nose at the beginning of the action on September 17, 1862, at Antietam. The horse ran over some steep rocks and fell, bruising Doubleday so that he was not able to hold the reins in his hands for a time. Later in September he became ill, he thought, because the dead animals on the field caused sickness and malaria. Doubleday was sitting upon his horse at Gettysburg on July 3, 1863, when a shell fragment passed through the brim of his hat and struck him on the double fold of his coat collar at the back of his neck. He was knocked down on the neck of his horse as if hit by a club. For several weeks afterward he suffered from severe headaches. On July 5 he was relieved from duty with the Army of the Potomac and was to report for orders in Washington, D.C. He was brevetted major general in 1865 and, remaining in the army, was made colonel in 1867. After two years in Texas his surgeon recommended he leave and go north. For some years he had had irritability of the neck of the urinary bladder with enlargement of the prostate, which caused him to have urgency and frequency of urination. By 1873 he was considerably weakened by the condition, which had become associated with some bleeding.[1] Doubleday died January 26, 1893, at Mendham, New Jersey, and was buried in Arlington National Cemetery.

DEATH CERTIFICATE: Cause of death, aortic stenosis. Length of sickness, two years.

1. *OR,* vol. 19, pt. 1:226; vol. 27, pt. 1:260, 262, pt. 3:543; *OR Suppl.,* vol. 1, pt. 1:199; WPCHR, vol. 604; U.S. Army, CWS, roll 8, vol. 13, report 5, pp. 309–611; LR, ACP, 4583, 1872, fiche: 000097.

NEAL DOW • *Born March 20, 1804,* in Portland, Maine. A businessman, politician, and strong prohibitionist, he was commissioned colonel of the 13th Maine Volunteers in November 1861. He was promoted to brigadier general to rank from April 1862. In the assault upon Port Hudson on May 27, 1863, he received a contused wound of the right arm and a gunshot wound of his left thigh. The ball struck the front of his thigh in the middle, passed backward and inward, and came out at the apex of Scarpa's Triangle (triangular area bounded superiorly by the inguinal ligament, laterally by the sartorius muscle, and medially by the adductor longus muscle). Dow was carried to a small farmhouse not far from the field. When the building was needed to be used for a hospital two weeks later, he was transferred to another farmhouse about two miles in the rear. He remained there for three weeks until he was captured by a body of Confederate cavalry. He was taken first to Jackson, Mississippi, then to Montgomery, Alabama, and finally to Libby Prison in Richmond. He was sent back to Montgomery for two months and then returned to Libby Prison, where he slept without bedding on the crowded floor. As a consequence of his poor health, he was unable to participate in a prisoner escape in February. He was exchanged in March 1864 with his health broken by a severe chronic cold, bronchitis, and a cough. In November 1864, following a leave, Dow had to admit that he was permanently disabled and forwarded his resignation. He continued his anti-liquor activities in the United States and in Europe. The scar on his thigh where the ball had entered was adherent, tender, and painful in 1877. In addition to disability from his wound he still had chronic bronchitis with a productive cough.[1] Died October 2, 1897, in Portland, Maine, and was buried there in Evergreen Cemetery.

1. *OR*, vol. 26, pt. 1:68, 124; vol. 33:559–60; U.S. Army, CWS, roll 4, vol. 6, report 11, pp. 377–88; RVA, Pension SC 147,693.

ALFRED NAPOLEON ALEXANDER DUFFIÉ • *Born May 1, 1835,* in Paris, France. As a graduate of the French military college of St. Cyr he served in Africa and Europe, was wounded eight times, and was awarded four military decorations. He came to the United States in the autumn of 1859 with the hope that the change in climate would help his asthma. When the Civil War began, he was in Saratoga, New York, receiving medical treatment. He resigned his commission in the French army and in August 1861 was appointed captain of the 2nd New York Cavalry, which he commanded at Second Bull Run. During the crossing of the Rappahannock River at Kelly's Ford on March 17, 1863, Duffié's horse was shot, and Duffié was thrown into the river, severely bruising one of his legs. However, he did not leave his troops. His promotion to brigadier general ranked from June 1863. Captured by Confederate partisans in October 1864, he was paroled at the end of February 1865. After his exchange in April, he had no further command and was discharged in August. He still suffered from asthma and desired a change in climate, which he hoped would benefit his health. He was appointed United States consul at Cadiz, Spain, in May 1869. In 1877 he went to Canterets in the Pyrenees to take its waters as a remedy for his asthma but had no improvement. He died at Cadiz on November 8, 1880. According to his wife, he died from consumption. In December his body was brought back to the United States, and he was buried at Staten Island, New York.[1]

1. *OR*, vol. 25, pt. 1:52; U.S. Army, CWS, roll 1, vol. 2, report 41, pp. 589–97; *MOLLUS* 5:335–68, 6:313–48; RVA, Pension WC 655,771.

EBENEZER DUMONT • *Born on November 23, 1814,* in Vevay, Indiana. Served in the Mexican War. A lawyer and politician in Indiana, he entered Federal service as a colonel of the 7th Indiana Volunteers in April 1861. The following September he was promoted to brigadier general of volunteers. In October 1861 at Elkwater, [West] Virginia, he contracted diarrhea with a low form of fever and had to leave his command. His physician reported he would never regain his health, and Dumont continued to have diarrhea for the rest of his life. He had a medical leave starting in June 1862, which was extended. His surgeon stated that he suffered from great prostration from his arduous labor. Although he returned to duty in September, he was sick most of the time and was not able to be in the field. After a sick leave at home from December 12 to January 16, 1863, due to disease of the stomach and duodenum, he returned to duty before he had fully recovered. Dumont's resignation was accepted in February 1863 so he could take a seat in Congress. He returned to the practice of law and engaged in politics. At one point his physician suggested he leave the law and take up farming to help his condition. His attending physician reported that his death resulted from the prostration produced by the diarrhea.[1] Died April 16, 1871, at Indianapolis and was buried there in the Crown Hill Cemetery.

1. OR, vol. 20, pt. 2:138; RVA, Pension WC 193,576; U.S. Army, CWS, roll 2, vol. 3, report 46, pp. 1299–323.

ABRAM DURYÉE • *Born on April 29, 1815,* in New York City. As a member of the militia he was injured by stones and more or less disabled during the Astor Place riots on May 10, 1849. When the Civil War started, he recruited a regiment of volunteers, which entered Federal service as the 5th New York. His promotion as brigadier general of volunteers ranked from August 1861. While serving near Baltimore in 1861 he was violently thrown from his horse. The accident produced a severe contusion of his hip and the lower part of his back that was followed by swelling and erysipelas. He was confined to his quarters in Baltimore for about a month. Duryée received a slight wound and a severe contusion of the right chest under the arm from a shell at Second Bull Run on August 30, 1862. His wounds were dressed in an ambulance during the retreat. As a result of his injuries, one surgeon said Duryée developed a hernia. Another suggested it was produced when his horse threw him. Regardless of the cause, he was compelled to wear a truss for the rest of his life. At Antietam on September 17, 1862, he was slightly wounded. At the end of the war he was brevetted a major general of volunteers. Duryée returned to New York where he served as police commissioner and as a dockmaster. In 1887 he suffered from a double hernia and rheumatism in the joints of his right arm and shoulder, supposedly resulting from the contusion received at Second Bull Run. On May 26, 1887, he had a stroke. Afterward his left arm and leg were entirely useless, and he never left his room again. Unable to dress, feed, or help himself in any way, he required constant attention. He died September 27, 1890, in New York and was buried in Green-Wood Cemetery, Brooklyn.[1]

DEATH CERTIFICATE: Cause of death, left hemiplegia, sequential cerebral apoplexy of nearly three-and-one-half years; contributing cause, cerebral hemorrhage.

1. OR, vol. 2:89; vol. 12, pt. 2:345, 384; U.S. Army, CWS, roll 4, vol. 6, report 20, pp. 435–67; ibid., roll 8, vol. 14, report 2, pp. 9–13; RVA, Pension WC 285,398; Richard Moody, *The Astor Place Riot.*

Isaac Hardin Duval • *Born September 1, 1824,* at Wellsburg, [West] Virginia. Duval had been a hunter, trapper, guide, and businessman before the Civil War. In June 1861 he was mustered into Federal service as a major of the 1st [West] Virginia Infantry. Duval was severely wounded in the foot at Port Republic on June 8, 1862, but was able to return to duty in July. During the Battle of Cedar Mountain on August 9, 1862, he was run over and his head was injured. In the middle of September the suffering from his head injury was so intense that at times he was unable to perform his duty and considered resigning. However, he was appointed colonel that month. On March 9, 1863, he received a sick leave because of hemorrhoids and constipation. He had another sick leave from October 29 to December. At the Battle of Winchester, Virginia, on September 19, 1864, Duval was wounded by a musket ball in his left thigh but did not leave the field until after the battle. His promotion as brigadier general ranked from that month. He received a leave on a surgeon's certificate of disability. By the middle of October the wound was slowly improving, but he had developed an abscess on his head. He had a medical leave for twenty days starting February 12, 1865. He was at Staunton, Virginia, on May 17, 1865, when an attempt was made to assassinate him. However, he was not hurt. He was discharged with a brevet as major general in 1866.[1] Following the war he was a politician and office holder. Died July 10, 1902, at Wellsburg, West Virginia, and was buried there.
DEATH CERTIFICATE: No cause of death listed.

1. CSR; *OR,* vol. 43, pt. 1:25, 55, 116, 363; vol. 46, pt. 3:1174; RVA, Pension WC 568,778; U.S. Army, CWS, roll 6, vol. 10, report 54, pp. 547–49; *MOLLUS* 1:157–58.

William Dwight • *Born July 14, 1831,* in Springfield, Massachusetts. Depending on the source, he either resigned or was discharged from USMA before graduation. While at West Point he was treated for excoriatio five times, cephalalgia and contusio each four times, odontalgia three times, catarrhus, morbi. varii., rheumatism, phlegmon, and luxatio twice each, and febris ephemeral and opthalmia each once. Dwight was in the manufacturing business when the Civil War started. He was appointed a lieutenant colonel of the 70th New York in June 1861. At Williamsburg, Virginia, on May 5, 1862, he received multiple wounds. First, he was wounded in the right leg, which he considered only a scratch. Soon afterward he received two more wounds. One ball entered his thigh near the hip, passed downward, and was later extracted from just above the knee. The other ball entered his abdomen just below the navel, passed through his body, and made its exit near his left hip. Temporarily unconscious, he was left for dead. Taken prisoner, Dwight was carried from the field to Williamsburg by his own men, who were also prisoners. He was exchanged on November 15, 1862, and his promotion as brigadier general of volunteers ranked from that month. While near Port Hudson, Louisiana, in May 1863 he developed rheumatism of his lower extremities, which continued to intermittently bother him for the rest of his life. After arriving in New Orleans in February 1864, he was for some weeks prostrated by a fever. He assumed command of his brigade on March 26 and served in the Shenandoah Valley. After his discharge from the army in January 1866, he suffered from recurrent attacks of rheumatism of his lower extremities at least six times a year. Each attack either confined him to his room for three or four weeks or rendered him so lame that he could walk only with great pain and difficulty.[1] Died April 20, 1888, in Boston and was buried there in Forest Hills Cemetery.

DEATH CERTIFICATE: Immediate cause of death, cirrhosis of liver.

1. CSR; *OR*, vol. 11, pt. 1:460, 482–83; vol. 46, pt. 2:762; WPCHR, vols. 607, 608; U.S. Army, CWS, roll 7, vol. 12, report 1, pp. 1–416; RVA, Pension SC 164,095.

ALEXANDER BRYDIE DYER • *Born on January 10, 1815,* in Richmond, Virginia. Graduated from the USMA in 1837. As a cadet he was treated for diarrhea, sore throat, wound, sore feet, influenza, strain, boil, and abscess each one time. Served in the Florida and Mexican wars. Dyer performed ordnance duties before and during the Civil War. In September 1864 he was promoted to brigadier general in the Regular Army and was made chief of ordnance. After the war he continued in the same position until 1869, when his health began to deteriorate. He became sick on January 4, 1872, and continued in poor health for the rest of his life. He died in the hospital at the Washington Arsenal on May 20, 1874, and was buried in the Arlington National Cemetery. Hospital records listed the cause of death as Bright's disease. The adjutant general reported that the cause of death was hypertrophy and dilatation of the heart with granular disease of the kidneys.[1]

1. WPCHR, vol. 602, 603; RVA, Pension WC 165,711.

E

AMOS BEEBE EATON • *Born May 12, 1806,* in Catskill, New York. Graduated from the USMA in 1826. He served in the Florida and Mexican wars. His major service was in the commissary department, and he was appointed commissary general of the U.S. Army, ranking from June 1864. He remained in this position until he retired in 1874. Eaton died on February 21, 1877, at New Haven, Connecticut, and was buried there in Grove Street Cemetery. He was sitting with his wife in the lecture room of the Yale School of the Fine Arts awaiting the beginning of a lecture when he was suddenly stricken.[1]

DEATH CERTIFICATE: Cause of death, primary, weakness with irritability of the pneumogastric nerves, causing occasional functional disturbance of the lungs and heart, especially of the former; immediate, cardiac syncope, suspending almost immediately the action of the heart and lungs and the consciousness.

1. LR, ACP, 1041, 1844, fiche: 000098.

JOHN EDWARDS • *Born October 24, 1815,* in Louisville, Kentucky. Prior to the war he lived in Indiana, California, and Iowa. He was a lawyer, politician, and founder of a newspaper. In August 1862 he was appointed colonel of the 18th Iowa Infantry, and in September 1864 he was promoted to brigadier general of volunteers. He served mainly on garrison duty but had some field duty in the West. During his service in the field he contracted rheumatism in his hips and the joints of his lower limbs and catarrh in his head. Edwards was treated in the field and in hospitals in Springfield, Missouri, and at Fort Smith, Arkansas. He was discharged from the service in January 1866. Following the war he resumed his law practice and was a politician and clerk in the auditor's office. He died April 8, 1894, in Washington, D.C., and was buried in Arlington National Cemetery.[1]

DEATH CERTIFICATE: Cause of death, rheumatism, cystitis, and asthenia.

1. RVA, Pension WC 420,650.

OLIVER EDWARDS • *Born on January 30, 1835,* in Springfield, Massachusetts. At the start of the Civil War he left his foundry business in Illinois and returned to Massachusetts. He entered Federal service as first lieutenant and adjutant of the 10th Massachusetts Infantry. Early in December 1861 he was in poor physical condition as the result of a previous attack of typhoid fever and a subsequent relapse. In July 1862 he was at Harrison's Landing, Virginia, and had intermittent fever. He was given a sick leave to return to his home. He was commissioned colonel of the 57th Massachusetts in September 1862 and brigadier general of volunteers in May 1865.[1] During this time he saw action at Fredericksburg, Chancellorsville, Gettysburg, Spotsylvania, in the Shenandoah Valley, and at Appomattox. After the war, he served as postmaster and superintendent of a manufacturing company. He died April 28, 1904, at Warsaw, Illinois, and was buried in Oakland Cemetery.

DEATH CERTIFICATE: Cause of death, capillary bronchitis.

1. CSR.

THOMAS WILBERFORCE EGAN • *Born June 14, 1834,* in Watervliet, New York. Egan entered Federal service with the 40th New York in April 1861 and was commissioned lieutenant colonel of the unit in July. He was wounded in the left side of his scalp over the frontal bone at the Battle of Fair Oaks on June 1, 1862. In November he obtained a disability leave because over the previous six months he had had difficulty performing his duties due to diarrhea and bleeding piles. He returned to duty in March 1863 and served at Chancellorsville. While at Petersburg on June 16, 1864, Egan received a penetrating wound in the area of the right kidney from a shell fragment. This resulted in a slight paralysis of his legs. In September he returned to duty and was promoted to brigadier general of volunteers. He was wounded by a minié ball in his right forearm at Petersburg on November 14, 1864. This wound produced partial paralysis of his arm. He was taken on the USA Steamer *Ben Deford* from City Point, Virginia, to Washington, D.C., where part of his recovery was spent in the Metropolitan Hotel. His promotion as brevet major general ranked from October 1864, and he was separated from the army in January 1866. Egan held the position of deputy collector in the New York Customs House for six years. In November 1868 he still suffered from his last two wounds. The wound in his back produced stiffness and pain in the right leg, and in wet or damp weather he was entirely disabled. His arm remained paralyzed, and bone fragments continued to be discharged from the wound. He was scarcely able to write or use his arm in any way. By 1886 he required regular aid and attendance.[1] He died in obscurity, in a charity hospital on February 24, 1887, in New York. Buried in Cypress Hills National Cemetery, Brooklyn, New York.

1. CSR; *OR*, vol. 40, pt. 1:22, 221, 391; vol. 42, pt. 2:117, 594, 1019, pt. 3:617; vol. 46, pt. 2:707; RVA, Pension SC 95,437; RAGO, entry 534.

ALFRED WASHINGTON ELLET • *Born October 11, 1820*, at Penn's Manor, Pennsylvania. He was a practicing civil engineer prior to the Civil War and in August 1861 was appointed a captain of the 59th Illinois Infantry. Along with his brother Charles, he purchased vessels for the U.S. government, and they carried out active naval actions against the Confederates on western rivers. His promotion to brigadier general of volunteers ranked from November 1862, and he resigned his commission in December 1864. Ellet returned to civil engineering but became a prominent civic leader and organizer of a bank in Kansas. By 1892 he was disabled from the destruction of the mitral valve of his heart from acute rheumatism, albuminuria, and a paralytic stroke involving his whole left side.[1] Died January 9, 1895, at El Dorado, Kansas, and was buried in the local cemetery.

1. RVA, Pension WC 477,814.

WASHINGTON LAFAYETTE ELLIOTT • *Born March 31, 1825*, at Carlisle, Pennsylvania. Served in the Mexican War. He entered the USMA but did not graduate because he left to undertake the study of medicine. Elliott was directly commissioned as a second lieutenant into the army in May 1846. While in Mexico he was sick from January to March 1847 and in April was on his way to Philadelphia for the benefit of his health. He was on recruiting duty until July 1848. In September 1861, after service in the Regular Army, he was commissioned as colonel of the 2nd Iowa Cavalry. He served at New Madrid, Island No. 10, and Corinth. In June 1862 he was made a brigadier general of volunteers. He was wounded in the left arm at the Second Battle of Bull Run, August 30, 1862, and returned to duty in September. He fought at Chancellorsville, Gettysburg, and in East Tennessee. After service in the Atlanta campaign he commanded a division in the Battle of Nashville. In 1866 he received brevet promotions to major general in both the Regular Army and volunteers. Elliott remained in the army with the rank of major. He was on sick leave from September 15, 1876, until he retired as a colonel in March 1879. He had developed heart disease from rheumatism. He died in San Francisco on June 29, 1888, and was buried there in the Presidio.[1]

DEATH CERTIFICATE: Cause of death, organic disease of the heart.

1. OR, vol. 51, pt. 1:1098; U.S. Army, CWS, roll 1, vol. 2, report 28, pp. 433–47; RVA, Pension 29,749.

WILLIAM HEMSLEY EMORY • *Born on September 7, 1811,* in Queen Annes County, Maryland. Graduated from the USMA in 1831. He resigned his commission in 1836 and was reappointed in 1838. Served in the Mexican War. Emory was involved in surveying and mapmaking when the Civil War started. He was commissioned a brigadier general of volunteers in March 1862 and served on the Peninsula. In April 1863 he had a severe attack of "gravel" (renal calculus), which was mistakenly diagnosed as neuralgia of the testes. He left Alexandria, Louisiana, with an aide-de-camp in May 1863 to visit New Orleans for surgical care. In June he was placed in command of the defenses of New Orleans. On September 20 he sailed from New Orleans on a surgeon's certificate of disability and reached New York by the end of the month. He returned in November and served on court-martial duty. He was a corps commander in the Red River campaign and in the Shenandoah Valley. On July 14, 1864, he had to halt at Potomac Crossroads because of a sharp attack of cholera morbus. He remained in the army until 1876 when he was retired as a brigadier general in the Regular Army. Over the years he continued to have episodes of intense pain produced by renal calculus. Died December 1, 1887, at Washington, D.C., and was buried in the Congressional Cemetery. According to his attending surgeon, Emory died from renal cirrhosis, a form of Bright's disease.[1]

1. OR, vol. 15:307; vol. 26, pt. 1:336; vol. 37, pt. 2:312; U.S. Army, CWS, roll 1, vol. 1, report 51, pp. 939–73; RVA, Pension WC 241,344.

GEORGE PEABODY ESTEY • *Born on April 24, 1829,* in Nashua, New Hampshire. Army records list him as *Este,* however. He left his law partnership and was commissioned lieutenant colonel of the 14th Ohio in April 1861. He was in [West] Virginia, at Mill Springs, and in the Tullahoma campaign. Estey was severely bruised on the leg by a bullet on July 9, 1864, near Vining's Station during the

Atlanta campaign.[1] He was in the March to the Sea and the Carolinas campaign. He was commissioned brigadier general of volunteers in June 1865 and resigned his position in December. Estey returned to the practice of law. Died February 6, 1881, in New York City and was buried in the Nashua Cemetery. The cemetery marker spells his name *Estey*.

DEATH CERTIFICATE: Cause of death, apnea, pneumonia and edema of the lungs of two days' duration.

1. *OR*, vol. 38, pt. 1:740.

HENRY LAWRENCE EUSTIS • *Born on February 1, 1819*, in Fort Independence, Boston, Massachusetts. Graduated from the USMA in 1842. After performing engineering duties, he resigned from the army in 1849 to become a professor of engineering at Harvard. In August 1862, despite his poor health, he was appointed colonel of the 10th Massachusetts Volunteers. He served at Fredericksburg, Chancellorsville, Gettysburg, and in the Gettysburg campaign. He was promoted to brigadier general to rank from September 1863. His health breaking down, he finally resigned in June 1864 and resumed his professorship at Harvard. It is not clear if he resigned because of health reasons, because he "ate opium," or to prevent charges being brought against him. For the two years prior to his death he was in failing health due to lung disease. Not wanting to desert his students, he first rode the short distance to his classes and then had his students come to him. His physicians ordered him to the South in December 1884, but the change of climate was not helpful, and he returned to his residence on January 7 in a hopeless condition.[1] Died at Cambridge, Massachusetts, on January 11, 1885, and was buried in Mount Auburn Cemetery.

DEATH CERTIFICATE: Immediate cause of death, disease of liver and lungs.

1. *OR*, vol. 36, pt. 1:96; *Boston Daily Advertiser,* Jan. 12, 1885.

CHARLES EWING • *Born March 6, 1835*, in Lancaster, Ohio. He left his law practice in St. Louis and in May 1861 was commissioned captain of the 13th U.S. Infantry. During the spring and summer of 1863 he was bothered by a cold and a severe pain in his throat. The condition affected his voice when he gave commands, and he was often seen spitting blood. Ewing treated himself with various medications and wore a bandage around his neck almost all of the time. He was slightly wounded in the hand on May 19, 1863, at Vicksburg, and another bullet went through his hat. Ewing was on William T. Sherman's (his brother-in-law) staff at Chattanooga, in the Atlanta campaign, the March to the Sea, and in the Carolinas. In March 1865 he was commissioned brigadier general of volunteers.[1] After a short period in the Regular Army, he resigned in 1867 and started a law practice. He died June 20, 1883, at Washington, D.C., and was buried in Arlington National Cemetery.

DEATH CERTIFICATE: Cause of death, pneumonia, typhoid pneumonia. Duration of last sickness, twelve days.

    1. *OR*, vol. 24, 2:264; RVA, Pension XC 2,664,560; Heitman, *Historical Register and Dictionary* 2:21.

HUGH BOYLE EWING · *Born October 31, 1826,* in Lancaster, Ohio. He entered but did not graduate from the USMA. While at the academy, he was treated for catarrhus eight times, cephalalgia four times, vulnus laceration twice, and once each for nausea, obstipatio, contusio, febris intermittent, phlegmon, pyrosis, ophthalmia, excoriatio, and an abscess. Ewing was practicing the law when the Civil War started. In August 1861 he was made colonel of the 30th Ohio Volunteers. In early October 1862, after Antietam, he obtained a sick leave because of chronic dysentery, which had bothered him for the previous three months. He was promoted to brigadier general of volunteers in November 1862. Ewing served at Vicksburg, Chattanooga, and in North Carolina. In the middle of June 1864, he had an attack of rheumatism. In August and during the fall of 1865 he was treated for inflammatory rheumatism and was frequently confined to his chair or room. After being mustered out of the army in January 1866, he was rarely free for more than a day or two from pain from the rheumatism and was bedridden for periods of eight to forty days. By February 1879 he had weakness, debility, lumbago, inflammatory swelling of his feet and knees, and sand in his urinary bladder. He died June 30, 1905, near Lancaster, and was buried in that city. Record of death, probate court: Cause of death, old age.[1]

    1. CSR; WPCHR, vols. 605, 606; U.S. Army, CWS, roll 3, vol. 4, report 8, pp. 169–206; RVA, Pension WC 682,514.

THOMAS EWING, JR. · *Born on August 7, 1829,* in Lancaster, Ohio. He was a lawyer and a member of the Kansas state supreme court in 1861. After resigning his position on the court, he became colonel of the 11th Kansas Cavalry in the autumn of 1862 and brigadier general in March 1863. He was at Prairie Grove and later commanded the District of the Border. In November 1863 he was sick with chills and fever. During the spring of 1864 he suffered with neuralgia and a boil on his neck. Breveted a major general, he resigned in February 1865. He returned to the practice of law and took up politics. He left his home in New York City on January 20, 1896, to go to his office. As he was crossing Third Avenue at 18th Street to get to the elevated station, an uptown cable car came along, and he stopped to let it pass. When the car had gone by, he started across the avenue and failed to notice a southbound car coming. The gripman was unable to put on the brakes in time to avoid an accident. Ewing was struck by the car and thrown several feet; he landed heavily on his head. He was picked up and carried to the sidewalk. A policeman called an ambulance and, after his head was dressed, he was taken home. The wound was severe and the scalp was lacerated. Although the physicians did not think it was serious, he died the next day and was buried in Oakland Cemetery, Yonkers, New York.[1]

DEATH CERTIFICATE: Shock from fracture of skull caused when accidently struck by 3rd Ave. cable car.

1. *OR*, vol. 22, pt. 2:702, 708; Jay Monaghan, *Civil War on the Western Border, 1854–1856*, 298; *New York Times*, Jan. 21, 1896.

F

LUCIUS FAIRCHILD • *Born December 27, 1831,* in Franklin Mills (present day Kent), Ohio. Fairchild was a clerk of a county circuit court and enlisted as a private at the start of the Civil War. In August 1861 he was made lieutenant colonel of the 2nd Wisconsin. At the Battle of Gainesville, Virginia, on August 28, 1862, he was lying ill in a wagon in the rear of the Union column but immediately joined his regiment when the firing started. During the fighting his horse was killed and his field glasses were shot away. Although sick in the hospital with severe indisposition on September 17, 1862, he got up and hastened to join the regiment upon the first indication of their being engaged in battle. On the first day at Gettysburg, July 1, 1863, his left arm was fractured just above the elbow by a minié ball. Supporting his wounded arm with his other hand, he attempted to walk back to Gettysburg, but two of his men had to support him and took him to the rear until they found a stretcher. The regiment's surgeon gave him morphine and bandaged his arm. He was taken to the home of Rev. Charles F. Schaeffer, the principal of the Lutheran Theological Seminary in Gettysburg. That afternoon, under the influence of chloroform, the arm was amputated about six inches below his shoulder. The amputated arm was buried in a tin box in the garden of the Schaeffers' home. The surgeon had him up and walking within a few hours. The next day a Confederate cavalry officer came to the door and, seeing his condition, gave him his parole. For the next few days he was always attended by a member of his regiment. There was no suppuration, and the stump was covered with adhesive plaster. As soon as he had sufficiently recovered, he returned home; he had been given the ball and two pieces of the bone above the elbow to take with him. The ligatures had not sloughed out by early August much to the local surgeon's surprise. The missing arm always seemed to be present and there was constant throbbing pain "between the fingers, the palm, under the finger nails and in the joints of the fingers" in the absent hand. There was also a severe itching sensation that he would try to scratch only to find the limb absent. His family brought in the best doctors of Wisconsin and even took him to specialists in Chicago. Fairchild was promoted brigadier general of volunteers to rank from October 1863 but saw no more service. He resigned in November. For the rest of his life he was deeply involved in politics and veterans' affairs. During January 1864 he had some type of accident that interrupted his recovery. By June he was prematurely white-haired. Even when the stump had healed, he found that pinning his empty sleeve was painful and "the arm tired of being so constantly in the same position." Giving into a superstition of the time that "the arm which is buried is cramped or crooked," thus causing him pain, he had the Schaeffers disinter the box containing the arm. Shortly after receiving it in an express package, he noticed that the pain in his "arm" gradually subsided. He was elected secretary of state of Wisconsin and in 1866 was elected governor. On the evening of July 1, 1866, while taking a stroll in his garden, a man jumped out and struck him across the forehead with a "slung-shot." Fairchild took out his pistol but the gun would not discharge. It was not clear if the attack was prompted by political motives or by a young lady who was trying to blackmail him. At forty years old he looked much older, his face edged by deep lines probably secondary to the constant pain. While consul at Liverpool, England, in 1877 he was incapacitated for a month by an episode of bronchitis. He died May 23, 1896, at Madison, Wisconsin, and was buried there in Forest Hill Cemetery.[1]

DEATH CERTIFICATE: Primary cause of death, chronic nephritis. Secondary, arteriosclerosis. Duration of disease, about two years.

1. CSR; *OR*, vol. 27, pt. 1:256, 273; *OR Suppl.*, vol. 3, pt. 1:542; RVA, Pension WC 678,639; U.S. Army, CWS, roll 8, vol. 13, report 3, pp. 227–43; *MSHW*, vol. 2, pt. 2:749; *MOLLUS* 4:189; Henry Sandford to Mrs. J. Fairchild, July 5, 1863; Charlie to mother, July 6, 8, 12, 1863; Sally Fairchild to Cassias, July 19, 1863; Sarah to Cash, Aug. 10, 1863; S. S. Schaeffer to "my friend," Feb. 9, Mar. 25, Apr. 11, 1864, Wisconsin MSS, Fairchild Papers Correspondence; Sam Ross, *The Empty Sleeve*, 44, 49–53, 63, 81, 158–59, 165.

ELON JOHN FARNSWORTH • *Born on July 30, 1837,* in Green Oak, Michigan. In 1861 he enlisted in the 8th Illinois Cavalry and by December was a captain. He became a brigadier general of volunteers to rank from June 1863. Farnsworth was killed on July 3, 1863, at Gettysburg. He was wounded five times and his body was found in the rear of the position held by the enemy's second line. Although there were Confederate reports that he shot himself in the head rather than surrender, there was no such wound described when his body was discovered.[1] His body was buried in Rockton, Illinois.

1. *OR*, vol. 27, pt. 1:916, 993, 1005, 1013; *SHSP* 4:177, 6:182; *CV* 16:119; *Battles and Leaders* 3:394–96.

JOHN FRANKLIN FARNSWORTH • *Born on March 27, 1820,* in Eaton, Quebec, Canada. A prewar lawyer and politician, he was made colonel of the 8th Illinois Cavalry in September 1861. He served on the Peninsula and at Antietam. During the summer and fall of 1862, he developed varicosities of the veins of his left foot, leg, and groin. He had a sick leave in October. His promotion to brigadier general ranked from November. His limb was swollen and painful, and for a long time the surgeon bandaged the entire leg, from the foot to the torso every

morning before Farnsworth mounted his horse. Later, even this did not provide relief. At the Battle of Fredericksburg in December 1862 he had to command from an ambulance, unable to ride his horse. In the latter part of the
month, he was given sick leave because of phlebitis. He went to New York for
treatment but never recovered enough to return to duty. In February 1863 there
was inflammation of the veins and a tendency for abscesses. Having been elected
to Congress, he tendered his resignation, which was accepted in March 1863.
After the war he had continued problems with his leg. The druggist who helped
him dress the limb stated it was frequently ulcerated, and Farnsworth was repeatedly confined to his house. He was able to remain in Congress until 1873,
when he returned to his law practice. In 1880, the physician who had seen him
in 1862 reexamined him and reported that the varicosities were larger and the
leg volume had increased. Farnsworth died in Washington, D.C., on July 14,
1897, and was buried in St. Charles, Illinois.[1]

DEATH CERTIFICATE: Cause of death, primary, pulmonary tuberculosis; immediate, exhaustion. Duration about one year.

1. *OR*, vol. 19, pt. 2:431; RVA, Pension SC 173,849.

EDWARD FERRERO • *Born January 18, 1831*, in Granada, Spain. His parents brought
him to the United States when he was a young child. When the Civil War started,
he was lieutenant colonel of a militia regiment and was mustered into the volunteer service as colonel of the 51st New York in October 1861. He served in the
North Carolina expedition, at Second Bull Run, Antietam, Fredericksburg,
Vicksburg, and Knoxville. In September 1862 he was promoted to brigadier
general of volunteers. He severely sprained his right ankle on January 15, 1863,
and received a leave of absence. At the time of the Battle of the Crater on July
30, 1864, Ferrero was supposedly exhausted and obtained a stimulant in the
form of rum from the surgeon. However, a court of inquiry concerning the
affair found that he spent most of his time in a bomb-proof and had not commanded his troops. Despite his poor showing, he was breveted major general
of volunteers in December.[1] After the war he followed his father's profession as
a dance instructor. He died December 11, 1899, at New York City and was buried
in Green-Wood Cemetery, Brooklyn.

DEATH CERTIFICATE: Cause of death, pulmonary edema, cardiac.

1. *OR*, vol. 40, pt. 1:119; RVA, Pension WC 673,787.

ORRIS SANFORD FERRY • *Born August 15, 1823*, at Bethel, Connecticut. A lawyer
and politician, he was commissioned colonel of the 5th Connecticut in July
1861. During the fall of 1861 he had a malarial or typhomalarial fever. It did not
wholly disable him from duty until about October 15. On October 26 he was
taken by carriage to a private residence near Rockville, Maryland, where he
remained until mid-November, then returned to duty only partially improved.

Soon afterward, Ferry went home on sick leave. He rejoined his regiment in December in a much better condition. He served in the Shenandoah Valley and on the Peninsula. In March 1862 he was promoted brigadier general of volunteers. He was admitted to the hospital because of a fever in January 1863, and during the following spring and summer he was very yellow and apparently had jaundice. He was greatly prostrated and suffered from pain in the top and back of his head. His symptoms increased in severity until autumn, when he noted improvement. Again in 1864 and 1865, while with the Army of the James, he suffered intense pain in his head and back, particularly when riding, and had a sallow or bilious appearance. He was elected U.S. senator from Connecticut in 1866. In the spring of the same year he developed obscure symptoms, including paralysis of the muscular tissue of the bladder. In 1868 he demonstrated lack of coordination, which was stated to signify sclerosis of the spinal cord. His attending physician later reported in retrospect that he had well-developed symptoms of Progressive Locomotor Ataxia (late form of syphilis involving spinal cord and sensory nerve trunks). His condition was further complicated by gastric disorders, neuralgia, and slight malarial attacks.[1] He died November 21, 1875, at Norwalk, Connecticut, and was buried in the Norwalk Cemetery. DEATH CERTIFICATE: Cause of death, spinal complaint.

1. CSR; U.S. Army, CWS, roll 1, vol. 1, report 57, pp. 1009–27; RVA, Pension WC 191,405; RAGO, entry 534.

FRANCIS FESSENDEN • *Born on March 18, 1839,* in Portland, Maine. A new lawyer, he was commissioned a captain in the 19th U.S. Infantry at the outbreak of the Civil War. At Shiloh on April 7, 1862, he received a severe gunshot wound near the elbow joint and had to leave the field. He remained on sick leave until August 1862 and, although not fully recovered, was ordered on recruiting service in Indianapolis. Near Cane River or Monett's Crossing, Louisiana, on April 23, 1864, a minié ball badly shattered his right leg. A blanket was placed under him and the wound was dressed by the surgeon. Six days later he entered St. James Officers' Hospital in New Orleans. The tibia was fractured irregularly for two and one-half inches at the upper part of the middle third; two pieces of bone were entirely detached. The fibula was not fractured. A flap amputation at the upper third of the lower leg was performed on April 30 using chloroform. At the time of the operation, the periosteum was found to be detached with infiltration of pus between the integuments down to the ankle joints. Later examination of the surgical specimen demonstrated that the bones of the tibia were stripped of periosteum and were evidently dead for a distance of several inches above and below the splintered area. One of the fractures ran directly across the nutrient foramen, and the artery to the bone had been ruptured at this point. This had resulted in considerable hemorrhage, and the blood had infiltrated through the calf of the leg. Fessenden's constitutional condition was good and he progressed favorably. He left the hospital May 18, 1864. In October he was a member of a military commission. He obtained a five days' leave in August 1865 to visit Philadelphia and have repairs made to his artificial leg. He had been promoted to brigadier general of volunteers in May 1864 and to major general in November 1865.[1] After his discharge, Fessenden returned to his law practice. He died in Portland, Maine, on January 2, 1906, and was buried in that city.

DEATH CERTIFICATE: Cause of death, septicemia from osteomyelitis of stump of leg.

1. *OR*, vol. 34, pt. 1:190, 207, 246, 434; U.S. Army, CWS, roll 4, vol. 6, report 29, pp. 545–75; *MSHW*, vol. 2, pt. 3:513, case 754; *MOLLUS* 16:142.

JAMES DEERING FESSENDEN • *Born September 28, 1833*, at Westbrook, Maine. A member of his father's law firm at the start of the war, he recruited a company of men who would become part of the 2nd Regiment of U.S. sharpshooters. His major service was as a staff officer in South Carolina and during the Atlanta campaign. In January and February 1862 he was sick and away from his command. His promotion to brigadier general ranked from August 1864, and he was discharged in January 1866.[1] Fessenden returned to the practice of law and took up politics. He died in Portland, Maine, November 18, 1882, and was buried there.

1. CSR.

CLINTON BOWEN FISK • *Born December 8, 1828*, at York, New York. He was involved in the insurance business at the start of the war. In September 1862 he was appointed colonel of the 33rd Missouri Infantry and two months later was made a brigadier general of volunteers. He was brevetted major general in March 1865. Following the war, he worked for prohibition and the rights of black people. He was assistant commissioner of the Freedmen's Bureau for Kentucky and Tennessee and founded Fisk University. He gave the chief address at his mother-in-law's funeral in Michigan and while there contracted la grippe. On May 24, 1890, he returned to his residence in New York City and never left his apartment again. The condition developed into catarrhal fever, which in turn became rheumatic fever. His wife and daughter took care of him, and on some days his condition appeared to improve. On the Saturday before he died his condition became worse. That night his physicians had a consultation and determined that fatty degeneration of the heart had been for some time an obscure but positive condition, aggravated now by the rheumatic fever. They held little hope for his recovery. His physician stayed with him and supposedly saved his life when the first heart failure occurred.[1] He died on July 9, 1890, and was buried in Coldwater, Michigan.

DEATH CERTIFICATE: Chief cause, heart failure; contributing cause, rheumatic endocarditis following remittent and rheumatic fevers, of six and one-half weeks' duration.

1. Alphonso A. Hopkins, *The Life of Clinton Bowen Fisk,* 306–13.

MANNING FERGUSON FORCE • *Born December 17, 1824,* in Washington, D.C. He was practicing law in Ohio when the war started, and he entered the Federal service as a major of the 20th Ohio Volunteers. Force was at Fort Donelson, Shiloh, and Vicksburg. He was promoted brigadier general in September 1863. On November 13 he was treated for hemorrhoids and returned to duty the following day. In the Battle of Atlanta, July 22, 1864, while trying to aid a wounded officer of his staff, he received a gunshot wound of the face. The minié ball entered just below the lateral corner of his left eye and passed out about an inch in front of the right temporomaxillary articulation. Bones were fractured and blood gushed from his nose and mouth. He was admitted to a general field hospital and transferred on the July 27 to the No. 17 general hospital in Nashville, Tennessee. He had developed an abscess in the area of the wound. On July 30 he was admitted to the officers' general hospital in Louisville, Kentucky, and he was sent home on sick leave on August 2. On August 20, the motion of his jaw and the sensation of the left side of his face were impaired but improving. The external wound was healed and there was only slight discharge from the posterior nares. He returned to duty in October and was in the March to the Sea and the Carolinas campaign. Force had an outstanding career after the war as a lawyer, judge, and writer. His attending physician, who took care of him for the ten years before his death, noted the following changes in his condition: There was disturbed speech and twitching of the muscles of the face and neck. For the last three years of Force's life there was a general alteration of the sensations in his arms, hands, and the upper portion of his body. This was so marked that he could not recognize any object by tactile sensation. The abnormal sensation gradually increased in severity and he had little muscular control. Following a fall a year and a half before he died, he could not rise and had to be carried home. He failed to regain control of his legs and gradually lost all use of his right leg. There was also loss of control of the rectum and bladder and a disturbance in the function of erectile structures. The reporting physician stated that his neurologic changes were related to Force's facial wound, but his wife's pension was rejected because the examining physician did not feel his problems were service-related. Force died May 8, 1899, at the Ohio Soldiers' and Sailors' Home at Sandusky, Ohio, where he was commandant, and was buried in Spring Grove Cemetery, Cincinnati, Ohio. According to the attending physician, Force's death was due to the destructive changes of his nervous structures.[1]

1. *OR,* vol. 38, pt. 1:109, pt. 3:549, 565, 572; RVA, Pension WC 495,143; U.S. Army, CWS, roll 8, vol. 14, report 7, pp. 351–595; RAGO, entry 534; LR, CB, roll 258, F146, 1866; *MOLLUS* 10:306.

JAMES WILLIAM FORSYTH • *Born on August 8, 1835,* in Maumee, Ohio. Graduated
from the USMA in 1856. While a cadet he was seen at the hospital for excoriatio
four times, diarrhea twice, and once each for morbi. varii., clavus, febris intermittent tertian, contusio, and catarrhus. Following graduation from West Point,
he served in the Washington Territory until the start of the war. He spent most
of his wartime service on staff duties with McClellan and Sheridan, and in May
1865 he was commissioned brigadier general of volunteers. Following the war
he remained in the army. He was frequently hospitalized at Fort Riley, Kansas:
January 17–20, 1889, with influenza, and from July 23 to August 2, 1891. He was
sick in June 1892. He had phlegmonous inflammation from June 11–18, 1893. He
was made a brigadier general, U.S. Army, in 1894. He was hospitalized with
acute bronchial catarrh from December 11–14, 1895, and with acute tonsillitis of
both tonsils from September 25–28, 1896. He retired from the military in May
1897. Died at Columbus, Ohio, on October 24, 1906, and was buried there in
Greenlawn Cemetery. According to the local commanding officer, Force died
of paralysis.[1]

1. WPCHR, vols. 608, 609; LR, ACP, 5398, 1872, fiche: 000101.

JOHN GRAY FOSTER • *Born May 27, 1823,* in Whitefield, New Hampshire. Graduated from the USMA in 1846. He was wounded in the leg during the Battle of
Molino del Ray on September 8, 1847. He returned to the United States and
arrived in Washington, D.C., on February 1, 1848. On February 15 he took a post
at Nashua, New Hampshire, and returned to active duty in December. He was
serving as an engineer when the war started, and in October 1861 he was promoted to brigadier general of volunteers. He was a division commander in
Burnside's North Carolina expedition. In May 1863 he was not well. On December 11, 1863, he assumed command of the Army of the Ohio. On December
13–14 he was confined to his quarters in Knoxville, Tennessee, because the pain
in his previously wounded leg was aggravated by his journey from Lexington.
On December 17, Gen. J. G. Parke offered to send an ambulance for him. The
same leg was fractured on December 23 when his horse fell upon a ledge of
rock. Completely disabled by this accident, he requested to be relieved of command. Unable to take the field on January 25, 1864, because of his disabled leg,
he wanted an operation to obtain relief. His knee joint was becoming more
painful. Still suffering from his injuries, he was relieved of comand on February
9 and went to Baltimore. He remained on sick leave until May when he took
command of the Department of the South. In February 1865 he went to Baltimore and apparently had surgery on his leg, but details are not available. Foster
was on sick leave until May 1, 1865, when he returned and was placed on court-
martial duty in Washington, D.C., until June 27. He remained in the army and
served in the engineers. From 1871 until just before his death he was assistant to

the chief of engineers in Washington. Foster was sick from August 24 until he died September 2, 1874, in Nashua, New Hampshire. He was buried there in the Nashua Cemetery. According to his wife, he died of consumption.[1]

1. OR, vol. 18:688; vol. 31, pt. 1:283, 286–87, 330; pt. 3:384, 401, 503; vol. 32, pt. 1:131, pt. 2:208; vol. 47, pt. 2:18, 178, 338, 423; U.S. Army, CWS, roll 1, vol. 2, report 48, pp. 671–92; ibid., roll 4, vol. 7, report 18, pp. 303–6; LR, ACP, 3547, 1874, fiche: 000044.

ROBERT SANFORD FOSTER • *Born on January 27, 1834,* in Vernon, Indiana. A tinner prior to the war, he entered Federal service as a captain of the 11th Indiana in April 1861. He passed through grades and was promoted brigadier general of volunteers to rank from June 1863. His major service was in the Shenandoah Valley, on the Peninsula, during the siege of Charleston, and as a division commander at Petersburg. In the summer of 1863, he contracted diarrhea with subsequent development of piles and disease of his stomach and liver. At the same time he had the onset of rheumatism. His illness, he speculated, was due to the bad food and water. He was not hospitalized but taken by ambulance to the headquarters at Suffolk, where he was confined to his bed for several days. The diarrhea and rheumatism continued for the rest of his life. He resigned in September 1865 and held various civic and Federal positions in Indiana. A severe attack of acute articular rheumatism in 1870 confined him to bed and degenerated into a subacute form. In 1888 Foster had a prolonged attack of rheumatism, which lasted for three months and confined him to bed.[1] Died March 3, 1903, in Indianapolis, Indiana, and was buried in Crown Hill Cemetery.

1. RVA, Pension SC 866,293.

WILLIAM BUEL FRANKLIN • *Born February 27, 1823,* at York, Pennsylvania. Graduated from the USMA in 1843. Served in the Mexican War. He performed engineering duties before the Civil War and was in charge of the construction of the Capitol dome and Treasury addition. Franklin was commissioned brigadier general of volunteers in May 1861 and was at First Bull Run. At Harrison's Landing in the summer of 1862 he received ten days' sick leave. He was a corps commander at Antietam. His performance at Fredericksburg was sharply criticized, and in January 1863 he was relieved from duty in the Army of the Potomac. Franklin had just arrived at the front at Mansfield, Louisiana, April 8, 1864, when his horse was shot from under him and he was wounded in the leg. Although he continued on the field, within a few days he was suffering so much he could not get in the saddle. On the first of May he left his command for New Orleans. He went to New York on sick leave in June and then to his home in Maine. After visiting U. S. Grant's headquarters in July he was captured by Confederate troops on the railroad train between Baltimore and Philadelphia. The following night he escaped and returned home. He was still disabled, however, and his sick leave was extended in August.[1] At the end of the war he resigned all of his commissions and became a businessman and engineer. Died on March 8, 1903, at Hartford, Connecticut, and was buried in York.

DEATH CERTIFICATE: Cause of death, senile dementia, several years' duration.

1. CSR; *OR*, vol. 21:1005; vol. 34, pt. 4:531; vol. 40, pt. 3:456; vol. 41, pt. 2:496; U.S. Army, CWS, roll 1, vol. 2, report 35, pp. 505–23; ibid., roll 5, vol. 9, report 22, pp. 571–77.

JOHN CHARLES FRÉMONT • *Born on January 21, 1813,* at Savannah, Georgia. Before the Civil War he had a varied and colorful career as an army engineer, frontiersman, and politician. His appointment by President Abraham Lincoln as major general in the Regular Army ranked from May 1861. After a lackluster military service, he resigned in June 1864. Following the war he was a politician but lost his financial holdings and to some extent was dependent on others for his livelihood. Died July 13, 1890, in New York City and was buried in Rockland Cemetery, Piermont-on-the Hudson, New York.

DEATH CERTIFICATE: Chief cause, (1) hemorrhage from the stomach; (2) Peritonitis of three days' duration; contributing, heat of July 8.

WILLIAM HENRY FRENCH • *Born January 13, 1815,* in Baltimore, Maryland. Graduated from the USMA in 1837. At West Point he was treated for a toothache twice and once each for headache, boils, eruptio, cold, diarrhea, vertigo, influenza, wound, and cynanche tonsillitis. Served in the Florida and Mexican wars. Stationed at Eagle Pass, Texas, at the start of the Civil War, he took his troops overland and then by ship to Key West, Florida. He was promoted to brigadier general of volunteers to rank from September 1861 and major general from November 1862. He was on the Peninsula and at Antietam, Fredericksburg, Chancellorsville, and Mine Run, where he was a corps commander. French was sick and on leave from December 23 to January 13, 1863. He was discharged from the volunteer service in May 1864 and was made colonel of the U.S. Fourth Artillery. Died May 20, 1881, at Washington, D.C., and was buried in Rock Creek Cemetery. He died at his residence of apoplexy, according to the attending physician.[1]

1. CSR; WPCHR, vols. 602, 603; U.S. Army, CWS, roll 1, vol. 1, report 5, pp. 47–93; LR, ACP, 3318, 1877, fiche: 000031.

JAMES BARNET FRY • *Born on February 23, 1827,* at Carrollton, Illinois. Graduated from the USMA in 1847. At West Point he was treated for catarrhus three times, cephalalgia twice, and for hordeolum (localized infection of eyelid) once. He had garrison duty in Mexico City. Although he commanded a battery of light artillery at the start of the Civil War, his career was subsequently devoted to staff service. During the last year of the war he was provost marshal general of the United States. He had passed through grades to that of brigadier general and held position of provost marshal general by April 1864. At the end of the war he remained in the army. Apparently he had been ill in May 1877, as the Division medical director wrote Fry and stated that if he understood Fry's case properly, it would be useless for him to continue the use of any medicine. He recommended that for the restoration of his health he needed active and constant exercise in the open air in some healthy part of the country. He suggested that Fry try to go on an expedition out on the plains and be in the field for several months. In November 1878 Fry was hospitalized at the post hospital for dyspepsia. He went on sick leave in April 1879 and the next month requested an extension on surgeon's certificate of disability. His surgeon reported that he was suffering from hyperemia of the membranes of the brain induced by long and continued mental labor. Also, he had chronic congestion of the internal tissues of the eye tending to glaucoma or permanent destruction of vision. Fry reported back for duty in December. He was hospitalized again in November 1880 with acute capillary bronchitis. When he was ordered to New Orleans in December, he replied that since his health was already bad, the climate there would finish him. His poor health continued, and he applied for retirement on July 1, 1881, after thirty years' service. He died July 11, 1894, in Newport, Rhode Island, and was buried in the churchyard of St. James the Less, Philadelphia, Pennsylvania. Cause of death, apoplexy.[1]

1. WPCHR, vol. 605; LR, ACP, 2910, 1871, fiche: 000046; RAGO, entry 534; Deaths registered in the City of Newport for the year ending December 31, 1894.

SPEED SMITH FRY • *Born on September 9, 1817,* in what is present-day Boyle County, Kentucky. Served in the Mexican War. A county judge at the start of the Civil War, Fry was appointed colonel of a militia unit in July 1861 and in October colonel of the 4th Kentucky Infantry. He was slightly wounded at Logan Cross Roads, Kentucky, on January 19, 1862, and served at Shiloh and Stones River. In March 1863 he was promoted to brigadier general of volunteers. In April he contracted influenza, which severely affected his head and throat and caused deafness in both ears. He felt this was the result of having to sleep upon the wet ground without a tent or cot. In May he was awaken by a noise and a pain in his right ear. He soon discovered it was caused by a large bug that had entered his ear. He called the surgeon, who failed to extricate the bug but did kill it with the use of laudanum and oil. The next day he went to the medical director, who removed the bug with a small stick, and he received a medical leave. Fry performed garrison duty toward the end of the war and was mustered out of Federal service in August 1865. He could not hear a watch ticking close to the right ear and could barely hear it when held close to the left ear. There was a distressing roaring and buzzing sound, most marked in the right ear. By 1885 he was told not to attempt any further treatment of his ears. He had been trying warm water and pure castile soap injected into the ear without benefit. He had to abandon his law profession because he could not hear the witnesses. At the time of his death, he was superintendent of the Soldiers' Home near Louisville.[1] Died August 1, 1892, near Louisville, Kentucky, and was buried in Danville, Kentucky.

1. CSR; *OR*, vol. 7:81; RVA, Pension Speed S. Fry.

JOHN WALLACE FULLER · *Born July 28, 1827,* at Harston, Cambridgeshire, England. He was operating a publishing business at the start of the Civil War. Probably because he had experience as an officer of militia, he was appointed colonel of the 27th Ohio Volunteers in August 1861. He was at New Madrid, Island No. 10, Iuka, and Corinth. On August 15, 1862, a surgeon reported that Fuller was suffering with great nervous frustration and debility consequent upon climatic influences and his deranged digestive organs. He had been affected to some degree by this condition for a number of weeks, but it had grown worse for the previous few days. The surgeon recommended a change of diet and climate. He was promoted to brigadier general of volunteers in January 1864 and served in the Atlanta campaign, the March to the Sea, and the Carolinas campaign. After receiving the brevet of major general, he resigned in August 1865.[1] Fuller was engaged in the wholesale boot and shoe business for the rest of his working days. Died March 12, 1891, at Toledo, Ohio, and was buried in Woodlawn Cemetery in that city.

DEATH CERTIFICATE: Cause of death, immediate cause, dilation of right heart, three weeks' duration.

1. CSR.

G

WILLIAM GAMBLE · *Born on January 1, 1818,* at Duross, County Tyrone, Ireland. Gamble enlisted in the Regular Army in 1839 and rose to the rank of sergeant-major by the time of his discharge in 1843. At the start of the Civil War he was engaged as a civil engineer. He was made a lieutenant colonel and then, in December 1862, colonel of the 8th Illinois Cavalry. He received a gunshot wound during the fighting at Malvern Hill on August 5, 1862. The minié ball entered at a point about two inches below his right nipple, passed upwards and backwards through the lung, and lodged halfway through the right scapula. A surgeon later cut the bullet out on the field. By January 1863, in spite of his wound, he was back in brigade command. He was at Gettysburg and in the early phases of the Overland campaign. Over the next few years he had frequent hemorrhage from his lungs. He was brevetted brigadier general of volunteers to rank from December 1864. Following the war, he remained in the army and was appointed major of the Eighth Cavalry in 1866. While accompanying his regiment to California via the Central American Transit route, he contracted cholera and died in Virgin Bay, Nicaragua, on December 20, 1866. By December 27, twenty-six of his men had died from the disease.[1] He was buried there in Virgin Grove Cemetery.

1. RVA, Pension SO 112,730; RG 94, Letters Received by Adjutant General's Office, Jan. 14, 1867, NA, Washington, D.C.

JAMES ABRAM GARFIELD • *Born November 19, 1831,* in Cuyahoga County, Ohio. He was employed driving dray horses that pulled canal barges between Cleveland and Pittsburgh in the summer of 1848. In October he contracted the ague and went home to bed. Vigorous treatment with calomel did not help. Finally the fever broke in January. Early that year he enrolled in school. A member of the Ohio senate at the start of the Civil War, he was made a lieutenant colonel in August 1861 and colonel of the 42nd Ohio in December. He was at Shiloh, Corinth, and Chickamauga. Garfield's military career was punctuated by frequent periods of ill health, particularly diarrhea. In June 1861, while at home, he had some problem with his arm. The limb had improved by the time he returned to duty in July but still caused him pain with movement. In August and again in October he had diarrhea, and the medicine given to him by his doctor made him sick, causing vomiting and purging. His promotion to brigadier general of volunteers ranked from January 1862. That month he had diarrhea, and in February he developed a severe cold and fever. When Garfield was exposed to smallpox he was immediately vaccinated. Soon afterward he contracted camp fever and "dried up the pustule before it had matured." He developed a rheumatic type of pain through all of his bones. In spite of his poor condition, he kept moving his brigade forward. In April he had bloody dysentery and suffered with a severe and painful attack of the piles. It was very hard for him to ride his horse. After a period of relatively good health, the diarrhea associated with fever returned in June. He lost weight and was confined to his bed in camp for a few days. To remove the bile from his system he took a purgative medicine. He theorized that the two weeks of breathing the air that came from the large Rebel camp with all its sickness and offal had half poisoned his system. His health had improved by late in the month. He was on court-martial duty during the trial of John Basil Turchin until July when he awoke with a headache, fever, diarrhea, jaundice, and severe fits of vomiting. His surgeon gave him a powerful emetic, which brought forth floods of "irrepressible bile." He remained on court-martial duty as long as he could, although he had to be carried to the court on a litter and was required to spend part of the time on a cot. In August he went home on leave but had a prolonged trip due to a delay caused by his illness. His skin was yellow and he had lost forty-three pounds. He arrived in Washington, D.C., on September 19 and his activities were limited due to a sprained ankle and his weakness. In October he had a recurrence of diarrhea, which continued into the next month. He was also lame and nearly laid up with a corn on his foot. To correct his habit of stooping he wore a shoulder brace. By the middle of the month he had a dull headache, kind of a slow fever, and pain in his bones. He had been told that everyone who came to Washington from the North had to go through a period of seasoning to the bilious fever. By late December Garfield's health was fine, his bowels reliable. His health continued to be good until he arrived at Murfreesboro, Tennessee, in late January 1863, when he developed a severe inflammatory sore throat and diarrhea. In an attempt to control the diarrhea he tried a period of fasting. Again his health improved, and he did reasonably well until May, when he was sick for a few days. His surgeon said it was an attack of bilious remittent fever, probably occasioned by malaria. He had general body pain and could not find a comfortable position. By the end of the month he had relapsed, but this time he had a severe attack of vomiting. His surgeon brought him a hair mattress, sheets, a pillow, and mosquito bars to help make him comfortable. During late June he was in better health but believed he was inclined to torpidity of the liver. The first of August he had a return of his piles along with fever and diarrhea. He was not able to sit up or put on his clothes for a week. His appetite was poor and he was fearful of a return of the jaundice. Again he treated himself by starvation. His cot was placed in a railroad car and he was transported to Stevenson, Alabama, where he found a room away from the camp. By following rigid rules, Garfield slowly improved to the point where he could sit up and walk in the yard for short periods. In September 1863 he was worn down with fatigue and diarrhea, and a boil he had broken when he rode on it. Throughout 1864 he kept his rectal ointment ready.[1] After he returned to civilian life he served in the House and Senate before being elected president of the United States. His gastrointestinal symptoms were diagnosed as neuralgic dyspepsia in 1873 and his physician recommended a diet of raw beef, stale bread, and milk. During the summer of 1875 he had a severe recurrence of his hemorrhoids, which did not respond to the usual medical treatment. He had surgery, but rather than hemorrhoids the surgeon found a rectal ulcer. Following the surgery he was bedridden for the rest of the summer. Four months after his July 2, 1881, inauguration as president of the United States, he was mortally wounded in the Washington railroad depot by Charles Julius Guiteau. Using a .44 caliber revolver, the British Bulldog, Guiteau fired into Garfield's back from less than a yard away. Guiteau then took two steps forward and fired once more as the president was half twisting and half falling. Garfield lay in a pool of vomit, bathed in sweat, and his pulse was faint and irregular. One bullet had merely grazed his arm while the other had entered about four inches to the right of the spine, fractured the eleventh rib, and went into his body. After Garfield was given aromatic spirits of ammonia and a small amount of brandy he seemed to improve. He was placed on a mattress, and doctors probed the wound before he was carried upstairs. Garfield complained of pain in his ankles and in the right side of his scrotum. Mattresses were removed from a Pullman car and put into an express wagon so he could be taken back to the White House. On arrival there, he was carried to an upstairs bedroom. He continued to vomit every half hour; although his vital signs diminished, he remained alert. Morphia was administered, and a number of doctors probed the wound with their fingers and probes but were unable to locate the bullet. That night Garfield was given morphine and rested well between vomiting episodes. One-eighth of a grain of morphine along with one-eightieth grain of atropine was given by hypodermic injection. The next day his temperature began to rise and his abdomen became distended. He received constant attention: he was shifted in bed fifteen to twenty times a day to prevent bedsores; his numb feet were rubbed; and he was fed and cleaned. On July 4, two surgical specialists arrived from New York and Philadelphia; after probing and examining the wound they agreed with the patient's treatment. The next day his vomiting ceased and oral feeding was started using lime water and fresh milk. A cow had been put out to pasture on the White House lawn for this purpose. He had a normal bowel movement on the sixth. Morphine injections were reduced on the eighth and stimulants in the form of rum were given. The wound was discharging laudable pus. His temperature began to rise and fall in an irregular fashion and he was started on five grains of quinine sulfate each day because of a diagnosis of malaria. By July 12 the wound was discharging healthy pus and was dressed "antiseptically" with carbolic acid twice a day. His condition was unchanged from July 13–21. The next day spicules of bone and fragments of clothing were noted in the discharging pus. A circumscribed area of induration appeared in the right groin on the twenty-third and the next day a drainage incision, three inches long, was made below the wound using a director probe. An irrigating catheter was passed through the incision for a distance of seven inches. At the time this track was considered to be the true course of the missile. Also, Alexander Graham Bell had constructed a metal detector that seemed to substantiate this location. Garfield was able to preside over a brief bedside cabinet meeting on July 29. By July 31 he appeared to be doing well, and the two openings continued to drain large amounts of "laudable pus." The morphine and quinine were discontinued on August 5. Because of continued vomiting, proctoclysis (liquid feedings by enema) was started on the fifteenth. His right parotid gland became swollen and painful on the eighteenth. A catheter was passed twelve and one-half inches into the suspected track of the ball toward his groin on August 20. Viscous material was collected from his throat on the twentieth, oral feedings were discontinued, and the enema feedings were increased. The parotid swelling was incised without anesthesia on August 24, and it was estimated he had lost eighty pounds. He developed bronchitis on August 25. Pus began to drain from the right external auditory meatus the next day through two sinuses that appeared spontaneously in the internal canal. On August 28 additional discharging sinuses appeared just below the right ear. Another incision and drainage of the parotid gland was made on August 30. The next day a spontaneous opening from the parotid abscess developed in Garfield's mouth and irrigating fluid passed into his throat. The summer tem-

perature in Washington was high and caused him great discomfort. Navy engineers had invented and installed an air-conditioner, which provided some relief. On September 6 he was moved by train to the cooler climate at the Franklin
Cottage at Elberson, New Jersey. The journey by train of over two hundred
miles lasted seven hours. On September 10 he was able to sit up at intervals but
developed bronchopneumonia. His condition remained the same over the next
week, but on the seventeenth he had a severe chill. He became weaker and more
febrile. Before he died he had a temperature of 108.8° with tachycardia and chest
pain. He died September 19 at Elberon, New Jersey, and was buried in Lake
View Cemetery, Cleveland, Ohio. The autopsy findings were as follows:

There was bilateral bronchopneumonia. About a pint of bloody fluid was
present in the abdomen. The ball had entered the body 3 ½ inches to the right
of the vertebral spine, fractured the eleventh rib, passed obliquely to the left
and forward, passed through the body of the first lumbar vertebra, and lodged
in the adipose tissue just below the lower border of the pancreas. The ball was
encysted and rested 2½ inches to the left of the spinal column and behind the
peritoneum. Between the fractured first lumbar vertebrae and the ball was a
blood-filled cavity produced by a rent ⁴/₁₀ of an inch long in the splenic artery,
about 2½ inches from the coeliac axis. On the right side of the spinal column
the track of the bullet was greatly dilated and filled with pus. This collection
had burrowed behind the right kidney, down between the peritoneum and the
right iliac fossa, and into the right groin. The surgeons performing the autopsy
stated that the splenic artery had initially been injured when he was shot and
had slowly leaked blood for weeks. They speculated the cause of death was a
sudden bleeding episode. However, his severe malnutrition, bronchopneumonia, abdominal abscess, and general septic condition probably played a major
role in his death.[2]

1. OR, vol. 20, pt. 2:330; U.S. Army, CWS, roll 4, vol. 7, report 47, pp. 739–811; Allan Jay Peskin,
"James A. Garfield, 1831–1863" (diss.), 19–20, 231–32, 243; James A. Garfield, The Wild Life of the
Army: Civil War Letters of James A. Garfield, 22, 28, 39, 62, 64, 67–68, 71, 83–84, 86, 105–6, 110–11, 115–
16, 119, 124–25, 127, 133–34, 137–38, 144, 156, 172, 180–81, 183, 203, 223–25, 259, 261, 269–70, 284, 291–93,
296–98.

2. Allan Peskin, Garfield, 373, 392, 433, 596–607; Stewart A. Fish, "The Death of President Garfield,"
Bulletin of the History of Medicine 24 (1950): 378–92.

KENNER GARRARD • Born September 30, 1827, in Bourbon County, Kentucky.
Graduated from the USMA in 1851. At the academy he was treated for obstipatio,
cephalalgia, and catarrhus one time each.[1] He was captured by Confederate
forces at San Antonio in April 1861 and was exchanged in August 1862. In September he was appointed colonel of the 146th New York and in July 1863 was
promoted to brigadier general of volunteers. He served at Fredericksburg,
Chancellorsville, Gettysburg, in the Atlanta campaign, and at the Battle of Nashville. He was brevetted brigadier and major general in the Regular Army in

March 1865 and resigned in November 1866. Garrard returned to his home in Cincinnati and engaged in business and civic affairs. Died May 15, 1879, in the Grand Hotel at Cincinnati and was buried in Spring Grove Cemetery. Burial records: Cause of death, hernia.

1. WPCHR, vols. 606, 607.

THEOPHILUS TOULMIN GARRARD • *Born on June 7, 1812*, at the Union Salt Works near Manchester, Kentucky. Served in the Mexican War. In September 1861 he was appointed colonel of the 7th Kentucky (Union) Infantry; his promotion to brigadier general ranked from November 1862. About the end of March 1863, while at Millikens Bend, he lost the central vision of his left eye. The surgeon who examined him reported there was some obscure disease in the posterior chamber of his eye and advised consultation. In July 1863 he reported to the medical director at Cincinnati for treatment of his eye, which had been impaired by a rupture. Garrard remained there until September 10, the condition being pronounced incurable. On September 12 he left for Memphis, Tennessee, and was assigned to duty in Kentucky to construct military roads. Mustered out of the service in April 1864, he farmed and operated his salt works. He had lost all sight in his left eye and the vision of the right eye was so poor that he was not able to attend to any business that required use of his eyes. He had no additional medical problems except for a short episode of abdominal pain in August 1879 that resolved spontaneously.[1] Died March 15, 1902, near Manchester, Kentucky, in the same house in which he was born. He was buried in the cemetery at Garrard, Kentucky.

1. U.S. Army, CWS, roll 5, vol. 8, report 13, pp. 631–51; RVA, Pension SC 204,498.

JOHN WHITE GEARY • *Born December 30, 1819*, at Mount Pleasant, Pennsylvania. A contusion from a spent ball in September 1847 at Chapultepec disabled him for a time. His health deteriorated while governor of the Kansas Territory, and he resigned in March 1857. He was farming in Pennsylvania at the outbreak of the Civil War. In June 1861 he was appointed colonel of the 28th Pennsylvania and brigadier general of volunteers in April 1862. During a skirmish at Bolivar Heights on October 16, 1861, a piece of shell struck him on the front of his leg below the knee. Although it cut to the bone he continued on the field, and it subsequently healed rapidly. At Cedar Mountain on August 9, 1862, he was wounded twice, first slightly in the left foot and then severely in the left elbow. He remained on the field until that evening when he was compelled to retire due to exhaustion produced by pain and blood loss. A conical musket ball had shattered the olecranon and outer condyle of the left elbow, flattening itself against the latter. There had been considerable bleeding, and the joint was swollen and tender. After his wound was dressed at the division field hospital, he was sent to Culpeper and then to Washington. The battered projectile and some bone splinters were extracted and the limb was put up in a felt trough or angular splint. A large fenestra was cut out opposite the wound and the arm was kept at rest at an angle of 130 degrees. Initially there was considerable inflammatory reaction and copious suppuration. At the end of five weeks the inflammation had diminished and passive motion was started cautiously. Geary returned with his arm in a bandage and assumed brigade command in late September. On October 9, 1862, his arm was still weak and he had a large painful boil. By the middle of the month he had four "volcanic" boils; however, his arm seemed to improve. Although still weak, his arm was more supple on November 11, 1862. During January 1863 he had severe carbuncles on his back. At Chancellorsville on May 3, 1863, a cannonball hit him in the chest and knocked him unconscious. Unable to speak, he gave up his command for a day. He could not speak above a whisper for weeks. After Gettysburg he saw service at Chattanooga and in the March to the Sea. In late August 1863 he was unwell for several days but was able to discharge his duties. Although he had regained his strength by September, he was sick again in November. On December 12, 1863, he had diarrhea, which he had had previously. Because his original vaccination for smallpox did not have an effect, he was vaccinated again in May 1864. Geary was brevetted major general to rank from January 1865 and left the army in 1866. He was elected governor of Pennsylvania and died soon after his second term. He died suddenly on January 18, 1873, at Harrisburg, Pennsylvania, while fixing breakfast for his youngest son. He was buried in the Harrisburg Cemetery. Rumors were that he was poisoned by the chemicals he used to maintain the black color of his beard![1]

1. CSR; *OR*, vol. 12, pt. 2:134, 137, 158, 161, 325; vol. 19, pt. 2:436; vol. 25, pt. 1:759; U.S. Army, CWS, roll 3, vol. 4, report 16, pp. 497–521; *MSHW*, vol. 2, pt. 2:830, case 1741; RAGO, entry 623, "File D"; Paul Beers, "A Profile: John W. Geary," *CWTI* 9 (June 1970): 11–16; Wilcox, *Mexican War*, 461, 685; John White Geary, *A Politician Goes to War*, 19–20, 55, 58, 60, 62–63, 86, 111–12, 135, 146, 159–60.

GEORGE WASHINGTON GETTY • *Born October 2, 1819*, in Georgetown, D.C. Graduated from the USMA in 1840. As a cadet he was treated for nausea twice and fever once. Served in the Mexican and Florida wars. A captain in the Regular Army when the Civil War started, he was appointed lieutenant colonel in the volunteer service in September 1861. He served on the Peninsula, at Antietam, Fredericksburg, Suffolk, and Gettysburg. He had a leave for the benefit of his health the last of July 1862. Getty was promoted to brigadier general of volunteers to rank from September and was ordered to report for duty in October. He was absent on sick leave late in September 1863 and returned the next month. He was severely wounded through the shoulder at the Wilderness on May 6, 1864, but refused for some time to leave the field. On May 12th he was a patient at Fredericksburg. He returned in June and was assigned to garrison duty. In August 1864 he was brevetted major general of volunteers and in the regular service in March 1865. Getty remained in the army and was appointed colonel of the 38th Infantry in 1866. In June 1883 he applied for three months' leave from Fort Monroe, Virginia, because he suffered from catarrh aggravated by the atmosphere of the location. He was on sick leave from July 10 to October 2, 1883, when he was retired due to age. He died at Forest Glen, Maryland, on October 1, 1901, and was buried in Arlington National Cemetery. His attending physician reported the primary cause of death was senility and the immediate cause was an enlarged prostate with cystitis.[1]

1. CSR; *OR*, vol. 19, pt. 2:381; vol. 29, pt. 2:230; vol. 36, pt. 1:126, 190, 678; pt. 3:758; WPCHR, vol. 604; LR, ACP, 3456, 1886, fiche: 000104; Stevens, *Sixth Corps*, 341.

JOHN GIBBON • *Born April 20, 1827,* in Philadelphia, Pennsylvania. Graduated from the USMA in 1847. According to Gibbon, an incorrect date was used for his birth when he entered the U.S. Military Academy. As a cadet he was treated for catarrhus twice and wound incision and nausea each once. Served in the Mexican and Florida wars. He had sick leave from August 31, 1859, to March 29, 1860. A captain of artillery in 1861, he was made a brigadier general of volunteers in May 1862. He was at Second Bull Run and Antietam. At the Battle of Fredericksburg on December 13, 1862, he was wounded in the right wrist, and a bone of the hand was broken by a piece of shell. After going to the rear and having his wound dressed, he went to Aquia Creek by boxcar and to Washington by steamer. When he was able to travel he went to Baltimore. His wound healed slowly but he was able to rejoin the army in March 1863. On the afternoon of July 3 at Gettysburg Gibbon was severely wounded. The bullet entered in the middle of his left arm near the shoulder and passed backward, fracturing the upturned edge of the scapula. He was taken by ambulance to the hospital at Rock Creek and was then transported by ambulance to Westminster, Maryland, where he arrived the next morning. He was cared for at a relative's house until that afternoon when he was placed in a boxcar with other wounded. That night the car was left a few miles out of town in the pouring rain, and the next day the wounded were taken to Baltimore. The wound healed slowly, and when he was fit for light duty he was sent to take charge of a draft rendezvous in November. He rejoined the army in March 1864. Affected by the intense heat, dust, and bad water, he had sick leave for a few days in August. He remained in the army and served primarily against the Indians. Fighting like a private with a rifle in his hand, he was wounded by a ball in his thigh at Big Hole Pass, Montana, in the action with Nez Perce Indians on August 9, 1877. He was able to take his troops back to Deer Lodge, Montana, and he had sick leave from August to September 24, 1877. Gibbon was made a brigadier general in the Regular Army in 1885 and retired in 1891. He died on February 6, 1896, in Baltimore, Maryland, and was buried in Arlington National Cemetery. According to the officer of the post, he died from pneumonia.[1]

1. CSR; *OR*, vol. 21:58, 92, 455, 480; vol. 25, pt. 2:176; vol. 27, pt. 1:75, 117, 375, 417, 421; vol. 42, pt. 1:218; vol. 51, pt. 1:1111, 1122; WPCHR, vol. 605; U.S. Army, CWS, roll 1, vol. 1, report 34, pp. 549–62; LR, ACP, 127, 1879, fiche: 000105; John Gibbon, *Personal Recollections of the Civil War*, 104–6, 159, 168, 170–71, 184, 254; *MOLLUS* 21:299.

ALFRED GIBBS • *Born April 22, 1823*, in what is present-day Astoria, New York. Graduated from the USMA in 1846. He was slightly wounded April 17, 1847, at Cerro Gordo. He was wounded again in a skirmish with Apaches at Cook's Spring (Sierra de los Miembres), New Mexico, on March 9, 1857. Gibbs was captured by Confederate forces in July 1861 at San Augustine Springs, New Mexico, and was not exchanged for over a year. He was made colonel of the 130th New York Infantry in September 1862. In May 1863 he was given a leave because he was suffering from an attack of intermittent fever (quotidian). He had another sick leave in October because his health was impaired by remittent fever and he suffered from an old abdominal wound. In January 1864 Gibbs had a severe attack of rheumatic gout and was ordered to Washington for treatment. However, physically unable to travel, he was treated in camp, and by January 25th he was able to perform his duties. His promotion as brigadier general of volunteers ranked from October 1864. He served in the Shenandoah and at Appomattox. Following the war he remained in the army and had sick leave while at San Antonio, Texas, from December 1865 to the middle of February 1866. Some months before his death on December 26, 1868, at Fort Leavenworth, Kansas, he suffered with intermittent fever, chronic diarrhea, and hemorrhoids. He was buried in St. Mary's Cemetery at Portsmouth, Rhode Island. The attending surgeon reported that he died of congestion of the brain.[1]

1. CSR; RVA, Pension 137,047; Heitman, *Historical Register and Dictionary* 2:22; LR, CB, roll, 433, G92, 1869.

CHARLES CHAMPION GILBERT • *Born March 1, 1822*, at Zanesville, Ohio. Graduated from the USMA in 1846. Served in the Mexican War. Before the Civil War, he was a faculty member at the U.S. Military Academy and served on the frontier. A captain in the Regular Army, he was wounded in the shoulder on August 10, 1861, at the end of the Battle of Wilson's Creek. He accompanied the army on its retreat and obtained a sick leave. Although not fit for active duty, he was appointed acting inspector general on September 22. About the first of December, his wound having healed, he reported for full duty. He was at Shiloh and Perryville. In September 1862 he was appointed brigadier general of volunteers.

However, his appointment was not confirmed by the Senate, and when his commission expired in March 1863 he was not reappointed. The rest of the war he served on desk duties as a major. Gilbert remained in the army after the war. During August and September 1867 he was treated for gastric fever. Because of an attack of malaria, he had sick leave from November 12 to January 16, 1868. In June 1880 he applied for leave on surgeon's certificate. The surgeon reported that Gilbert was suffering from general debility and nervous prostration induced by malarial cachexia and chronic kidney disease. Also, the surgeon stated that he had suffered from the effects of the latter disease for the previous three years. Gilbert again requested leave in October 1884 because he was suffering from an impairment of nervous and vital forces as a result of both his age and his prolonged frontier service in a cold climate. He was sick from July to the middle of August 1885. He had sick leave on surgeon's certificate because of nervous prostration from October 20 until March 1, 1886, the date of his retirement. Died January 17, 1903, in Baltimore and was buried in Cave Hill Cemetery, Louisville, Kentucky. According to a family member he died from pneumonia.[1]

1. *OR*, vol. 3:79; U.S. Army, CWS, roll 2, vol. 3, report 5, pp. 123–37; LR, ACP, 1422, 1880, fiche: 000053.

JAMES ISHAM GILBERT • *Born on July 16, 1823,* in Louisville, Kentucky. Prior to the Civil War, Gilbert was a lumberman, Indian trader, merchant, dealer in real estate, and operator of a livery stable. He joined the service as colonel of the 27th Iowa Volunteers in October 1862. At Pleasant Grove, Louisiana, on April 9, 1864, he was slightly wounded in the left hand but remained in command until the fighting ceased. After serving in Nashville he was promoted to brigadier general of volunteers in February 1865. He was discharged in August and returned to lumbering and mining interests. He first engaged in the grocery business after he moved to Topeka, Kansas, in 1882, but because of poor health he sold the business and organized the Topeka Coal Economizing Company, of which he was president at the time of his demise. His death was very sudden; he had just taken a footbath and gotten into bed when he died. His death on February 9, 1884, in Topeka was caused by apoplexy or neuralgia of the heart, and he was buried in Aspen Grove Cemetery, Burlington, Iowa.[1]

1. *OR*, vol. 34, pt. 1:356; RVA, Pension SC 433,268; *Topeka Daily Commonwealth*, Feb. 12, 1884; *Daily Kansas State Journal*, Feb. 11, 1884.

ALVAN CULLEM GILLEM • *Born July 29, 1830,* at Gainesboro, Tennessee. Graduated from the USMA in 1851. While at West Point, he was treated once each for catarrhus, subluxatio, morbi. varii., dysentery, contusio, ophthalmia, obstipatio, and excoriatio. Served in the Florida wars. Prior to the Civil War he had frontier and garrison duty. During the war he was a quartermaster, commander of artillery, colonel of volunteer infantry, and adjutant general of Tennessee. His promotion as brigadier general of volunteers ranked from August 1863. He remained in the Regular Army after the war and carried out the reconstruction plan, served on frontier duty, and fought against the Modocs. At Benicia Barracks, California, on December 3, 1874, the surgeon certified that Gillem was afflicted with an abnormal action in his brain and spinal marrow from which he had suffered since the end of the war with the Modoc Indians. He was given a special order for a one-year leave of absence. His condition was such that a soldier had to accompany him from his station at Benicia Barracks to his home in Tennessee. The physician who took care of him the rest of his life reported that during that period he was bedridden and totally insane from softening of the brain, for which there was no cure. Gillem died on December 2, 1875, at the Soldiers' Rest near Nashville, Tennessee, and was buried in Mount Olivet Cemetery. The attending surgeon reported that he died from softening of the brain.[1]

1. WPCHR, vols. 606, 607; RVA, Pension Min. C. 183,081; *San Francisco Alta,* Dec. 13, 1875.

QUINCY ADAMS GILLMORE • *Born February 28, 1825,* in present day Lorain, Ohio. Graduated from the USMA in 1849. While a cadet, he was treated for ophthalmia ten times, cephalalgia nine times, catarrhus eight times, odontalgia three times, debility twice, and febris intermittent, febris continued, and morbi. varii. each one time. Commissioned into the Corps of Engineers after graduation from the U.S. Military Academy, he had duty as an instructor at West Point and as an engineer. His promotion to brigadier general of volunteers ranked from April 1862. While in command on Tybee Island on May 3 he developed malarial fever, and on the fourteenth he started for New York on sick leave. He went to Washington in June and had a return of fever. Gillmore returned in August and was on temporary duty mustering troops in New York. He was on sick leave in New York City because of chronic bronchitis from April until late May 1863. He was promoted to major general to rank from July 1863. Early on the morning of July 14, 1864, at Offutt's Cross Roads, Maryland, his foot was injured when his horse fell, and he could not put it on the ground or ride on horseback. The fall had produced a subluxation and contusion of the left ankle joint. In mid-August he had to use two crutches to move about. From September through November he was president of a board testing Adelbert Ames's wrought-iron cannon. After resigning from his volunteer position, Gillmore remained in the army as a major of engineers. In October and November 1882, he was not able to give proper attention to his official duties because of pain, and he expected to undergo a severe surgical operation. It is not clear what type of surgery was proposed or if he had undergone the procedure. In March 1883 it was recommended that he resume his duties. He was in Brooklyn in February 1885 and, when ordered to go to Washington on court-martial duty, was delayed by an attack of what he thought was malaria. He died April 7, 1888, in Brooklyn, New York, and was buried at West Point. In response to an official inquiry, a local officer reported his death was induced by chronic inflammation of the bladder following an operation for renal stones.[1]

DEATH CERTIFICATE: Cause of death, uremia, Bright's disease of eight years' duration.

1. *OR*, vol. 23, pt. 1:12; vol. 14:459; vol. 37, pt. 1:266, pt. 2:266, 303, 310–11, 314; WPCHR, vols. 605, 606, 607; U.S. Army, CWS, roll 7, vol. 12, report 1, pp. 1–416; LR, ACP, 5364, 1875, fiche: 000107; RVA, Pension C 324,697.

GEORGE HENRY GORDON • *Born July 19, 1823,* in Charlestown, Massachusetts. Graduated from the USMA in 1846. Gordon was slightly wounded on April 17, 1847, at Cerro Gordo. He was listed as sick in September 1847 and was wounded again on December 21, 1847, at the San Juan Bridge. He resigned from the army in 1854 and became a lawyer. Gordon was made colonel of the 2nd Massachusetts in May 1861 and was promoted to brigadier general of volunteers in June 1862. He served in the Shenandoah, at Antietam, and at Suffolk. From November 17, 1862, until the middle of January he was sick with typhoid fever. When he tried to go back to his command he had a relapse. It was not until February that his health permitted him to return to command. However, after a fortnight his fever compelled him to leave again in March, and he was not able to come back until the middle of April. He was attacked with violent congestive chills and fever in September 1864 and went north on sick leave. The surgeon reported he had anemia and debility as the result of malarial poisoning, and at the time he was suffering from an attack of intermittent fever. Gordon returned September 27 only to have a recurrence of the same symptoms on October 16. He was ordered north on leave and on November 5 was assigned to duty as chief of staff for Benjamin F. Butler in New York City.[1] Following the war he returned to his law practice and also authored a number of military books. He died August 30, 1886, at Framingham, Massachusetts, and was buried in Framingham Centre.

DEATH CERTIFICATE: Immediate cause of death, heart disease.

1. *OR*, vol. 12, pt. 3:409; vol. 18:659; vol. 25, pt. 2:272; vol. 27, pt. 3:779; U.S. Army, CWS, roll 1, vol. 1, report 36, pp. 765–73; ibid., roll 4, vol. 7, report 34, pp. 503–4; LR, CB, roll 164, G235, 1865; Heitman, *Historical Register and Dictionary* 2:23; "Official List of Officers who Marched with the Army under command of Major General Winfield Scott," USAMHI.

WILLIS ARNOLD GORMAN • *Born on January 12, 1816,* near Flemingsburg, Kentucky. Although listed as being slightly wounded at Buena Vista, in actual fact he had a fall from his horse on the battlefield on February 23, 1847, which increased a slight preexisting inguinal hernia to a scrotal type. In consequence he was unable to perform further field duty. Prior to the Civil War he was a lawyer and politician. He was a member of Congress from Indiana and was appointed governor of the Minnesota Territory. In April 1861 he was commissioned colonel of the 1st Minnesota Volunteers and was promoted to brigadier general to rank from September. Sick and unable to command in late June 1862, he remained with the army until it arrived at Harrison's Landing in July and then went to the hospital. He left the hospital on July 14 and resumed command of his brigade on July 17.[1] After serving at Antietam he was sent to Arkansas. Following his discharge from Federal service in May 1864, he returned to the practice of law. Died May 20, 1876, at St. Paul, Minnesota, and was buried there in Oakland Cemetery.

DEATH CERTIFICATE: Cause of death, debility.

1. *OR,* vol. 11, pt. 2:87; vol. 51, pt. 1:108; CSR, Mexican War; U.S. Army, CWS, roll 1, vol. 2, report 3, pp. 39–49; ibid., A. Sully report, roll 1, vol. 1, report 23, pp. 311–30; Wilcox, *Mexican War,* 664.

CHARLES KINNAIRD GRAHAM • *Born June 3, 1824,* in New York City. During the Mexican War he served in the navy. A lawyer and engineer before the Civil War, he constructed the dry dock at the Brooklyn Navy Yard. After the war started, he passed through grades from major to colonel of the Excelsior Brigade (74th New York). When the army reached Harrison's Landing, Graham was stricken with fever and was sent north to recover. He had camp dysentery from the last week of June 1862; by July 21 the surgeon reported it was approaching the typhoid form. He was much reduced in strength and was frequently delirious. On July 22 he was sent north on sick leave. While recovering, he was placed in charge of the recruiting service for the Excelsior Brigade in New York City, where he remained until October. His promotion as brigadier general of volunteers ranked from November 1862. He became ill again the same month with chronic diarrhea, supposedly from the exposure to camp life. He was compelled to return north to Washington. He rejoined his regiment in January and served at Chancellorsville. On July 2, 1863, at Gettysburg, Graham was severely wounded. A musket ball passed through both shoulders, and he received a contusion of the right hip from a piece of shell. Declining any assistance after he dismounted, he walked, apparently with little difficulty. He was captured on the battlefield and taken to Richmond. Imprisoned until September, he returned to his home in New York City on sick leave. He was suffering from cystitis and prostration caused by his wounds and from neglect and exposure. The physician prescribed tonics and generous amounts of food. During the winter of 1863–64 he had frequent attacks of rheumatism. He was brevetted major general in 1865 and returned to civil engineering. During the fall and winter of 1865 he was confined to his house by a violent attack of acute rheumatism. In the spring of 1867 he again had acute rheumatism, which was accompanied with pericarditis. His recovery was slow and he had repeated relapses during 1867 and 1868. The contractions of his muscles—the result of the rheumatism—produced permanent distention of his fingers and feet, causing partial luxation in many of his joints. In 1872 he had a particularly severe attack of rheumatism that affected several joints; it was complicated by endocarditis, pericarditis, pleurisy, and bronchial pneumonia. He was confined to his bed for four months. This attack left the fingers of Graham's right hand and the bones of his feet severely deformed. Also, his physician stated, this attack resulted in pleural and pericardial adhesions, causing pulmonary and cardiac dysfunction. Over the years his rheumatism continued unabated. The physician who saw him in 1876 reported that he was liable to serious attacks of rheumatism and other disorders arising from imperfect nerve force. From September 1879 to March 1880, as treatment for his rheumatism, he was administered forty galvanic baths for the purpose of increasing the circulation of his blood and checking the tendency toward paralysis.[1] Died April 15, 1889, at Lakewood, New Jersey, and was buried in Woodlawn Cemetery, New York.

DEATH CERTIFICATE: Cause of death, pneumonia. Length of sickness, twenty-two days.

1. CSR; *OR*, vol. 27, pt. 1:72, 499; vol. 29, pt. 2:470; RVA, Pension SC 168,879; U.S. Army, CWS, roll 1, vol. 2, report 34, pp. 491–503; RAGO, entry 534.

LAWRENCE PIKE GRAHAM · *Born on January 8, 1815,* in Amelia County, Virginia. Served in the Florida and Mexican wars. Graham was directly commissioned into the army in 1837 as a second lieutenant. Having been promoted to major in 1858, he was appointed a brigadier general of volunteers in August 1861. He became sick with typhoid fever on the Peninsula in the latter part of April 1862 and was placed in the hospital at Warwick Court House. Graham left on sick leave the first part of May and returned to Fair Oaks early in June. In September he was ordered to St. Louis to sit on the court-martial of Gen. Justus McKinstry. He was president of the court until October 18 when he had a violent hemorrhage and was dangerously ill for several months. He returned to Baltimore and sent monthly surgeon's certificates that he was not ready for the field but could do light duty. He assumed court-martial duty in February 1863. He was made colonel of the Fourth U.S. Cavalry in 1864 and was discharged from the volunteer service in August 1865. He remained in the army and served on the frontier until December 1870, when he retired. In late July 1905 he sustained a fracture of the left hip. Died September 12, 1905, in the Providence Hospital at Washington, D.C., and was buried in Arlington National Cemetery. According to hospital records he died from exhaustion and the result of the fracture.[1]

1. CSR; *OR*, vol. 11, pt. 1:390, 561; vol. 51, pt. 1:585; U.S. Army, CWS, roll 1, vol. 1, report 9, pp. 155–58; LR, CB, roll 474, G139, 1870.

GORDON GRANGER • *Born November 6, 1822,* in Joy, New York. Graduated from the USMA in 1845. Served in the Mexican War. Granger had duty in the mounted rifles on the frontier before the Civil War. In August 1861 he was appointed colonel of the 2nd Michigan Cavalry and served at Wilson's Creek, New Madrid, Island No. 10, and Corinth. He was commissioned brigadier general of volunteers in March 1862. On March 15 he was unable to leave his bed and asked that someone else be detailed for officer of the day. His promotion as major general ranked from September 1862. He commanded at the division and corps levels at Chickamauga, Chattanooga, Knoxville, and Mobile. In January 1864 he was too sick to visit Mayville, Tennessee, in person and had to send his inspector general instead. He remained in the army after the war and in 1866 was appointed colonel of the 25th Infantry. He had an episode of acute retinitis in January 1867. Granger had no lung problems until March 1872, when he was on a march with his troops in New Mexico. Following a heavy dust storm, he developed a severe cough with hemorrhage. By September he had chronic bronchitis with occasional hemoptysis. He was granted a thirty days' leave of absence on certificate of disability on December 6, 1872, but did not avail himself of the privilege. On May 2, 1873, an ophthalmoscopic examination of his left eye revealed retinitis and extensive hemorrhage into the retina from the choroidal vessels. Much of the blood had been absorbed, leaving a number of fixed opacities in the retina, and floating masses clouded the vitreous. There was almost total loss of vision in the left eye while vision of the right eye was normal. He also had consolidation of a portion of his left lung, associated with intermittent episodes of hemorrhage. The surgeon recommended he go to a better climate and a lower altitude. On May 19, 1873, he was granted a sick leave, which was extended by eleven months. Granger was unable to perform his duties in late 1874 and 1875. In June 1875 he had daily hemorrhage from his lungs and the last of the month had lost a gill (¼ pint) or more of blood. Granger had a stroke on November 19, 1875, which involved his left arm and left leg. He recovered sufficiently to attend to duty some weeks prior to his last illness. According to the chief medical officer, he had an attack of apoplexy January 10, 1876, at Santa Fe, New Mexico, and died the same day.[1] He was buried in Lexington, Kentucky.

1. CSR; *OR*, vol. 30, pt. 2:178; vol. 32, pt. 2:255, 423–34; pt. 3:171; LR, ACP, roll 43, 2153, 1874.

ROBERT SEAMAN GRANGER • *Born on May 24, 1816,* in Zanesville, Ohio. Graduated from the USMA in 1838. At West Point he was treated once each for diarrhea and headache. Served in the Florida and Mexican wars. During the Mexican War in 1848, he had chronic diarrhea and was quite sick. His health was failing when his company was ordered to the Rio Grande, and he was given leave to go north. He returned to Ohio, suffering with chronic intestinal disease, and recuperated under his mother's care. Granger had lost some thirty to thirty-five pounds and was compelled to eat the plainest of foods. He left in April 1849 to rejoin his troops, but when he arrived in New Orleans he was too ill to proceed and returned to Ohio. In August he was feeling better and planned to rejoin his regiment by September. In 1853 he developed symptoms that his surgeon later diagnosed as dyspepsia. The problem continued to bother him, and he obtained a leave from April through September 1855. In October he was placed on recruiting duty in Kentucky. From February until July 1858 he was on sick leave. Granger returned to duty in Texas where he was captured by the Confederates in April 1861 and was not exchanged until August 1862. In October he was commissioned brigadier general of volunteers. He was ill in March 1863 and again in November 1864. Brevetted major general in the regular service and promoted to lieutenant colonel of the Eleventh Infantry, he remained in the army after the war. He requested leave in August 1871 when his mother died because he was unwell and unfit for duty. During the summer of 1873 he requested to be put on the retired list or to be transferred out of the bad climate at Fort Vancouver, Washington Territory. He received medical leave from October to December 1873 because of chronic dyspepsia and retired from the army at his own request. According to his attending surgeon, prior to his death he had suffered with chronic nephritis for some time.[1] Died April 25, 1894, in Washington, D.C., and was buried in Zanesville, Ohio.

1. *OR*, vol. 23, pt. 2:117; vol. 39, pt. 3:651; WPCHR, vols. 603, 604; LR, ACP, 2556, 1873, fiche: 000108; Heitman, *Historical Register and Dictionary* 2:23.

LEWIS ADDISON GRANT • *Born on January 17, 1828*, in Winhall, Vermont. Grant left his law practice and in August 1861 was appointed major of the 5th Vermont. During January and February 1862 he was sick in quarters. He suffered from an attack of fever of the typhoid type at New Kent Court House, Virginia, during the middle of May 1862. In spite of his illness, he continued on duty until after the Division arrived at White House, Virginia, when he became prostrate with fever and was left there. About ten days later, in a weak and debilitated condition, he took command of the regiment. By July his surgeon stated that his diarrhea had become chronic. He was wounded at Fredericksburg in December 1862 but did not leave the field. Grant was at Chancellorsville, in the Shenandoah, and at Petersburg. His promotion to brigadier general of volunteers ranked from April 1864. On April 2, 1865, while on the Petersburg line, he was wounded in the head by a random minié ball and taken to the Turnbull house. The wound was apparently minor and he only relinquished command until nightfall.[1] Grant moved frequently after the war but finally settled in Minnesota. He died March 20, 1918, in Minneapolis and was buried there in Lakewood Cemetery.

DEATH CERTIFICATE: Cause of death, chronic interstitial nephritis, arteriosclerosis. Duration, several years; contributory, dilatation of heart, edema of lungs, duration seven days.

1. CSR; *OR*, vol. 46, pt. 1:571, 587, 954, 967–68, 971; RVA, Pension WC 855,737; *MOLLUS* 21:331, 26:403.

ULYSSES SIMPSON GRANT • *Born April 27, 1822*, in Point Pleasant, Ohio. Graduated from the USMA in 1843. Served in the Mexican War. As a young boy in Ohio he was sick with fever and ague for some time. While at West Point the riding master put him on a vicious horse and had him leaping the bar. The bar was moved up until it passed the "record," at which point the horse refused to jump. Grant urged the horse on; just as it was to jump, the girth broke, throwing him to the ground, stunned. The riding master gave him six demerits for dismounting without leave! In addition, while a cadet he was seen for a cold and sore throat each three times and sore feet once. For six months before his graduation he had a severe cough ("Tyler's grip") and was reduced in weight. In 1844 he kept a horse, rode outside most of the time, and recovered from his cough. Grant was part of the group of officers who suffered from snow blindness during a trip up Popocatepetl in Mexico in the spring of 1848. Grant resigned from the army in 1854 and had little success with a number of occupations. He had a fever, shivering, and a cough in the summer of 1858 and thought he had ague. In June 1861 he was appointed colonel of the 21st Illinois, and his commission as brigadier general of volunteers ranked from May. He commanded at Belmont and Forts Henry and Donelson. In March 1862 he had a cold with a headache and chest pain. On April 4, 1862, at Shiloh, his horse fell and pinned his leg under its body. His ankle was injured and the boot had to be cut off. He was unable to walk without crutches. On the night of April 7, his ankle was so swollen and painful that he was unable to rest. About midnight during a rainstorm he moved from beneath a tree to a log house on the bank of the Tennessee River. The house was being used as a hospital and all night the wounded were brought there. The sight was more than he could endure, and he returned to his place under the tree in the rain. For his meritorious service at Vicksburg he was appointed major general in the Regular Army in 1863. Grant was reviewing Nathaniel Banks's army a short distance above Carrollton, Louisiana, on September 4, 1863, when his horse shied at a locomotive and fell on him. He was carried to the St. Charles Hotel in New Orleans. He had swelling from his knee to the thigh, and it extended along the body up to his armpit. For over a week he lay in the hotel unable to turn himself because of the pain. On September 16 he returned to Vicksburg, able to give orders, but had to remain flat on his back in bed. Although still weak and in discomfort, he managed to get out of bed on September 25 and went about on crutches. In October Grant assumed command of the Department of the Tennessee, Cumberland, and Ohio. He still required crutches and had to be carried over places where it was not safe to cross on horseback. On the night of October 23, 1863, his horse slipped in coming down a mountain and further injured Grant's lame leg. He was made lieutenant general in March 1864 and given command of all the Union armies. He was effectively the commander of the Army of the Potomac in 1864–65. By April 30, 1864, his leg gave him little trouble except for occasional numbness. Afflicted with boils on May 9, he still rode out on inspections. On April 7, 1865, he had a severe headache. He was told to bathe his feet in hot water and mustard and to apply mustard plasters to his wrists and the back of his neck. However, the treatment produced little relief. Only after he received Robert E. Lee's letter concerning the surrender of Confederate forces did the headache stop. He was in Philadelphia, May 14–15, 1865, too ill to travel to Washington, D.C. On his arrival in Washington he was still sick.[1] After the war Grant was awarded the rank of full general in July 1866. In 1868 he was elected president of the United States, a position he held for two terms. Christmas Eve 1883 he slipped and struck his previously injured left leg against the curbstone. Although considered only a bruise and a shock to the sciatic nerve, he was laid up for weeks and afterward was lame. The leg pain recurred in a few months and he required crutches until June. During the summer of 1884, after Grant had eaten a peach, he suddenly got up and paced the floor saying that eating the fruit hurt his throat. In October he went to the doctor who found his soft palate inflamed, dark, and scaly, suggestive of an epithelial problem. The base of the right side of the tongue was somewhat rigid. For two months the doctor treated him by lessening congestion and the odors from the ulcerated area. Almost from the first, local applications of a cocaine solution were used to reduce pain. In addition, Grant gave up cigars and had a tooth extracted. By February 1885 the ulcer was more active and a biopsy was obtained. A histologic diagnosis of epithelioma or epithelial cancer was made. The possibility of surgery was considered but was rejected. There was further progression of the lesion and more tissue infiltration by March. He had occasional severe coughing spells due to the accumulation of material in his throat. One coughing episode produced hemorrhage. Morphine injections were used to allow him to sleep and brandy injections were used for a stimulant. In May his voice failed him, and it was suggested he move to the better climate of the mountains. His neck was swollen in June, and the ulceration on the back of the throat and tongue was more active. Nutrition was furnished by milk, eggs, and beef tea. No longer able to sleep lying down because it brought on coughing spells, he slept in a chair. Grant's condition deteriorated throughout July, and by the twenty-second his respiration was rapid, his pulse fast and small, and his limbs cold. Hot applications were applied to his feet and mustard to his stomach. Brandy was occasionally administered hypodermically. He died quietly on July 23, 1885, at Mount McGregor, New York.[2] He was buried in a mausoleum on Riverside Drive in New York City.

1. *OR*, vol. 24, pt. 3:372; vol. 30, pt. 1:39; pt. 3:661, 694, 732, 735, 840; vol. 46, pt. 3:1149, 1152, 1162; WPCHR, vol. 604; *Battles and Leaders* 1:467, 477; 3:684;4:731–32; Horace Porter, *Campaigning with Grant*, 3, 25, 88, 462–63, 468; William S. McFeely, *Grant: A Biography*, 106; Ulysses S. Grant, *Personal Memoirs of U. S. Grant*, 1:42–43, 57, 103, 181–84, 211, 334–35, 581–83; Cox, *Military Reminiscences*, 2:103; *MOLLUS* 10:346.

2. Thomas M. Pitkin, *The Captain Departs: Ulysses S. Grant's Last Campaign*, 23–26, 33–35, 44, 59, 61–62, 67, 69–70, 76, 79, 86, 133–39.

GEORGE SEARS GREENE • *Born on May 6, 1801,* in Apponaug, Rhode Island. Graduated from the USMA in 1823. He resigned his army commission in 1836 and entered civil engineering. Greene reentered the army in January 1862 as colonel of the 60th New York Infantry and was promoted to brigadier general of volunteers in April. In October he was granted a twenty-day sick leave. He was severely wounded on October 29, 1863, at the Battle of Wauhatchie, Tennessee. A ball had entered the left side of his upper jaw just under his nose and made its exit on the right side of his face. It carried away all the teeth of the upper jaw, crushed the bone, and cut the right salivary duct. Because of loss of blood and being unable to speak, Greene was forced to retire to the temporary field hospital. He was then moved to a hospital in Nashville. He was absent until December when he was detailed for general court-martial duty. In May 1864 he was relieved from this duty and was to report to New York for orders. He did not return to field duty until 1865, when he led a division in the Carolinas. Following his discharge from the service he returned to civil engineering. Over the years he was debilitated by malnutrition. His jaw wound had produced a salivary fistula, and an extensive surgical procedure by a prominent New York surgeon was required to close it. He continued to have great difficulty with it and required frequent medical attention. He was not able to masticate food well, and from time to time material impacted, causing inflammation of the antrum that produced a discharge and pain. Died January 28, 1899, in Morristown, New Jersey, and was buried in the Greene Family Cemetery, Warwick, Rhode Island.[1] DEATH CERTIFICATE: Cause of death, cardiac failure from age and athroma.

1. CSR; *OR*, vol. 19, pt. 2:436; vol. 31, pt. 1:95, 116, 120, 127, 129–30; vol. 37, pt. 1:435; RVA, Pension SC 161, 677; RAGO, entry 534; "Grave Matters" 5, no. 1 (1995): 6.

DAVID MCMURTRIE GREGG • *Born on April 10, 1833,* in Huntingdon, Pennsylvania. Graduated from the USMA in 1855. While at West Point, he was treated for eruptio five times, odontalgia three times, phlegmon twice, and once each for excoriatio and catarrhus. Prior to the Civil War he served on the frontier and was on garrison duty. In New York City, early in 1861, he became ill from eating too many oysters. On August 3, following his recovery, Gregg joined the cavalry as a captain. On October 12 he had a severe case of typhoid and was hospitalized in Washington. One night a trooper had to carry him out of the building when it caught on fire. In January 1862 he was made colonel of the 8th Pennsylvania Cavalry, and on July 24 he was able to rejoin his regiment. He served on the Peninsula, at Antietam, Chancellorsville, Gettysburg, and in the Overland campaign. In the middle of September 1862 he was in Philadelphia under medical treatment for diarrhea and remittent fever. The following month another surgeon stated he had intermittent fever. His appointment as brigadier general of volunteers ranked from November 1862. In February 1865 he resigned from both the regular and volunteer service. Gregg was a farmer in Delaware, United States consul at Prague for a brief period, and finally settled in Reading, Pennsylvania. He was ill the last four months of his life.[1] Died August 7, 1916, in Reading and was buried in the Charles Evans Cemetery.

1. CSR; WPCHR, vols. 608, 609; Milton V. Burgess, *David Gregg: Pennsylvania Cavalry Man*, 32–33, 113.

WALTER QUINTIN GRESHAM • *Born March 17, 1832*, at Lanesville, Indiana. A lawyer and politician before the Civil War, he raised a company of troops, and in March 1862 he was made colonel of the 53rd Indiana. His major service was at Vicksburg and in the Atlanta campaign. In October he had neuralgia of the stomach and obtained a leave. He was present sick in February 1863. Although still sick in March, he was on duty in Memphis, Tennessee, as president of a court-martial. A surgeon's certificate dated April 8 stated that Gresham was suffering from chronic inflammation of the stomach and the duodenum. He returned to his home in Corydon, Indiana, where his surgeon reported that the inflammation of his intestinal tract was the result of a prior episode of typhoid fever and neuralgia of the stomach. In August 1863 he was appointed brigadier general of volunteers. Outside of Atlanta on July 20, 1864, his left tibia was badly shattered three and one-half inches below the knee by a sharpshooter. He was carried from the field on a stretcher, and an operation performed that night included the removal of bone fragments. Gresham was taken to New Albany, Indiana, where he remained under the care of a physician. He was still confined to his room in May 1865 because the wound continued to discharge and healing was not complete enough for the limb to bear weight. In April 1866 he was mustered out of the service. The wound was still open the next month, and he was not able to walk without a cane and a crutch. He took up the practice of law at New Albany, Indiana, as soon as he could maneuver on crutches. In September 1873 the cicatrix covering the wound was still imperfect and tender. The limb was edematous and very weak because of the great loss of bone and the poor union. He still required a cane. Two years later the leg was unchanged, still painful and edematous. By September 1877 there was more atrophy of the leg, and the knee and ankle joints were stiff.[1] He died May 28, 1895, in the Arlington

Hotel at Washington, D.C., and was buried in Arlington National Cemetery. DEATH CERTIFICATE: Cause of death, primary, acute pleurisy with effusion; immediate, supervening acute pneumonia of the right lung, four weeks' duration.

1. CSR; *OR*, vol. 38, pt. 3:39, 543, 580, 590, pt. 5:208; RVA, Pension WC 426,353; U.S. Army, CWS, roll 6, vol. 10, report 29, pp. 155–83; LR, ACP, I-125, 1863; *MOLLUS* 10:296.

BENJAMIN HENRY GRIERSON • *Born on July 8, 1826,* in Pittsburgh, Pennsylvania. He was eight years old when his horse bolted and threw him to the ground. While he was getting up, he was kicked in the face and received a deep gash. For two weeks he was unconscious, and his eyes were bandaged for eight weeks. He could see from one eye, but it took months before he could use the other. The long scar on the right side of his face was later covered by his beard. A music teacher and merchant, he joined the Federal service as an aide-de-camp to Benjamin M. Prentiss. Grierson was commissioned major of the 6th Illinois Cavalry in October 1861 and colonel the following April. On September 6, 1862, during a Confederate attack on their camp near Olive Branch, Mississippi, his clothes were pierced by bullets and two fingers of his left hand were bruised. He was appointed brigadier general of volunteers to rank from June. In April 1863 he led his famous cavalry raid through Mississippi. At Vicksburg on July 20, 1863, he received a serious injury to his right knee when he was kicked by a horse. His high cavalry boots prevented a more serious injury. Although unable to ride on horseback for the rest of the year, he remained on duty using crutches. Even riding in a carriage caused pain. He was given a leave from September 21 to October 31, 1863, on a surgeon's certificate. During May 1864 he was under treatment for piles. His commission as major general of volunteers ranked from May 1866, and he resigned from the volunteer service the next month. He was appointed colonel of the Tenth Cavalry and served mainly on the frontier. During the fall of 1866 he underwent an examination by a board of officers, and it was reported that he had a stomach disorder, a problem he had when under stress. On July 5, 1867, he was admitted to the post hospital at Fort Leavenworth, Kansas, but the diagnosis was not noted. He had recurrent episodes of digestive complaints, and for ten years after the injury to his knee he required the use of crutches and a cane. Promoted to brigadier general in April 1890, he retired a few months later. In the summer of 1907 he developed the flu and had a stroke from which he never recovered. His memory was impaired, and for the next four years his condition deteriorated so that he was confined to his bed. In the summer of 1911 his speech was incoherent.[1] He died August 31, 1911, in Omena, Michigan, and was buried in Jacksonville Cemetery at Jacksonville, Illinois. DEATH CERTIFICATE: Cause of death, senile debility and paralysis. Duration, four years; contributory, age.

1. *OR*, vol. 17:55–57; vol. 30, pt. 3:439; U.S. Army, CWS, roll 6, vol. 10, report 53, pp. 511–46; ibid., roll 3, vol. 4, report 15, pp. 481–93; RAGO, entry 534; Bruce Jacob Dinges, "The Making of a Cavalryman: Benjamin M. Grierson and the Civil War along the Mississippi, 1861–1865" (diss.), 13–14, 191–92, 461–62, 483; William H. Leckie and Shirley A. Leckie, *Unlikely Warriors: General Benjamin Grierson and His Family*, 71, 144, 249, 306.

CHARLES GRIFFIN • *Born December 18, 1825,* in Granville, Ohio. Graduated from the USMA in 1847. At West Point he was seen for catarrhus twice and once each for odontalgia, cephalalgia, otitis, and excoriatio. He had gotten as far as Louisville, Kentucky, on his way to Mexico, when his surgeon advised him in September 1847 to return to Cincinnati because of quotidian fever. While in New Orleans in February 1848 he had intermittent fever and inflammation of the bowels and was given three months' sick leave to go home. He returned to duty at Tampa Bay, Florida, in June 1848. In 1860, after service on the frontier, he was appointed to instruct artillery tactics at the military academy. He organized a field battery at the beginning of the Civil War and, because of his conduct at First Bull Run and on the Peninsula, was promoted to brigadier general of volunteers to rank from June 1862. He was at Second Bull Run, Fredericksburg, Chancellorsville, and in the major campaigns against Lee's army in 1864–65. He had a sick leave during June and July 1863 and returned to duty in August. Griffin was commissioned major general of volunteers in April 1865 and remained in the Regular Army as a colonel. According to the surgeon general's office, he became ill with yellow fever on September 9, 1867, while in Galveston, Texas, and died there on September 15.[1] He was buried in Oak Hill Cemetery, Georgetown, D.C.

1. CSR; WPCHR, vol. 605; RVA, Pension WC 110,213; LR, CB, roll 43, G216, 1863.

SIMON GOODELL GRIFFIN • *Born August 9, 1824,* in Nelson, New Hampshire. Before the Civil War Griffin was a teacher, farmer, politician, and lawyer. In 1861 he was elected a company captain in the 2nd New Hampshire and fought at First Bull Run. After passing through grades, he was promoted to brigadier general of volunteers, ranking from May 1864. He served in the Carolina Expedition, at Second Bull Run, Antietam, Fredericksburg, Vicksburg, and Petersburg. While in the service he had evidence of malarial poisoning. Discharged from the army in August 1865, he engaged in politics, manufacturing, and land speculation. In January 1892 he was totally disabled by the consequent infirmities of age.[1] Died January 14, 1902, at Keene, New Hampshire, and was buried there at the Woodland Cemetery.

DEATH CERTIFICATE: Cause of death, polyuria (diabetes insipidus of six months' duration); contributing cause, age and exhaustion.

1. RVA, Pension SC 934,079.

WILLIAM GROSE • *Born on December 16, 1812,* near Dayton, Ohio. Grose left his position as a common pleas judge and was appointed colonel of the 36th Indiana Volunteers in October 1861. In the middle of January 1862 he had the onset of bilious remittent fever. He was wounded in the left shoulder blade by a small ball during the Battle of Shiloh on April 7, 1862. In the advance on Corinth, Mississippi, on May 30, when the nearby artillery was fired, he received a shock to his head, particularly the left side and left ear. On December 31, 1862, during the Battle of Stone's River, he again felt a pressure in his left ear from the heavy firing. He began several months of medical treatment in August but remained on duty and was at Vicksburg. At the Battle of Chickamauga on September 20, 1863, he was wounded at the junction of his neck and left shoulder by a piece of shell. He was left sick at Chattanooga, Tennessee, on October 25. In December his surgeon diagnosed his condition, which had been intermittently symptomatic since the previous August, as iritatio spinalis and nephritis. Grose obtained a sick leave; after his return to duty, he requested another leave in April 1864 since his health was still not good. Grose served in the Atlanta campaign and at Franklin and Nashville. His promotion as brigadier general of volunteers ranked from July 1864. Brevetted major general to rank from August 1865, he resigned his commission in January 1866. Following the war he practiced the law and held state and Federal positions. In July 1890 he was suffering from rheumatism, particularly in his previously wounded left shoulder and arm. He could not raise the arm above the level of his shoulder without producing pain. A recent fall from a ladder upon a stone pavement had also injured his right knee. His hearing was poor, particularly in his left ear, and there was a constant bilateral roaring sound. He had to give up the legal profession because of his inability to hear.[1] Died July 30, 1900, in New Castle, Indiana, and was buried in South Mound Cemetery.

DEATH CERTIFICATE: Cause of death, senility.

1. CSR; RVA, Pension WC 525,208.

CUVIER GROVER • *Born July 29, 1828,* in Bethel, Maine. Graduated from the USMA in 1850. As a cadet he was treated for contusio four times, catarrhus three times, cephalalgia, vulnus laceration, odontalgia, and colica each twice, and cynanche parotides, vulnus incisum, rheumatism, phlegmon, and morbi. varrii. each once. After taking part in the Mormon expedition and serving on the frontier, he was appointed brigadier general of volunteers, ranking from April 1862. He was on the Peninsula, at Second Bull Run, and at Port Hudson. He received three injuries at Cedar Creek on October 19, 1864. He was wounded early in the day in the heel and the body but did not leave the field until after he received a contusion of the left forearm. Only simple dressings were used. On October 22 he was moved from the field hospital to a hospital in Winchester; two days later he was moved to a general hospital. Grover returned to his command in December. At the end of the war he was brevetted major general, U.S. Army, and in 1866 was appointed lieutenant colonel of the 38th U.S. Infantry. He was sick with progressive anemia in September 1884 and was on sick leave from March 1885 until his death. His surgeon reported that since Grover had not responded to therapy and had a doubtful prognosis, he should see a specialist. In May a diagnosis of pulmonary abscess was made. The next month he went to Atlantic City, New Jersey, in an effort to improve his health and died there June 6, 1885. He was buried at West Point. According to his attending physician, he died from hemorrhage from the pulmonary abscess.[1]

1. *OR*, vol. 43, pt. 1:32, 55, 133, 321, 324; WPCHR, vols. 605, 606, 607; U.S. Army, CWS, roll 3, vol. 4, report 22, pp. 709–11; RVA, Pension WC 219,207; RAGO, entry 534.

H

PLEASANT ADAM HACKLEMAN • *Born on November 15, 1814,* in Franklin County, Indiana. A practicing lawyer, he held various county and state positions in Indiana, and at the start of the Civil War he was appointed colonel of the 16th Indiana Infantry. In April 1862 he was promoted to brigadier general of volunteers. He was mortally wounded on October 3, 1862, at the Battle of Corinth. The ball hit him in the neck, severed the esophagus so he could not swallow, injured the trachea, and passed out on the opposite side near the spine. He died that night in a room at the Tishomingo Hotel in Corinth.[1] He was buried in Rushville, Indiana.

1. *OR*, vol. 17, pt. 1:155, 161, 175, 256–57, 273, 283; U.S. Army, CWS, roll 5, vol. 9, report 31, pp. 861–944; *MOLLUS* 12:189.

HENRY WAGER HALLECK • *Born January 16, 1815,* in Westernville, New York. Graduated from the USMA in 1839. He was seen for a cold four times and rheumatism once at West Point. During the Mexican War he was in California serving as an engineer. Afterward he studied the law, resigning his commission in 1854. He established a law practice in California and published books on the subject. Halleck was appointed major general in the regular service to rank from August 1861. In November 1861 he was appointed commander in the Department of the Missouri. In the middle of January 1862 he was sick in St. Louis with camp measles. At Corinth in June 1862, he was confined to his tent for several days with the "Evacuation of Corinth." His health was somewhat broken in early July, and by the end of August, utterly tired out, he was in Washington, D.C. He was appointed general-in-chief and served in this capacity until

March 1864, when he was made chief-of-staff after U. S. Grant was promoted to general-in-chief. In September 1864 he had his annual attack of "coryza" or "hay-cold," which affected his eyes to the point that he could scarcely see to write. Halleck remained in the army after the war and was appointed to command the Division of the South in 1869. He died January 9, 1872, at Louisville and was buried in Green-Wood Cemetery, Brooklyn, New York. According to the army surgeon general, Halleck died from softening of the brain superimposed on chronic organic disease of the heart and liver.[1]

1. *OR*, vol. 8:499, 511; vol. 11, pt. 1:103; vol. 17, pt. 2:9, 64; WPCHR, vol 604; William T. Sherman, *Memoirs of General William T. Sherman* 2:116; LR, ACP, 128, 1872, fiche: 000111.

JOSEPH ELDRIDGE HAMBLIN • *Born January 13, 1828,* in Yarmouth, Massachusetts. Previously employed in Boston, New York, and St. Louis, he entered Federal service in May 1861 as a first lieutenant and adjutant of the 5th New York Volunteers. He was made a colonel of the 65th New York in May 1863. Hamblin served on the Peninsula, at Antietam, Fredericksburg, Chancellorsville, and Gettysburg, in the Wilderness campaign, at Petersburg, in the Shenandoah, and at Appomattox. He was wounded twice at Cedar Creek on October 19, 1864, and had to be ordered to the rear. The severest wound was in his right leg and was complicated by an abscess in December. Hamblin reported back for duty on January 31, 1865, and was in command on February 13. His commission as brigadier general of volunteers ranked from May 1865.[1] Hamblin returned to the insurance business following the war. In 1867 he was made adjutant general and chief of staff of the New York National Guard. He died July 3, 1870, in New York City and was buried in Yarmouth, Massachusetts.

DEATH CERTIFICATE: Chief cause, peritonitis from colon. Secondary, perforation of bowel. Time from attack till death, five and a half days, after severe marching and exposure on a trip with a company of the Seventh Regiment.

1. *OR*, vol. 42, pt. 3:1029; vol. 43, pt. 1:131, 175, pt. 2:460; vol. 46, pt. 2:317, 551; LR, CB, roll 264, H11, 1866.

ANDREW JACKSON HAMILTON • *Born on January 28, 1815,* in Huntsville, Alabama. Hamilton, a lawyer, was a member of Congress from Texas when the Civil War started. An active opponent of secession, he had to flee Texas and went to Mexico in 1862. After his arrival in Washington he was appointed brigadier general of volunteers to rank from November 1862 and military governor of Texas. When his first commission as brigadier was not acted on by the Senate, he was reappointed in September 1863. His appointment as governor of Texas was ratified in June 1865. Following the war he reentered politics. He died April 11, 1875, in Austin, Texas, and was buried there in Oakwood Cemetery.

CHARLES SMITH HAMILTON • *Born November 16, 1822*, in Westernville, New York. Graduated from the USMA in 1843. During his time at the academy, he was seen for excoriatio twice and once each for ulcers, odontalgia, wound incision, and cephalalgia. Hamilton was badly wounded at Molino del Rey on September 8, 1847. He continued on the field, encouraging his men until they were beyond the reach of his voice. After recuperating in Mexico City, he returned in November and remained with his regiment until the end of the war. He resigned in April 1853 and took up farming and the manufacture of flour. In May 1861 he was commissioned colonel of the 3rd Wisconsin Infantry and brigadier general of volunteers six days later. He was ordered to Alexandria to take command of a division in March 1862. He lost the way to Harpers Ferry and became very wet; when he finally arrived, he boarded a cold train in his soaked condition and went to Alexandria. It was not until after he had boarded his troops on the transport that he was able to procure dry clothes. By the time they landed at Hampton Road he had lost his voice, and the medical director recommended that he relinquish his command. He went to the doctor's home and remained there for a couple of weeks with what he was told was diphtheria. After returning to his troops, he suffered during the following action with lumbago and stiff joints. A diagnosis of rheumatic disease of the heart was made in the summer. During the campaign of Corinth and Iuka in September and October, he had occasional palpitations of his heart during periods of excitement. On November 9, 1862, he reported that it was uncertain if he could ride. Arguments with his superiors prompted his resignation, which was accepted in April 1863. He returned to Wisconsin where he became a businessman. The occasional palpitations became a chronic irregularity of his heart action in 1877. Defects appeared in the sight of one of his eyes in the middle of 1884, and his ophthalmologist told him he had a hemorrhage from a retinal blood vessel. Starting in 1885 he had episodes of rheumatism, more in his legs than anywhere else. Early in 1886 he had a congestion of his brain that rendered him helpless and totally blind for a time. A severe episode of rheumatism in August 1887 confined him to his room. A physical examination in December revealed some impairment of the motion of his knees and shoulder joints, but aside from an occasional missed heartbeat, there were no abnormal heart sounds. In addition to the evidence of bleeding into the retinas there were bilateral cataracts. Vision in the left eye was limited to the perception of light and large objects, while vision in the right eye was reduced by half.[1] Died April 17, 1891, at Milwaukee, Wisconsin, and was buried there in Forest Home Cemetery.

DEATH CERTIFICATE: Cause of death, pneumonia and paralysis, duration ten days.

1. *OR*, vol. 17, pt. 2:330; WPCHR, vol. 605; LR, CB, roll 95, H556, 1864; RVA, Pension C 425,002; Heitman, *Historical Register and Dictionary* 2:24.

SCHUYLER HAMILTON • *Born July 25, 1822,* in New York City. Graduated from the USMA in 1841. At West Point he was treated for bile and rheumatism each three times, nausea, bruise, and headache each twice, and diarrhea, pain in side, cold, corn, sprain, sore throat, and poisoning each one time. He was severely wounded on two occasions in Mexico. His skull was fractured and he was hit by a ball in the abdomen at Monterey on September 21, 1846. Three weeks later he suffered sunstroke. At Mil Flores, Mexico, on August 13, 1847, he was wounded by a lance. The lance entered between the shoulder blades, passed through the lower lobe of the left lung, and came out under his left breast. The lance blade was bent at nearly a right angle with his body as the lancer dashed on with the shaft still in his hand. It was pried out by breaking two ribs. He had a sick leave from January 25 to March 7, 1847. Hamilton resigned from the army in 1855 and took up farming in Connecticut. In 1861 he reentered Federal service as a private in the 7th New York National Guard. After serving as a military secretary with the staff rank of colonel he was commissioned brigadier general of volunteers to rank from November 1861. He served at New Madrid, Island No. 10, and Corinth. On May 9, 1862, he became acutely sick. Ill through the military operations, he remained on duty but had to depend on his staff officers. He was granted a sick leave on June 12. In July his surgeon reported that Hamilton had been suffering from typhoid fever that resulted in chronic diarrhea and other grave disorders. In early November 1862 he reported for duty. He was ordered on December 14 to go to New York because of his failing health. His trip was delayed at Nashville and Louisville because of violent diarrhea, prostration, and severe cramps. The surgeon in New York who treated him in January and February 1863 stated that Hamilton had chronic dysentery, chronic enteritis, and impeded circulation of the liver with partial suspension of bile secretion. Hamilton resigned on February 27, 1863, because of ill health and disability. On July 13, 1864, the examining surgeon reported that Hamilton was totally disabled by chronic disease of the liver, which caused chronic duodenitis, chronic enteritis, and dysentery. These conditions were due to the effects of exposure to field service, malaria, and bad water.[1] Died March 18, 1903, in an apartment house in New York City and was buried in Green-Wood Cemetery, Brooklyn.

DEATH CERTIFICATE: Direct cause, syncope. Indirect, senescence, colitis and asthenia.

1. *OR,* vol. 10, pt. 1:724–25; vol. 20, pt. 2:177, 179; U.S. Army, CWS, roll 2, vol. 3, report 12, pp. 251–53; LR, ACP, 4635, 1871; RVA, Pension SC 36,161; RAGO, entry 534; WPCHR, vol. 604; Heitman, *Historical Register and Dictionary* 2:24.

CYRUS HAMLIN • *Born on April 26, 1839,* at Hampden, Maine. His father, Hannibal Hamlin, was senator from Maine and Lincoln's first vice president. He was practicing law in Maine when the Civil War started, and he entered Federal service in April 1862 as an aide-de-camp with the rank of captain. He was appointed colonel of the 80th U.S. Colored Infantry in February 1863 and was commissioned brigadier general of volunteers in December 1864. Following the war he remained in New Orleans and practiced the law. He died in New Orleans on August 28, 1867, probably from yellow fever, although his death certificate does not give a cause and his father reported that he died from malaria.[1] His remains were initially buried in Girod Cemetery, New Orleans, but within a few months he was moved to Mount Hope Cemetery, Bangor, Maine.

1. U.S. Army, CWS, roll 6, vol. 10, report 17, p. 85; Death certificate; *MOLLUS* 17:294; *New Orleans Daily Picayune*, Aug. 30, 1867.

WILLIAM ALEXANDER HAMMOND · *Born on August 28, 1828,* in Annapolis, Maryland. He graduated from medical school in 1848 and was appointed assistant surgeon in the Army Medical Corps the next year. Before the Civil War he had three rather extended sick leaves, but the exact diagnosis in each case was not reported. While on duty in New Mexico he went on sick leave from June 1852 to March 1853. He returned to duty in Florida but had to take a sick leave from July 1853 to February 1854. Hammond was at Fort Riley, Kansas, until October 1857, when he went on sick leave. He returned on October 3, 1859. In 1860 he resigned his commission and accepted a professorship at the University of Maryland. The following year he returned to the army.[1] In April 1862 he was appointed surgeon general with the rank of brigadier general. He quarreled with Secretary of War Edwin Stanton; when an acting successor was named, he requested a court-martial. Convicted of ungentlemanly conduct, he was dismissed from the service and returned to private practice. Died January 5, 1900, in Washington, D.C., and was buried in Arlington National Cemetery.

DEATH CERTIFICATE: Cause of death, fatty degeneration and dilation of the heart. Heart exhaustion after exertion. Duration of last sickness, thirty minutes.

1. LR, ACP, 2892, 1879, fiche: 000018.

WINFIELD SCOTT HANCOCK · *Born February 14, 1824,* in Montgomery Square, Pennsylvania. Graduated from the USMA in 1844. As a cadet, he was seen for sore feet three times. Served in the Mexican and Florida wars. He received a contusion below the knee from a musket ball at Churubusco on August 20, 1847, but did not leave the field. He was ill when the army reached Chapultepec on September 13, 1847, and was lying in his tent with chills and fever. After the battle started he wrapped himself in a blanket and went on the roof to watch the fighting. He recovered sufficiently to rejoin the army in the last days of the assault on Mexico City. Hancock left his position as chief quartermaster at Los Angeles and was appointed a brigadier general of volunteers to rank from September 1861. He was made a major general to rank from November 1862. On December 13, while at Fredericksburg, a ball went through his overcoat and grazed his abdomen. Although unhurt, he was struck with several small fragments of shell at Chancellorsville on May 3, 1863. Sitting on his horse at Gettysburg on July 3, he was hit in the front of the right thigh. Hancock initially reported that he had been shot with a tenpenny nail. In fact, he had been hit by a minié ball that had first passed through the pommel of his saddle and carried foreign material into his thigh muscles. A tourniquet was made from a handkerchief and was twisted with a pistol barrel to arrest the bleeding. On the field the surgeon probed the wound with his finger and removed the nail and pieces of wood. Hancock was transported by ambulance to Westminster, Maryland, and then to Baltimore by train on July 4. Next, he was taken to Philadelphia where he remained for a month before going to his father's house to recover. In spite of repeated attempts to remove the ball, it remained in place, and there was continued drainage. The ball had entered from the front and was lodged behind the bone. By having Hancock assume the same sitting position he was in when struck, a physician was finally able to follow the bullet track and extract the minié ball. The wound remained open in October but he was able to walk using a cane. He returned to the army in the latter part of December 1863 and resumed command of the Second Corps. After being in the field a few weeks, he was sent north on recruiting duty because of his unhealed wound. Although his wound was still open in March 1864, he was back at army headquarters and resumed command the next month. In May he requested to ride in a spring wagon when necessary since he had difficulty riding in the saddle. The first of June his activity had reopened the wound, so he poured water from his canteen over it. Bone fragments extruded from his wound. He relinquished command on June 17, 1864, and after he had partially recovered, he again resumed command on June 27. In August he was made brigadier general in the Regular Army. Because of continued suffering from his wound he received leave in November and went on recruiting duty. Until then he had distinguished himself as a corps commander in Grant's campaign against Petersburg. In February 1865 he returned to his command. He remained in the army with the rank of major general. In October 1868 his wound threatened to reopen. Hancock was Democratic nominee for president in 1880. In 1884 his leg was injured and an abscess formed, which healed poorly. The last of 1885 he was in poor health and remained at headquarters almost all the time, rarely going out. Although not feeling well on January 24, 1886, he left for Washington. Four days later a surgeon in Washington lanced a boil on the back of his neck. On his return to Governors Island it was noted by the department surgeon that he had developed a carbuncle. He was nourished with beef tea and milk. In addition, he was given hypodermic injections of brandy, whiskey, ether, and carbonate of ammonia, separately and combined. The carbuncle continued to grow, and on February 7 he was delirious. An outside consultant suggested he may have kidney disease, so an examination of his urine was performed. To the surprise of his attending physicians, it was found that he had diabetes mellitus.[1] He died on February 9, 1886, at Governors Island and was buried in Montgomery Cemetery in Norristown, Pennsylvania.

DEATH CERTIFICATE: Primary cause, malignant carbuncle. Secondary, diabetes.

1. *OR*, vol. 27, pt. 1:75, 117, 133, 353, 366, 375; vol. 29, pt. 1:246; vol. 33:640, 718; vol. 36, pt. 2:320, 485; vol. 40, pt. 1:178–79, 219, 307, pt. 2:162, 170, 467; vol. 42, pt. 3:705; WPCHR, vol. 604; U.S. Army, CWS, roll 1, vol. 2, report 19, pp. 221–29; ibid., roll 3, vol. 5, report 4, pp. 611–70; Tucker, *Hancock the Superb*, 41–42, 107, 123, 156–57, 165–67, 275, 309; David M. Jordan, *Winfield Scott Hancock: A Soldier's Life*, 146–48, 228, 313–15; *MOLLUS* 20:358; *New York Times*, Feb. 10, 1886.

JAMES ALLEN HARDIE • *Born on May 5, 1823*, in New York City. Graduated from the USMA in 1843. He spent the period of the Mexican War in San Francisco. Hardie was adjutant general of the Department of Oregon when the Civil War started. He was made lieutenant colonel and aide-de-camp to Gen. George B. McClellan. His appointment as brigadier general of volunteers ranked from November 1862 but his name was not submitted to the Senate for confirmation. Hardie suffered from some derangement of his digestive organs, which gave him torpidity of the liver. This condition continued into the winter of 1864–65. During this period he started complaining of a disorder of his brain, which produced sudden aberrations of his mind during the day and sleeplessness during the night. In March 1865 he received the brevets of brigadier and major general, U.S. Army. After the war he remained in the army and served as an inspector general. In July 1876 he was sent on an inspection tour in the Southern states and was affected by malaria. Following this, his health continued to gradually and perceptibly decline until his death. He died December 14, 1876, in Washington, D.C., and was buried in Mount Olivet Cemetery. According to the attending army surgeon, he died from jaundice resulting from organic disease of the liver.[1]

1. RVA, Pension WC 177,365; LR, ACP, 22, 1877, fiche: 000063.

MARTIN DAVIS HARDIN • *Born June 26, 1837*, in Jacksonville, Illinois. Graduated from the USMA in 1859. At West Point he was treated for phlegmon eight times, catarrhus six times, contusio four times, subluxatio three times, ophthalmia and diarrhea each two times, and morbi. varii. and colica each once. After service in Oregon, he entered the war as an aide to Henry J. Hunt. On August 30, 1862, at Second Bull Run, Hardin was wounded by a gunshot in the side. The ball struck on the left side of the thorax two or three inches below the clavicle, perforated the pectoral muscle, and exited out through the scapula. The ball did not go through the chest but swept around through the axilla and came out through the scapula; the lung was not involved. In September the arm and shoulder were markedly swollen. In January 1863 he went to Washington with the cold, livid, paralyzed arm hanging at his side and the wound discharging. His condition was further complicated by fever and catarrh the next month. Although still suffering from his wound he fought at Gettysburg in July. He was on sick leave from August 14 until December. He, along with some of his troops, was ambushed by guerrillas near Catlett's Station, Virginia, on December 14, 1863. Hardin was shot through the left arm; the humerus was shattered, requiring an amputation of the arm. In March 1864 he was ordered to assume command of the depot for drafted men at Pittsburgh, Pennsylvania. At the crossing of the North Anna River on May 23, 1864, he was knocked from his horse by the fire from an enemy battery and injured. He was made brigadier general of volunteers to rank from July 1864 and was assigned to command. In 1866 he was commissioned major of the Forty-Third Infantry. He retired from the army in 1870 because of his disabilities and his amputated arm.[1] He died December 12, 1923, in Saint Augustine, Florida, and was buried there in the National Cemetery.

DEATH CERTIFICATE: Cause of death, carcinoma of ileum.

1. CSR; *OR*, vol. 12, pt. 2:395; vol. 27, pt. 1:658–59; vol. 29, pt. 1:978; WPCHR, vol. 609; LR, CB, roll 501, R258, 1870.

ABNER CLARK HARDING • *Born February 10, 1807,* in East Hampton, Connecticut. Around 1851, failing eyesight compelled him to leave his law practice and enter business. He enlisted as a private when the Civil War started and shortly afterward was commissioned colonel of the 83rd Illinois. He was promoted to brigadier general to rank from March 1863, but the following June he was forced to resign because of his deteriorating eyesight. He died at Monmouth, Illinois, on July 19, 1874, and was buried there.

CHARLES GARRISON HARKER • *Born on December 2, 1835,* at Swedesboro, New Jersey. Graduated from the USMA in 1858. As a cadet he was treated for diarrhea four times, colica, catarrhus, and cephalalgia each three times, phlegmon and contusio each twice, and vulnus incisum, ophthalmia, nausea, odontalgia, and tonsillitis each once. He served on the frontier prior to the Civil War and was commissioned colonel of the 65th Ohio Infantry in November 1861. He served at Perryville, Stones River, and Chickamauga. In April 1864 he was promoted to brigadier general. On May 14, 1864, he was slightly wounded by a shell fragment in front of Resaca, Georgia, but he refused to leave the field. He was shot from his horse by a sharpshooter at Kennesaw Mountain on June 27, 1864. The ball fractured his right arm and entered his chest. He was admitted to the field hospital and died in a few hours.[1] His body was finally buried in the New Episcopal Cemetery at Swedesboro.

1. CSR; *OR*, vol. 38, pt. 1:91, 199, 293, 369, 888, pt. 4:611–12, 626; WPCHR, vol. 609; RAGO, entry 534.

EDWARD HARLAND • *Born June 24, 1832,* in Norwich, Connecticut. He left his law practice and entered Federal service as a company captain in the 3rd Connecticut Volunteers in May 1861 and fought at First Bull Run. In September he was made colonel of the 8th Connecticut. He served at North Carolina, Antietam, and Fredericksburg. His commission as brigadier general ranked from November 1862. Harland resigned in June 1865 and returned to Connecticut where he was a lawyer, politician, and bank president. He died in Norwich on March 9, 1915, and was buried there in the Yantic Cemetery.
DEATH CERTIFICATE: Primary cause of death, chronic emphysema, ten years' duration. Secondary, la grippe, five days' duration.

WILLIAM SELBY HARNEY • *Born on August 27, 1800,* in Haysboro, Tennessee. Served in the Florida and Mexican wars. In 1818 he was commissioned into the Regular Army as a second lieutenant. He rose through grades because of his service in Florida and Mexico, and in June 1858 he was promoted to brigadier general in the Regular Army. His Southern connections were regarded with suspicion by the higher command, and he was relieved of duty. In 1863 he was retired. He died May 9, 1889, in Orlando, Florida, and was buried in Arlington National Cemetery.

THOMAS MALEY HARRIS • *Born on June 17, 1817,* in Ritchie County in what is now West Virginia. Prior to the Civil War he was a practicing physician. He had hemorrhoids that became worse during his period of military service. In late 1861 he was appointed lieutenant colonel of the 10th West Virginia and in May 1862 became its colonel. He led the regiment in the Shenandoah Valley in 1862. In 1863 his digestion became weak and imperfect, and the action of his bowels was irregular, requiring frequent laxatives and purgatives. His evacuations became unhealthy, lacked consistency, and were too dark in color and too acid in character. This produced a tendency for his hemorrhoids to prolapse. His knee joint was dislocated in the winter of 1863–64 when his horse fell on an improvised bridge. Harris was too ill to travel in February 1864 but fought at Cloyd's Mountain in May. When his troops left on June 16 he remained in Virginia because of illness. In July he rejoined the army and served with Sheridan in the Shenandoah and then in the Petersburg campaign. On December 22, 1864, when his transport landed at City Point, he accidently stepped off of the gangplank and fell into the water. He was exhausted and chilled when he was finally pulled out of the ice-cold water with the help of a rope. Within a few days he had an attack of rheumatism, which confined him to his quarters for two weeks or more. The rheumatism continued for the rest of his life. He received the full rank of brigadier general in December 1864 and was mustered out in 1866. Harris returned to the practice of medicine, engaged in politics, and wrote medical articles. His hemorrhoids were finally cured by an injection of carbolic acid in

1883. For his various other symptoms he dieted carefully and took several preparations of pepsin for indigestion. He used tincture gentian compound and tincture cinchona compound as a heart stimulant; as a nerve tonic and cholegogue
he took tincture nux vomica and acid nitroprusside; for rheumatism he used a
whole round of rheumatic remedies, and for gout he had taken succus alternans,
syrupus sarsaparillae with potassium, iodide, and corrosive sublimate. By 1891
he was nearly blind, deaf, and badly crippled by rheumatism. In 1902 he had to
use a wooden frame to assist him in writing. Two years later he required a large
ear trumpet and walked with the aid of a cane. He became sick in August 1906
and was bedfast the next month. For the first time in several days he was able to
take some nourishment the day before he died.[1] Died September 30, 1906, at
Harrisville, West Virginia, and was buried in the city cemetery.

1. RVA, Pension WC 624,620; H. E. Matheny, *Major General Thomas Maley Harris*, 215, 221–22;
Steiner, *Physician-Generals*, 55–56.

WILLIAM HARROW • *Born on November 14, 1822,* in Winchester, Kentucky. He
practiced law before the Civil War and in April 1861 was made captain of an
Indiana militia company. His unit became a part of the 14th Indiana and he was
appointed through grades to colonel. On July 30, 1862, Harrow, who felt his
health had never been strong, was physically at a point where he was unfit for
his required duties and becoming more feeble. His surgeon's letter stated that
Harrow had hemoptysis and bronchitis along with many symptoms that indicated incipient tuberculosis. However, he served at Antietam. He was sick in his
quarters in November with bronchitis. His appointment as brigadier general of
volunteers ranked from that same month. Bronchitis still troubled him in December, and he suffered from neuralgia and an abscess of the face as well. He
went on a leave of absence, and during January 1863 he was on sick leave in
Washington. Although still too sick to fight, he resumed command of his brigade at Gettysburg. After service at Mine Run he commanded a division in the
Mine Run campaign. His resignation was accepted in April 1865. Harrow returned to Indiana and to his law practice and politics. He was killed September
27, 1872, in a railroad accident. Anxious to reach New Albany, Indiana, as soon
as he could, he had taken the accommodation train instead of the regular service. When the train reached the switch, twelve miles north of New Albany, it
hit a broken rail and precipitated the caboose car, in which Harrow was riding,
down a slight embankment. He was thrown out of the car, which then fell on
him, breaking his shoulder and hip and producing internal injuries. He arrived
at New Albany around six o'clock in the evening, insensible. Two doctors were
summoned, and he was soon able to speak. However, he died at eight o'clock
P.M.[1] Harrow was buried in Bellefontaine Cemetery, Mount Vernon, Indiana.

1. CSR; Tucker, *Hancock the Superb*, 142; RVA, Pension WC 405,741; *New Albany (Ind.) Ledger-
Standard*, Sept. 28, 1872.

JOHN FREDERICK HARTRANFT • *Born December 16, 1830,* near Pottstown, Pennsylvania. Giving up civil engineering, he became a lawyer the year before the beginning of the Civil War. Hartranft was colonel of a three-month regiment that entered Federal service as the 4th Pennsylvania Volunteers in April 1861. At the expiration of its service, on the eve of First Bull Run, the regiment left the field but Hartranft remained. In November 1861 Hartranft was commissioned colonel of the 51st Pennsylvania Regiment and led it in the North Carolina expedition. He developed severe diarrhea on July 10, 1862, near Jackson, Mississippi. He had to direct his troops from an ambulance. Unable to sit up and immobilized by a severe fever, he went into Jackson to recuperate. Diagnosed as having remittent fever, he was given a sixty-day sick leave to go home. His appointment as brigadier general occurred in May 1864. His wrist was slightly wounded by a minié ball near Peterburg on June 17, 1864. Discharged from service in 1866, he returned to politics in Pennsylvania. In 1873 he was discovered to have renal disease that progressed over the years; by 1889 he had fluid retention and pain. On the evening of October 11, 1889, he had weakness and severe chills. The pain became more intense, and he was unable to pass his urine on the morning of October 17, 1889. He went into coma and died that day in Norristown, Pennsylvania, and was buried in Montgomery Cemetery. The cause of death was recorded as Bright's disease and pneumonia.[1]

1. A. M. Gambone, *Major-General John Frederick Hartranft,* 80–82, 100, 281–83.

GEORGE LUCAS HARTSUFF • *Born May 28, 1830,* in Tyre, New York. Graduated from the USMA in 1852. While a cadet he was treated for diarrhea and catarrhus each five times, cephalalgia four times, excoriatio, morbus varii., and excoriatio each twice, and dysentery, odontalgia, subluxatio, contusio, and clavus each one time. Served in the Florida wars. While in Texas in the fall of 1853 he had yellow fever with black vomit. He was given a sixty-day leave that had to be extended for three months because he had not fully recovered. While serving in Florida he had dysentery. On December 20, 1855, near Fort Myers, Florida, he was wounded in a fight with the Seminoles. First, after everyone else was either dead or disabled, except for the two soldiers who loaded his weapons while he fired, he was hit in the left arm. Next, he was wounded in the left breast. Hartsuff told the two men to save themselves; in trying to find shelter for himself, he fell into a pond of water. Submerged almost to his head, it took him some time to get out of the water. He remained in the area for three days, mostly on his back without food or fresh water. The bullet remained in his chest for the rest of his life and supposedly contributed to his death almost twenty years later. In March 1856 he was on duty in the field. After two years in Florida he was sent north. On September 8, 1860, he was on board the steamer, *Lady Elgin,* on Lake Michigan between Chicago and Milwaukee when he almost drowned. It was a stormy night and the *Lady Elgin* was struck on its port side forward of the paddle box by a lumber-laden schooner, the *Augusta*. Her wheel was torn off and the cabin and hull were ripped open, which allowed water to put out the fire under the boilers, and she was helpless. At least 373 passengers were lost; Hartsuff was one of the 155 that was saved. He was brevetted captain in the adjutant general's department in 1861. He was on sick leave in October because of debility from remittent fever. In April 1862 he was appointed brigadier general of volunteers. In August, although prostrated by severe illness, he continued to perform his duty from an ambulance. However, he was so sick he could not keep anything down for days. After service at Second Bull Run, Hartsuff was severely wounded in the hip by a sharpshooter at Antietam on September 17, 1862. The minié ball entered opposite the inferior part of his left sacroiliac symphysis. He remained on his horse for a few moments and then, because of faintness, had to dismount. Putting his arms around the necks of two soldiers, he tried to walk back. Too faint, he had to be laid down. He was carried first on a blanket and then on a cot to an ambulance. In a little house a mile from the field, the surgeon examined and probed the wound. He tried to remove the bullet with forceps but could not find it. He speculated that it had penetrated the ilium and was in the pelvic cavity. Hartsuff was taken by ambulance to Middletown; that evening, still in the ambulance and under chloroform, he was examined by five surgeons. They also could not locate the bullet. Moved to Frederick City, he was again examined under chloroform without the bullet being found. President Lincoln visited him there at the Ramsey House on Record Street on October 4. After a month, he was taken by railroad car to Washington and was placed on a review board. In November his wound was discharging freely. By February 1863 he could walk with a cane rather than using crutches although the wound was still open and discharging. After administering chloroform, doctors surgically removed pieces of dead bone from under the fascia. This was followed with yet another examination using chloroform, but still the bullet was not located. He was placed on general court-martial duty in April 1863. Finally, the wound closed in May, and Hartsuff returned to duty. During August the wound became tender, and a small opening appeared. It did not have any discharge and soon closed. A similar lesion was present the next month. Although still unable to ride or to walk without a cane, he was put on a review board in October. In November 1863 there was free discharge from the wound. He could ride only a few minutes without some pain associated with numbness about the hip and leg. He was first ordered to Cincinnati as president of a court-martial board and then was sent to Wilmington, Delaware, for a retirement examination. The examination revealed a cicatrix of the left upper portion of his chest from the old Florida gunshot wound. The ball had passed through the fleshy part of the proximal arm into the upper and outer edge of the thorax. Over the lumbar region near the left sacroiliac junction there was a second cicatrix. On December 17 he was placed on a board to revise the rules and articles of war. On March 12, 1864, he sustained an accident to his tibia. Apparently he had no or poor treatment of the injury. When he was examined sixteen days later, the physician reported he had sustained a laceration of his leg over the flexor muscles of the foot. By that time the deep fascia was sloughing. Erysipelas had developed in the lower portion of the wound and his condition was complicated with a constitutional tendency to rheumatism. He was able to travel in April. Following the war, he went back to the adjutant general's department as a lieutenant colonel. In 1870 he still had rheumatism in the area of his prior wounds and retired the following year because of his disability. Before his death he made a number of trips to New York for medical treatment of an affection of his throat. He moved to New York City and on May 9, 1874, he developed a cold. By the tenth he was too sick to leave his bed and the following day developed pneumonia. Delirious, he rapidly grew worse and died on May 16. A postmortem examination was conducted with the following findings: The scar in the lung made by the Florida wound was found and it was ascertained that the pneumonia began in that area and had entirely absorbed the lung. The surgeon hypothesized the wound was probably the origin of the pneumonia and the immediate cause of death. Neither bullet was located![1] He was buried at West Point.

1. CSR; OR, vol. 12, pt. 2:383, 345; vol. 19, pt. 1:56, 121, 171, 190, 259; vol. 23, pt. 2:220; vol. 31, pt. 1:260; vol. 52, pt. 1:357; U.S. Army, CWS, roll 1, vol. 1, report 56, pp. 1005–8; LR, ACP, 2557, 1871, fiche: 000113; RAGO, entry 534; WPCHR, vols. 606, 607, 608; Charles M. Scanlan, *The Lady Elgin Disaster*, 96–99; *Lady Elgin*, Ship Information and Data Record, Milwaukee Public Library; Heitman, *Historical Register and Dictionary* 2:24.

MILO SMITH HASCALL • *Born August 5, 1829,* in Le Roy, New York. Graduated from the USMA in 1852. During his period as a cadet he was seen for catarrhus and odontalgia eight times each, obstipatio, contusio, febris intermittent, and subluxatio three times each, excoriatio and morbi. varii. each twice, and ophthalmia, clavus, phlegmon, and colica one time each. He resigned from the military in 1853 and was engaged as an attorney, railroad contractor, and county clerk before the Civil War. In June 1861 he was appointed colonel of the 17th Indiana and his appointment as brigadier general of volunteers ranked from April 1862. At the time of the skirmish near Little Pond, Tennessee, on August 30, 1862, Hascall was confined to his room by severe illness, and another had command of his brigade. In September 1864, after serving in the Atlanta campaign, he reported his health had never been robust, and his resignation was accepted in October. Following the war, he engaged in the banking and real estate business. He died August 30, 1904, at Oak Park, Illinois, and was buried there in the Forest Home Cemetery. Burial permit: Cause of death, cirrhosis of the liver.[1]

1. OR, vol. 16, pt. 1:905; vol. 38, pt. 2:577; WPCHR, vols. 606, 607, 608; RVA, Pension VA XC 2,681,666.

JOSEPH ABEL HASKIN • *Born on June 21, 1818,* in Troy, New York. Graduated from the USMA in 1839. As a cadet he was treated for a cold three times and once for a headache. Storming Chapultepec on September 13, 1847, he was wounded and taken into Mexico City where his left arm was amputated at the shoulder. He continued having trouble with the stump, and it did not completely heal until the bullet was removed nine years later. Haskin performed recruiting duties, was a quartermaster, and served on garrison duty before the Civil War. On January 10, 1861, he was forced to surrender the U.S. government property at Baton Rouge to a larger Rebel force. From 1862 until 1864, Haskin was in charge of the northern defenses of Washington, D.C. He developed a cough in 1863 that gradually increased in frequency but did not keep him from his duty. He was promoted to brigadier general of volunteers ranking from August 1864. Haskin remained in the army with the rank of lieutenant colonel and was retired December 15, 1870, for disability from the loss of his arm. It is not stated how the diagnosis was made, but a surgeon reported that in 1864 he had found well-marked indications of pulmonary disease; by 1872 the disease had rapidly progressed. Haskin died on August 3, 1874, in Oswego, New York. He was buried there in Riverside Cemetery, but his remains were later moved to Arlington. The attending physician reported he died from consumption.[1]

1. WPCHR, vol. 604; LR, CB, roll 25, H208, 1863; RVA, Pension Old War 27,654; Heitman, *Historical Register and Dictionary* 2:24; U.S. Army, CWS, roll 5, vol. 8, report 1, pp. 1–41.

EDWARD HATCH • *Born on December 22, 1831* in Bangor, Maine.[1] He left his lumber business in Iowa and in August 1861 was commissioned a captain of the 2nd Iowa Cavalry. He was injured when a shell fragment struck his abdomen and caused paralysis of his bowels and urinary bladder. He was having less trouble by the middle of January 1862, except that his bowels would become painful when he was on horseback. At the May 9 engagement at Farmington, Mississippi, he was slightly wounded in the foot. The following month he was made colonel of his regiment. He was at New Madrid, Island No. 10, and Corinth. Hatch was shot through the right lung at Moscow, Tennessee, on December 4, 1863. Fired at close range, the conical ball struck his chest on a level with and about an inch to the outside of the right areola area and penetrated the intercostal space, pleura, and lung. It made its exit through the back part of the thorax, fracturing the fifth rib and passing through the right scapula at a point equal distance from its apex and borders. The scapula was elevated at the time he was hit because he had his arm above his head. The division surgeon treated him at Moscow until December 24, when he was moved to Memphis. Upon his arrival, he was still expectorating frothy blood, had difficulty breathing, and was almost speechless. The treatment of the wound consisted of perfect rest, cold-water dressings, anodynes, and a generous allowance of a nourishing diet. His recovery progressed well without complications; however, for more than a year the arm was almost useless. Late in January 1864 he went on medical leave to Philadelphia and Washington. While recovering from his wound, he was placed in command of the cavalry depot at St. Louis. His promotion as brigadier general of volunteers ranked from April 1864. In June 1864 he was ordered to Memphis and then to the field in July. By October 1864, up to some fifty-three fragments of necrosed bone had been removed from the posterior wound. He was at the Battle of Nashville. He remained in the army, was commissioned a colonel in 1866, and spent most of his remaining service on the frontier. By the middle of 1870 he had no problems from his wound except for the usual aches and pains associated with any previous wound and an occasional sense of suffocation, as though there was not enough room in his lungs to breath. A finger could easily push the overlying tissue through the hole in the scapula, and the perforation appeared to be between an inch and an inch and a half in diameter and nearly round. While stationed at Fort Robinson, Nebraska, he fractured his right femur on March 27, 1889. After a good night's sleep, he awoke on the morning of April 11 feeling well and intending to get into a wheelchair within two weeks. That evening as the gun was fired for reville he called out twice. The nurse found him very pale, with his hand on the back of his head, and saying, "Oh, oh." When the attending surgeon arrived, Hatch was dead. The physician stated that Hatch died from a blood clot on his brain.[2] He was buried in the National Cemetery at Fort Leavenworth, Kansas.

1. LR, ACP, 5556, 1875, fiche: 000114.

2. CSR; *OR*, vol. 31, pt. 1:577, 587, 594, pt. 3:336; vol. 39, pt. 2:162; LR, ACP, 5556, 1875, fiche: 000114; U.S. Army, CWS, roll 5, vol. 8, report 1, pp. 1–41; B. J. D. Irwin, "Three Cases of Penetrating Gunshot Wound of the Thorax, with Perforation of Lungs; Recovery," *American Journal of Medical Science,* new series, 40 (1875): 404–7.

JOHN PORTER HATCH • *Born on January 9, 1822,* in Oswego, New York. Graduated from the USMA in 1845. Served in the Mexican War. After being on garrison duty, he was acting as chief commissary in the Department of New Mexico when the Civil War started. He was commissioned brigadier general of volunteers to rank from September 1861. Hatch was slightly wounded at Second Bull Run on August 30, 1862, but able to return to duty the next day. He was severely wounded while on horseback at the Battle of South Mountain on September 14, 1862. A musket ball passed through the calf of his right leg, and he had to be taken to the rear. He went on sick leave to Oswego, New York. In October his recovery was retarded by an attack of intermittent fever, and he was confined to his bed for two months. His limb discharged unhealthy matter from several points down as low as the top of the heel. The surgeon who examined him theorized that a portion of his boot or of his pantaloons had been carried into the wound. No foreign substance was found on probing, and the surgeon stated it would have to be discharged spontaneously. Although his leg was still swollen and tender, Hatch had recovered sufficiently to report to Washington. He was placed on court-martial duty in February 1863 and remained in that position until July, when he was ordered to Philadelphia to relieve the commander of the Draft Rendezvous. In January 1864 he had command of the cavalry depot in St. Louis, and at the end of the war he was in charge of the District of Charleston. He remained in the military with his old rank of major and served on the frontier. In 1886 he retired with the rank of colonel. He died April 12, 1901, in New York City and was buried in Arlington National Cemetery. According to the post hospital assistant surgeon, the immediate cause of death was cardiac dilatation.[1]

1. CSR; *OR*, vol. 12, pt. 2:253, 346, 369; vol. 19, pt. 1:28, 52, 170, 184, 216, 220; U.S. Army, CWS, roll 1, vol. 1, report 44, pp. 873–83; LR, ACP, 133, 1886, fiche: 000069.

HERMAN HAUPT • *Born March 26, 1817,* in Philadelphia, Pennsylvania. He graduated from the USMA in 1835. Within three months after graduation he resigned from the military. During the winter of 1840–41 he developed ague while surveying along the Susquehanna River and had to remain at home for several months. A railroad engineer before the Civil War, he entered Federal service as a colonel to rank from April 1862. Although appointed brigadier general of volunteers in September 1862, he did not accept the commission. He returned to civilian life in September 1863 and pursued an outstanding career as an engineer. In December 1905, while walking to the train station to return to Philadelphia, he had a heart attack and collapsed. He was taken back to his room and his son was called. The next day his son placed him in a wheelchair and took him back to the railroad station to go to Philadelphia. He died on the train in the Jersey City train yard on December 14, 1905. Haupt was buried in West Laurel Hill Cemetery, Philadelphia.[1]

DEATH CERTIFICATE: Cause of death, heart failure, heart disease.

1. James A. Ward, *That Man Haupt: A Biography of Herman Haupt,* 16, 247.

JOHN PARKER HAWKINS • *Born September 29, 1830,* in Indianapolis. Graduated from the USMA in 1852. Hawkins was treated while at West Point for catarrhus three times, cephalalgia and clavus twice each, and vertigo, obstipatio, morbi. varii., odontalgia, diarrhea, phlegmon, and clavus each one time. While on a hunt on the Republican Fork of the Kansas River in January 1854, he and his group were caught in a severe snowstorm. His left ear was badly frostbitten, and he was very concerned about it at the time. However, it peeled and returned to normal. He served on the frontier until the Civil War, when he joined the Commissary Department. He was ill in May 1863 and on the fifteenth went north on sick leave. He returned in August, restored in health and able to take any amount of exercise. That same year Hawkins was promoted brigadier general of volunteers and commanded a brigade of Negro troops.[1] Following the end of the war and his discharge from the volunteer service, he returned to his position as a captain in the subsistence department. Hawkins rose to brigadier general in December 1892 and headed the subsistence department until his retirement in 1894. Died February 7, 1914, in Indianapolis and was buried there in Crown Hill Cemetery.

DEATH CERTIFICATE: Cause of death, chronic parenchymatous nephritis; contributory, edema of lungs.

1. *OR*, vol. 24, pt. 1:93; WPCHR, vols. 606, 607, 608; U.S. Army, CWS, roll 2, vol. 3, report 47, pp. 167–67 ½; John P. Hawkins to Mag. (sister Margaret) and Thos. (Thomas Speed), Jan. 18, 1854, and John P. Hawkins to Rose, Aug. 9, 1863, Hawkins-Canaby-Speed Papers, USAMHI.

JOSEPH ROSWELL HAWLEY • *Born on October 31, 1826,* in Stewartsville, North Carolina. Before the Civil War, he was a lawyer, politician, and newspaper editor. He joined the Federal service in April 1861 as a company captain in the 1st Connecticut Volunteers and fought at First Bull Run. He later served in Florida, in the siege of Charleston, and in the Petersburg campaign. On May 9, 1864, Hawley was compelled by illness to turn over his command, and the next morning he went back to the camp. He had almost daily pain from rheumatism, and by August his surgeon recommended he take a leave. In September he was made brigadier general of volunteers and the next month he returned to duty and resumed command. He was discharged in 1866 and was elected governor of Connecticut. For the rest of his life he pursued politics and was a U.S. senator at the time of his death on March 18, 1905, in Washington, D.C. He was buried in Cedar Hill Cemetery, Hartford, Connecticut.[1]

DEATH CERTIFICATE: Cause of death, primary, chronic gastritis of one year duration; immediate, exhaustion.

1. CSR; *OR*, vol. 36, pt. 2:50; vol. 42, pt. 1:103; vol. 51, pt. 1:1238.

JOSEPH HAYES • *Born September 14, 1835,* at South Berwick, Maine. He followed a varied career prior to the Civil War, as a banker in Wisconsin, a civil engineer in Iowa, and a real estate broker in Boston. He entered Federal service as major of the 18th Massachusetts in August 1861 and rose to colonel by March 1863. The first of August 1862, near Harrison's Landing, Virginia, he was prostrate with a severe attack of fever with diarrhea. He was unable to perform any duties for over a week. He was at Antietam, Fredericksburg, and Chancellorsville. At Gettysburg on July 2, 1863, he was positioning skirmishers when his horse fell and rolled over on his leg. The bone was probably cracked rather than fractured. On September 24, 1863, near Culpeper, Virginia, Hayes was thrown from his horse and knocked insensible; the horse was going at full speed when it stumbled, causing the bridle to break. Hayes's right shoulder was dislocated, and he received severe contusions of his head and body. He was given a leave to recover. However, he never regained full use of his right arm and could not place it behind his head. During the action in the Wilderness on May 5, 1864, he was wounded on the head by a bullet and was left on the field. Subsequently, he was taken to a hospital in Annapolis and then to Washington where the surgeon cut out the bullet from his neck. He was treated from May 16 to June 18, 1864, and then returned to duty. His promotion as brigadier general of volunteers ranked from May. At Petersburg, Virginia, in August 1864 he was captured. While a prisoner he was admitted to the Confederate hospital at Danville, Virginia, on November 30, 1864, with chronic diarrhea. He was sent back to the prison on December 15. Returning to civilian life after the war, he again followed a number of professions and was a broker, head of a coal company, and had mining interests. In later years, Hayes's old head wound was reported to have made him a periodic dipsomaniac. An examination on March 24, 1906, revealed a scar on his head from the bullet wound and the scar on his neck where the surgeons had extracted the bullet. The leg that had been injured at Gettysburg was fractured on two occasions following the war and required further treatment. By 1906 the leg was markedly weakened and had not fully recovered.[1] He died in a private sanitarium in New York City on August 19, 1912, and was buried in South Berwick, Maine.

DEATH CERTIFICATE: Pneumonia, bronchial.

1. CSR; *OR*, vol. 36, pt. 1:576, pt. 2:818; RVA, Pension C 2,490,959.

RUTHERFORD BIRCHARD HAYES • *Born October 4, 1822,* in Delaware, Ohio. At the age of nineteen, he had a severe cough. He had recurrent episodes of tonsillitis at age twenty-five and developed a peritonsillar abscess in 1849. Following cathartics, cod-liver oil, and rest, it drained spontaneously. A lawyer and politician, he was made major of the 23rd Ohio in June 1861. At Giles Court House on May 10, 1862, he was slightly wounded in the right knee by a shell. He said it was only a scratch, just enough to draw blood and spoil his pants. He was severely wounded below the left elbow at South Mountain on September 14, 1862. The ball fractured one of the bones in his forearm and opened a large vessel. He fell to the ground vomiting. He had one of the soldiers twist a handkerchief around his arm to arrest the bleeding. When his troops fell back, he was left on the ground and had to call to his men to come back after him. He was taken to the field hospital where the regimental surgeon released the tourniquet, dressed the wound, and gave him oral opium and brandy. He was transported by ambulance to Middletown, Maryland, where his brother-in-law, a physician, took care of him. Although he had an open comminuted fracture, he received conservative treatment and within a few days did not have pain except when he moved the arm. On July 24, 1864, while at Winchester, his head and shoulder were injured by a musket ball. While galloping rapidly, his horse was shot from under him at Cedar Creek on October 19 and the resulting fall disabled his ankle. After getting another horse, he continued on the field, although later he was hit in the head by a spent ball and was slightly stunned. In October 1864 he was appointed brigadier general and in June 1865 resigned to take his place in Congress.[1] He was elected nineteenth president of the United States in 1876. During the time he was president he gained weight and, except for occasional headaches, enjoyed good health. The dull headaches occurred at night and disappeared when he arose in the morning. They reminded him of the ones he had had when he had taken quinine. Following one term in office he retired to private life. After a trip to Columbus and Cleveland, he boarded the train on January 10, 1893, to return to his home in Fremont, Ohio. After complaining of being cold, he was taken back to the waiting room in the station where stimulants were administered; he soon felt well enough to reboard the train. It was not long before he was seized with a violent sensation of pain in his chest, which lasted until after he returned home. The train was met at the depot by a carriage and the family physician. He was taken to Spiegel Grove, his estate, and the physician remained with him most of the night and the greater part of Sunday. The following Tuesday, January 13, he died of neuralgia of the heart or angina pectoris and was buried in Oakwood Cemetery, Fremont. His body was later moved to the state park built on his former estate.[2]

1. *OR*, vol. 19, pt. 1:460–61, 467; vol. 43, pt. 1:366; R. B. Hayes listing of his wounds, Rutherford B. Hayes Civil War Records Misc., Rutherford B. Hayes Presidential Center, Spiegel Grove, Fremont, Ohio; Rutherford B. Hayes, *Diary and Letters of Rutherford B. Hayes*, 266–67, 354–55, 528; *MOLLUS* 4:239; Rudolph Marx, *The Health of the Presidents*, 221–30.

2. Rutherford B. Hayes, *Hayes: The Diary of a President*, 114–15, 175–76, 243–44; *Fremont (Ohio) Democratic Messenger*, Jan. 26, 1893.

ISHAM NICHOLAS HAYNIE • *Born on November 18, 1824,* at Dover, Tennessee. Served in the Mexican War. Haynie graduated from law school in 1852 and was judge of the court of common pleas at Cairo, Illinois, when the Civil War started. He recruited the 48th Illinois Infantry, which he led at Forts Henry and Donelson. Haynie was severely wounded in the left thigh at the Battle of Shiloh on April 6, 1862. He resigned in March 1863 when his appointment as brigadier general of volunteers was not acted on by the Senate.[1] He returned to the practice of law in Illinois. He died May 22, 1868, in Springfield, Illinois, and was buried there in Oak Ridge Cemetery. Interment book, Cause of death, congestion of liver.

1. CSR; *OR*, vol. 10, pt. 1:116, 133.

ALEXANDER HAYS • *Born on July 8, 1819,* in Franklin, Pennsylvania. Graduated from the USMA in 1844. Hays was wounded in the leg at Resaca de la Palma on May 9, 1846. The wound made him unfit for arduous service and, after being on recruiting duty, he rejoined the army at Vera Cruz. In 1848 he resigned from the army; he was in Pittsburgh at the start of the Civil War following a period in California. Hays went back into the army as captain of the 16th Infantry and then became colonel of the 63rd Pennsylvania Volunteers, which was on the Peninsula. A surgeon's certificate of July 29, 1862, reported that he had amaurosis (blindness) of his right eye and partial paralysis of the left arm, from which he had suffered for the previous six weeks. He was given a leave and returned the next month. At the battle of Second Bull Run, August 29, he was wounded in the leg. In September he was promoted to brigadier general of volunteers. By the end of September the wound was still open and he was absent until January 1863. Hays was division commander at Gettysburg. On November 7 he was laid up with rheumatism but got up, mounted his horse, and went with the troops. Hays was killed by a bullet through his head at the Wilderness on May 5, 1864. He fell from his saddle and the troops carried his body to the rear.[1] He was buried in Allegheny Cemetery, Pittsburgh.

1. CSR; *OR*, vol. 12, pt. 2:417, 422; vol. 21:953; vol. 36, pt. 1:2, 64, 122, 190, 325–26, 480; vol. 51, pt. 1:970; LR, ACP, 2650, 1882, fiche: 000115; RAGO, entry 534; Lymon, *Meade's Headquarters,* 42.

WILLIAM HAYS • *Born May 9, 1819,* in Richmond, Virginia. Graduated from the USMA in 1840. He was seen twice for sore feet while at the academy. Served in the Mexican and Florida wars. He was wounded at Molino del Rey on September 8, 1847. He had sick leaves from November 12, 1855, to December 17, 1856, and from May 10, 1858, to April 30, 1859. Hays was engaged in garrison duty until the start of the Civil War. After service in the defense of Washington and with artillery units, Hays was promoted to brigadier general of volunteers in December 1862. He was on the Peninsula and at Antietam and Fredericksburg. He was injured May 3, 1863, at Chancellorsville when his horse fell, and he was taken prisoner. Paroled two days later, he was back at Gettysburg in July. Hays had sick leave and was on court-martial duty from August 16 to October 27. In September he had an abscess on the scar just below the right clavicle. From November 1863 until February 1865 he acted as a provost marshal of the southern district of New York. Back in the field for Petersburg and Appomattox, he was relieved of his command in April 1865 when he and his headquarters staff were found asleep. He remained in the army after the war but remained a major until he died. During October 1872 he was confined to his room in New York City because of general anasarca due to valvular disease of the heart. By December his anasarca had improved.[1] He died on February 7, 1875, at Fort

Independence, Boston Harbor. Initially buried in Yonkers, New York, his body was later moved to West Point.

DEATH CERTIFICATE: Immediate cause of death, disease of heart, due to congestion of lungs and liver, fourteen days' duration.

1. *OR*, vol. 25, pt. 1:177, 307, 375–76; RVA, Pension WC 175,483; LR, ACP, 5430, 1872, fiche: 000116.

WILLIAM BABCOCK HAZEN • *Born on September 27, 1830,* in West Hartford, Vermont. Graduated from the USMA in 1855. While a cadet he was treated for excoriatio seven times, cephalalgia six times, catarrhus five times, contusio four times, catarrhus and subluxatio twice each, and febris intermittent, odontalgia, debility, and clavus once each. He was wounded in a fight with the Comanches on November 3, 1859, near the headwaters of the Llano River, Texas. The bullet went through his hand and lodged in his right side between the sixth and seventh ribs. After four days on the field, he was taken by horseback to Fort Inge, Texas, where he was able to obtain medical care. The lack of early treatment, blood loss, and infection delayed his recovery. In December he was accompanied to San Antonio by a surgeon who was ordered to remain with him until he could be left alone. He remained under treatment until January 28, 1860, when he went on sick leave. The bullet remained embedded in his back, and he returned to duty as an instructor at West Point in February 1861 with his wound still unhealed and his arm in a sling. In later years when Hazen tried to obtain the surgeon's certificate from Fort Inge he was informed that it along with other records had been surrendered to the Confederates. He was made colonel of the 41st Ohio in October 1861. In May 1862 he obtained sick leave because of malaria and did not return to duty until July. James A. Garfield thought that he looked healthy and was simply pretending. Hazen was at Shiloh and Perryville. At Stones River on December 31, 1862, his shoulder was bruised by a ball. At Chickamauga in September 1863 he was struck twice but not injured. Hazen was at Chattanooga, Knoxville, Atlanta, the March to the Sea, and in the Carolinas. He was promoted to brigadier general in April 1863 and major general in April 1865. He remained in the army and in July 1866 was appointed colonel. The symptoms from his old Indian wound continued. In May 1872, the ball in his back, after having been encapsulated for so long, suddenly, either from the degeneration of the walls of the sac or from some accidental cause, evacuated from its bed. It had given rise to great nervous derangement and even to partial paralysis of his lower extremities, especially the right leg. In October he still had pain and partial paralysis in his back and lower extremities and required a sick leave until May 23, 1873. He had deafness in July 1875 from the chronic inflammation of his internal ear, which had been present for several years. He had further sick leaves from October 1875 to April 1876 and from March 27 to May 22, 1882. He was appointed chief signal officer with the staff rank of brigadier general in 1880. In 1884 he developed diabetes mellitus. Died January 16, 1887, in Washington, D.C., and was buried in Arlington National Cemetery. The attending surgeon reported that his death was due to coma from diabetes mellitus.[1]

1. *OR*, vol. 20, pt. 1:547; vol. 30, pt. 1:765; LR, CB, H1207, 1863; U.S. Army, CWS, roll 1, vol. 2, report 31, pp. 465–77; WPCHR, vols. 607, 608, 609; RVA, Pension WC 232,850; LR, CB, H1207, 1863; Heitman, *Historical Register and Dictionary* 2:24; Hazen, *Narrative*, 1, 50, 77, 433–35; Garfield, *Wild Life of the Army*, 103–4.

CHARLES ADAM HECKMAN • *Born on December 3, 1822*, in Easton, Pennsylvania. In November 1847 he left Vera Cruz for New Orleans on a surgeon's certificate of disability and was subsequently discharged. Heckman was a railroad conductor when the Civil War started, and in October 1861 he entered Federal service as lieutenant colonel of the 9th New Jersey. He was in the Carolinas campaign and later in the Army of the James. His promotion to brigadier general of volunteers ranked from November 1862. He was captured at Drewry's Bluff on May 16, 1864, and when he reached Libby Prison he refused to be searched and wanted to fight. Threatened with the "black hole," he capitulated. He was paroled at Charleston Harbor, South Carolina, on August 3, 1864. During the time he was a prisoner, he suffered from exposure and poor food. He also contracted a bad cold, which supposedly produced kidney disease. He was disabled from active duty by a fall from his horse and resigned May 25, 1865. After he returned to civilian life, he became a public utility contractor and later a train dispatcher. In applying for a pension in May 1886 he reported he had suffered with the following diseases: neuralgia of the head and heart; congestion of the liver and congestive chills; inflammation of kidneys and bladder causing frequent discharge of urine; and great bodily suffering with nausea and physical helplessness. Heckman held a number of positions but because of his poor health had difficulties performing the work. In 1882 he had to resign from his last position.[1] Died January 15, 1896, in Germantown, Pennsylvania, and was buried in Easton, Pennsylvania.

DEATH CERTIFICATE: Cause of death, chronic suppurative nephritis.

1. *OR*, vol. 36, pt. 2:16, 117, pt. 3:31; RVA, Pension WC 440,215.

SAMUEL PETER HEINTZELMAN • *Born on September 30, 1805*, in Manheim, Pennsylvania. Graduated from the USMA in 1826. Served in the Mexican and Florida wars. In May 1861 he was promoted to brigadier general of volunteers and to major general to rank from May 1862. At the Battle of Bull Run on July 21, 1861, he was severely wounded in the right elbow. With his arm in a sling, he rode up and down the field in an effort to restore order. He was sent to Centreville and then to Washington on sick leave. Heintzelman was able to return in August to limited duty. In late May 1862 he was sick. He received a severe contusion of his left wrist by a spent ball at the Battle of Glendale on June 30, 1862. Heintzelman remained on the field; however, this injury disabled his arm for several weeks. In October 1863 he was unfit for active duty for a short time. For the remainder of the war he served in command of portions of the Washington defenses, the Northern Department, and on court-martial duty. He remained in the army and retired in 1869 with the rank of major general. He died May 1, 1880, in Washington, D.C., and was buried in Forest Lawn Cemetery, Buffalo, New York. According to the attending surgeon's statement, he died of dropsy superinduced by dilatation of the heart, resulting from partial consolidation of the right lung in consequence of pleurisy contracted in the line of his duty in June 1862.[1]

1. *OR*, vol. 2:315, 323, 410; vol. 11, pt. 2:100, 102; vol. 29, pt. 2:309–10, 313, 323; *OR Suppl.*, vol. 2, pt. 1:41; U.S. Army, CWS, roll 3, vol. 4, report 12, pp. 267–81; RVA, Pension WC 192,257; Oliver Otis Howard, *Autobiography of Oliver Otis Howard* 1:161.

FRANCIS JAY HERRON • *Born February 17, 1837*, in Pittsburgh, Pennsylvania. He was a banker in Iowa when the Civil War started and was mustered in as captain of the 1st Iowa in time for service at Wilson's Creek. At the Battle of Pea Ridge, Arkansas, on March 7, 1862, he was severely wounded and captured. A cannonball had struck his horse in the left front shoulder; after passing through the horse, it struck Herron. He was taken to Van Buren, Arkansas, and placed in the hospital. The Confederate surgeon who examined him found that Herron had a compound fracture of the right internal malleolus and partial dislocation of the ankle joint. The surgeon placed the fractured bones in apposition and then reduced the dislocation. Herron was taken to Fort Smith and exchanged three weeks later. The Confederate surgeon accompanied him approximately one hundred miles to the Federal lines. Herron reached St. Louis about the first of May after being carried sixteen days in an ambulance. He then went on sick leave. Herron was commissioned brigadier general of volunteers and in the middle of July reported back for duty. His appointment as major general of volunteers ranked from November 1862. Early in January he became ill with a fever and rode in an ambulance for a number of days. He was able to sit up by January 20. On March 30 he was ordered to assume command of the Army of the Frontier and was at Vicksburg near the end of the siege. On September 21, during the expedition to the Red River, he was taken ill with fever and was confined to his bed. On October 5 he was given a sick leave and did not return to his command on the Rio Grande until January 3, 1864. He resigned from the army in June 1865. Herron held various state and federal positions in Louisiana until Federal troops were removed in 1877, after which he went to New York. In November 1875, the former Confederate surgeon who had first cared for Herron's wounded ankle in 1862 treated him for an attack of acute arthritis in the same joint. In early 1876 he had been confined to his bed and was compelled to use crutches for about seven weeks. In March his ankle was stiff and very tender and he could not bear full weight on the leg.[1] He died January 8, 1902, at his residence in New York City and was buried in Calvary Cemetery, Long Island City, New York.

DEATH CERTIFICATE: Chronic pyelitis, nephritis and renal insufficiency.

1. CSR; *OR*, vol. 8:261, 267; vol. 22, pt. 2:35, 185; vol. 26, pt. 1:321, 327, 723; vol. 34, pt. 2:13; U.S. Army, CWS, roll 2, vol. 3, report 37, pp. 1129–43; *MOLLUS* 10:350; RVA, Pension SC 142,525.

EDWARD WINSLOW HINCKS • *Born on May 30, 1830,* in Bucksport, Maine. He was a member of the Massachusetts legislature in 1855. In August 1861 he was made colonel of the 19th Massachusetts Infantry. On June 30, 1862, in the action at Glendale, he was severely wounded. A bullet had passed through the upper portion of his right thigh and he received a severe contusion of his right ankle. Unable to continue, he was sent to the rear. After a leave of absence, he returned August 8 to Harrison's Landing. Although not recovered from his wounds, he was immediately assigned to command. On September 3, entirely prostrated from the effects of his wounds and the severities of the campaign, he was relieved from his brigade command. Hincks resumed command again in a few days. At Antietam on September 17, 1862, he was wounded twice. One bullet passed through his right arm, badly fracturing the radius. Another ball—perhaps the same one—entered his abdomen on a level with the umbilicus and three inches above the middle of the crest of the right ilium. It traversed the colon and emerged a little to the right of the lumbar vertebrae. Hincks lay upon the field unattended until about noon of the following day. When found, he was taken to a vacant house and finally to a field hospital. On September 21, fecal material began to escape from the exit wound. Symptoms of peritonitis on the twenty-sixth were treated by complete rest, morphia, and cold-water dressings. Impacted feces in the lower part of the descending colon were removed mechanically. On October 12 he was moved to the hospital in Baltimore where he remained for four weeks until he was taken to Boston. In a few weeks the dejections resumed their natural channel and the fistulous orifice healed soundly. His promotion to brigadier general of volunteers ranked from November 1862. He reported to Washington for light duty on March 23, 1863, and was placed on court-martial duty. On June 9 he was directed to report to the medical director at Boston for treatment. He was assigned to duty as provost marshal general of New Hampshire on July 4. Hincks resumed command of troops in April 1864 but by May was too ill to perform his duties. On the assault on Petersburg on June 15, he was thrown by the fall of his horse, received a severe concussion, and suffered continued pain in the area of his abdominal wound. Also, he had attacks of neuralgia that were aggravated by malarial influences. In July he was placed on court-martial duty. After the war he remained in the army and in 1866 was commissioned a lieutenant colonel. During the summer of 1869 he had a severe illness compounded by neuralgia and malarial influences, and he applied for sick leave in July. Hincks was placed upon the retired list for wounds received in action on December 15, 1870. Whenever he became constipated there was acute pain in the inguinal area. Use of the right hand and wrist produced pain. The fingers could not be sufficiently closed to grasp any small article, but he could grasp with moderate firmness any article an inch and a half in diameter.[1] He was the first governor of the National Home for Disabled Volunteers at Hampton, Virginia, and then governed at Milwaukee, Wisconsin, until 1880. Hincks died in Cambridge, Massachusetts, on February 14, 1894, and was buried in Mount Auburn Cemetery.

DEATH CERTIFICATE: Immediate cause of death, cirrhosis of liver.

1. CSR; *OR,* vol. 19, pt. 1:307, 323; vol. 33:947; vol. 36, pt. 2:594; vol. 40, pt. 2:459–60, 577, pt. 3:18, 68, 70; vol. 43, pt. 2:127; vol. 51, pt. 1:996; U.S. Army, CWS, roll 1, vol. 2, report 24, pp. 341–83; LR, CB, roll 477, H380, 1870; *MSHW,* vol. 2, pt. 2:78.

ETHAN ALLEN HITCHCOCK • *Born May 18, 1798,* at Vergennes, Vermont. Graduated from the USMA in 1817. Served in the Mexican and Florida wars. When at Corpus Christi on his way to Mexico, he took a very large quantity of quinine at the suggestion of a physician, and later supposed this might have predisposed him to his subsequent medical problems. During 1845 he developed diarrhea and by March 1846 he had been sick for twelve months. When the troops marched, he had to accompany them the first few days riding in an ox wagon on a bed set upon boxes of ammunition. When they camped opposite the city of Matamoros he was too weak to sit up. His bones ached, but weakness was his main complaint. In April he had a sick leave and tried to travel back on horseback, but because he was so ill he made most of the trip in a wagon. The next month a surgeon suggested that he may have a fistula in ano or an exaggerated case of piles. Hitchcock used a looking glass to examine the area and found a discolored projection as large as a walnut to the right side of the anus. In St. Louis, Dr. Beaumont said that the projection filled with coagulated blood should be cut off, but Hitchcock wanted to wait. Finally on May 9, one hemorrhoid was punctured but it recurred. He continued to have symptoms, and on the twelfth the surgeon operated on the two external hemorrhoids. With a large fishhook-like instrument, he snagged each projection, and then, using a sharp knife, excised a portion of each. A piece of raw cotton, covered with cold cream, was placed over the wound and held in place by a bandage between his legs that was secured to a cotton strip around his waist. There were two internal hemorrhoids, and the surgeon proposed operating on them as well. In August 31, 1846, Hitchcock still had diarrhea and debility, but an examination by a "celebrated" surgeon did not reveal any remaining rectal disease. He was better and ready to return to duty by the end of September. However, in October he had a relapse of his diarrhea but was able to return to duty. He fought at Molino del Rey in September 1847. During November, after having occupied a cold, damp building with brick floors that never dried after being washed, he became sick and developed pain in his right shoulder. The pain left but recurred in June 1848 in his right arm around the elbow. Pain continued over the next six months, migrating between his shoulders and then to the left arm, associated with numbness in the two forefingers of his left hand. He consulted a surgeon who said he had "incipient paralysis" and should go home. He arrived back to duty in early 1849, and in March his surgeon recommended he go to Arkansas Springs for the water. When Hitchcock dropped his left hand to his side, he soon had tingling sensations and worried that it was a forerunner of paralysis. Following two months of the water treatments, he could recognize little change. As an experiment more than from faith, he resorted to a galvanic instrument twice a day for ten minutes each time. Within ten days all of his bad symptoms went away, but subsequently, over time, they returned in a less severe form. In June 1849, he applied for a twelve-month leave to go to Europe, and he took his galvanic machine with him. Systematically, he tried the Turkish baths in Europe with only minimal slow improvement. He noted that whenever he threw his head back, as in a barber's chair, his arms became almost paralyzed and the terrible prickling sensations extended to his tongue. His symptoms continued after his return to America in October 1850, and he resigned from Federal service in 1855 when an extension to a sick leave was refused. In early 1862 he was approached about reentering Federal service but felt the state of his health was too poor; however, he accepted an appointment as major general in February. He left St. Louis for Washington on March 7 and had a severe nosebleed on the way, the sixth or seventh he had had over the previous three weeks. On his arrival in Washington on the tenth, he was unable to see the secretary of war, who was having a meeting with the president. He returned to his hotel and had another profuse nosebleed. A physician was called, and the bleeding was finally stopped when some powder was placed on lint and applied. Weakened, he had to go to bed, and the secretary of war visited him in his hotel room that evening. By May 1862, his health and strength had declined since his arrival in Washington, and he felt unequal to the duties of his commission. He had a slight fever every day, was subject to headaches, had lost his appetite, and was barely able to reach his room from the lower story of the hotel. From May through October 1862 he was on a medical leave of absence in Morristown, New Jersey. He was finally mustered out in September 1867. The next year in June he was at Hot Springs, Arkansas, and after faithfully trying the water with limited benefit he sought permission to again visit the waters in Europe.[1] He died August 5, 1870, at Sparta, Georgia, and was buried at West Point.

1. LR, ACP, 3864, 1893, fiche: 000070; "Description of an illness he had after leaving Mexico," Ethan Allen Hitchcock Papers; Ethan Allen Hitchcock diaries, Book 46, pp. 2–3, 13, 28, 31, 33, 37, 42, 67, 70, 75, 91–93, 95, 122–26, 129–30, 134–36, 155; Book 47, pp. 39, 88; Book 53, pp. 1–2, 5, 7, 9, 13, 27, 64, 76–77; Book 55, p. 120; Book 77, p. 199, Gilcrease Museum, Tulsa, Okla.

EDWARD HENRY HOBSON · *Born on July 11, 1825,* in Greensburg, Kentucky. Served in the Mexican War. A prominent merchant and banker before the Civil War, he was made colonel of the 13th (Union) Kentucky Infantry in January 1862. At Spring Hill, Tennessee, about the last of March, his horse fell with its entire weight upon him, severely crushing his right leg and ankle. He was injured so badly that although he would not leave his command, he was compelled to be carried and treated in an ambulance. At Shiloh in April he again took command. His promotion to brigadier general of volunteers ranked from November 1862. In August 1863 he had medical leave and did not return to command until the following January. He received a gunshot wound in his left arm on June 11, 1864, at Keller's Bridge, Kentucky, but did not mention it in his official report. The injury paralyzed his arm, causing it to drop powerless at his side. The wound was dressed and liniments applied by his family servant. He went home on leave for further treatment and was discharged in August 1865. After the war, he entered politics and held state and federal positions. His leg remained swollen and his arm was disabled more or less for the rest of his life.[1] Died September 14, 1901, in Cleveland, Ohio, and was buried at Greensburg, Kentucky.

DEATH CERTIFICATE: Cause of death, gastritis. Duration, two days.

1. RVA, Pension SC 253,943; LR, CB, roll 96, H586, 1864.

JOSEPH HOLT · *Born January 6, 1807,* in Breckinridge County, Kentucky. After a career as a lawyer, commonwealth's attorney, and newspaper editor, he was quite wealthy. He went into partial retirement in 1842 to recover from tuberculosis. In 1857 he became commissioner of patents under President James Buchanan. Two years later he entered the Cabinet as postmaster general and in 1860 became secretary of war. President Lincoln appointed him colonel and judge advocate general of the army in September 1862 and brigadier general in June 1864. In this position he carried out the constitutionally questionable policies of the government in dealing with political and wartime prisoners.[1] He died on August 1, 1894, in his Washington, D.C., residence, and was buried in the family cemetery at Holt, Breckinridge County, Kentucky.

DEATH CERTIFICATE: Cause of death, primary, fracture of neck of femur, caused by fall; immediate, exhaustion. One week duration.

1. LR, CB, roll 96, H834, 1864.

JOSEPH HOOKER • *Born November 13, 1814,* in Hadley, Massachusetts. Graduated
from the USMA in 1837. During his term at West Point he was treated once each
for fever, debility, diarrhea, toothache, influenza, catarrhus, sore feet, and a cold.
Served in the Mexican War. In May 1853 he resigned his commission and took
up business in Oregon and California. He was appointed brigadier general of
volunteers to rank from May 1861, major general of volunteers in May 1862, and
brigadier general in the Regular Army in September 1862. He served on the
Peninsula, and at Antietam on September 17, 1862, he was wounded in the foot.
Hooker was on horseback, standing in the stirrups with his weight on his right
foot, which was turned outward when it was struck. Weak from the loss of
blood, he was removed from the saddle before he could fall, unaware that he
had been struck. He was placed on a stretcher and taken to the Pry house on the
left bank of the Antietam Creek. The ball had hit the inner side of the foot
inferior to the middle of the scaphoid bone. It passed between the first and
second layers of the plantar muscles, almost transversely across the plantar
portion of the foot, and emerged inferior to the anterior border of the cuboid
bone. Surprisingly, the bones of the foot were uninjured. Warm-water dressings were applied, and although there was no constitutional disturbance on the
next morning, the foot was hot and inflamed. Using a syringe, the surgeon
thoroughly washed out the wound with warm water and substituted cold for
warm-water dressings. The next day Hooker was comfortable, the appearance
of the foot had improved, and the inflammatory signs were gone. A lotion of
plumbi (lead) instead of cold-water dressings was ordered because it would be
more likely to allay any irritation that might arise. Before Hooker left for Washington, he was advised by his surgeon to resume the use of tepid water as soon
as all tendency to active inflammation was gone. He was hospitalized at the
Insane Asylum in Washington because the other hospitals were full. He returned
to duty in November but was still unable to mount his horse unaided. On November 25, he requested that the surgeon reexamine him. The newly formed
cicatrices were somewhat tumified and painful to pressure. By the end of the
month there had been further improvement, although his step lacked its former
full motion. After Fredericksburg, Hooker was named commander of the Army
of the Potomac. On the morning of May 3, 1863, at Chancellorsville, he received
a very severe contusion from the column of a building, which fell against him
when hit by a cannon shot. He was unconscious for a short time. When he
recovered, he mounted his horse but developed acute pain; becoming faint, he
had to be taken from his horse. Finally, after some brandy, he was able to remount his horse and go to the rear. At about 10 o'clock he was lying in a tent
some 600 to 800 yards to the rear. Later in the day, on horseback, he joined Gen.
Darius N. Couch. His right side was discolored and partially paralyzed for weeks
afterward. In July 1864 he left the Army of the Potomac for service as a corps
commander at Chattanooga and on the Atlanta campaign. During a reception

for U. S. Grant in November 1865, Hooker had a stroke and lost the use of his right side. He was taken to his residence and had a slow, partial return of function. In the summer of 1866, he had recovered enough to take a new post and was transferred to Detroit. Early the next year he had another stroke and retired from the army as a major general in 1868. He frequently traveled, although he had to use a cane and be assisted when he left home. He died October 31, 1878, in Garden City, New York, and was buried in Cincinnati. According to the surgeon and medical director, he died of paralysis of the heart.[1]

1. *OR,* vol. 19, pt. 1:30, 57, 170, 182, 189, 275; vol. 25, pt. 2:377–78; WPCHR, vols. 602, 603; U.S. Army, CWS, roll 1, vol. 2, report 47, pp. 651–69; ibid., report of D. M. Couch, roll 5, vol. 9, report 6, pp. 39–115; *MSHW,* vol. 2, pt. 3:60; LR, ACP, 91, 1892, fiche: 000119; *MOLLUS* 18:225; *Battles and Leaders* 3:220–21; Paul E. Steiner, *Medical-Military Portraits of Union and Confederate Generals,* 166–68; Walter H. Hebert, *Fighting Joe Hooker,* 142–43, 164, 152, 171, 213–15, 224, 287, 293–96.

ALVIN PETERSON HOVEY • *Born September 6, 1821,* near Mount Vernon, Indiana. Before the war he was a lawyer, a member of the Indiana supreme court, and a U.S. district attorney. He was appointed colonel of the 24th Indiana at the outbreak of hostilities and brigadier general of volunteers in April 1862. He was at Shiloh and Vicksburg and in the early stages of the Atlanta campaign. At the end of the war he was in command of the District of Indiana. He returned to Indiana politics; in 1872, when the report of his Civil War service was requested, his response was delayed because of a broken wrist.[1] He served in Congress and died while governor of Indiana in the Denison Hotel, Indianapolis, on November 23, 1891. He was buried in Bellefontaine Cemetery, Mount Vernon, Indiana. DEATH CERTIFICATE: Immediate cause, collapse, due to la grippe and failure of circulation and respiratory functions.

1. LR, CB, roll 26, H557, 1863; U.S. Army, CWS, roll 4, vol. 7, report 46, pp. 627–735.

CHARLES EDWARD HOVEY • *Born on April 26, 1827,* in Thetford, Vermont. Prior to the war he had an outstanding record as an educator and school administrator. He organized the 33rd Illinois Infantry and was commissioned colonel in August 1861. Near Cache River, Arkansas, on July 7, 1862, he was slightly wounded. His promotion as brigadier general to rank from September was not acted on by the Senate and expired in March 1863. During the Battle of Arkansas Post on January 11, 1863, he was wounded twice by shell fragments. His right arm was struck about midway between the elbow and the wrist, while the second wound was about two inches below the left knee. The arm wound was chiefly a deep flesh wound and the muscles were badly torn. The leg wound mainly involved the bone, although the skin and muscles were cut away. He remained on the field and where he temporarily, along with a staff officer, cared for his wounds. Later the wounds were dressed by a surgeon, and Hovey remained with his command. He tendered his resignation in June 1864 and was granted a leave of absence. From about May to December 1866 he had malarious poison of a virulent character and of an intermittent type, which was associated with chronic diarrhea that seemed to thwart every effort to overcome it. He was treated for the same problems the following summer but appeared much weaker than before. An examination in 1879 revealed an ugly scar on his leg, measuring two inches long by a half an inch wide. The skin had grown upon or over the injured part of the bone. He died at Washington, D.C., on November 17, 1897, and was buried in Arlington National Cemetery.[1]

DEATH CERTIFICATE: Cause of death, Bright's disease, exhaustion. Duration, seven months.

1. CSR; *OR,* vol. 17, pt. 1:706, 758; RVA, Pension WC 475,671.

OLIVER OTIS HOWARD · *Born November 8, 1830,* in Leeds, Maine. Graduated from the USMA in 1854. At the academy in February 1851, he was exercising with a horizontal bar when it turned, causing him to fall on his head. The injury was complicated by an attack of erysipelas. In addition, while he was a cadet he was treated for excoriatio eight times, phlegmon five times, catarrhus three times, contussio and vulnus incisum two times each, and rheumatism, hemorrhoids, ophthalmia, diarrhea, cephalalgia, and subluxiatio once each. During the summer of 1859 he had an attack of severe rheumatism that lasted about a week. In May 1861 he was elected colonel of the 3rd Maine.[1] On June 6, 1861, at the New York Armory, he was standing on the limber of a gun carriage and fell off. Although he landed on his feet, his heavy saber struck his left big toe and crushed the nail. This injury bothered him the rest of his life. Late the same month, while in Washington D.C., Howard had "something like cholera." Initially unconscious, he was treated in his tent, but later he was cared for in the home of a friend's parents. He went back to camp on July 5 and took part in the battle of First Bull Run. His appointment as brigadier general of volunteers ranked from September 1861. On June 1, 1862, at the Battle of Fair Oaks, he was wounded twice in the right arm. First, a small Mississippi rifle ball hit him in the forearm. The arm was bound up by a handkerchief, and he continued in the battle. His horse's leg was broken and, on dismounting, he received the second wound in his elbow. The surgeon bound up his arm behind a large tree stump, and Howard walked to the rear. When he was examined it was found that the first ball had just grazed the ulna. The second ball had passed through the humerus between the condyles, fractured the head of the ulna into multiple fragments, and lodged in the elbow joint. He was informed that his arm had to be amputated but that they must wait for six hours until reaction had set in. Howard occupied the Negro cabin at the Courtney house while waiting for the surgery. He was put on a stretcher, and a tourniquet was placed around his arm near the shoulder. Four stout men carried him to the amputating area where the tourniquet was loosened and chloroform administered. A flap amputation at the middle third of the shaft of the humerus was performed. The next day he set out on a leave of disability and rode to Fair Oaks Station beside the ambulance driver. He had a rough three-hour trip by freight car to White House Landing, where he boarded the steamer *Nelly Baker*. There were three or four ladies on board serving as nurses, and the surgeon redressed his arm. When Howard arrived in Baltimore he was put in the back of a hack and taken from the wharf to the railroad station. He remained briefly in the Astor House in New York City and then went home by steamer and railroad car. He was confined to his room for only three days. Ten days after his arrival he attended a meeting in Portland, Maine. On July 4, after speaking in Livermore, Maine, he slipped while going down the stairs. He tried to obtain support with his missing hand and drove the stump into the ground. A sole-leather protector prevented serious damage. He was absent until August 27 and was at Antietam early in September. The first week of October 1862 he developed a slow fever and on medical advice went on leave. His recovery was rapid, and he returned on November 5 in time for Fredericksburg. At Chancellorsville on May 2, 1863, his horse reared up, bruising Howard's leg and scratching his hand. In June he had a short period of fever but did not leave his command. He fought at Gettysburg. In September he had an inflammation of a tooth but did well on doses of opium. The next month he developed a cold and was absent on sick leave from October 17 to November 6, 1863. He was at Chattanooga and served in the Atlanta campaign as a corps commander and as commander of the Army of the Tennessee. At Pickett's Mill on May 27, 1864, his left foot was bruised by a shell fragment, which cut through the sole of his boot and through the upper leather. That night, in pain, he sat among the other wounded in a forest glade. At the end of the war he was promoted to brigadier general in the Regular Army. He was made first commissioner of the Freedmen's Bureau but his administration of the bureau was poor. His main contribution after the war was to help establish Howard University. He was promoted to major general in 1886 and retired in 1894. Died in Burlington, Vermont, on October 26, 1909, and was buried in Lake View Cemetery. According to a family member, he died of angina pectoris.[2]

1. WPCHR, vols. 607, 608, 609; LR, ACP, 638, 1872, fiche: 000058; Howard, *Autobiography* 1:54, 97.

2. *OR*, vol. 11, pt. 1:769–70, 783; vol. 19, pt. 2:433; RAGO, entry 623; Robert Hubbard to Nelie, Sept. 26, Oct. 19, 1863, bound book of typed copies, Robert Hubbard Letters, USAMHI; John Alcott Carpenter, "An Account of the Civil War Career of Oliver Otis Howard. Based on his Private Letters" (diss.), 21, 86; U.S. Army, CWS, roll 1, vol. 1, report 46, pp. 893–901; LR, ACP, 638, 1872, fiche: 000058; *MSHW*, vol. 2, pt. 2:726, case 402; RAGO, entry 623, "File D"; *Battles and Leaders* 4:308; Howard, *Autobiography* 1:128, 137, 246–55, 310, 386.

ALBION PARRIS HOWE • *Born March 13, 1818,* in Standish, Maine. Graduated from the USMA in 1841. While at West Point he was treated twice for pain in his back and once each for fever, bile, cold, and an inflamed eye. Served in the

Mexican War. Prior to the Civil War, he was an instructor at West Point and had frontier and garrison duty. He served as an artillery officer when the war started and was made a brigadier general to rank from June 1862. He served on the Peninsula and at Antietam, Fredericksburg, Chancellorsville, Gettysburg, and Mine Run. In 1863 he was placed in command of the artillery depot and of the Office of the Inspector of Artillery at Washington and remained in this position until 1866. Following the war he remained in the army and retired as colonel of the Fourth Artillery in 1882. During the summer of 1875 he had a bad fever and almost died. In August of the following year he had a medical leave because of continued pains and weakness of his back and lower limbs. He developed hemorrhoids in 1877. Died January 25, 1897, in Cambridge, Massachusetts, and was buried in Mount Auburn Cemetery, Cambridge. The attending physician said the cause of death was a "general giving out of the vital powers."[1]

1. WPCHR, vol. 604; LR, ACP, 3996, 1882.

JOSHUA BLACKWOOD HOWELL • *Born on September 11, 1806,* near Woodbury, New Jersey. A prewar lawyer and brigadier general of Pennsylvania Militia, he entered Federal service as colonel of the 85th Pennsylvania in November 1861. He was at New Bern and Charleston. Howell had a forty-day sick leave starting on August 9, 1862. On the night of August 16, 1863, a shell penetrated the splinter-proof shelter containing the telegraph instruments in front of Fort Wagner, South Carolina, and he was injured by the explosion. This produced a concussion, while the shell fragments bruised his head. He was sent north on sick leave in September and had returned by late October. In the middle of June 1864 he was ill due to general debility and residual injury to his brain, and he left on sick leave on July 28. He returned the next month. Near Petersburg on September 12, 1864, he was mortally injured when his horse reared and fell on him, inflicting injuries that rendered him speechless. He was moved into a vacant tent at the Tenth Corps headquarters. The next day he was suffering from violent contusions of his stomach and head and was taken to the hospital of the 85th Pennsylvania Volunteers. He never recovered enough to be able to talk intelligently after his injury and died on September 14.[1] He was buried in Eglington Memorial Gardens at Clarksboro, New Jersey. Seven months later he was posthumously named a brigadier general to rank from the date of his fatal accident.

1. CSR; *OR,* vol. 28, pt. 1:288, 343; vol. 38, pt. 2:302; vol. 40, pt. 2:153, pt. 3:584; RVA, Pension C 32,540.

ANDREW ATKINSON HUMPHREYS • *Born on November 2, 1810,* in Philadelphia. Graduated from the USMA in 1831. Served in the Florida wars. Broken in health from the exposure and fatigue endured in the Indian campaigns, he reached

Charleston, South Carolina, on September 25, 1836. His resignation from the
U.S. Army that same month was accepted. Soon afterward he had an attack of
"Florida illness" and was nursed back to health by his mother. He improved
slowly and was apparently in good health by May 1837. Humphreys reentered
the service as a first lieutenant, Corps of Topographical Engineers, to rank from
July 1838. In 1849 his health suffered from office work and he went on field duty.
He become seriously ill while working upon the Mississippi River and left New
Orleans in September 1851 on a surgeon's certificate of disability. He arrived at
Philadelphia late in the month. The fresh air, good nourishment, and rest recommended by his surgeon improved his health to some degree. However, he
was on sick leave from December 1, 1851, to May 2, 1853. He traveled on special
duty to Europe in May to improve his health, and to examine ways to protect
the Delta rivers from inundation. His headaches went away and he gained weight.
After he returned in July 1854, he was assigned to special service. His poor health
and the warm weather in May and June of 1861 prevented him from entering
any work in the field. He returned in October and was assigned to special duty
on the first of December. In March 1862 he was made a colonel of volunteers
and in April, brigadier general. He had some unspecified illness in June. He
returned to Washington City the last of August and was confined to his house
for a few days by sickness. He was promoted major general of volunteers in July
1863. Also, that summer he felt his position as chief of staff for Gen. George G.
Meade had allowed him to improve his health, so he continued in this position
until November 1864. He then assumed a corps command for the campaigns in
Virginia. In June 1865, because of his poor health as the result of his service on
the Gulf, he did not desire duty in Florida and turned down an offer to go there.
Made brigadier general, U.S. Army, and chief of engineers in August 1866, he
was mustered out of volunteer service the next month. His attending physician
from 1876 until his death stated that his headaches and nervous disturbances
indicated nerve exhaustion due to his duties, which had caused a great strain
on his intellectual powers. Humphreys was present sick from July to October
1878 and from February until June 1879, when he retired from active service at
his own request. Humphreys had at times suffered from attacks of lumbago. On
the day he died, December 27, 1883, in Washington, D.C., he had a similar attack. That evening he had been reading in the parlor and was found dead in his
chair. He was buried in the Congressional Cemetery in Washington.[1]
DEATH CERTIFICATE: Cause of death, atheroma of the coronary arteries of the
heart, syncope.

1. *OR*, vol. 11, pt. 1:153; vol. 12, pt. 3:640; vol. 49, pt. 2:1027; RVA, Pension WC 225,371; LR, ACP, 120, 1884, fiche: 000121; U.S. Army, CWS, roll 1, vol. 1, report 35, pp. 565–764; Henry H. Humphreys, *Andrew Atkinson Humphreys*, 43–45, 54, 60, 141–42, 155, 158, 167, 207, 325.

HENRY JACKSON HUNT • *Born September 14, 1819,* at Detroit, Michigan. Graduated from the USMA in 1839. Served in the Mexican War. As a child, he had a

number of respiratory infections, and by his teenage years he was deaf in one ear. While a cadet he was treated once each for a cold and diarrhea. He was slightly wounded by two spent balls during the attack on Molino del Rey on September 8, 1847, but remained on the field. In 1852 he developed headaches that were to remain with him for years. Until the start of the Civil War, Hunt had routine duty, except for his participation in the revision of the system of light artillery tactics. He played an active and important role in the development of Union artillery and was made brigadier general of volunteers in September 1862. He was at First Bull Run, Malvern Hill, Antietam, and Fredericksburg. On July 3, 1863, while at Gettysburg, his wounded horse fell on him and he was slightly injured. In the middle of the month he was incapacitated by overexertion and sunstroke. He continued as chief of artillery until June 1864 when he was placed in charge of all siege operations on the Petersburg line. He remained in the army after the Civil War and reverted to his rank of lieutenant colonel of the Third Artillery. From 1871 through 1881 he had episodes of migraine headache and rheumatism. During March 1873, unable to travel and suffering with a severe paroxysmal cough, he asked for an extension of his sick leave. He retired from the army in 1883. In the spring of 1887 he had increased difficulty with his rheumatism and gout, and his legs and ankles were grossly swollen. His migraine headaches continued, and he was totally deaf. He took large amounts of carbonate of lithium to ease the pain. He died at the Soldiers' Home in Washington, D.C., on February 11, 1889, and was buried there. The attending surgeon listed the cause of death as pneumonia.[1]

1. OR, vol. 40, pt. 3:219; WPCHR, vol. 604; LR, ACP, 3456, 1871, fiche: 000057; Edward G. Longacre, *The Man Behind the Guns*, 25, 53–54, 176, 205, 240, 252–53, 276; Heitman, *Historical Register and Dictionary* 2:25.

LEWIS CASS HUNT • *Born on February 23, 1824*, at Fort Howard at Green Bay, Wisconsin. Graduated from the USMA in 1847. He was treated at the Cadet Hospital for cephalalgia, phlegmon, and catarrhus five times each and once for contusio. Served in the Mexican War. While in Mexico he contracted diarrhea. In September 1854, his surgeon certified that moderate travel was required to improve his chronic diarrhea. He was promoted to captain, Fourth Infantry, in 1855. During the first half of 1857 he traveled in France, Italy, Austria, and Germany, where he was seen by a number of physicians who prescribed medicinal waters and baths for his diarrhea. The diarrhea improved but left him with weak bowels. As colonel of the 92nd New York, he was badly wounded in the groin by a rifle ball on May 31, 1862, during the Battle of Seven Pines. Hunt was given a leave and returned to his regiment in September for service in North Carolina. He was promoted to brigadier general of volunteers in November 1862. In the middle of May 1863, after being hospitalized for two weeks because of chronic diarrhea, he was sent north on leave. In July he was ordered to establish the Draft Rendezvous Camp at New Haven, Connecticut. Following the war, he was promoted lieutenant colonel in the Regular Army in 1868 and served throughout the West. In 1875 he developed eczema, which became chronic and was particularly bad in the winter months in the Dakotas. In November 1877 he went on sick leave because of his skin condition and returned in December when his regiment was ordered to San Antonio. Because of his eczema as well as carbuncles on the back of his neck and on the base of his skull, he required a leave in August 1879. His chronic diarrhea became worse after he left Texas in September 1880, and in December he went to Ann Arbor, Michigan, on sick leave. By the middle of 1882, he had improved but still had "weakness of his bowels" and needed to take astringent medications. He had to manage his activities and did not go to social events where a speedy exit could not be accomplished. By October he had noted that when his diarrhea occurred, his eczema was better, and when his diarrhea improved, his eczema was worse. He received homeopathic treatments and nux vomica and thought he was improving. Hunt remained most of the next year at Ann Arbor on medical leave. In November 1883 he developed itching of his hands, face, eyes, ears, scrotum, and inner portion of his thighs. This was associated with swelling and exudation of the fingers, upper portions of the hands and wrists, and the eyes and ears. He stated it looked like poison ivy. It finally spread over all his body and left permanent marks in the areas where the skin had been the most affected. Hunt reported this was similar to an attack he had seven years before while at Fort Totem, Dakota. He was using cold cream on his skin at night. A further extension of his leave was denied in February 1884, although he was confined to his home and complaining of great thirst. Hot sulphur spring waters were advised by his physician. While stationed at Vancouver Barracks in 1885, his diarrhea became so severe that he had to be hospitalized at San Diego, California, in November. In July 1886 he was confined to his bed with chronic diarrhea and did not want to go back to Vancouver. He stated he would rather retire or have sick leave. Hunt's retirement was refused and he was ordered to Fort Union, New Mexico, where he arrived thoroughly exhausted. Six days after his arrival on September 6, 1886, he died from the effects of the diarrhea, according to the post commander.[1] He was initially interred in the post cemetery, but later his remains were moved to the National Cemetery at Fort Leavenworth, Kansas.

1. CSR; OR, vol. 11, pt. 1:927; WPCHR, vols. 605, 606; U.S. Army, CWS, roll 2, vol. 3, report 51, pp. 1381–83; LR, ACP, 3918, 1877, fiche: 000064.

DAVID HUNTER · *Born July 21, 1802,* in Washington, D.C. Graduated from the USMA in 1822. Served in the Mexican War. Following duty on the frontier and in Chicago, he resigned in 1836. After six years of speculating in real estate in Chicago, he returned to the army in March 1842 as a major and paymaster. His association with Abraham Lincoln on the inaugural train to Washington helped him obtain his brigadier stars in May 1861. On July 21, 1861, at First Bull Run, he was wounded in the neck. He left the field in an ambulance and was taken to

Centreville, Virginia. In August 1861 he was promoted to major general of volunteers and was back in command the next month. He retired in 1866 with the rank of colonel and the brevets of brigadier and major general, U.S. Army. Hunter died at his residence in Washington, D.C., on February 2, 1886.[1] He was buried in Princeton, New Jersey.

DEATH CERTIFICATE: Cause of death, immediate, angina pectoris, onset sudden.

1. *OR*, vol. 2:315, 334, 384, 395, 746; LR, ACP, 1396, 1886, fiche: 000122; U.S. Army, CWS, roll 5, vol. 9, report 29, pp. 643–741; RVA, Pension WC 224,525.

STEPHEN AUGUSTUS HURLBUT • *Born November 29, 1815,* in Charleston, South Carolina. Served in the Florida wars. After practicing the law in South Carolina, he moved to Illinois in 1845 and became involved in politics. In July 1861 he was appointed a brigadier general of volunteers and was made a major general in September 1862. He commanded a division at Shiloh and Corinth. During the middle of December he had erysipelas about his face and eyes. Unfit for field duty, he could do office work. Gen. Henry W. Halleck prevented him from obtaining a leave until January 10, after which he was absent for a month. In July 1863 he resigned because he felt his health was failing but later withdrew the resignation. He was discharged from the service in June 1865.[1] Charges of drunkenness and corruption marred his postwar years, as it did his wartime service, but he still won two terms in Congress and became minister to Columbia and Peru. He died at the ministry in Lima, Peru, on March 27, 1882, and his body was returned to Belvedere, Illinois, where he was buried.

1. *OR,* vol. 17, pt. 2:508, 553; vol. 24, pt. 3:44; LR, CB, roll 26, H407, 1863.

RUFUS INGALLS • *Born on August 23, 1818,* at Denmark, Maine. He graduated from the USMA in 1843. At the academy he was treated for diarrhea twice and once each for a cold, burns, sore feet, and sore hands. Served in the Mexican War. At the start of the Civil War he was appointed chief quartermaster of the Army of the Potomac. Ingalls was sick in August 1862 and his work was impaired. He was promoted to major the same year and brigadier general of volunteers to rank from May 1863. On September 5, 1864, he obtained a sick leave. He remained in the army after the war and in 1866 was made assistant quartermaster general with the rank of colonel. Ingalls was appointed quartermaster general of the U.S. Army in February 1882 and retired the next year. He died at the Grand Hotel, New York City, on January 15, 1893, and was buried in Arlington National Cemetery.[1]

DEATH CERTIFICATE: Chief cause, fatty degeneration of the heart; contributing cause, syncope.

1. *OR,* vol. 11, pt. 1:85; vol. 19, pt. 2:173; vol. 42, pt. 2:631: WPCHR, vol. 604; LR, ACP, 2163, 1878, fiche: 000065.

J

CONRAD FEGER JACKSON • *Born on September 11, 1813,* in Alsace Township, Pennsylvania. He served in the Mexican War. Before the Civil War, he worked for the Reading Railroad and was a member of a militia company. Jackson was mustered into Federal service as colonel of the 9th Pennsylvania Reserves (38th Pennsylvania Infantry) and served on the Peninsula. He was promoted brigadier general to rank from July 1862. On August 30 after Second Bull Run, he was sick and had to leave the field. He was killed instantly by a bullet through his head at Fredericksburg on December 13, 1862. Both Jackson and an aide were shot and killed at the same time. Their bodies were not reclaimed for three days and were received under a flag of truce.[1] Jackson was buried in Allegheny Cemetery, Pittsburgh.

1. *OR,* vol. 12, pt. 2:395; vol. 21:59, 139, 451, 512, 522; RVA, Pension C 3,292.

JAMES STRESHLY JACKSON • *Born September 27, 1823,* in Fayette County, Kentucky. Served in the Mexican War. He practiced law and was a congressman when he resigned in December 1861 to become colonel of the 3rd Kentucky (Union) Cavalry. In July he was appointed brigadier general of volunteers. At the Battle of Perryville on October 8, 1862, Jackson was standing beside one of his batteries when he was hit in the right chest by two bullets. He tried to speak but died in a few minutes.[1] Jackson was buried in Riverside Cemetery, Hopkinsville, Kentucky.

1. *OR,* vol. 16, pt. 1:1050.

NATHANIEL JAMES JACKSON • *Born July 28, 1818,* at Newburyport, Massachusetts. A trained machinist, he was superintendent of a mill in Maine when the war started. Jackson was a member of a state militia group and entered Federal service as a colonel of the 1st Maine. On June 27, 1862, at the Battle of Gaines' Mill, Virginia, Jackson was wounded above the right elbow by a shell fragment. He was taken to the hospital at Annapolis, Maryland, for treatment. Jackson was given a leave on account of disability on July 6. At Crampton Gap, Maryland, on September 14, 1862, he received a wound in his knee from a musket ball. This wound did not disable him, and he was treated in camp. He was made a brigadier general that month. On April 17, 1863, while crossing a swamp at night near Chancellorsville, Virginia, his horse slipped, and Jackson's right thigh was fractured. It was an oblique fracture of the lower third of the femur. He was admitted to the Georgetown Seminary Hospital the next day and remained there through July. From August 1863 to September 1864 he was on duty at the Draft Rendezvous, Riker's Island, New York. In November he assumed command of the First Division, Twentieth Corps, and participated in the Savannah campaign. At some point during the march from Atlanta to Savannah in early December he received a slight flesh wound above the right internal malleolus from a pistol shot. It apparently caused little disability, and he did not mention it in his report on the campaign. He was mustered out of service in August 1865. By February 1878 he had limited motion and enlargement of his right knee. Two healed scars from gunshot wounds were present. One was at the outer edge of the right patella and the other was five inches above the internal malleolus. There was a three-inch-long scar from the right elbow joint, which ran along the inner side of the humerus. He had lost half of his hearing in his right ear, and there was loss of sensation in his right forearm and hand. An examination in 1886 revealed that the upper portion of the previously fractured femur overlapped the lower portion, and the right thigh was three-fourths of an inch shorter than the left. The area of the fracture and the leg below were enlarged and the motion of the knee joint reduced by half. He was very lame and was unable to stoop to the floor. In October 1891 he had a stroke. There was improvement by the next year, but he required constant attention. Died April 21, 1892, at Jamestown, New York, and was buried in Newburyport.[1]

DEATH CERTIFICATE: Cause of death, cerebral hemorrhage.

1. CSR; *OR*, vol. 11, pt. 2:434, 449–50; vol. 25, pt. 1:676; vol. 39, pt. 3:742; vol. 44:216; U.S. Army, CWS, roll 3, vol. 4, report 6, pp. 145–52; RVA, Pension SC 152,097.

RICHARD HENRY JACKSON • *Born July 14, 1830,* at Kinnegad, Westmeath County, Ireland. Served in the Florida wars. Jackson entered the U.S. Army as a private in 1851 and, after passing through enlisted ranks, was commissioned a brevet second lieutenant by examination in 1859. He had been treated for intermittent fever in October 1857, constipation in February 1858, and diarrhea in April. Jackson was not made a brigadier general of volunteers until May 1865, but he had served in Florida, South Carolina, and in the Petersburg campaign. In February 1866 he was discharged from volunteer service and resumed his regular rank as captain. In May 1871 he requested a six-month leave to go to Europe for the benefit of his health and business. During August 1884 he had "neuralgia of the membranes of the brain complicated with rheumatism" and was on sick leave from August 12 to September 11. In February 1885 he was treated for vertigo. On July 30, 1885, Jackson was commanding the Guard of Honor for the remains of Gen. U. S. Grant at Mount McGregor, New York, when he was struck by lightning. Injured with a contusion of his neck, face, and body, he was on sick leave until September. The last of the year, he was treated for acute dyspepsia. For a number of years he had chronic inflammation of the neck of his urinary bladder and prostatic enlargement associated with frequent urination and constant pain. However, it did not interfere with his duties until May 1891. He was admitted to the hospital at Station McPherson, Atlanta, Georgia in June, and was

off duty until September. An episode of epidemic catarrh resulted in another hospitalization for two weeks in January 1892. A lieutenant colonel, he was hospitalized at Station McPherson on November 9, 1892, and died there on November 28.[1] He was buried in the National Cemetery at West Point.
HOSPITAL CARD: Cause of death, acute inflammatory rheumatism. Complication, inflammation of the meninges of the base of the brain.

1. LR, ACP, 1928, 1879, fiche: 000123; RVA, Pension C 419,019.

CHARLES DAVIS JAMESON • *Born on February 24, 1827,* in Orono, Maine. A prosperous businessman and commander of a state militia regiment at the start of the Civil War, he was elected colonel of the 2nd Maine. His promotion as brigadier general ranked from September 1861. At the Battle of Seven Pines on May 31, 1862, his horse was killed and fell on Jameson's leg. The horse was lifted off of him, and he was helped away from the field. Soon afterward he contracted a fever, took a leave of absence, and returned to Maine. According to his attending physician, he died in his residence on November 6, 1862, at Oldtown, Maine, of typhoid fever.[1] He was buried in Riverside Cemetery, Stillwater, Maine.

1. OR, vol. 11, pt. 1:814; vol. 25, pt. 2:141, 187; RVA, Pension WC 30,508.

ANDREW JOHNSON • *Born December 29, 1808,* in Raleigh, North Carolina. Johnson was elected to Congress in 1843 and served in this capacity for ten years. While a member of Congress he broke his right wrist in a railroad accident. The fracture was poorly set, making it painful for him to write afterward. He was governor of Tennessee from 1853 to 1857 and United States senator from 1857 to 1862. In March 1862 he was appointed military governor of Tennessee and brigadier general of volunteers. Chronic diarrhea and a high fever afflicted him in 1864. He resigned from the army in March 1865 to accept the position of vice president of the United States. He gave a rambling inaugural speech, supposedly due to the large glass of alcohol his doctor had recommended for his diarrhea and abdominal cramps. After the assassination of President Abraham Lincoln he became seventeenth president of the United States. While president, his chronic dysentery continued, and he had trouble with kidney stones. After he returned to Tennessee in 1869, he had an episode of malaria. When an epidemic of cholera occurred in Tennessee in 1873, he did not flee, as many did, but remained to help the sick. He contracted the disease and was weakened by the episode for the rest of his life. On July 30, 1875, near Elizabethton, Tennessee, while with his granddaughter, he had a stroke, which resulted in left-sided paralysis. Following a second stroke the next day, bleeding was performed, but he succumbed and was buried in the Andrew Johnson National Cemetery in Greeneville.[1]

1. Marx, *Health of the Presidents,* 195–203.

RICHARD W. JOHNSON • *Born February 27, 1827,* near Smithland, Kentucky. Graduated from the USMA in 1849. While at West Point, he was treated for odontalgia, catarrhus, cephalalgia, and clavus twice each and contusio, boil, excoriatio, rheumatism, and diarrhea once each. Johnson spent his service on the frontier before the Civil War and was made a brigadier general of volunteers in October 1861. He was captured and exchanged in 1862, then served at Stones River, Chickamauga, Chattanooga, and in the early stages of the Atlanta campaign. He was ill with bronchitis, intermittent fever, and diarrhea at Columbia, Tennessee, and was on sick leave from March 29 to April 13, 1862. Because of what his surgeon termed as a long-continued bilious derangement connected with fever of a remittent type, he received another sick leave from September 29 to November 15, 1863. In October, while on leave, he developed diarrhea. Johnson was struck by part of a shell on the right side during the Battle of New Hope Church, Georgia, on May 27, 1864. Severely bruised and already in poor health, he had to give up his command and leave the field. During July he was having severe pain of the right side between the costal margin and the hip. He reported back for duty in late August and resumed command. Following his last injury he was never physically able to be in the field, although he continued on duty for the rest of the war. His surgeon reported that in October 1866 he had been treating Johnson for congestion and defective action of the liver, secondary to his injury. He retired as major general in 1867 because of disability from wounds.[1] After returning to civilian life, Johnson was an educator and author. He died April 21, 1897, in St. Paul, Minnesota, and was buried there in Oakland Cemetery.

DEATH CERTIFICATE: Cause of death, acute pneumonia.

1. CSR; *OR,* vol. 10, pt. 1:306; vol. 38, pt. 1:93, 195, 523–24, 561–62, 596; WPCHR, vols. 605, 606, 607; U.S. Army, CWS, roll 1, vol. 1, report 18, pp. 277–83; ibid., roll 4, vol. 7, report 35, pp. 511–14; RG 94, Office of the Adj. General, Records and Pensions Office, Military Officers Personnel File, R & P 481,455; RVA, Pension, C 495,026.

PATRICK HENRY JONES • *Born on November 20, 1830,* in County Westmeath, Ireland. He left his law practice in June 1861 and was mustered into Federal service as a second lieutenant of the 37th New York. During May and June 1862 he had an attack of malaria. He was sick in a hospital in Washington, D.C., from September 26 to October 31, 1862. In October he was made colonel of the 154th New York. At Chancellorsville on May 2, 1863, he was slightly wounded in the right hip and captured. On May 15 he was paroled, and in July he was hospitalized in Washington, D.C. In August he had an episode of amaurosis (blindness); after being hospitalized at Annapolis, Maryland, he returned to duty in September. He was on detached service in charge of paroled prisoners in October and was back to duty in November. He had sick leave in February 1864. Although not well in May, he was with his command for the Atlanta campaign. On May 8,

1864 at Mill Creek Gap, Georgia, he received a contusion of his side and was seriously injured when his horse fell over a cliff. After being discharged from the hospital, he reported that he was fit for duty on June 7. During the last six months of 1864, he had chronic diarrhea. His surgeon stated that he needed a change of climate and mode of living, so in December Jones went north on leave. His promotion to brigadier general ranked from that month. In April 1865 he rejoined his brigade at Goldsboro, North Carolina, and resigned in June. He mainly practiced the law after the war. In later years, his physician blamed his deafness on his exposure to cannon fire and his chronic malaria and diarrhea to his service in the swamps along the Chickahominy River. In addition, he had almost constant pain in the area of the right sciatic nerve, secondary, the surgeon suggested, to his wound in the gluteal region. Usually every spring and fall he had attacks of chills and fever, which would last approximately a week or two and would confine him to his bed. For his episodes of jaundice he took calomel, followed by citrate of magnesia and some type of patent Indian medicine. On examination in October 1886, the scar where the bullet had entered was about two inches below the trochanter major and was the size of a ten-cent piece. The exit scar was about four inches back and an inch below the first scar. There was enlargement of his liver and spleen by percussion, his skin looked anemic, the conjunctiva were yellowish, and he was emaciated. In August 1898 his liver and spleen were still enlarged, and he appeared more emaciated and debilitated. Some weeks before his death he developed severe gastroenteritis. The condition did not respond to therapy, and he could not control his bowels. He could not eat solids and took only scalded milk with some brandy.[1] Jones died July 23, 1900, at Port Richmond, Staten Island, and was buried there in St. Peter's Cemetery.

DEATH CERTIFICATE: Direct cause, cardiac failure. Indirect cause, gastroenteritis.

1. CSR; *OR*, vol. 38, pt. 1:98, pt. 2:204; vol. 47, pt. 1:589, 699; RVA, Pension C 584,171, 2 parts.

HENRY MOSES JUDAH • *Born June 12, 1821,* in Snow Hill, Maryland. Graduated from the USMA in 1843. He was treated one time each for a toothache, nausea, rheumatism, headache, cold, and constipation while a cadet. Served in the Mexican War. Prior to the Civil War he had sick leaves from July 5, 1852, to June 19, 1853, and from May 31 to July 9, 1856. The surgeon who took care of him reported later that he had contracted inflammatory rheumatism during these years of service, which frequently attacked the pericardium of his heart and later produced enlargement and valvular disease of that organ. After service on the West Coast, he returned to the East in 1861 and was made a brigadier general of volunteers in March 1862. He had a sick leave from June 16 to July 16, 1862. He relinquished command, went on sick leave September 20, and returned in October. In August 1863 he applied for a sick leave for the purpose of having a surgical operation performed. No other details are available. He returned on

September 12 and reported at Knoxville, Tennessee. In May 1864, he was granted
a leave because of an episode of typhoid fever. He had routine administrative
duties for the rest of the war.[1] When peace came, he reverted to the rank of
major and commanded a garrison in New York. Died January 14, 1866, at
Plattsburg Barracks, New York, and was buried at Westport, Connecticut, in
Kings Highway Cemetery.

1. *OR*, vol. 38, pt. 1:112, pt. 2:511, pt. 4:247; U.S. Army, CWS, roll 1, vol. 2, report 7, pp. 83–86;
WPCHR, vol. 604; LR, ACP, 260, 1876, fiche: 000124; RVA, Pension, C 85,096.

K

THOMAS LEIPER KANE • *Born on January 27, 1822,* at Philadelphia. Prior to the
Civil War he studied the law, joined the Mormons, and founded a village in
Pennsylvania, which was given his name. Kane entered the war as a lieutenant
colonel of the 13th Pennsylvania Reserves (42nd Pennsylvania Volunteers). He
was ill and unfit for duty on December 2, 1861, but continued on the field. On
December 20 at Dranesville, Virginia, he was wounded by a ball in the right
side of the face. The ball passed through the right cheek, struck the superior
maxillary bone, knocked out one molar tooth and, passing across the other
side, knocked out two upper molars. The malar branch of the facial nerve and
infraorbital nerve on the left side were damaged. After being treated in camp,
he was taken to Washington, D.C., on December 24 for treatment. Within a few
weeks, his face wound produced neuralgia and difficulty with his vision, which
added to his suffering. On June 6, 1862, near Harrisonburg, Virginia, he was
wounded below the right knee. Faint from shock and loss of blood, he was left
on the field. When he tried to sit up after the fight was over, he was struck in the
middle of his chest by the butt end of a Confederate's rifle, knocked unconscious, and captured. Paroled in a few days, he was examined in Philadelphia by
a surgeon on June 19. The wound in his leg had been treated poorly and was in
bad condition. The surgeon opened the wound and removed a portion of a
split pistol ball along with spicules of bone and shreds of clothing. The ball had
entered about two and one-half inches below the knee and about three quarters of an inch from the crest of the tibia and passed to the other side. After
striking the bone it must have split, one fragment passing out on the outer side
of the calf and the other passing downwards, lodging in the belly of the tibialis
anteriors muscle. The lower end of the sternum had been broken by the rifle
butt. Kane was in Philadelphia on July 8, 1862, and was unable to travel because
of his wound and camp diarrhea. On his return to the army in August, he had
to be assisted to mount and dismount his horse and could not walk without
crutches. His appointment as brigadier general of volunteers ranked from September. That same month, he had boils and an abscess of his wound. Even after
the wound appeared to heal, it continued to intermittently open and suppurate

over the next two years. While crossing the Rapidan River on the night of April 28–29, 1863, his horse stumbled, and Kane was drenched and developed pleurisy. In late May, in addition to the pleurisy, he developed pneumonia. He was so sick that he had to be carried by stretcher to Aquia Creek, where he took a boat to Washington, D.C., and then went to a hospital in Philadelphia. Still ill, and since communication with the army at Gettysburg was cut off, he had to make his way through Confederate lines in citizen's dress. He finally reached the battlefield in an ambulance and resumed command of his brigade on the morning of July 2, 1863. Before long, however, his wound reopened, and he was so ill he gave up command and went back to Philadelphia for treatment. He resigned from the army for reasons of poor health in November 1863. He had pains in his depressed sternum, ulceration of the upper jaw, altered vision, and was spitting up blood. After he returned to civilian life he attended to land in northwestern Pennsylvania, was president of the board of public charities, and served as a railroad president. When he was examined in 1882 there was a small cicatrix over the right upper maxilla, and the roof of the mouth was dark red to purple with a tender spot. The sternum was depressed an inch in depth, and there was a loud systolic murmur over the whole precordium, loudest in the area of the apex. Breath sounds over the left infraxillary area were altered. He had markedly decreased vision. Kane died December 26, 1883, in his residence at Philadelphia and was buried in Laurel Hill Cemetery.[1]

DEATH CERTIFICATE: Cause of death, pneumonia, acute lobar.

1. CSR; *OR*, vol. 5:474, 480; vol. 12, pt. 1:18, 676, 712; vol. 27, pt. 1:846, 848–49; RVA, Pension, C 208,488.

AUGUST VALENTINE KAUTZ • *Born January 5, 1828,* in the province of Baden, Germany. Served in the Mexican War. Graduated from the USMA in 1852. On October 25, 1855, during a fight with Indians at Grave and Cow creeks, Oregon, a bullet hit him in the right chest. He probably would have been killed but for two books in his pocket. The ball passed through the corner of one book but was stopped by the second and only knocked him down. He was wounded in the leg on March 1, 1856, at Muckleshute Prairie, Washington Territory. In May 1861 he was made a captain and served in the defenses of Washington. He had an attack of acute rheumatism and was on sick leave from November 12–22. Kautz went to New York City to avail himself of the electrical baths in that city. Subjected to a severe snowstorm in late March 1862, he became ill and was confined to the hospital at Fortress Monroe from April 1–29 with orchitis. He was premature in rejoining his regiment on the Peninsula and had a relapse on May 4. By May 10 he was able to ride and joined his regiment. During June and July he had periods when he was not well, and he remained in his tent and took quinine. In September 1862 he was appointed colonel of the 2nd Ohio Cavalry volunteer regiment. Throughout 1863 he had episodes of rheumatism, ague, colds, and headaches. He was appointed a brigadier general of volunteers in May 1864 and served in the Petersburg campaign. In the middle of October he had malarial fever, which did not respond to therapy. He obtained a leave on October 24 and returned in the middle of the next month. After the war he remained in the U.S. Army, reaching the rank of brigadier general in 1891. On leave in Karlsbad, Bohemia, in July 1883, he reported that he was under medical treatment but did not describe his condition. While president of a court-martial in Washington state in February 1887, he had a sudden attack of gastrointestinal dyspepsia and obstinate constipation. In the spring and fall of 1890, the spring of 1893, and from June to September 1895, he had a flare-up of symptoms, suggesting an ulcer. Died September 4, 1895, in Seattle, Washington, and was buried in Arlington National Cemetery. At postmortem examination there was a perforated duodenal ulcer within an inch of the pylorus and scars from old gastric disease.[1]

DEATH CERTIFICATE: Simple chronic ulcer of duodenum.

1. *OR Suppl.*, vol. 2, pt. 1:112–17, 126, 131; U.S. Army, CWS, roll 6, vol. 10, report 31, pp. 189–209; "Daily Journal 1863," August Valentine Kautz Papers, USAMHI; RVA, Pension C 429766; Crook, *George Crook*, 29; Heitman, *Historical Register and Dictionary* 2:26.

PHILIP KEARNY • *Born on June 2, 1815,* in New York City. Served in the Mexican War. Having inherited a fortune in 1836, he did not have to work, so he engaged in military activities. He was commissioned a second lieutenant in the Regular U.S. Army in 1837. In 1839 he attended the French Cavalry School at Saumur and served with the Chasseurs d'Afrique in Algiers in 1840. His left arm was shattered by grapeshot on August 20, 1847, at Churubusco, Mexico. He was carried to the rear, and the arm was amputated above the elbow. Following an absence on account of his wound, he had recruiting duty from May 1848 until August 1851. After rejoining his regiment in October 1851, he resigned. During the early part of 1854, Kearny was almost killed when his horse fell with him through a rotting bridge. He served in Napoleon III's Imperial Guard during the Italian War. When the Civil War started he returned home from Europe and was made a brigadier general to rank from May 1861. In April 1862 his health had improved, and he no longer had irregularities of his pulse, which had bothered him in the past. At the Battle of Charles City Cross Roads on June 30, 1862, a shell burst over his head; small fragments hit Kearny on the breast without causing injury. In August he suffered from the heat, and he was weak from having eaten little for ten to twelve days. He was well when in the saddle, but once he dismounted he felt tired and weak and had to lie down on his back. At Chantilly on September 1, 1862, he inadvertently rode into Confederate lines and, lying low on his horse, was killed instantly by a rifle ball. The ball entered his body through the gluteal muscles at a point a little back of the articulation of the left hip joint. The ball impinged on the bones of the pelvis, penetrated the os innominatum, and passed through the abdominal viscera to just above the umbilicus and lodged between the skin and the sternum. It formed a distinct and discolored tumor just above the center of the chest.[1] He was first buried in Trinity Churchyard, New York City, but later his remains were removed to Arlington National Cemetery.

1. *OR,* vol. 12, pt. 3:586, 805, 807, 811; vol. 25, pt. 2:141; LR, ACP, 1505, 1877, fiche: 000126; Philip Kearny, *Letters from the Peninsula: The Civil War Letters of General Philip Kearny,* ed. William B. Styple, 13–14, 47–48, 123, 152, 156, 181.

WILLIAM HIGH KEIM • *Born June 25, 1813,* near Reading, Pennsylvania. A politician, he participated in state military affairs prior to the Civil War. He was commissioned major general of Pennsylvania militia in April 1861. In December he was appointed a brigadier general of volunteers. During the Battle of Williamsburg, Virginia, on May 5, 1862, he was so sick he was barely able to sit on his horse. Three days later he made his report, which was incomplete "owing to severe indisposition." He arrived in Harrisburg, Pennsylvania, on May 14 and died four days later. According to his wife, he died from typhoid fever, while his son reported that he died from camp fever. He was buried in Charles Evans Cemetery, Reading.[1]

1. *OR,* vol. 11, pt. 1:561–62, pt. 3:186; RVA, Pension WC 348.

BENJAMIN FRANKLIN KELLEY • *Born on April 10, 1807,* in New Hampton, New Hampshire. A freight agent for a railroad, he helped recruit the 1st [West] Virginia in May 1861. His appointment as brigadier general of volunteers ranked from the same month. While leading the ninety-day regiment, he was severely wounded in the chest by a pistol shot at the Battle of Philippi, West Virginia, on June 3, 1861. He had been striking with his sword at one of the retreating Rebels while going down the town's street when the man turned and shot him. He was carried into the town where he received surgical care. The next day Gen. George B. McClellan ordered his surgeon to go to Philippi to take care of him. He arrived to find that that Kelley had lost considerable blood and was still bleeding profusely. The ball had passed through the right shoulder below the collarbone and struck near the middle of the flat part of the shoulder blade, breaking and bulging it out so there was a rounded enlargement on the back part of the bone. The surgeon felt the blood loss was more capillary than large vessel and dressed the wound. The next day Kelley was sent to Grafton; by the first of August, he had partially recovered and was given command of the District of Grafton. During an examination that fall, the surgeon found a large mass that extended some distance below the lower part of the shoulder blade. He opened it and a large quantity of matter was discharged, along with a musket ball and a quantity of fragments of clothes and lining. The external wound healed, but the remaining tissue mass was painful. He was relieved of command at his own request on January 10, 1862. Kelley remained under treatment until he had recovered enough to take the field. On April 1, 1862, he was appointed to the command of the Railroad District of the Mountain Department. He had a severe cold on January 7, 1864. He was captured by Confederate partisans in February 1865 and, after his release, resigned from the army in June. During his remaining years he held a number of Federal positions. Exercise produced uncontrollable twitching in his side, while cold weather caused difficulty breathing. He had neuralgia, rheumatism, and loss of power in his right arm. He died July 16, 1891, in Oakland, Maryland, and was buried in Arlington National Cemetery. Physician's affidavit: Died of disease of the right lung caused by a gunshot wound which passed through the upper part of the lung.[1]

1. *OR*, vol. 2:65; vol. 5:552; vol. 33:362; vol. 51, pt. 1:513, 564; *OR Suppl.*, vol. 1, pt. 1:112; U.S. Army, CWS, roll 1, vol. 2, report 52, pp. 719–49; RVA, Pension, C 315,028; *MOLLUS* 24:124.

JOHN REESE KENLY • *Born January 11, 1818,* in Baltimore, Maryland. Served in the Mexican War. A practicing lawyer and militia member in Baltimore, he was commissioned colonel of the 1st Maryland (Union) Infantry in June 1861. Kenly was knocked senseless from his horse by a pistol shot while riding to Winchester on May 23, 1862. He was captured and that night was carried into Front Royal. After a few days he was returned to Winchester and paroled on June 4, his wound having made him unfit for the Confederate forces to take him with them. He returned to his home in Baltimore, and when he was officially exchanged in August he started reorganizing his old regiment. That same month he was made a brigadier general of volunteers and served in both the Bristol campaign and in the early stages of the Overland campaign. Kenly was brevetted major general in 1865 and was discharged in August.[1] He died at Baltimore on December 20, 1891, and was buried in Green Mount Cemetery. Burial records: Cause of death, pneumonia.

1. *OR*, vol. 12, pt. 1:527, 535, 537, 558, 564; U.S. Army, CWS, roll 1, vol. 1, report 32, pp. 409–512.

JOHN HENRY KETCHAM • *Born December 21, 1832,* in Dutchess County, New York. Before the war he was a farmer and politician. In October 1862 he entered Federal service as colonel of the 150th New York. Within a short time he was brevetted brigadier general of volunteers. Ketcham was at Gettysburg and in the Atlanta campaign. He developed some deafness from cannon fire in July 1864. On December 21, 1864, soon after he rejoined his regiment at Argyle Island in front of Savannah, Georgia, he received a flesh wound. The ball entered just below and back of the left trochanter, passed through the muscle of the thigh and the scrotum near the testicle, and then exited below the buttocks. He was treated in a house used as part of the field hospital in the city of Savannah until his wounds were nearly healed. Ketcham was on sick leave until March 1865 when he resigned his commission in order to take a seat in Congress. For the rest of his life he held political positions. He had diminished hearing that was more marked in his left ear. The strength of the left thigh was decreased and the right testicle was atrophied.[1] He died in a private hospital in New York City on November 4, 1906, and was buried in Valley View Cemetery, Dover Plains, New York.

DEATH CERTIFICATE: Exhaustion, hemiplegia following cerebral apoplexy.

1. CSR; *OR*, vol. 44:209, 219, 237, 247; RVA, Pension C 184,652.

WILLIAM SCOTT KETCHUM • *Born July 7, 1813,* at Norwalk, Connecticut. Graduated from the USMA in 1834. During the time he was at West Point he was treated twice for a cold and once each for a wound, neck pain, headache, and catarrhus. He served in the Florida wars and on the frontier after graduation, reaching the rank of lieutenant colonel by 1861. He was made a brigadier of volunteers to rank from February 1862. Ketchum primarily had staff duties and was concerned with inspection, recruiting, and auditing. Following the war he spent four years on special service in the adjutant general's office in Washington, D.C., before retiring in December 1870. Ketchum died in Baltimore on June 28, 1871. Elizabeth G. Wharton, the owner of a boarding house, was suspected of killing him. A trial was held. The prosecution theorized that Mrs. Wharton was in debt to Ketchum and had invited him to her house for the purpose of poisoning him. She was supposed to have accomplished this by means of tartar emetic. On June 24, 1871, Ketchum had come from Washington to stay at Mrs. Wharton's house in Baltimore. He ate a hearty meal that evening, his first of the day, and went to bed. During the night he was sick and got very little sleep. On June 25 he visited with friends and ate with them. That evening, again at Mrs. Wharton's, he had a glass of lemonade, to which he added brandy. Later he suffered some slight vomiting and purging. Sick on June 26, he remained in his room all day, although he took each of his meals. A physician was called in the afternoon, and he found Ketchum sitting up and vomiting into a jar held between his knees. Regarding the case as an attack of cholera morbus, he ordered Ketchum to bed and directed him to take a mixture of limewater and creosote every two hours. His health improved, Ketchum told his physician on the next day, June 27, that he planned to return to Washington. However, throughout the day he became drowsy, had to be aroused, and appeared to be under the influence of some narcotic. A vial was discovered in his room, and he admitted to taking some laudanum. That evening he was found on a lounge sleeping heavily and breathing deeply. On the morning of June 28 he was still lying on the lounge. The physician was called again and discovered him in a semicomatose state, very difficult to arouse, and giving inarticulate answers. When Ketchum was touched, a slight convulsive tremor passed over him from head to foot. His face had a purplish tinge and his arms and legs were stiff and rigid. His pupils were not contracted but insensitive to light. Treatment consisted of application of ice to his head for the first hour; then he was given forty drops of tincture of gelsemium in a small amount of water. The gelsemium was repeated in two hours, and about one o'clock in the afternoon he had a convulsion characteristic of opisthotonos. The doctor returned to administer chloroform by inhalation to control the spasms and also to obtain a catherized urine specimen to test for albumin, as he suspected uremia. However, the urine examination was not remarkable. Afterward, Ketchum was given thirty grains of chloral hydrate mixed in a small amount of milk; administering it to him was difficult due to the violence of the convulsions. Ketchum bit the spoon so hard that his middle front tooth was loosened. No benefit was derived from the treatment, and he died about 3:00 P.M. in a convulsion. A limited autopsy was performed the next day, and only the brain and contents of the abdomen were examined. Again, nothing remarkable was found. The attending physician had not considered poisoning until the last hour of Ketchum's life. His suspicions were raised when a tumbler of milk punch with some white sediment was found in another room. A few days later he was informed that at least twenty grains of tartar emetic were found in the stomach contents. Because of a strong prejudice in the public mind against Mrs. Wharton in the city of Baltimore, the trial was moved to Annapolis. It terminated on January 24, 1872, after fifty-two days of a very involved and convoluted trial. Ketchum's body was disinterred for examination twice, the second time without knowledge of the defense. This time the liver and other viscera were analyzed. At the end of the trial Mrs. Wharton was judged not guilty. Some of the most prominent symptoms of tartar emetic poisoning were absent. The tests employed to determine the presence of tartar emetic and its possible amount were shown to be fallacious, and the whole chemical evidence was discredited. The glass of milk punch was not intended for the general but for another person in the house.[1] He was buried in Rock Creek Cemetery, Georgetown, D.C.

1. WPCHR, vols. 601, 603; John J. Reese, "A Review of the Recent Trial of Mrs. Elizabeth G. Wharton on the Charge of Poisoning General W. S. Ketchum," *American Journal of Medical Science* 63 (Apr. 1872): 329–55.

ERASMUS DARWIN KEYES • *Born May 29, 1810,* in Brimfield, Massachusetts. Graduated from the USMA in 1832. He was treated once for a wound and once for a cold while at West Point. An instructor at the military academy after graduation, he was also an aide and military secretary to Winfield Scott. He was promoted to colonel of the 11th Infantry in May 1861 and brigadier general to rank from the same month. He was on the Peninsula and at Gettysburg. Due to a controversy with Gen. John Adams Dix as well as his poor health, he resigned in May 1864.[1] He moved to San Francisco and became a wealthy, prominent businessman. Died in Nice, France, on October 14, 1895. He was finally buried at West Point.

1. WPCHR, vol. 601; LR, CB, roll 102, K173, 1864.

JAMES LAWLOR KIERNAN • *Born October 26, 1837,* at Mount Bellew, County Galway, Ireland. He graduated from medical school and practiced in New York. After serving as a surgeon of the 6th Missouri (Union) Cavalry during the first part of the war, he apparently preferred to fight and was appointed major of the unit. On March 7, 1862, at the Battle of Pea Ridge, he was wounded when a musket ball passed through his right leg and fractured the tibia. He was treated from March 9–25 in Cassville and from March 27 to April 30 at Jefferson Hospital at St. Louis. On May 6, 1863, his regiment was ordered to recapture some ambulances taken by the enemy near Port Gibson, Mississippi. During the skirmish he was thrown from his horse and was wounded in the left shoulder and lung. Left for dead in a swamp, he was captured. Despite his wounds, he was able to escape. He was treated at the U.S. general hospital at Grand Gulf, Mississippi, from May 10 to June 2. Kiernan was appointed brigadier general of volunteers in August 1863. During autumn of that year, while in Louisiana, he contracted malaria. In November he received a sick leave because of the malaria, and his wound had reopened. He resigned from Federal service on February 3, 1864, due to failing health. He served at a consular post in China for a short time and then returned to the practice of medicine in New York. By October 1868, the gunshot wound to the chest had healed, but the bullet remained in place, impeded respiration, and caused occasional hemorrhage. The wound of the leg had also healed, and he had frequent congestive chills. Died November 27, 1869, in New York City and was buried in Green-Wood Cemetery, Brooklyn. The surgeons who took care of him at the time of his death reported he died from "congestion of lungs" brought on by his chest wound and malaria.[1]

1. CSR; RVA, Pension WC 143,386; Steiner, *Physician Generals,* 58.

HUGH JUDSON KILPATRICK • *Born on January 14, 1836,* near Deckertown, New Jersey. Graduated from the USMA in 1861. While at West Point he was treated for phlegmon six times, cephalalgia four times, nausea three times, contusio, ophthalmia, subluxatio, and diarrhea twice each, and otitis, otalgia, cholera morbus, catarrhus, excoriatio, and rheumatism once each. In May 1861 he was made a captain of the 5th New York Infantry. During the skirmish at Big Bethel, Virginia, on June 10, 1861, he was wounded in the thigh by grapeshot. The shot had first torn the insignia off the shoulder of a nearby officer. Kilpatrick remained on the field until the end of the fighting; then, unable to walk, he was assisted off of the field by three men. On July 1 he went to New York and remained there for the rest of the month to recover and recruit. He returned to duty in the middle of August. He was made a lieutenant colonel of the 2nd New York Cavalry in September 1861. While advancing on Fredericksburg on April 19, 1862, he was slightly wounded in the knee. Throughout 1863 he complained frequently of pain in his back and kidney area, particularly after periods of exertion. During such episodes he had to travel stretched out in an ambulance. He was promoted to brigadier general in June. In the middle of July 1863, after Gettysburg, he obtained a leave of absence because of the pain in his side. He rejoined his troops on August 4. On May 13, 1864, on the road to Resaca, a Confederate jumped up from ten feet away and shot Kilpatrick. The minié ball entered the inner side of the left thigh in its upper third, passed behind the femoral artery and femur, and passed out on the opposite side close to the sciatic nerve. The muscles of the posterior part of the thigh were severely lacerated. The wound was dressed on the field, and he was sent to the rear. He went back to duty in late July after recuperating at West Point, Georgia. On his return, and for many months afterward, he was unable to ride much on horse-back because of pain and soreness caused by the pressure of the saddle on the area of the wound. He continued to have difficulty walking because of the con-tracted leg muscles, and he had numbness of the whole limb while sitting. Fre-quently he had to travel in a carriage. The last of 1865 he resigned all of his commissions and accepted the appointment as minister to the Republic of Chile. After an unsuccessful campaign to be elected to Congress, he was reappointed minister to Chile. On December 4, 1881, he died in Santiago, Chile. He was entombed in the parochial church of Sagrario, Santiago de Chile, and was ulti-mately buried at West Point. The cause of death according to his attending physician was nephritis (Bright's disease).[1]

1. CSR; *OR*, vol. 2:89–90; vol. 27, pt. 1:1004; vol. 38, pt. 1:102, pt. 2:747, 858, 889, 895; vol. 51, pt. 1:69, 376; WPCHR, vol. 609; U.S. Army, CWS, roll 2, vol. 3, report 25, pp. 677–707; RVA, Pension WC 208,359.

NATHAN KIMBALL • *Born November 22, 1822*, in Fredericksburg, Indiana. Kimball practiced medicine before and after the Mexican War. At Monterey, Mexico, on December 27, 1846, he developed bloody flux, which led to chronic inflammation of the bowel and incapacitated him for service. At Buena Vista in February 1847 he was wounded twice by bullets. Kimball applied for a pension because of the disabilities incurred during the Mexican War, but by July 1851 his health had improved so much that he did not pursue it further. In June 1861 he was made colonel of the 14th Indiana and brigadier general in April 1862. He was in [West] Virginia, in the Shenandoah, and at Antietam. At Fredericksburg on December 13, 1862, he was severely wounded by a canister ball through his right thigh and a shell fragment that struck his right groin. The thigh wound involved exten-sive tissue damage, whereas the groin injury was less severe. After being treated by the division surgeon, he was taken the next day, first by boxcar and then by steamer, to Washington, D.C. Following his return to duty, he was en route to Vicksburg when his wound became so painful that, upon reaching Indianapo-lis, he required a further extension of his leave. He finally arrived at Vicksburg in March 1863, but the thigh wound did not heal for eight more months. Kimball was relieved from field duty on July 31 at his own request. On August 4 he was ordered to Memphis where he became ill and received further sick leave. He was unable to go on horseback because the wound was at the point of greatest pressure on the saddle. In the middle of September 1863 he was assigned to command and was mustered out in August 1865. He served as state treasurer of Indiana and for a term in the legislature. In 1873 he was appointed surveyor general of the Utah Territory. By February 1896 his family physician reported that for the previous three years Kimball had suffered from "physical exhaustion and enervation resulting in great chronic vital depression of the entire system." Because of his condition Kimball required the aid and attendance of another person.[1] Died January 21, 1898, at Ogden, Utah, and was buried in Weber, Utah.

1. *OR*, vol. 21:51, 74, 131, 287, 290, 292; U.S. Army, CWS, roll 2, vol. 3, report 30, pp. 859–911; RVA, Pension SC 160,586; Gibbon, *Personal Recollections*, 104–5.

JOHN HASKELL KING • Born on February 19, 1820, at Sackets Harbor, New York. Served in Florida and at Vera Cruz during the Mexican War. He was appointed a second lieutenant of the First U.S. Infantry in 1837 and by 1846 was a captain. King was on duty in Texas at the start of the Civil War and was able to bring regular troops east. He continued to command regular troops at Shiloh and Corinth, and his appointment as brigadier general of volunteers ranked from November 1862. He was wounded at Stones River on December 31, 1862, and had to go to the hospital. After Chickamauga, in November 1863, he took sick leave. He served in the Atlanta campaign and was brevetted major general in the Regular Army on March 13, 1865, and in the volunteers on May 31, 1865. At the end of the war he was promoted to colonel of the Ninth Infantry and served on the frontier until he retired in 1882. He died April 7, 1888, at his residence in Washington, D.C., and was buried in Arlington National Cemetery. An army surgeon reported the cause of his death as pneumonia.[1]

1. CSR; *OR*, vol. 20, pt. 1:380, 395, 398; vol. 31, pt. 2:459; LR, ACP, 1976, 1882, fiche: 000129.

RUFUS KING • *Born January 26, 1814,* in New York City. Graduated from the USMA in 1833. As a cadet he was treated twice for a headache and once each for a sore throat, a wound, and a cold. He resigned from the service three years after graduation to become a civil engineer and also engaged in newspapers, politics, and education. King was appointed brigadier general of volunteers to rank from May 17, 1861. He had an epileptic seizure on August 23, 1862, and was hospitalized. After a poor military performance at Second Bull Run and because of his ill health he resigned in 1863.[1] Following short periods as U.S. minister to Rome and with New York customs, he retired to private life in 1869. He died October 13, 1876, in New York and was buried in Grace Churchyard, Jamaica, Long Island.

1. *OR*, vol. 12, pt. 2:253, 338; WPCHR, vol. 601; RAGO, entry 534; Steiner, *Physician-Generals*, 126, 130; Wallace J. Schutz, *Major General John Pope and the Army of Virginia*, 127.

EDMUND KIRBY • *Born March 11, 1840,* at Brownville, New York. Graduated from the USMA in 1861. While he was at West Point he was treated for phlegmon, contusio, and diarrhea twice each and cephalalgia, excoriatio, nausea, and catarrhus once each. By the end of April 1862 he had recovered from a bout of typhoid fever. He was at First Bull Run, the Seven Days, Antietam, and Fredericksburg. On May 3, 1863, Kirby was in command of an artillery battery at Chancellorsville, when his left thigh was struck by two round balls from a spherical case shot. He ordered one of the guns to be taken off the field before he was moved. After he was examined at the brigade hospital, he was sent to Washington, D.C., and arrived there on the fifth. The balls had entered his thigh about two inches above the condyles, producing a comminuted fracture of the lower third of the femur. On May 10, using a tourniquet and chloroform as the anesthetic, the leg was amputated at the middle third of the thigh by the circular method. One ball was found embedded in the medullary canal of the femur and the other in the vastus externus muscle. The operation was followed by an increase of his fever, which rapidly assumed the typhoid type. He survived the operation for only a few days and died of pyemia on May 28, 1863.[1] President Lincoln made him a general the day of his death in Washington. He was buried at Brownville, New York.

1. *OR*, vol. 25, pt. 1:251, 310, 314; WPCHR, vol. 609; *MSHW*, vol. 2, pt. 3:280; Howard, *Autobiography* 1:214.

EDWARD NEEDLES KIRK • *Born February 29, 1828,* in Jefferson County, Ohio. He was practicing the law at the start of hostilities. After helping raise the 34th Illinois Infantry, he was commissioned its colonel in September 1861. At Shiloh on April 7, 1862, he was severely wounded in the shoulder and taken to Louisville, Kentucky. In a few days he developed diarrhea. Kirk was taken to his home in Sterling, Illinois, and in August his condition was further complicated by pyemia. He was made brigadier general of volunteers in November. At Stones River on December 31, 1862, he was wounded in the hip and taken to the hospital in an ambulance. Kirk would not allow the attendants to take him out of the ambulance because he said if they remained there any longer they would be captured. The minié ball had lodged in the side of his spine next to the sacrum. He lingered for nearly seven months. According to his wife and attending physician, he died on July 21, 1863, in the Fremont House in Chicago.[1]

1. CSR; *OR*, vol. 10, pt. 1:106, 304–5; vol. 20, pt. 1:208, 255, 296, 301, 320; *CV* 3:162; RVA, Pension WC 38,050.

JOSEPH FARMER KNIPE • *Born March 30, 1823,* in Mount Joy, Pennsylvania. Served in the Mexican War. Employed by a railroad when the Civil War started, he was commissioned colonel of the 46th Pennsylvania Volunteers in August 1861. The first of May 1862 he developed diarrhea, which lasted for a few weeks and produced debility. On May 25, 1862, at Winchester, Virginia, he was wounded in the right shoulder and right knee. Back on duty, he was wounded twice at Cedar Mountain on August 9 and had to be carried off the field. One was a scalp wound while the other, in the palm of his right hand, was from a piece of shell. His promotion as brigadier general of volunteers ranked from November 1862. In the summer of 1863 he developed rheumatism. He had a sick leave in Washington in late May but was back to duty in June. During the middle of the month he developed malarial fever, which continued into July. He was slightly wounded in the left shoulder at Resaca, Georgia, on May 15, 1864, but apparently did not leave the field. He commanded a division of cavalry at Nashville. Following the war, Knipe was appointed a postmaster in Pennsylvania and then held a number of state and federal positions. An examination in March 1884 revealed a scar on the outside of his right hand across the carpal joint of the little finger, which was numb. There was a two-inch "L"-shaped scar in the right frontal area of his head that extended back to the parietal area. This scar was associated with neuralgia of the scalp and eye. He was disabled as a consequence of his old shoulder and knee wound. By 1896 these symptoms seemed to have improved, and he had only limited loss of motion in the injured joints. However, he continued to have headaches and neuralgia.[1] Died August 18, 1901, in Harrisburg and was buried in Old Harrisburg Cemetery.

DEATH CERTIFICATE: Cause of death, cancer. Duration of last illness, two years.

1. CSR; *OR*, vol. 12, pt. 1:607, pt. 2:148, 152, pt. 3:252; *OR Suppl.*, vol. 3, pt. 1:628; RVA, Pension SC 342,802; LR, CB, roll 102, K247, 1864; RAGO, entry 534.

WLADIMIR KRZYZANOWSKI · *Born July 8, 1824*, in the Prussian Polish city of Raznova. He helped recruit Poles and Germans into the 58th New York Volunteers in 1861. In January 1862 he was sick in Washington, D.C. At Second Bull Run on August 30 his horse was shot and he fell off onto his head. Stunned, he struggled to his feet and continued in the fight. Soon afterward his unit was assigned to the defenses of Washington and he was able to go on sick leave to visit his wife. His appointment as brigadier general in November 1862 was not acted on by the Senate and expired in March. He was at Chancellorsville, and at Gettysburg on July 1, 1863, his horse was shot from under him again and he was violently thrown to the ground. The full weight of the horse fell on his left chest and body, rendering him unconscious for a time. In addition, his lower extremities were injured. He had difficulty breathing and was treated by the assistant surgeon before returning to battle. He had occasional pulmonary hemorrhages, and his subsequent asthma attacks started after this injury. In August 1863 he had a severe attack of bronchitis and an affection of the liver. He went on sick leave in early September and rejoined his brigade in a few weeks as it changed trains in Alexandria. He was at Chattanooga and in the early stages of the Atlanta campaign. He was brevetted brigadier general of volunteers in March

1865 and was discharged the following October. Krzyzanowski was appointed special inspector in Panama and left on November 20, 1878, for Aspinwall. In the summer of 1880 he was ill and required a sick leave. He left Aspinwall in June 1880 and arrived in New York on June 15. In August 1881, following his return to Panama, he was prostrate with fever. Late that year his wife became sick and returned north. He arrived home in January 1882, unfortunately, after his wife had died. He returned to Panama again and in the summer had a return of "Panama fever." In June he received a one-month leave of absence and left Panama, after which his service in that country was terminated. He arrived in New York Harbor in late July 1882 afflicted by asthma, fever, and depression. In October 1883, Krzyzanowski was made special agent for the U.S. Treasury Department in Customs District No. 2 at New York City. His asthma attacks increased in frequency and severity, and he had to take several days' sick leave. In 1885 his illness made his life more difficult. In August and December new respiratory attacks confined him to his bed for long periods, and he requested transfer to a more healthy, drier climate. He was too sick to travel when ordered in January 1886 to report to Tucson, Arizona. A surgeon examined him in May and described the scar of a saber cut on the anterior surface of the left wrist, one and a half inches long and one-fourth to one-half inch wide and adherent to the tendons. It was the residual of one of the wounds incurred before he had come to America. He appeared weak and anemic, and examination of the urine demonstrated large amounts of albumin. An examination in September revealed a chronically thickened right pleura, some compensation emphysema on the left side, disturbed respiration, and slight cyanosis. The signs of pleural thickening were so marked that a number of doctors over the years used needles to ascertain if there was fluid. Results were negative. After slight improvement, his asthma returned, accompanied by pleurisy, uremia, and chronic Bright's disease. By the end of the year he was confined to his bed. He had increasingly painful headaches, respiratory discomfort, and diarrhea, and his blood pressure rose. He had sharp pains in his chest every time he moved and continued to endure the pain through December and January. He had a severe pulmonary hemorrhage on January 26, 1887, and died on January 31 in New York. He was buried in Arlington National Cemetery.[1]

DEATH CERTIFICATE: Cause of death, chronic Bright's disease, pleurisy, and uremia.

1. CSR; RVA, Pension WC 405,884; James S. Pula, *For Liberty and Justice: The Life and Times of Wladimir Krzyzanowski*, 53, 58, 121–23, 207, 209, 212–14, 224–27.

L

FREDERICK WEST LANDER • *Born on December 17, 1821,* at Salem, Massachusetts. Lander performed a number of surveys for the railroads before the Civil War.

After serving as an aide to Gen. George B. McClellan, he was commissioned brigadier general of volunteers to rank from May 1861. He was wounded in the calf of the leg during a skirmish at Edwards Ferry (Ball's Bluff), Maryland, on October 22, 1861. A few minutes later, he and his aide rode up to a surgeon, whom the aide asked to examine Lander. When the surgeon pulled the boot-strap out of the hole where it had been carried by the ball, the general swore "a blue streak" and vowed he would go to the ferry before having anything done. The surgeon later reported that he was rather glad to get him off of his hands. Relieved of his command and on medical leave, he was in Washington, D.C., the next month. On February 14, 1862, he applied for relief from command since his health was too broken for him to do any serious work. Two weeks later he was mortally stricken by a "congestive chill." After sleeping under the influence of morphine injections for twenty hours, he died on March 2, 1862, at Camp Chase, Paw Paw, Virginia.[1] He was buried in the Broad Street Burial Ground in Salem, Massachusetts.

1. CSR; *OR,* vol. 5:66, 338, 406, 647; vol. 51, pt. 1:531, 544–46; *MOLLUS* 26:279.

JACOB GARTNER LAUMAN • *Born January 20, 1813,* in Taneytown, Maryland. Lauman was a businessman in Iowa and entered Federal service as colonel of the 7th Iowa Infantry in July 1861. During the late summer and fall of 1861 he had chronic diarrhea and malarial fever. The assistant regimental surgeon treated him in camp. Lauman was still sick when he went into the battle of Belmont, Missouri, on November 7, 1861. He sustained a wound in his left thigh when a minié ball entered from the front and passed close to the femur. He was assisted to the rear of the tents where he remained a short time. He was placed on an artillery gun and taken further to the rear. He was still able to take part in the retreat back to the boats. The surgeon stated the wound was slow to heal be-cause of the debilitated condition of Lauman's system caused by his prior sick-ness. He went on sick leave to his home in Burlington, Iowa, rejoined his regi-ment in January 1862, and served at Fort Donelson. In March he was commis-sioned brigadier general of volunteers and commanded a brigade at Shiloh. During the spring of 1863 he had a slight stroke. He was home on leave in July after Vicksburg and returned in September. Lauman again went home on fur-lough in January, and on February 9, 1864, he had a severe second stroke. Lauman never recovered enough to return to the field or even to attend to his private affairs. He was mustered out of service in August 1865. He was frequently confined to bed, but at intervals he was able to walk a short distance with the assistance of a cane and a friend. Finally, he developed almost complete paralysis of his left side.[1] He died February 9, 1867, at Burlington and was buried in Aspen Grove Cemetery.

1. CSR; *OR,* vol. 3:272, 277, 280, 297; U.S. Army, CWS, roll 3, vol. 4, report 9, pp. 207–14; ibid., roll 6, vol. 10, report 15, p. 81; RVA, Pension WC 204,126.

MICHAEL KELLY LAWLER • *Born on November 16, 1814,* in County Kildare, Ireland. Served in the Mexican War. He was a successful farmer, businessman, and militia officer, and his regiment, the 18th Illinois, entered Federal service in early 1861. When he joined the service he was five feet, nine inches tall and weighed three hundred pounds. On February 15, 1862, in an assault on Fort Donelson, a musket ball passed through his left forearm, cutting some of the muscles. He lost the use of the thumb and forefinger of the hand and in later years could not grasp a hatchet or hairbrush. Being left-handed, he had difficulty using his right hand. Also, during the bombardment of the fort, he sustained damage to his ears and head. These injuries produced bilateral deafness and supposed brain damage that was later suggested to contribute to his death. Lawler went home on sick leave and returned to his unit in April. His promotion as brigadier general of volunteers ranked from November 1862. He went on leave on surgeon's certificate on March 10, 1863, and returned on March 30 to fight at Vicksburg. On July 4 a surgeon examined him and reported that Lawler had hepatitis and diarrhea. He obtained a sick leave from July 18 to August 16. The division surgeon certified on December 15, 1863, that Lawler was disabled from fever and his advanced years, making it necessary for him to return home. The physician at Equality, Illinois, on January 31, 1864, reported that the leave should be extended because he had severe tonsillitis in connection with a bronchial inflammation. Lawler reported for duty in February. After the war he returned to his farm and engaged in raising horses. He had difficulty from a stomach condition, which was described as a nervous stomach. The doctor advised him to chew tobacco for the condition, although until this time he had never used tobacco in any form. Early in January 1882 his health began to fail. He died July 26, 1882, near Equality and was buried in the nearby Hickory Hill graveyard.[1]
DEATH CERTIFICATE: Cause of death, softening of the brain.

1. CSR; *OR,* vol. 7:176, 186; vol. 24, pt. 2:615; vol. 34, pt. 2:452; U.S. Army, CWS, roll 2, vol. 3, report 9, pp. 181–221; ibid., roll 8, vol. 14, report 9, pp. 639–61; RVA, Pension WC 208,905; William T. Lawler, *The Lawlers, from Ireland to Illinois,* 7–8.

JAMES HEWETT LEDLIE • *Born on April 14, 1832,* in Utica, New York. A civil engineer by training, he was involved in railroad construction when the war started. He entered military service as a major of the 19th New York Infantry, later named the 3rd New York Artillery. Ledlie was appointed brigadier general in December 1862. Not confirmed by the Senate, his commission expired in March 1863. He was reappointed in October and later confirmed. In May 1864 he was treated for malarial fever. At the time of the fight at the Crater on July 30, Ledlie asked his surgeon for stimulants, stating that he had malaria and had been struck by a spent shell. Ledlie's poor performance at the Crater was severely criticized. He was granted a leave on August 4 on account of physical disability. He returned to duty on December 8, 1864, and the next day was ordered to return to his home and await further orders. He resigned in January 1865. Purportedly he had contracted diarrhea, an enlarged liver, and hemorrhoids. From 1869 until his death, he suffered from rheumatism, diarrhea, and malaria. Mrs. Ledlie cautioned their laundress to thoroughly dry and air his flannel clothing because of his chills and fever. From April 1877 to June 1881, liver pads or mustard plasters were used frequently, and he was seen shaking and trembling as if he were having a chill.[1] Died at the St. Marks Hotel in New Brighton, Staten Island, on August 15, 1882, and was buried in Forest Hill Cemetery, Utica.

DEATH CERTIFICATE: Cause of death, cholereticemia (increased bile in the blood), cirrhosis of liver.

1. *OR*, vol. 40, pt. 1:75, 119, 123; vol. 42, pt. 1:44, 72, pt. 2:44, pt. 3:867, 896; RAGO, entry 534; RVA, Pension WC 253, 231.

ALBERT LINDLEY LEE • *Born on January 16, 1834*, in Fulton, New York. He resigned his position as a judge and entered the Federal service as major of the 7th Kansas Cavalry in October 1861. His promotion to brigadier general of volunteers ranked from November 1862. In a general assault on Vicksburg on May 19, 1863, a musket ball entered his right cheek and passed out the back of his neck. He received a leave of absence and returned to command in July. Unwell in March 1864, he was utterly prostrated and unable to do his duties again in November.[1] Following the Civil War, he traveled and conducted business in New York. He died December 31, 1907, in a hotel in New York City and was buried in Mount Adnah Cemetery in Fulton, New York.

DEATH CERTIFICATE: Cause of death, chronic nephritis; contributory, grippe of ten days' duration.

1. *OR*, vol. 25, pt. 2:18, 231–32; vol. 34, pt. 2:572; vol. 41, pt. 4:653, 665; U.S. Army, CWS, roll 2, vol. 3, report 48, pp. 1349–57.

MORTIMER DORMER LEGGETT • *Born on April 19, 1821*, near Ithaca, New York. Prior to the Civil War he was a lawyer and educator. After serving as a civilian aide to Gen. George B. McClellan, he was commissioned colonel of the 78th Ohio in January 1862. His promotion as brigadier general of volunteers ranked from November 1862. At Vicksburg in the crater at Fort Hill on June 25, 1863, a piece of wood splintered by a solid shot struck him from the left shoulder to the right hip. Unconscious, he was carried back a few yards and awoke while the surgeon was removing pebbles and gravel from his flesh and dressing his wound. When the dressing was removed the next day, it was found that the skin and muscles of the abdomen were torn and there was protrusion of bowel at his umbilicus. For several days he vomited blood. Although not a drinker, he did take some alcohol for this injury. The hernia bothered him for the rest of his life but did not keep him from duty. In August 1864, after service in the Atlanta campaign, he was given a disability leave. In January 1865 he was sent home because of severe chronic diarrhea and returned by March. Leggett resigned in September, returned to the practice of the law, and later entered business. For years after the war he continued to suffer with the diarrhea and umbilical hernia. He died in Cleveland on January 6, 1896, and was buried in Lakeview Cemetery. According to his wife, he died from apoplexy superimposed on blood poisoning.[1]

DEATH CERTIFICATE: Cause of death, apoplexy.

1. CSR; *OR,* vol. 38, pt. 1:109, pt. 5:634; vol. 47, pt. 1:207; RVA, Pension WC 464,512; Steiner, *Physician-Generals,* 68–72.

JOSEPH ANDREW JACKSON LIGHTBURN • *Born September 21, 1824,* at Webster, Pennsylvania. Unsuccessful in his attempt to enter West Point, he served in the Regular Army as an enlisted man from 1846 until 1851. He was made colonel of the 4th West Virginia Infantry in August 1861. Lightburn was appointed a brigadier general of volunteers in March 1863 and served at Vicksburg. Near Knoxville, Tennessee, in December, he had the onset of asthma and was treated by the regimental surgeon until February 1864. He went home on sick leave on February 2 and rejoined his regiment a month later. He fought at Chattanooga, and on August 19, 1864, in front of Atlanta, Lightburn was wounded in the head by a rifle bullet. The ball struck him on the left of the frontal bone and passed back around his skull for about four inches. He was admitted the next day to a hospital and was treated with a simple dressing. On August 24 he left for the North to recover. Afterward, he reported back in September and was assigned to duty as president of an examining board. In 1867, following the war, he was ordained a Baptist minister and followed this profession until his death. Lightburn continued to have asthma and headaches over the area of the wound, associated with altered vision. He died May 17, 1901, in Lewis County, West Virginia, and was buried on Broad Run in that county. According to his wife, he died of asthma and heart trouble.[1]

1. *OR,* vol. 38, pt. 1:104, pt. 3:184, pt. 5:604–5, 610; vol. 43, pt. 2:28; RVA, Pension WC 527,406; U.S. Army, CWS, roll 1, vol. 2, report 55, pp. 763–73; ibid., roll 7, vol. 11, report 5, p. 527; RAGO, entry 534.

HENRY HAYES LOCKWOOD • *Born August 17, 1814,* in Kent County, Delaware. Graduated from the USMA in 1836. While at West Point, he was treated for a headache nine times, a cold five times, a sore throat and toothache twice each, and once each for diarrhea, sick stomach, epistaxis (nosebleed), fever, and influenza.[1] Served in the Florida wars. During the Mexican War he served aboard the frigate *United States* and took part in the capture of Monterey, California. Afterward, he was an instructor at the U.S. Naval Academy until he was appointed colonel of the 1st Delaware Infantry in May 1861. The following August he was made brigadier general of volunteers and was a brigade commander at Gettysburg. Lockwood resigned in 1865 and returned to duty at the U.S. Naval Academy and the Naval Observatory in Washington. He died in Georgetown, D.C., on December 7, 1899, and was buried at Annapolis.

DEATH CERTIFICATE: Cause of death, primary, interstitial nephritis; immediate, convulsion. Duration, some months.

1. WPCHR, vols. 602, 603.

JOHN ALEXANDER LOGAN • *Born on February 9, 1826,* in southern Illinois. Served in the Mexican War. In Santa Fe during the winter of 1847–48, he contracted measles and was very ill for weeks. By the following spring he had recovered. He was a congressman from Illinois when the Civil War started. He recruited the 31st Illinois and was made its colonel in September 1861. In February 1862 he developed rheumatism after sleeping on the ground. He fought at Belmont, and at Fort Donelson on February 15 he was wounded twice. The first ball struck his left shoulder. He went to the rear and had the wound bandaged, then returned to the regiment. A second shot hit the pistol on his belt and nearly broke his ribs. Although barely able to stay in the saddle, he remained on the field. Weak from loss of blood, his prognosis uncertain, he was put in a cot in Grant's headquarters' boat, the *New Uncle Sam.* Later Logan's wife joined him at Fort Donelson, where they stayed for two weeks before sailing back to southern Illinois. Unable to put his arm, which required a sling, into a coat sleeve, he returned at the end of March wearing new brigadier general stars. Following a period of illness, he returned to duty in April 1862. On May 3 he deferred assuming command of his brigade because of ill health and took command about two days later at Corinth. During February 1863 he had another acute attack of rheumatism. Logan later reported that he had been wounded at Vicksburg but did not give a specific date. He was supposedly sitting in a chair, leaning back with his right foot up against the ridgepole of the tent when he was wounded. The bullet struck the leg of the chair just at the top and produced a flesh wound of his posterior thigh. The surgeon dug the ball out and bandaged the wound. However, at Logan's request, the surgeon did not say anything about it. Logan could not get into the saddle for some days, but all that anyone else knew about the event was that the chair had been hit. Although his health had been impaired since the beginning of the Vicksburg campaign, he remained on duty until July 20, 1863, when his poor health prompted orders returning him to Illinois. In December he reported for duty and assumed command of the Fifteenth Corps. On May 20, 1864, during the Atlanta campaign, a ball struck his right shoulder but did not produce a wound. A shot passed through the muscle of his arm just above the elbow on May 30 at Dallas, Georgia, and he had to carry his arm in a sling for a couple of weeks. He was ill and worn out in July but continued on duty. On July 22, after the death of James B. McPherson, Logan took temporary command of the Army of the Tennessee. While on home leave in November 1864 he developed a severe inflammation of the throat and could not return until December 4. He was at Savannah and in the Carolinas. After the war he returned to politics. Congressman Logan was sick December 7, 1868, and did not make the opening roll call, but he was in the House in January. In December 1873, Logan arrived with his family for the opening of the new congressional session. However, illness had left him weak, and he was confined to a room at the Palmer House in Chicago from the last of November to the first of December 1875. He could not walk alone because of inflammatory rheumatism and was intermittently incoherent from the effects of the opiates he received. Since he was unable to attend the opening of the congressional sessions, he remained in Chicago and did not reach Washington until the first of the year. He was still not well when he answered the first roll call in January. Weak and exhausted from the campaign trail and crippled by his rheumatism, he was in bed during the winter of 1880. Again he was unable to answer the opening roll call in December. Logan left Washington, D.C., and was at Hot Springs, Arkansas, in April and May 1881 for treatment of his rheumatism. The spa waters and his medications appeared to help. In 1881 he was a candidate for vice president of the United States. At Moline, Illinois, in mid-September 1886, he spoke in the rain and was soaked. He was chilled and bedridden with what was called "a bilious attack aggravated by a cold." Although afflicted with an acute attack of rheumatism, he answered the December 6, 1886, roll call. Two days later he had neuralgia of the sciatic nerve and another bout of rheumatism. His last day in the Senate was December 9. On December 15 he was sitting in his room with his swollen right hand wrapped in cotton-batting. For his arthritis, Logan used three types of therapy. First, he took the prescriptions recommended by his physician. Second, he received massages from a gentleman who stated he could rub rheumatism out through the soles of the feet or through the ends of the fingers, according to the location of the point affected. Third, he slept every night with a brick-sized block of sandstone, which had alleged curative powers. Within a day or two he contracted a cold that resulted in a relapse, and the rheumatic affection extended to his hips and lower extremities as well as to both arms. The episode was attended at times by a high fever and nervous prostration, during which periods he had delirium. Toward the end he was confined to bed with his wife in attendance. He lay with his legs drawn up and so rigid that it was difficult to move them, since even slight changes of position produced great agony. On December 24 he seemed better; his limbs lost their rigidity and the muscles relaxed. He became semiconscious and was only aroused with difficulty. He died peacefully on December 26, 1886. His remains were deposited in the mausoleum of a friend until a monument could be erected in the Soldier's Home Cemetery. Following its completion, his remains were reinterred there.[1]

DEATH CERTIFICATE: Cause of death, primary, acute rheumatism with rheumatic fever, duration December 12 to December 26. Immediate, congestion of brain, duration, December 12 to December 26.

1. CSR; *OR*, vol. 7:177; vol. 10, pt. 1:755, 759; vol. 24, pt. 3:47, 537; vol. 31, pt. 3:353; vol. 38, pt. 3:86; vol. 39, pt. 3:751; vol. 45, pt. 2:46; vol. 52, pt. 1:18; RVA, Pension WC 242,791; William Gene Eidson, "John Alexander Logan: Hero of the Volunteers" (diss.), 9–10, 100, 102–5, 123, 162–63; George Francis Dawson, *Life and Services of Gen. John A. Logan*, 448–49, 451–52, 458–61; *MOLLUS* 14:148, 159; James Pickett Jones, *John A. Logan: Stalwart Republican from Illinois*, 33, 80, 85, 88, 141, 154–55, 221–23, 270, 362–63.

ELI LONG • *Born on June 16, 1837,* in Woodford County, Kentucky. Graduated from the USMA in 1855. Long was treated at West Point for phlegmon eleven times, excoriatio six times, contusio three times, and for hemorrhoids, ophthalmagia, obstipatio, morbi. varii., tonsillitis, cephalalgia, and subluxatio once each. The last part of November 1857 he was sick at Fort Leavenworth, Kansas. The next month he made a trip of some five hundred miles, escorting the mail from Fort Riley to the crossing of the Arkansas River and back. He was ill the whole time and had to remain in his ambulance during more than half of the trip. In the winter of 1858–59 he was severely frostbitten while on a two-hundred-mile journey. According to medical records he had the following conditions in 1860: May 10–15, contusion; October 1–5, dysentery; October 6–9, haemorrhoids; and October 22 to November 5, haemorrhoids. A captain at Stones River on December 31, 1862, he was wounded in the left shoulder by a ball. He returned to duty as colonel of the 4th Ohio Cavalry in February 1863 and served in the Tullahoma campaign and at Chickamauga. Long was slightly wounded by a pistol shot in his left side at Farmington, Tennessee, in a running fight on October 7, 1863, but remained with his troops. On August 21, 1864, near Lovejoy's Station, Georgia, he was wounded in the right thigh and the right forearm. Severely injured, he rode his horse to the rear, supported on either side by two mounted orderlies. The following month he was promoted brigadier general of volunteers. He returned from sick leave in November and was at the Battle of Nashville. At Selma, Alabama, on April 2, 1865, he was wounded by a bullet on the left side of the top of his head. His skull was indented, and the wound produced a severe concussion associated with paralysis of his tongue, the right side of his face, and his right arm. On April 25 he was sent first to Louisville, Kentucky, and then to New York for treatment. Long retired from the army in 1867. In the summer of 1876 he still had partial paralysis of his right arm associated with atrophy of his right shoulder.[1] He died in the Presbyterian Hospital, New York City, on January 5, 1903, and was buried in Hillside Cemetery, Plainfield.

DEATH CERTIFICATE: Cause of death, enlarged prostate gland and endarteritis, operation for prostatic enlargement.

1. CSR; *OR*, vol. 30, pt. 2:671, 687, 691; vol. 38, pt. 2:840–41, 844, pt. 5:629; vol. 49, pt. 1:343, 351, 361,

390, 403, 406, 439, pt. 2:444; LR, ACP, 289, 1876, fiche: 000134; RVA, Pension WC 558,792; U.S. Army, CWS, roll 3, vol. 4, report 23, pp. 713–31; WPCHR, vols. 608, 609; "Synopsis of the Military Career of Brevet Maj. Gen. Eli Long, U.S.V.," Eli Long Papers, USAMHI; *MOLLUS* 6:269, 15:75.

CHARLES RUSSELL LOWELL • *Born January 2, 1835,* in Boston. Lowell had a Harvard education and travelled abroad for a number of years. When the Civil War started, he was managing an ironworks. In May 1861 he received a commission as captain in the 3rd U.S. Cavalry. He was commissioned colonel of the 2nd Massachusetts Cavalry in May 1863. Early in the day at Cedar Creek, Virginia, on October 19, 1864, he was wounded in the arm but refused to leave the field. Later, at the head of his brigade, he sustained a wound to his lung. He died the following day at Middletown, Virginia, and his commission as brigadier general ranked from the day of his mortal wound. He was buried in Mount Auburn Cemetery, Cambridge, Massachusetts.[1]

  1. CSR; *OR*, vol. 43, pt. 1:54, 96, 136, 434, 450–51; RVA, Pension C 120,052.

THOMAS JOHN LUCAS • *Born September 9, 1826,* in Lawrenceburg, Indiana. Served in the Mexican War. A watchmaker by trade, he was made lieutenant colonel of the 16th Indiana in 1861. In December 1862 Lucas had the onset of chronic diarrhea and was almost incapacitated by it in January. On January 10 he was on the steamer *J. C. Snow,* too sick to go out with his regiment. Near Vicksburg on April 18, 1863, he was shot in the left leg but remained on the field. During the general assault on Vicksburg on May 22, he was shot in the leg, jaw, and nose, destroying the division of his nose. He received a sick leave on June 9 and went home. His condition was complicated the last of the month with chronic diarrhea and a tendency to inflammation of the bowels. The following August he returned to duty and the next month was appointed a member of a military commission that met at Indianapolis, Indiana. In November 1864, after service in the Red River campaign, he was made brigadier general of volunteers. Following the war he held various Federal positions. From 1865 until his death he was under medical treatment for chronic catarrh, diarrhea, and continued problems with his wounds.[1] He died November 16, 1908, in Lawrenceburg and was buried in Greendale Cemetery in Dearborn County, Indiana.
DEATH CERTIFICATE: Cause of death, senility; contributory, chronic bronchitis. Duration, years.

  1. CSR; *OR*, vol. 17, pt. 1:730; RVA, Pension SC 279,626.

NATHANIEL LYON • *Born on July 14, 1818,* in what is now Eastford, Connecticut. Graduated from the USMA in 1841. At West Point he was treated for headaches twice and once each for toothache, bile, and chapped. Served in the Florida and Mexican wars. He was wounded September 13, 1847, at Chapultepec. The slight wound did not incapacitate him at the time, but later it became inflamed, forcing him to leave duty for a couple of days. Lyon had dental problems as early as 1855 and by 1861 wore false teeth. In April 1861 he had a marked fever but continued on duty. As commander of the St. Louis arsenal, Lyon frustrated the secessionists' plans for the city and was promoted from captain to brigadier general of volunteers in May. At Lindell Grove, Missouri, on May 10, he swung to the ground from his horse and was immediately kicked in the stomach by an aide's horse. He fell to the ground unconscious but recovered within thirty minutes. At Wilson's Creek on August 10, 1861, he received three wounds. First, he was wounded in the outer part of his right calf and then was grazed on the right side of his head. After a handkerchief was wrapped around his head, he walked slowly to the rear and remounted another horse. Charging the enemy, he was struck in the chest by a ball from a squirrel rifle and killed. The ball entered below his fourth rib and exited from the right rear of his body just below the shoulder blade. Lyon's body was taken to the rear and placed in a wagon. A sergeant, not realizing who Lyon was since he was dressed in a captain's uniform, had the body removed so the wagon could be used for the wounded. When the army retreated the corpse was not retrieved. When discovered by Confederate troops, his body was taken to Price's headquarters. It was later turned over to Dr. S. H. Melcher, who took it to the Ray house. An escort was assembled, and the remains were taken to Springfield. When the Confederates left Springfield, the corpse was again left behind. No metallic coffin was available, and an attempt to embalm the body was unsuccessful because the large heart wound did not allow retention of the fluid. On August 11 in Springfield, the construction of a walnut coffin encased in zinc was ordered. The body was taken to a nearby farmhouse and placed in the icehouse. On the evening of August 13 the corpse was buried in a cornfield on the farm. A week later an ambulance arrived bearing a large iron coffin. On the night of August 22, the remains, which had been exhumed, were placed in the coffin and the coffin packed in ice. The ambulance arrived in St. Louis on August 26 to retrieve the corpse. The coffin was placed on a train and finally buried in a cemetery below the nearby village of Phoenixville, Connecticut, on September 5.[1]

1. *OR*, vol. 3:54, 61–62, 67, 77; WPCHR, vol. 604; Heitman, *Historical Register and Dictionary* 2:29; Christopher Phillips, *Damned Yankee*, 56, 121, 154, 189–90, 254–56, 258.

WILLIAM HAINES LYTLE • *Born on November 2, 1826*, in Cincinnati, Ohio. Served in the Mexican War. A lawyer and politician, he was appointed major general of Ohio militia in 1857. In May 1861 he was commissioned colonel of the 10th Ohio. On September 10, 1861, at Carnifex Ferry, [West] Virginia, he was badly wounded by a ball from a squirrel rifle, which killed his horse and passed through his leg, missing all vital structures. He fell from his horse within thirty yards of the Confederate front. He had sick leave and went to Cincinnati, Ohio, by steamer. During the Battle of Perryville on October 8, 1862, he was wounded and left on the field. While sitting on a rock, he was captured by Confederate troops and taken to a hospital. His wound was marked by a ragged half-inch tear on the right side of his face in front of the ear. Two physicians examined him, and one found that the ball had passed from the rear and had lodged in the soft parts near the point of his chin. In November 1862 he was promoted brigadier general of volunteers, although not officially exchanged until the following February. He was wounded on September 20, 1863, at the battle of Chickamauga. Taken to a field hospital at Crawfish Springs, he died the same day.[1] He was finally buried in Spring Grove Cemetery, Cincinnati.

1. CSR; *OR*, vol. 5:134–37; vol. 16, pt. 1:1033, 1047, 1127, pt. 2:592, 609; vol. 30, pt. 1:145, 175, 491, 581, 583, 587, pt. 2:304, 330; vol. 32, pt. 3:498; *CV* 5:248–49, 466, 9:423; *MOLLUS* 1:24–25, 28–29, 9:71.

M

JOHN MCARTHUR • *Born on November 17, 1826,* in the parish of Erskine in Renfrewshire, Scotland. Before the Civil War, he ran an ironworks and participated in a Chicago militia company. In May 1861 he entered service as a colonel of the 12th Illinois Volunteers. While returning to camp near Caseyville, Illinois, on June 10, 1861, his horse became unmanageable and threw him, dislocating his right shoulder. He was treated by the regimental surgeon. After service at Forts Henry and Donelson he was promoted brigadier general of volunteers in March 1862. McArthur was wounded by a ball in his right foot at Shiloh on April 6, 1862, but he returned to command on April 8 when Gen. W. H. S. Wallace was killed. He continued in command until April 18 when, relieved of duty, he went home on leave.[1] He was at Iuka, Corinth, Vicksburg, in the Atlanta campaign, and at the Battle of Nashville. Following the war his business efforts were a failure. He died May 15, 1906, in Chicago and was buried in Rosehill Cemetery.

DEATH CERTIFICATE: Cause of death, apoplexy, third or fourth stroke. Hardships and injuries sustained during service greatly impaired his constitution.

1. *OR*, vol. 10, pt. 1:101, 149, pt. 2:100; U.S. Army, CWS, roll 1, vol. 2, report 26, pp. 415–23; RVA, Pension WC 653,154.

GEORGE ARCHIBALD MCCALL • *Born on March 16, 1802,* in Philadelphia, Pennsylvania. Graduated from the USMA in 1822. Served in the Florida and Mexican wars. After being absent because of illness from May 8, 1828, to January 1829, McCall was with his regiment in Florida until June 1829. He was on sick leave from May 15, 1830, to April 1, 1831, due to an hepatic affection with the sort of general derangement of health produced by the influence of the hot and humid climate. He was sick again from August to September 7, 1845. Because of a severe hemorrhoidal condition and general neuralgia he obtained a sick leave from April 5, 1847, to March 25, 1850, and was confined to his bed for some months. He resigned from the army in April 1853 because of chronic neuralgia. McCall was commissioned major general of Pennsylvania Volunteers in May 1861 and two days later was made a brigadier general of U.S. Volunteers. Although in good health in the middle of May 1862, his health was impaired by an hepatic derangement and miasmatic fever by June 4. On June 30, 1862, he was wounded, possibly by Union fire, and captured at New Market, Virginia. He was imprisoned in Libby Prison in Richmond and exchanged in August. The miasmatic fever returned on August 21 and continued at intervals during the next months. His surgeon speculated his hepatic derangement and general debility were due to his miasmatic fever and confinement at Richmond. McCall became so debilitated that he could not stay in the saddle. After his exchange, he was on sick leave until March 31, 1863, the day his resignation was accepted, because of repeated attacks of intermittent fever and neuralgia. His physician attributed McCall's continued illness to brain trouble with a disturbed action of his heart. He was unable to withstand prolonged effort; little exertion was sufficient to prostrate him and bring on an attack of insensibility that seemed dependent upon congestion of the brain. The surgeon classified his problem as "essential vertigo." He further stated that his disturbed condition in the brain arose from a feeble, somewhat enlarged heart and also from sclerosed blood vessels due to a "lowered basal motor action" producing impaired nutrition of the brain substance. According to his family physician, McCall's fatal attack of apoplexy arose from cerebral hemorrhage. This was dependent directly upon the degenerative changes in the cerebral vessels and indirectly upon the relaxation of the vessels from vasomotor depression.[1] Died at Belair, Pennsylvania, on February 25, 1868, and was buried in Christ Church Cemetery, Philadelphia.

1. OR, vol. 11, pt. 2:32, 93, 164, 228, 384, 392, 418; vol. 12, pt. 3:335, 463; vol. 51, pt. 1:74; RVA, Pension WC 212,340; RAGO, entry 534.

GEORGE BRINTON McCLELLAN • Born December 3, 1826, in Philadelphia, Pennsylvania. Graduated from the USMA in 1846. At the Battle of Contreras, Mexico, on August 19, 1847, he had two horses shot from under him, and he was struck by grapeshot. The projectile hit his sword, resulting in bruising. In 1848 he had an episode of dysentery and malaria; after being hospitalized for over a month, he returned to duty in November. In later years when similar symptoms recurred he referred to them as his "Mexican complaint." Following his return to the north, he had a subluxation of an unspecified site in August 1849 and received ten days of treatment at the post hospital at West Point. He received laudanum in 1853 for chills, fever, and pain in his jaw. He resigned in 1855 and became chief engineer of the Illinois Central Railroad. President of the Ohio and Mississippi Railroad when the war began, he was made major general of Ohio Volunteers in April 1861. Within a few weeks, President Lincoln appointed him major general in the Regular Army. He was victorious at Rich Mountain and named to command the Army of the Potomac. In August he was sick for a week with what was possibly a recurrence of malarial fever. He had an attack of typhoid on December 23, 1861, and was treated by three homeopathic physicians from New York. He was not able to appear before the Joint Committee on the Conduct of the War until the middle of January. On March 19, his horse fell into a hole at the wharves at Alexandria and he was slightly hurt. On May 22, 1862, during the Peninsular campaign he developed dysentery. He remained sick in his tent until May 29 when he became worse and finally called for his surgeon. McClellan was in bed for several days because of pain and he was not thinking clearly. He arose from his sickbed and went to the field on the evening of May 31. After returning from the field on June 1, he was completely exhausted and was not able to ride for ten days. At Alexandria on August 27 he had a sudden attack of indisposition for which he drank brandy. Again in September 1862, after the Battle of Antietam, he had diarrhea that lasted a few days. Early in September 1864 he caught a cold and had a return of his "Mexican complaint." On November 7, 1862, he was removed from command. He was nominated for president by the Democratic party in 1864. Early in October 1885 he had an episode of chest pain that was diagnosed as angina pectoris. He appeared to improve but on the evening of October 28 had a recurrence of the pain.[1] Died October 29, 1885, at Orange, New Jersey, and was buried in Riverview Cemetery, Trenton.

DEATH CERTIFICATE: Cause of death, angina pectoris. Length of sickness, six weeks.

1. *OR*, vol. 7:524, 526, 531, 926; vol. 19, pt. 1:219; vol. 51, pt. 1:713; *OR Suppl.*, vol. 2, pt. 1:23, 72; Richard Allan McCoun, "General George Brinton McClellan; from West Point to the Peninsula; the Education of a Soldier and the Conduct of War" (diss.), 82; Steiner, *Medical-Military Portraits*, 10–14; Stephen W. Sears, *George B. McClellan: The Young Napoleon*, 15, 22, 100, 136–37, 192, 194–96, 319–22, 400–401; Ward, *That Man Haupt*, 98.

JOHN ALEXANDER MCCLERNAND • *Born on May 30, 1812*, near Hardinsburg, Kentucky. Served in the Black Hawk War. A lawyer and politician, he was a member of Congress at the start of the Civil War. He was appointed a brigadier general of volunteers to rank from May 1861. During the Battle of Belmont, Missouri, on November 7, 1861, his horse was wounded, and McClernand's head was grazed by a ball. He was at Fort Donelson and Arkansas Post, and served as a corps commander at Vicksburg until he ran afoul of Grant and was relieved. On May 1, 1864, he was ill, probably with malaria, and resided in a house in Alexandria, Louisiana, for two or three days. Unable to continue on active duty, he turned over the command to Gen. M. K. Lawler. He was admitted on May 15 to the USA hospital steamer *Laurel Hill* with a diagnosis of chronic diarrhea and went to the St. James General Hospital in New Orleans. His surgeon reported in late June that he had ulceration of his bowels. McClernand went to Illinois to recover, but continued poor health forced him to resign in November 1864. Following the war, McClernand returned to private life and politics. He died September 20, 1890, in Springfield, Illinois, and was buried there in the Oak Ridge Cemetery. Burial records state that the cause of death was old age.[1]

1. *OR*, vol. 3:280; vol. 34, pt. 1:276, pt. 2:134, pt. 3:457, 519; vol. 53:507; RAGO, entry 534; LR, CB, roll 109, M1310, 1864; Secretary of Oak Ridge Cemetery Board.

ALEXANDER McDOWELL McCOOK • *Born April 22, 1831,* in Columbiana County, Ohio. Graduated from the USMA in 1852. While at West Point he was treated twice each for cephalalgia and catarrhus and once each for hemorrhoids and pertussis. After garrison and frontier duty, he was an instructor at West Point when hostilities started. He was commissioned colonel of the 1st Ohio Volunteers in April 1861, brigadier general of volunteers in September, and major general in July 1862. McCook was sick on December 28, 1862. He served at First Bull Run, Shiloh, Corinth, Perryville, Stones River, Tullahoma, and Chickamauga. He remained in the army as a captain and was promoted to lieutenant colonel in 1867. He was treated for "roteln" (German measles) from March 11–15, 1889. He was made major general in 1894 and retired in 1895. During 1900 he was ill with malaria. On May 23, 1903, his physician was called to see him because of a derangement of his stomach that was associated with slight dizziness. When his physician returned on the twenty-seventh, McCook had suffered a small stroke with slight loss of the power of his right hand. The weakness gradually increased with each day, and by the thirty-first he had lost control of his right hand and foot and had motor aphasia. After slight improvement on June 12, he had a second cerebral hemorrhage, became unconscious, and lived for only half an hour. He died in Dayton, Ohio, and was buried in Cincinnati. According to his attending physician, the cause of death was cerebral apoplexy. Contributing factor, malaria.[1]

1. *OR*, vol. 20, pt. 2:269; WPCHR, vols. 606, 607; LR, ACP, 3660, 1874, fiche: 000059; RVA, Pension WC 574,443.

DANIEL McCOOK, JR. • *Born on July 22, 1834,* at Carrollton, Ohio. A law partner with W. T. Sherman and Thomas Ewing in 1860, he was a captain of the 1st Kansas Infantry in the summer of 1861. In July 1862 he was commissioned colonel of the 52nd Ohio. He was too sick on October 29, 1862, to march with his command, and the medical director recommended that he be allowed to return to Louisville, Kentucky, for treatment. He returned to the field and, after being ill for many months, he requested sick leave on December 19, 1863. His surgeon found that the lower one-third of his right lung was hepatized, apparently from a previous pneumonia. The next month he was under treatment for pneumonia in Washington, D.C. He was severely wounded on June 27, 1864, at Kennesaw Mountain, Georgia, and was sent to the hospital. In July he went on sick leave to his brother's home in Steubenville, Ohio, where he died on the seventeenth from effects of his wound. He was made brigadier general of volunteers the day before he died.[1] He was buried in Spring Grove Cemetery, Cincinnati.

1. CSR; *OR*, vol. 38, pt. 4:609, 611–12, 626; *MOLLUS* 4:266.

EDWARD MOODY MCCOOK • *Born June 15, 1833,* in Steubenville, Ohio. He left his law practice in Kansas and in May 1861 was appointed a lieutenant of cavalry in the Regular Army. McCook served at Perryville, Chickamauga, in the Atlanta campaign, and in the raid on Selma, Alabama. He was wounded in the forehead early in December 1862. By December 12 the wound was complicated by erysipelas, worsening his condition. In January 1864 McCook was so ill that another had to take his command. After passing through grades, he was made a brigadier general of volunteers in April 1864. Following his arrival near Louisville, Kentucky, in November 1864, he was confined to bed most of the time with inflammation of the lungs. He was absent on sick leave during January and February 1865. McCook resigned from the army in 1866 and served as United States minister to Hawaii and territorial governor of Colorado. He left public life in 1875 and became an influential and rich businessman. Died September 9, 1909, in Chicago and was buried in Union Cemetery, Steubenville, Ohio. Burial records: Cause of death, chronic nephritis.[1]

1. CSR; *OR*, vol. 32, pt. 1:85; vol. 45, pt. 1:85, 1024, 1062, 1093; vol. 49, pt. 1:799; Union Cemetery Allocation, Steubenville, Ohio.

ROBERT LATIMER MCCOOK • *Born on December 28, 1827,* in New Lisbon, Ohio. He was practicing law in Ohio when hostilities started, and he was made colonel of the 9th Ohio Volunteers in May 1861. McCook was at Carnifix Ferry in September 1861 and was wounded in an engagement at Logan's Cross Roads near Mill Springs, Kentucky, on January 19, 1862. He was shot through his right leg below the knee while three other balls passed through his horse. He was able to go on foot during the subsequent advance and proceeded with his troops to Somerset, Kentucky. He had a short sick leave in Cincinnati during February and was promoted brigadier general the next month. On the road between Hazel Green, Alabama, and Winchester, Tennessee, on August 5, 1862, he was sick and was riding in an ambulance some distance ahead of the brigade with a small escort. He had stopped to see about a camping ground for his command when the party was attacked by a band of guerrillas. One member rode up to the ambulance and shot McCook in the abdomen.[1] McCook's men carried him to a nearby house where he died on August 6, 1862. He was buried in Spring Grove Cemetery, Cincinnati.

1. CSR; *OR*, vol. 7:77, 81, 94; vol. 16, pt. 1:838–40.

IRVIN MCDOWELL · *Born October 15, 1818,* at Columbus, Ohio. Graduated from the USMA in 1838. As a cadet, he was treated for a cold twice and a sore throat and swollen face once each. Following his graduation, he was an instructor at West Point. He served in the Mexican War and was in the office of the adjutant general of the army when the Civil War broke out. In May 1861 he was appointed a brigadier general in the Regular Army. At Bull Run in July 1861, McDowell had an upset stomach from eating bad fruit and had to travel by buggy. In March 1862 he was made a major general of volunteers. He was sick April 29, 1862, but had recovered by the next day. He was reviewing the 1st Rhode Island Cavalry on June 18, 1862, when his horse was frightened, threw him off, and then fell on him. McDowell was badly injured and delirious for some time. By June 20 he felt better and stayed on to participate in Second Bull Run. He remained in the army following the Civil War and was made a major general in the Regular Army in November 1872. He retired in June 1882. He died on the night of May 4–5, 1885, in San Francisco and was buried at the Presidio. According to the medical director, the cause of his death was cancer of the pyloric end of the stomach.[1]

1. *OR,* vol. 12, pt. 3:410; vol. 51, pt. 1:71, 79; WPCHR, vols. 603, 604; LR, ACP, 5806, 1872, fiche: 000140; Manly Wade Wellman, *Giant in Gray,* 60.

GEORGE FRANCIS MCGINNIS · *Born March 19, 1862,* in Boston, Massachusetts. McGinnis was manufacturing hats in Indianapolis when the war started. He enlisted as a private in the 11th Indiana, a three-month regiment, and was made a lieutenant colonel within a few days. In August 1861 he was appointed colonel of the regiment when the unit was mustered in for three years. His promotion to brigadier general of volunteers ranked from November 1862. As he was not confirmed, he was reappointed from March 1863. On July 5, after Vicksburg, he had to be relieved of brigade command because of illness, and he did not recover sufficiently to resume command again until August 22. On November 3, 1863, during the battle at Grand Coteau, Louisiana, he was ill and was unable to take the field. On June 25, 1864, there was a question as to whether he should be relieved because of poor health. He was very sick on June 22, 1865, but no specific diagnosis was recorded for his continued illness.[1] After the war he returned to Indiana and held county and state offices. Died May 29, 1910, in Indianapolis and was buried in that city's Crown Hill Cemetery.

DEATH CERTIFICATE: Cause of death, uremia, nephritis; contributory, exhaustion.

1. *OR,* vol. 26, pt. 1:358; vol. 34, pt. 4:544; vol. 48, pt. 2:970; U.S. Army, CWS, roll 1, vol. 2, report 37, pp. 533–51.

JOHN BAILIE MCINTOSH • *Born on June 6, 1829,* at Fort Brooke, Florida. During the Mexican War he was a midshipman. He was engaged in business in New Jersey at the beginning of the Civil War and joined Federal service as a second lieutenant of the 2nd Regular Cavalry in June 1861. He was on the Peninsula and at Antietam, Chancellorsville, and Gettysburg. In November 1862 he was made colonel of the 3rd Pennsylvania Cavalry. He was severely injured on December 25, 1862, near Hartwood Church at the Potomac Creek bridge. Sent home on leave, he was back the next month. Although off duty from illness, he joined his brigade on the field for the Battle of Kelly's Ford, Virginia, on March 17, 1863. On reaching Geiselman's Woods on July 2, McIntosh, who was already exhausted, became very sick and was taken by a surgeon to the Geiselman's house for a short time. On October 1, 1863, at Catlett's Station, he was severely injured when his horse fell on him, and he was sent to Washington on a certificate of disability. He was put in command of the Cavalry Depot at Camp Stoneman in the middle of the month. He rejoined the army in May 1864 and was promoted brigadier general of volunteers in July. At the Battle of Winchester, Virginia, on September 19, 1864, he was wounded in the right leg. On the field that night, he had an amputation six inches below the knee. The next day he was at Harpers Ferry in good spirits, but he never again engaged in field duty. He was in New Jersey in January 1865 with his stump still unhealed and suppurating. McIntosh was on court-martial duty from February 8 to March 1. He remained in the army and in 1866 was made a lieutenant colonel. In January 1870 he requested retirement since his hip was bothering him. The examining board in May found that he was suffering from severe and almost constant neuralgic pains in his right thigh and hip. He retired as a brigadier general in 1870. For the last eighteen months of his life he was afflicted with valvular disease of the heart "resulting from irregularity of circulation produced by loss of his limb." In addition he developed angina pectoris.[1] He died on June 29, 1888, in New Brunswick, New Jersey, and was buried in Elmwood Cemetery.

DEATH CERTIFICATE: Cause of death, cardiac disease and angina pectoris.

1. CSR; *OR,* vol. 25, pt. 1:52; vol. 43, pt. 1:518, pt. 2:124; U.S. Army, CWS, roll 4, vol. 6, report 3, pp. 169–99; RVA, Pension WC 365,589; LR, ACP, 4214, 1873, fiche: 000141; *Battles and Leaders* 3:399; *MSHW,* vol. 2, pt. 3:471.

THOMAS JEFFERSON MCKEAN • *Born on August 21, 1810,* in Burlington, Pennsylvania. Graduated from the USMA in 1831 but resigned from the army in 1834 to become a civil engineer and politician in Iowa. He served in the Mexican War as an enlisted man. His appointment as brigadier general of volunteers ranked from November 1861. During the summer of 1862 he was having trouble with his feet; although not fit for field duty, he served at Corinth. McKean had sick leave on May 18, 1863, and returned on June 1. His Civil War service consisted mainly of being commander of a number of military districts, and he was discharged in August 1865. When McKean returned from the army, his family physician noted a decided change in his physical condition and reported that he was affected with diarrhea. McKean had symptoms of general paralysis that gradually increased, and he was totally helpless for several months before his death. Died April 19, 1870, at Marion, Iowa, and was buried in Oak Shade Cemetery. The attending physician reported the cause of death was softening of the brain and general paralysis.[1]

1. U.S. Army, CWS, roll 4, vol. 7, report 53, pp. 883–86; RVA, Pension WC 148,235; LR, CB, roll 282, M875, 1865.

RANALD SLIDELL MACKENZIE • *Born July 27, 1840,* in Westchester County, New York. Graduated from the USMA in 1862. At the age of three he had a slight sunstroke; physicians later suggested it might have contributed in later years to his mental problems. While at the academy, he was treated for catarrhus, excoriatio, and contusio each twice and cephalalgia and colica once each. Following his graduation, he was commissioned a second lieutenant of engineers. He was wounded in both shoulders in the action at Second Bull Run on August 29, 1862. The bullet had entered under the skin of the right shoulder and, passing under the skin, exited from the left shoulder. He was picked up from the field and taken to Centreville the next day and then to a hospital in Washington. He had a sick leave until October 19 but served at Fredericksburg and Chancellorsville. At Gettysburg in July 1863 he had a minor wound. He served with the Engineers Battalion in the Army of the Potomac until June 1864. Mackenzie was wounded in the right hand and lost two fingers at Petersburg, Virginia, on June 22. He was absent on sick leave until July 9 and was made colonel of the 2nd Connecticut Heavy Artillery the same month. His leg was skinned by a shell at the Battle of Winchester on September 19, 1864. After tying a handkerchief around the leg, he remained on the field. Later he was wounded a second time. At Cedar Creek, Virginia, on October 19, he was hit twice in the leg. The first was a grazing shot and the second was a wound. Soon afterward a piece of shrapnel struck him in the chest, knocking the wind out of him and temporarily paralyzing his arms. He declined to leave the field and, placed back on his horse, continued to give commands. After a sick leave at home, Mackenzie returned in the middle of November. He was appointed brigadier general of volunteers in December 1864. Following the war, he remained in the army and was made colonel of the Fourth Infantry in March 1867. His service was primarily on the frontier fighting Indians. Because he had lost two fingers on his right hand the Indians called him "Bad Hand." He received his last wound in an Indian fight at Blanco Canyon, Texas, on October 15, 1871. (Other sources report that this occurred on October 19.) An arrow went to the bone through the front of his right mid-thigh. He was taken to the rear, where a surgeon cut out the arrow and dressed the wound. He continued on the field, but the leg wound became worse, and he had to join the other disabled men at Duck Creek on October 29. On November 8 he arrived at Fort Richardson with the wound still opening on occasions. He developed acute rheumatism on July 20, 1873, which involved particularly the fascia and aponeuroses of his right shoulder and arm. The front of his right chest, his legs, and his left forearm were also involved. The reaction finally settled in his right knee joint and the surrounding structures. He was sick at Fort Clark, Texas, from August 6 to September 7, 1873. By September 12, the fever and constitutional distress along with much of the local pain, heat, and redness had in a great measure subsided. There was more or less tumefaction and a tendency to thickening and consolidation of the involved parts. In addition, his general system had lost functional vigor. He obtained a leave and, after being in Washington, D.C., during December, he returned in January 1874. In the autumn of 1875 at Fort Sill, Oklahoma, he had a bad accident. When his horse started suddenly, he fell from a wagon and landed on his head. For two or three days he remained in a stupor. Late in 1882 he had more trouble with his rheumatism, and he grew despondent over what he considered unfair treatment by his superiors. On October 30, 1883, he arrived back at San Antonio, Texas. Soon afterward he started exhibiting signs of mental changes and displayed eccentricity, drank excessively, and considered marriage. On the night of December 18 he was injured in a fight in San Antonio. The next day he had mental aberrations and, unable to exercise command, was placed on sick report. His violence and delusions varied from day to day. Three physicians decided that his condition was hopeless. On December 26, accompanied by a doctor, two orderlies, his two aides, and his sister, Mackenzie left on a train for the East. At midnight on December 29 he arrived at the Bloomingdale Asylum in New York. There was no improvement in his condition, and in February 1884 his case was diagnosed as general paralysis of the insane with a poor prognosis. His mental condition was not due to drinking, but his drinking had been a symptom of the disease. In March 1884 he was retired because of disability with the rank of brigadier general. Discharged from Bloomingdale in June, Mackenzie went to Morristown, New Jersey. He was moved again in 1886 to New Brighton, Staten Island, and attended by his sister. Died January 19, 1889, at New Brighton and was buried at West Point. According to his attending physician, the immediate cause of death was general paresis. Later historians, who assumed that everything called general paresis was due to a syphilitic infection, attributed his condition to this agent. More recently, it has been suggested that his mental problem was due to post-traumatic stress disorder and dementia. All such speculations about a retrospective diagnosis without actually seeing and examining the patient are just that: speculations.[1]

1. CSR; *OR*, vol. 42, pt. 3:1029; vol. 43, pt. 1:33, 131, 175; WPCHR, vols. 609, 610; LR, ACP, 3877, 1873, fiche: 000137; Ernest Wallace, *Ranald S. Mackenzie on the Texas Frontier*, 6–10, 54–55, 66, 170, 190–94; Charles M. Robinson, III, *Bad Hand: A Biography of General Ranald S. Mackenzie*, 15–18, 20,

22–26, 336; Heitman, *Historical Register and Dictionary* 2:29; Lessing Nohl, "Bad Hand: The Military Career of Ranald Slidell Mackenzie, 1871–1889" (diss.), 329–30.

JUSTUS MCKINSTRY • *Born July 6, 1814,* probably in Columbia County, New York. Graduated from the USMA in 1838. While at West Point, he was treated for a wound twice and once each for a cold, diarrhea, sore eyes, and a headache. Served in the Mexican War. His prewar career was as a quartermaster. In September 1861 he was made brigadier general of volunteers. McKinstry's illegal dealings with various contractors while quartermaster led to his arrest and dismissal in January 1863. Following his discharge he held minor business positions. Died in St. Louis on December 11, 1897, and was buried in Highland Cemetery, Ypsilanti, Michigan. Burial records: Cause of death, senile debility.[1]

1. WPCHR, vols. 603, 604; Highland Cemetery Association, Ypsilanti, Mich.

NATHANIEL COLLINS MCLEAN • *Born on February 2, 1815,* at Ridgeville, Ohio. He left his Ohio law practice and in 1861 was commissioned colonel of the 75th Ohio. He suffered from jaundice and debility in July 1862 and required a leave the next month. His promotion as brigadier general ranked from November 1862. He served at Chancellorsville, at New Hope Church, and in the Carolinas. McLean's military service in the field was long criticized by his superiors, and he finally resigned in April 1865.[1] He returned home, resumed his law practice, and later took up farming. Died at Bellport, Long Island, on January 4, 1905, and was buried there.

DEATH CERTIFICATE: Cause of death, chief cause, bronchitis; contributing, pulmonary congestion.

1. CSR; RVA, Pension, C 623,476.

JAMES WINNING MCMILLAN • *Born April 28, 1825,* in Clark County, Kentucky. Served in the Mexican War. Engaged in business in Indiana at the start of the war, he was appointed colonel of the 21st Indiana in 1861. In the parish of East Baton Rouge, Louisiana, on June 10, 1862, he received multiple gunshot wounds. One ball penetrated the right side of the abdomen, lodged probably near the spine, and was never removed. He was also shot through the left hand and arm. His entire treatment was performed in his quarters, so he was never hospitalized. His promotion as brigadier general ranked from November 1862. At the Battle of Winchester, Virginia, on September 19, 1864, he was struck on the head by a piece of shell, which apparently caused little difficulty. On October 26 he went on sick leave due to a fistula in ano, which he had had for thirteen months, and was back in December. In March 1865, he had a twenty-day sick leave because of subacute rheumatism and the effects of malarial poisoning. McMillan resigned his commission in May 1865. His family physician reported in 1872 that he had pain in his right hip and leg, probably from the retained ball. In addition, he also had "superficial deposits of seropurulent matter probably from pyemia caused by irritation from the ball." An examination in 1873 revealed that the well-healed scar of the entrance of the bullet was at a point 8¼ inches to the right and one inch above the umbilicus. Atrophy of the right leg and hip was present. There was still suppuration along with adherent scars on his scalp in 1874 from his old head wound. In 1875 he was appointed a member of the review board in the Washington pension office. The physician who took care of him in Washington reported that there was continuous necrosis of the bones of his skull, and the continued hip and leg pain at times required the use of anodynes.[1] He died at his residence in Washington, D.C., on March 9, 1903, and was buried in Arlington National Cemetery.

DEATH CERTIFICATE: Cause of death, primary, general debility, many years duration; immediate, exhaustion.

1. CSR; *OR*, vol. 15:58; RVA, Pension, C 824,361.

JOHN MCNEIL • *Born February 14, 1813,* in Halifax, Nova Scotia. A member of the Missouri legislature in 1844–45, he was president of an insurance company in St. Louis when the war started. McNeil was captain of a volunteer company early in 1861, colonel of the 3rd Missouri Infantry in May, and colonel of the 2nd Missouri State Militia Cavalry in June 1862. His commission as brigadier general of volunteers ranked from November. On May 15, 1863, he was wounded when one of his staff accidently shot him with a pistol. He returned in July when ordered to take command of the district of Southwest Missouri. His resignation was accepted April 22, 1865.[1] After returning to St. Louis he held a number of county and federal offices. Died June 8, 1891, in St. Louis and was buried there in Bellefontaine Cemetery.

DEATH CERTIFICATE: Cause of death, heart failure.

1. *OR*, vol. 48, pt. 2:160; U.S. Army, CWS, roll 2, vol. 3, report 16, pp. 429–57.

JAMES BIRDSEYE MCPHERSON • *Born November 14, 1828,* near the present town of Clyde, Ohio. Graduated from the USMA in 1853. As a cadet, he was treated at the hospital for rheumatism four times and once each for luxatio, catarrhus, phlegmon, diarrhea, excoriatio, and odontalgia. He was sick in the summer of 1854. He served as an engineer prior to the war and was promoted to first lieutenant in August 1861. Sick with a throat ailment at Fort Donelson during February 1862, he was sent to St. Louis for treatment. There were conflicting reports as to whether this was an infectious problem or a cystic tumor that produced pressure on his trachea and interfered with his respiration. He was a staff officer at Shiloh, and in October 1862 he was made a major general of volunteers. He commanded the Seventeenth Corps at Vicksburg and on March 26, 1864, was named to command the Army of the Tennessee. On July 22, 1864, he was killed in the opening minutes of the Battle of Atlanta. The ball had struck McPherson in the back, ranged diagonally forward, and came out at the left breast, passing near the heart and apparently through the lung.[1] He was buried near his boyhood home in Clyde.

1. OR, vol. 7:944; vol. 38, pt. 3:23, 28, 39, 54, 122, 395, 476, 556; WPCHR, vol. 608; Steiner, *Medical-Military Portraits*, 190–214; MOLLUS 10:311–43; Sherman, *Memoirs of General William T. Sherman* 2:78.

JASPER ADALMORN MALTBY • *Born on November 3, 1826*, in Kingsville, Ohio. He was severely wounded at Chapultepec during the Mexican War. A gunsmith and businessman, he entered the 45th Illinois Volunteers and was appointed lieutenant colonel in December 1861. At Fort Donelson on February 15, 1862, Maltby was wounded by two musket balls: one that went through both thighs and one that hit above the elbow. He was back on duty the following May and led a brigade at Vicksburg. On May 13, 1863, he was so sick that he had to ride in an ambulance. However, as soon as the enemy was known to be in force he mounted his horse and assumed command of his regiment. When Fort Hill was blown up on June 25, 1863, he was hit on the head and on his right side by a piece of timber, inflicting internal injuries and breaking several ribs. Following this injury, he developed an internal abscess as frequently as once every three months. Maltby was promoted to brigadier general in August 1863 and was discharged in January 1866. He had an intra-abdominal abscess in August 1867. While on duty as military mayor of Vicksburg in September 1867 he was very weak, barely able to sit up, and transacted work in spite of constant pain in his left side. The side was tender and had the appearance of another abscess beginning to form. Maltby was up and attending business at Vicksburg for a few hours before his death. Suddenly seeming to lose consciousness, he sank down and died on December 12, 1867. It was speculated that he died of yellow fever; however, his last symptoms do not support such a diagnosis, and his wife made a good case against the diagnosis. Either a cardiovascular event or something related to his long-term intra-abdominal infection would seem more probable.[1] He was buried in Greenwood Cemetery, Galena, Illinois.

1. CSR; OR, vol. 7:178, 197; vol. 24, pt. 1:708; RVA, Pension WC 181,619.

JOSEPH KING FENNO MANSFIELD • *Born on December 22, 1803*, in New Haven, Connecticut. Graduated from the USMA in 1822. He was wounded at Monterey, Mexico, on September 21, 1846. In 1853, he was appointed to the staff rank of colonel in the inspector general's department. He was promoted in May 1861 to brigadier general in the Regular Army. He was mortally wounded on September 17, 1862, at Antietam. His horse was shot first and then he was wounded, but the injury was not observed by his men. Mansfield attempted to ride over a rail fence but the wounded horse would not jump it. He dismounted and led the horse over. When the wind blew his coat aside it was observed that his front was covered with blood. He was too weak to mount another horse and asked to be taken off of the field. His men carried him off the field on their muskets until a blanket was procured. An ambulance was found, and he was taken to the rear where he died the next day.[1] He was buried in Indian Hill Cemetery, Middletown, Connecticut.

1. *OR*, vol. 19, pt. 1:30, 56, 179, 198, 270, 275, 485, 492; vol. 25, pt. 2:140, 186; *OR Suppl.*, vol. 3, pt. 1:563; Heitman, *Historical Register and Dictionary* 2:30; *Battles and Leaders* 2:640–41.

MAHLON DICKERSON MANSON • *Born February 20, 1820,* in Piqua, Ohio. Served in the Mexican War. Although he had studied medicine, he was a politician and druggist at the start of the Civil War. He joined the Federal service as a captain of the 10th Indiana in April 1861 and became its colonel in May. On September 21, 1861, he was riding down the street in New Albany, Indiana, when his horse slipped. He was thrown, and his left wrist was dislocated and the radius was fractured. He sent for a physician, who dressed his arm and put it in a sling. Obstinate diarrhea, nausea, and irritability of his stomach started in the middle of January 1862 and was treated in camp. The condition did not respond to therapy, and on March 19 he finally requested medical leave. During that month Manson was promoted to brigadier general. He was ordered to report for duty in May. While trying to get through Confederate lines during the night of August 29, 1862, at Richmond, Kentucky, he was wounded. The ball entered his right anterior thigh about five inches below the hip joint and was never removed. Soon afterward, his horse was killed; it fell on him, severely injuring his chest. Captured shortly afterward, he was paroled the next day. In August 1863, following a cold, he had the onset of rheumatism. He used a cane and had to be helped onto his horse. For the rest of his life he was never free from rheumatism. At Resaca, Georgia, on May 14, 1864, he had just stepped out of the works when a shell exploded near him. Stunned, he was taken to a private house on the field. The explosion had produced a concussion of his brain and had injured his right shoulder joint. At the time, there was temporary paralysis of the arm. The surgeon stayed with him until May 16, when Manson was taken to Dalton on the way to a general hospital in Knoxville. He continued to suffer from the effects of the concussion and remained in the hospital until August, when he returned to light duty. Finally, he was brought home on a cot and resigned from Federal service in December 1864. As a result of his continued illness, he was in St. Joseph's Infirmary in Louisville, Kentucky, from December 1, 1864, to March 1865. He had a fever of the typhoid type, delirium, and was confined to his bed for part of the time. It was determined that the fever was the result of a large abscess secondary to the injury. The abscess was under the right pectoral muscle, extended over the entire right side of his chest, and passed over his shoulder and down the arm to a point midway between the shoulder and elbow. When it was opened through an incision in the axilla, immense quantities of purulent matter were discharged. Following the war, he held various elected and appointive positions despite his physical problems. For the next thirty years he suffered from rheumatism and required the use of liniments and medications. For some months after he returned home he had to be waited on constantly. Crippled and hardly able to get around, he was at times so stiff that he could not put on his stockings, vest, or coat without help. He had shortness of breath, weakness, dizziness, and pain in his limbs. In March 1871 an examining surgeon found that Manson had partial paralysis of his right arm with atrophy, and his ability to raise the arm was limited. The old fracture and dislocation of the left wrist impaired pronation and supination. By 1874 he was unable to use his right arm to feed himself. He had constant pain in his right shoulder in 1875 and occasionally lost the use of his right leg while walking. He had a stroke between 1881 and 1884. In April 1886, an examination revealed the following: There was paralysis of his right arm. He suffered pain in the right arm and shoulder all the time and, as a result, did not sleep well. There was partial ankylosis of the right shoulder, atrophy of the right arm, a half-inch shortening of the right humerus, and associated loss of force and motion. There was a scar on the anterior and outer aspect of right thigh at about the middle point. Atrophy of the thigh was accompanied by loss of force and motility, with a tendency for the leg to evert. A tumor the size of a hen egg protruded from his umbilicus with a strong impulse felt on coughing, and had been present since his horse fell on him. By June 1887 he could not raise his right arm to a right angle with his body on account of partial ankylosis of the shoulder joint. On inspection, the right shoulder drooped lower than the left. There was loss of sensation of the right arm and decreased power of grasping. The left wrist had not properly been reduced. He had a second stroke about two or three years before his death but recovered to some extent. On February 1, 1895, he was on a train returning home when he became sick and had to be taken off at Frankfort, Indiana. Upon arrival at the Crutler House, his pulse was rapid, his temperature normal, and his heart action feeble. He had numerous bowel movements and could not retain his urine. He complained of pain in his breast and abdomen and died in Frankfort on February 4, 1895.[1] He was buried in Oak Hill Cemetery, Crawfordsville, Indiana.

DEATH CERTIFICATE: Cause of death, heart failure caused by rheumatism.

1. CSR; *OR*, vol. 16, pt. 1:914; vol. 38, pt. 1:113, pt. 2:678–79, 714, 716, 724; vol. 52, pt. 1:275; RVA, Pension XC 940,665.

RANDOLPH BARNES MARCY • *Born on April 9, 1812,* at Greenwich, Massachusetts, a town that no longer exists. Graduated from the USMA in 1832. Served in the Mexican War. During the Utah expedition in 1857–58 he suffered the "pains of a dozen deaths" due to the terrible conditions but he conducted the party to New Mexico. His men had no food for thirteen days except for their underfed mules. He served on the frontier and wrote a book on travel in the West. When the war began he was a paymaster. In May 1861 he became chief-of-staff to his son-in-law, George B. McClellan. Marcy was appointed an inspector general of the Regular Army with the rank of colonel in August 1861. In September 1861 he was appointed brigadier general of volunteers, but the Senate failed to confirm him and his appointment expired in March 1863. He reported for duty on January 1, 1862, after having restored his health from an undefined sickness. He was promoted to inspector general of the U.S. Army in December 1878 with the rank of brigadier general and retired in 1881. Died at his residence at West Orange, New Jersey, on November 22, 1887, and was buried in Riverview Cemetery in Trenton.[1]

1. LR, ACP, 5556, 1887, fiche: 000138.

GILMAN MARSTON • *Born on August 20, 1811,* at Oxford, New Hampshire. A lawyer and politician, he led the 2nd New Hampshire at the start of the war. On July 21, 1861, at the battle of First Bull Run, a musket ball fractured his right arm near the shoulder. After his wound was dressed, he remained in the saddle, and his horse was led by his orderly. Home on leave, he reported from New Hampshire in September that, although the bone seemed to have united, he still had little use of the arm. On December 15, 1861, he was wounded by a pistol accidently discharged by an officer's servant. There is no evidence that he missed duty from this injury. His promotion as brigadier general of volunteers ranked from November 1862. In June 1864 he was at Cold Harbor. He was ill on October 3, 1864, and, after turning over his command, went on leave. In April 1865 he resigned and returned to the practice of the law.[1] Died at Exeter, New Hampshire, on July 3, 1890, and was buried there.
DEATH CERTIFICATE: Cause of death, uremia.

1. CSR; *OR,* vol. 2:396, 399; vol. 51, pt. 1:1187–88; Sommers, *Richmond Redeemed,* 532.

JOHN HENRY MARTINDALE • *Born on March 20, 1815,* in Sandy Hill, New York. Graduated from the USMA in 1835. While at West Point, he was treated for a cold twice and for a sore throat, bronchitis, headache, debility, colica, influenza, and a toothache once each. Martindale resigned his commission in 1836 and practiced the law until the start of the Civil War. In August 1861 he was commissioned brigadier general of volunteers and in the spring of 1862 led a brigade on the Peninsula. He was sick with typhoid fever in early July 1862 and on July 11 left his brigade. During August through October he was absent sick in Washington. Following his recovery, he was assigned to other duties, and by March 1863 had still not resumed his command. He led a division at Cold Harbor, Bermuda Hundred, and Petersburg. In July 1864, Gen. Benjamin F. Butler reported that Martindale's health was so bad that he should not be assigned to command of the Tenth Corps. Because of his poor health he resigned in September 1864.[1] He returned to the practice of law in New York. Died in Nice, France, on December 13, 1881, and was buried in Batavia, New York.

1. CSR; *OR*, vol. 11, pt. 2:295; vol. 19, pt. 2:527; vol. 40, pt. 3:376; vol. 51, pt. 1:863; WPCHR, vols. 601, 602, 603.

JOHN SANFORD MASON • *Born August 21, 1824,* in Steubenville, Ohio. Graduated from the USMA in 1847. As a cadet, he was treated for catarrhus three times, cephalalgia twice, and obstipatio once. He served in Mexico until November 1847 when he had to take a sick leave. In March 1848 he went on recruiting service. In July he was confined to his bed in Smithfield, Ohio, with yellow fever. He arrived at Fort Adams, Rhode Island, in late September 1848 and, while living in the casemate quarters, suffered poor health due to a fever. He received a sick leave and returned to duty in the spring of 1849. The following fall his health deteriorated again when he had to live in the casemate quarters. He was stationed at Fort Vancouver, Washington, when the Civil War started. Mason was appointed colonel of the 4th Ohio Volunteer Infantry in October 1861. He served in West Virginia and on the Peninsula. In June 1862 he had the onset of diarrhea and bronchitis, with pain and tenderness in the region of the apex of his left lung, together with spasmodic asthma. By October 1862, the diarrhea had become chronic, and he was absent sick in Ohio from October 16 to November 6. He was promoted brigadier general in November and led a brigade at Fredericksburg. In January 1863 he received a leave on surgeon's certificate. On expiration of his leave he reported for duty in April, but because of continued ill health, his leave was extended. Still too sick to take the field, Mason spent the rest of the war in Ohio, California, and Nevada on muster and recruiting duty. He was promoted to major of the Seventeenth Infantry in 1864. He remained in the army and served on the frontier. Mason had severe physical changes starting in October 1869 while at Fort Bayard, New Mexico. He was on sick leave from August 1870 until May 1872, and over the next few years each surgeon made a different diagnosis. His surgeon reported in June 1870 that his symptoms for the previous eight months suggested congestion of the brain with a tendency to white softening. The surgeon who took care of him in September 1871 stated that he suffered from a cerebral affection whose character was obscure. In May 1872, the surgeon expanded the findings and stated that Mason's condition was probably due to an embolism. His problem was attended with frequent attacks of vertigo and a partial loss of sensation in his hands and legs. The surgeon theorized that the condition had been aggravated over the previous eighteen months by Mason living at a high elevation. After returning to duty at Fort Garland, Colorado, for a few weeks in May 1872, he went on sick leave again. His attending surgeon in July 1873 reported that the diagnosis was a slight "compression of the brain" and stated that he should not be at a high altitude. In October 1875 a surgeon stated he had partial anaemia of the brain accompanied with severe and paroxysmal headaches and occasional congestion of the blood vessels to the head. The latter was caused by the increased arterial pressure due in a great measure to the high altitude at which he had been residing. His problems continued, and he retired in 1888.[1] Mason died at his residence on November 29, 1897, in Washington, D.C., and was buried in Arlington National Cemetery.

DEATH CERTIFICATE: Cause of death, primary, general paralysis (paresis); immediate, edema of lungs and heart failure. Duration, several years.

1. CSR; *OR*, vol. 23, pt. 2:169, 218; vol. 50, pt. 2:675; WPCHR, vol. 605; RVA, Pension WC 466,809; LR, ACP, 2232, 1871; U.S. Army, CWS, roll 4, vol. 6, report 26, pp. 505–19.

CHARLES (KARL) LEOPOLD MATTHIES • *Born May 31, 1824,* in Bromberg, Prussia. After serving in the Prussian army, Matthies came to the United States in 1849. A businessman in Iowa, he entered Federal service as a captain in the 1st Iowa Volunteers in May 1861. He served at Island No. 10, Corinth, Iuka, and Vicksburg. On October 13, 1862, Matthies received a leave of absence on surgeon's certificate because of a bilious attack and went to Iowa to recover. Afterward he returned to his command on November 11. Having passed through grades, he was promoted to brigadier general of volunteers to rank from that month. During the last of December he was hospitalized in Memphis, Tennessee, and returned in January 1863. At Missionary Ridge on November 25, 1863, he was wounded in the head and was unconscious for a few minutes. He was compelled to leave the field and relinquish his command. He remained hospitalized near Chattanooga, Tennessee, until December 6 when he received a leave of absence and returned to Iowa. After recovering from his wound, he returned to his command at Huntsville, Alabama, in February 1864. He resigned in May.[1] Died October 16, 1868, in Burlington, Iowa, and was buried there in Aspen Grove Cemetery.

1. CSR; *OR*, vol. 31, pt. 2:69, 88, 648, 653; vol. 32, pt. 2:497; U.S. Army, CWS, roll 2, vol. 3, report 3, pp. 95–197.

GEORGE GORDON MEADE • *Born December 31, 1815,* in Cadiz, Spain. Graduated from the USMA in 1835. Cadet Meade was treated for a headache six times, a cold three times, and once each for a sore hand, a sore throat, a boil, a fever, rheumatism, nausea, influenza, a wound, and vomiting. Served in the Florida and Mexican wars. In April 1836, Meade was an invalid because of recurrent attacks of fever and was unfit for arduous field duties in Florida. A change of climate was recommended, and he was assigned to duty transporting the Seminoles, who were to be resettled. The group left Tampa by schooner and were transferred at New Orleans to flatboats for the trip up the Mississippi and Arkansas rivers. After reaching Little Rock on June 1, they went by foot overland into Indian Territory. His health improved during the trip but he resigned his commission in 1836 to become a civil engineer. In 1842 he rejoined the army corps of engineers. During the cold October weather in 1845 he undertook a survey of the inner waterway running to Point Isabel, Texas, and on his return was jaundiced. He continued to be ill into December, and the surgeon recommended that he go home on leave. In August 1861 he was made a brigadier general of volunteers. He was severely wounded twice at Frayser's Farm, Virginia, on June 30, 1862. Faint and suffering, he could scarcely maintain his saddle and rode slowly to the rear. The pain became worse, forcing him to dismount. When his two-wheeled mess wagon passed, he was placed in the cart and arrived at Haxall's Landing after midnight. That night he was put in Gen. Seth Williams's tent. The surgeon examined him and found that he had received a gunshot wound of his right forearm and a wound on the right side of his back, just above the crest of the ilium. The parts were swollen due to the length and severity of his trip to the rear. Probing for the ball in his back was impossible because the pain was so severe. The surgeon reported that the ball may have gone through the right kidney because of the location of the external wound. Meade did pass blood in his urine, so the urinary tract must have been injured. On July 1 he was carried down the James River in a hospital transport. He arrived at Fortress Monroe on the Hampton Road and was transferred to a boat headed for Baltimore. After his arrival there, he was put on a boat for Philadelphia, where he arrived on July 4. The arm wound healed rapidly, but he was confined for a few weeks by the body wound. He returned to duty on August 12, still much prostrated from the effects of his wounds, but served at Second Bull Run, Antietam, and Fredericksburg. In the middle of January 1863 he had a cold followed by pneumonia and was confined for nearly three weeks. When he left for Washington in February he was still not well. After leading the Fifth Corps at Chancellorsville he was named commander of the Army of the Potomac on June 28, 1863, less than a week before Gettysburg. His appointment as a brigadier general in the Regular Army ranked from July 1863. For the rest of the war he was army commander, although for most of the time he was effectively Grant's subordinate. His friends noted in October that his hair and beard were turning prematurely grey. Meade had pneumonia in January 1864 and went to Philadelphia to recover. He returned in late February. He was quite sick again on April 1, 1865, and for the next few days had chills followed by a cough and fever. He had to be transported in an ambulance. He remained in the army after the war and held department and division commands. An episode of pneumonia in May 1866 confined him to bed for three weeks. In April 1869 he had a bout of pneumonia, but this time it was associated with prominent jaundice. While taking a walk on October 31, 1872, he developed a severe pain in his side. He went home and was put to bed with pneumonia and jaundice. He died at his Philadelphia residence on November 6, 1872, and was buried in Laurel Hill Cemetery. Autopsy findings demonstrated he had pneumonia accompanied by enlargement of the liver from congestion. On the surface of the liver was a well-defined scar corresponding to the external skin scar and marking the course of a bullet. The attending surgeons stated that the old liver wound was a factor in Meade's repeated episodes of jaundice.[1]

DEATH CERTIFICATE: Cause of death, pneumonia.

1. CSR; *OR*, vol. 11, pt. 2:32, 228; vol. 27, pt. 1:769; vol. 29, pt. 2:598; vol. 33:448, 506, 541; vol. 46, pt. 3:423; RVA, Pension WC 219,235; LR, ACP, 11, 1885, fiche: 000144; WPCHR, vols. 601, 602, 603; Freeman Cleaves, *Meade of Gettysburg*, 14, 20, 40, 68–69, 71, 202, 219–20, 313, 317, 322, 324, 329–30; Lymon, *Meade's Headquarters*, 345, 348.

THOMAS FRANCIS MEAGHER • *Born on August 3, 1823,* in Waterford, Ireland. Because of his participation in various subversive groups, Meagher was expelled from Ireland by British authorities. He ultimately reached New York in the early 1850s. He organized a militia company in 1861, which became a part of the 69th New York Militia. At First Bull Run, Virginia, on July 21, 1861, he was knocked senseless on the field. A U.S. trooper galloped by, grabbed him by the back of the neck, put him across his saddle, and carried him a few hundred yards to the rear. When Meagher was able to get on his feet he walked back toward Centreville, Virginia, until he was picked up by an artillery wagon. While crossing a stream, one of the wagon's horses was shot, and Meagher was pitched into the water. The next winter he organized the Irish Brigade and was appointed brigadier general of volunteers to rank from February 1862. Toward the end of the Battle of Antietam on September 17, his horse was wounded and fell on him. Because of the severe shock, he had to be carried off the field. The next day he was able to return to duty. At the Battle of Fredericksburg, December 13, 1862, he was lame due to an ulcer of his left knee, which made it difficult for him to walk or ride. He had concealed the ulcer for days. On December 22 he went on sick leave and accompanied the body of a friend back to New York. Although he rose from his bed to go to the funeral, he was confined to bed for some weeks afterward. He resumed command of his brigade on February 18, 1863. In April the surgeon treated him for sciatica. Meagher resigned in 1865 and was appointed territorial secretary of Montana. On July 1, 1867, after being sick with severe diarrhea for three days, he found a place to sleep on a steamboat that had been moored on the Missouri River at Fort Benton, Idaho. He went ashore to a trading post in the afternoon and remained seated in a back room for several hours with his head on his hands. Frequently he had to rush out to the woods in back to relieve himself. The proprietor urged him to take the only remedy available, a glass of blackberry wine. This was repeated three times during his long ordeal at the trading post. Toward nightfall he went to the boat and retired to his stateroom. About 10:00 P.M. the sentry saw someone in white underclothes go to the stern. Realizing that this was the location of the temporary accommodations, and thinking one of the officers had a "short call," the sentry about-faced and started back the other way. He soon heard a splash. Meagher had fallen overboard, and in spite of the use of boats and buoys flung into the swollen and rapid river, his body was never found.[1]

1. OR, vol. 19, pt. 1:59, 279, 295, 298; vol. 21:228, 242; RVA, Pension WC 231,360; RAGO, entry 534; Michael Cavanagh, Memoirs of Gen. Thomas Francis Meagher, Comprising the Leading Events of His Career, 397–98, 474, appendix, 10–12.

MONTGOMERY CUNNINGHAM MEIGS • Born May 3, 1816, in Augusta, Georgia. Graduated from the USMA in 1836. He was treated at the Cadet Hospital for a sprained ankle twice and one time each for a headache and a pain in his side. Prior to the Civil War he had a prominent role in the construction of the Potomac Aqueduct and additions to Federal buildings in Washington, D.C. In the middle of 1860, Meigs stated that the rheumatism, which had bothered him for years and made writing difficult, might be helped by the climate of Tortuga. He was made quartermaster general of the U.S. Army in May 1861 with the rank of brigadier general and served as quartermaster general until his retirement. In November 1866 he was bothered by swelling of his legs, dyspepsia, and a fast pulse that increased with the slightest exertion. His brother, a physician, examined him and stated that the symptoms were due to many years of exertion. A severe cold in December further complicated his condition. He went to his office as usual on January 2, 1867, but was not able to remain very long. He went to the office again on January 3 but became tired with only minor exertions. On January 6 he remained in bed all day with a feeble pulse, cough, and headache. His physician stated he had a mild attack of typhoid fever. By the end of the month he was able to get out of bed. After recovering enough to travel, he returned to Philadelphia where his brother examined him and reported that he had emphysema. His father, also a physician, stated he could find no evidence of emphysema. A year's leave in Europe appeared to improve his health. He retired from the army in 1882. In May 1891 he reported his health was good except for rheumatism in his knee and twinges in other parts of his body. Steambaths appeared to control the symptoms. On occasion he also saw double.[1] Died at his residence in Washington, D.C., on January 2, 1892, and was buried in Arlington National Cemetery.

DEATH CERTIFICATE: Cause of death, primary, epidemic influenza, about a week; immediate, pneumonia.

1. WPCHR, vols. 602, 603; Russell F. Weigley, "M. C. Meigs, Builder of the Capitol and Lincoln's Quartermaster General: A Biography" (diss.), 313, 660–61, 663–65, 706.

SOLOMON MEREDITH • *Born May 29, 1810,* in Guilford County, North Carolina. A county sheriff and member of the state legislature, he was appointed colonel of the 19th Indiana at the start of the Civil War. Because of a fall during the Second Bull Run campaign on August 29, 1862, and the subsequent fatigue and exposure from the marches, he was unable to take command in the middle of September. Promoted brigadier general in October, he reported back the next month and was assigned to duty. He served at Chancellorsville, and at Gettysburg on July 1, 1863, he received severe internal injuries when his wounded horse fell with him. He also sustained contusions of his scalp, chest, and thigh. Meredith was absent sick from July to October 1863. On October 17 he was ordered to report to the adjutant general in Washington. In November he was ordered to return to the Army of the Potomac. He had a pleurisy-type of chest pain in late November and early January. During January and February 1864 he was absent on sick leave in Indiana. He suffered from general nervous prostration resulting from past exposure but more especially from the head wound received at Gettysburg. In addition, he had pain and soreness of his left breast, a cough, bloody expectorate, and difficulty breathing because of two fractured ribs. One surgeon suspected he had tuberculosis.[1] He remained in the army after the war and retired in 1869 to raise livestock. Died October 2, 1875, near Cambridge City, Indiana, and was buried in Riverside Cemetery.

1. CSR; *OR*, vol. 19, pt. 1:251; vol. 27, pt. 1:254, pt. 3:777; vol. 29, pt. 2:414; vol. 51, pt. 1:951, 1105; RAGO, entry 534; U.S. Army, CWS, Abner Doubleday, report 5, roll 8, vol. 13, p. 627; Pension of Sullivan Amory Meredith RVA, WC 787,534.

SULLIVAN AMORY MEREDITH • *Born in Philadelphia on July 4, 1816.* Engaged in business in Philadelphia at the start of the Civil War, he was commissioned colonel of the 10th Pennsylvania Militia. Near Gainesville, Virginia, on August 28, 1862, he was seriously wounded by a minié ball through the right breast and upper third of the arm. He had a medical leave in Washington and Philadelphia. In November, still suffering from his wounds, he had an acute attack of rheumatic gout. He was absent on sick leave until January 1863. Having been promoted brigadier general of volunteers in November 1862, he was appointed a member of a military commission at Washington in February. After his discharge in August 1865, he moved to Buffalo, New York, in 1866 and was involved in the wholesale drug business. Died December 26, 1874, in Buffalo, New York, and was buried there in Forest Lawn Cemetery. Burial records: Cause of death, heart disease.[1]

1. CSR; *OR*, vol. 12, pt. 2:370, 373–74; U.S. Army, CWS, roll 4, vol. 6, report 28, pp. 537–43; RVA, Pension WC 878,534; Register of St. Luke's Church, Buffalo, N.Y.

WESLEY MERRITT • *Born June 16, 1834,* in New York City. Graduated from the USMA in 1860. Merritt had a number of medical problems while at West Point.

He was treated for catarrhus nine times, diarrhea seven times, cephalalgia six times, odontalgia five times, contusio four times, excoriatio, nausea, and febris intermittent tertian three times each, phlegmon twice, and clavus, vulnus incisum, ophthalmia, subluxatio, headache, neuralgia, and tonsillitis once each. In February 1862 he was made aide-de-camp to Gen. Philip Cooke and later to Gen. George Stoneman. At Brandy Station, Virginia, on June 9, 1863, he received a scalp wound from a saber. His thick hat and the handkerchief he used as a sweatband prevented more serious injury. Merritt was promoted brigadier general of volunteers in June 1863. He was on sick leave in December 1864 and returned the next month. Following the end of hostilities, he was made lieutenant colonel of the 9th Cavalry and was advanced through grades to major general in 1895. At Fort Davis, Texas, in July 1867, he and many of his men had dysentery. The illness continued through the summer, and in October he was too sick to inspect the command. He went on sick leave in November and remained absent until June 1868. On January 30, 1869, he sustained a comminuted fracture of the ulna and radius of the left arm when the wheels of a spring wagon ran over his arm. The arm was set by an inexperienced surgeon, and recovery was slow. He returned to duty in June, but in August his hand and arm were still stiff. In September he went to Austin, Texas, for medical consultation on his arm. His last major service was as commander of the Philippine expedition in 1898–99. He retired in June 1900. His health started to decline in 1906, and he became more senile. His nurse accompanied him on his visits to Illinois and various spas in Virginia. Died December 3, 1910, at one of the resorts at Natural Bridge, Virginia, and was buried at West Point. The adjutant general's office reported he died from arteriosclerosis.[1]

1. CSR; WPCHR, vol. 609; RVA, Pension WC 951,774; RAGO, entry 534; Don E. Alberts, *Brandy Station to Manila Bay: A Biography of General Wesley Merritt,* 46, 190, 196, 201, 324.

NELSON APPLETON MILES • *Born August 8, 1839,* near Westminster, Massachusetts. Prior to the war he worked in a store and was a night student. He was commissioned first lieutenant in the 22nd Massachusetts Volunteers in September 1861. His appointment as lieutenant colonel of the 61st New York ranked from May 1862. A ball grazed his heel at Seven Pines on June 1, 1862, and the next day he was limping around the camp with a bandaged foot. He was promoted to colonel after Antietam. During the Battle of Fredericksburg, Virginia, on December 13, 1862, Miles was again wounded. A minié ball had entered the front of his throat and came out near his left ear. He held together the torn flesh with his hands and, seated on a stretcher, reported to Gen. O. O. Howard. Miles had to take a medical leave until February 1863, when he returned to duty. On the road from Chancellorsville toward Fredericksburg on May 3, 1863, he was severely wounded in the abdomen. A sharpshooter's bullet struck his metal belt plate and glanced into his body. Following this wounding he had a sudden sickening sensation and dropped his sword. Completely paralyzed below the waist, he rode back holding onto the pommel of the saddle with both hands. Soldiers took him off the horse and carried him on a blanket to the Chancellor house. Miles was placed on a table, and the wound was examined and dressed. The bullet had entered obliquely one or two inches below his umbilicus and fractured the margin of the pelvis. He remained in the house until it was struck by a bursting shell and set on fire. Taken out on a stretcher, he was carried about five miles to the woods, where he and the men rested that night. The next morning he was transported by ambulance over a rough corduroy road twelve miles to the Lacy House Hospital in Falmouth. From there he was taken to Washington where his brother met him and took him home. After two weeks he could slightly move the toes of his right foot. Broken bone fragments and the bullet were removed, and after several weeks he was able to return to the field. His commission as brigadier general of volunteers ranked from May 1864. In June 1864, outside of Petersburg, a bullet struck the shield of his sword, splitting it in two, and a small piece struck the side of his neck, only burning it a little. That summer his leg was stiff and caused considerable pain. In September some of the surgeons suggested that he undergo another operation to scrape the bone in his hip in order for it to heal. He could ride well and had pain only in damp weather. In October he was ill with a fever for a few days but slowly recovered. Miles remained in the army and had a notable record in the Indian wars. In 1895 he became general-in-chief of the army and served in the war with Spain. He retired in 1903. During the 1919 victory parade in Washington, he marched down Pennsylvania Avenue with the Medal of Honor group, collapsing from exhaustion at the foot of Capitol Hill. On May 15, 1925, he went with his grandchildren to the circus in downtown Washington. When the band played the national anthem he stood to salute, then fell over backwards. He was carried from the tent and died before he could be taken to the hospital. Buried in Arlington National Cemetery.[1]

DEATH CERTIFICATE: Cause of death, myocarditis, acute dilatation.

1. CSR; *OR*, vol. 11, pt, 1:766,770; vol. 21:230, 237; vol. 25, pt. 1:317, 320, 323, 332–33; vol. 27, pt. 2:214; Nelson A. Miles Papers, USAMHI; Nelson A Miles, "The Biggest Days of Battle," *Cosmopolitan Magazine* (1911): 408–21; Howard, *Autobiography* 1:342; *MOLLUS* 17:131; Nelson A. Miles, *A Documentary Biography of His Military Career, 1861–1903,* 34, 37, 318–19.

JOHN FRANKLIN MILLER • *Born on November 21, 1831,* at South Bend, Indiana. After practicing the law in California and Indiana, he was elected a member of the Indiana state senate in 1861. He was commissioned colonel of the 29th Indiana Volunteers in August 1861. In late December he received a leave because of illness, and in January he was home in South Bend. When he returned to duty the next month, he assumed brigade command at Shiloh and Corinth. Wounded on the morning of December 31, 1862, at Stones River, Miller received a leave of absence on January 8. On June 25, 1863, at Liberty Gap, Tennessee, he was wounded and one eye was destroyed. Sent to a field hospital initially, he was later sent to Nashville. By late November he had recovered enough to serve on a military commission. His promotion as brigadier general of volunteers ranked from January 1864.[1] Miller fought in the Battle of Nashville, resigned in September 1865, and went to California. He engaged in business until 1880 when he was elected to the U.S. Senate. Died March 8, 1886, in Washington, D.C., and initially was buried in Laurel Hill Cemetery, San Francisco. His remains were later moved to Arlington National Cemetery.

DEATH CERTIFICATE: Cause of death, primary, Bright's disease of kidneys, chronic. Certainly eight months and probably one year in duration; immediate, pulmonary edema and heart failure.

1. CSR; *OR*, vol. 23, pt. 1:484, 502–3, 506; U.S. Army, CWS, roll 6, vol. 10, report 1, pp. 1–33; *MOLLUS* 6:128.

STEPHEN MILLER • *Born January 7, 1816,* in Carroll, Pennsylvania. Engaged in business and politics in Minnesota when the Civil War started, Miller entered service as lieutenant colonel of the 1st Minnesota. He was at First Bull Run, and on October 1, 1861, he was violently thrown when his horse fell on the public road near Edwards Ferry, Maryland. He received several injuries and was confined to his bed for almost four months in Harrisburg, Pennsylvania, and Washington, D.C. His spine and kidneys were so severely injured that he continued to suffer afterward. In February 1862 he returned to duty, although feeble and emaciated. The next month he was again on sick leave, returning for duty on the Peninsula in April. In August 1862 he was made colonel of the 7th Minnesota and in October 1863 was promoted brigadier general. He had served prominently in suppressing the Sioux uprising in Minnesota. After his election as governor of Minnesota in January 1864, he resigned from the army. In June 1881 the physician who had been taking care of him reported that Miller suffered from kidney disease or an injury of "some kind to his kidney of a type that he could frequently only urinate with the aid of an instrument to draw the water from him." The trouble had been gradually increasing for the previous two years. For five months, Miller had been compelled to have one to two persons in constant attendance, and for the three months before his death he had generalized dropsy.[1] Died in Worthington, Minnesota, on August 18, 1881, and was buried in that city.

DEATH CERTIFICATE: Cause of death, mortification.

1. CSR; RVA, Pension SC 172,385.

ROBERT HUSTON MILROY • *Born on June 11, 1816,* near Salem, Indiana. Served in the Mexican War. Milroy was practicing law in Indiana when the Civil War started and entered Federal service as colonel of the 9th Indiana. In September 1861 he was appointed brigadier general of volunteers, and his commission as major general ranked from November 1862. He served in West Virginia, in the Shenandoah Valley, and at Second Bull Run. At Winchester, Virginia, on June 15, 1863, his horse was wounded by the explosion of a shell; while attempting to jump off, Milroy was thrown. He was jarred and sprained his left hip joint. In the excitement of the moment, he ignored his injury and mounted another horse. He experienced little inconvenience and was not confined to a hospital. After the war he was trustee of the Wabash and Erie Canal Company and in 1872 was made Indian agent in Olympia, Washington. His physicians in 1866 stated he had rheumatism of the hip and treated him with rest, cupping, and irritating plasters. In 1866–68 the hip joint became increasingly painful. His condition worsened over the years, and in 1875 his physicians confined him to bed and performed cupping, blistering, and extensions with only temporary relief. In 1875 Milroy began a two-year effort to cultivate a small farm, but his disability made it impossible. Examination of his hip in 1879 revealed extreme tenderness over and around the hip joint and severe pain in the head of the femur and acetabulum. Little pain was produced by extension of the limb, but the pain was severe in moving it away from the body. The physicians made a diagnosis of subacute or chronic inflammation in the acetabulum and ligaments. He walked with a limp and required a cane.[1] Died at Olympia, Washington, on March 29, 1890, and was buried there in the Masonic Cemetery.

1. *OR*, vol. 38, pt. 4:54; U.S. Army, CWS, roll 4, vol. 6, report 31, pp. 669–907; RVA, Pension WC 275,317.

ORMSBY MACKNIGHT MITCHEL • *Born July 28, 1809,* at the site of the present town of Morganfield, Kentucky. Graduated from the USMA in 1829. Mitchel served as an instructor at West Point for seven years; after resigning from the army, he engaged in teaching and astronomy. He was appointed brigadier general of volunteers in August 1861 and major general to rank from April 1862. He was placed in command of the Department of the South and the Tenth Corps at Hilton Head, South Carolina, in September 1862. The steamer *Delaware* had arrived at Hilton Head on August 26 after visiting various ports, including Key West, which had cases of yellow fever. The ship was quarantined for ten days. Three days later, after the passengers were allowed ashore, yellow fever broke out among the 7th New Hampshire volunteers who were on board. Mitchel became sick at Hilton Head on October 27 and had to give up his command. After being ill for only four days, he died of yellow fever at Beaufort, South Carolina, on October 30, 1862.[1] Buried in Green-Wood Cemetery in Brooklyn, New York.

1. CSR; *OR*, vol. 14:380–81, 384, 387–88.

JOHN GRANT MITCHELL • *Born on November 6, 1838,* in Piqua, Ohio. A law student, he enlisted in an Ohio unit and was made first lieutenant in July 1861. He passed through grades and in May 1863 was made colonel of the 113th Ohio. On

June 13, 1863, he had an attack of smallpox, and on June 25 he went to the general hospital No. 1 in Murfreesboro, Tennessee. By the end of July he still had not fully recovered, and his condition was further complicated by diabetes insipidus. A change of climate was recommended, and he was on sick leave in August. He served at Chickamauga, in the Atlanta campaign, at Nashville, and in the Carolinas. He was appointed brigadier general of volunteers in January 1865 and major general by brevet in March. Mitchell resigned in July and returned to his law practice in Ohio.[1] Died November 7, 1894, in Columbus, Ohio, and was buried in Green Lawn Cemetery.

DEATH CERTIFICATE: Cause of death, uremia; contributing, chronic cystitis.

1. CSR; RVA, Pension WC 648,807.

ROBERT BYINGTON MITCHELL • *Born April 4, 1823,* in Mansfield, Ohio. Served in the Mexican War. A lawyer and politician, he was commissioned colonel of the 2nd Kansas Infantry at the start of the war. At Wilson's Creek on August 10, 1861, he received a rifle shot in his left groin. The ball entered in the front, just above the head of the femur, exposed the femoral artery, passed through the pelvic bone, and came out posterior to the hip joint in two places. Nerves and ligaments of the hip were injured, and his kidneys were affected. He was treated in the New Court House Hospital in Springfield, Missouri, and then at a private home until October. His commission as brigadier general ranked from April 1862, and in July he was assigned to brigade command and led a division at Perryville. In October he still had lameness of his limb. During January and February 1863 he was sick at Nashville, Tennessee, with typhoid pneumonia or "winter fever." Following this illness, he had episodes of asthma the rest of his life. He was on sick leave until September 1863. He was at Chickamauga, but in November he was relieved from command of the cavalry, Department of the Cumberland, because he was incapacitated for field service by his wounds. He did not want a leave of absence but requested duty as commander of some post and was ordered to Washington for temporary duty. In February 1864 he was relieved from general court-martial duty and was ordered to report to the Department of Kansas for duty. In April 1864 he had an episode of erysipelas and was ill for several days. Mitchell was mustered out of the Federal service in January 1866 and became governor of the New Mexico Territory in June. Following the war, he continued to require treatment for his asthma, and at intervals he was confined to his bed. The attacks were occasionally associated with severe coughing and expectoration of offensive mucus.[1] Died January 26, 1882, at his residence in Washington, D.C., and was buried in Arlington National Cemetery.

DEATH CERTIFICATE: Cause of death, primary, asthma; immediate, pneumonia. Duration, two days.

1. OR, vol. 3:56, 67, 70, 83; vol. 17, pt. 2:105; vol. 30, pt. 1:892; vol. 31, pt. 2:62, pt. 3:222; vol. 34, pt. 2:848, pt. 3:241–42; RVA, Pension WC 196,683.

WILLIAM READING MONTGOMERY • *Born on July 10, 1801,* in Monmouth County, New Jersey. Graduated from the USMA in 1825. Served in the Florida and Mexican wars. He was wounded at Resaca de la Palma on May 9, 1846, and again at Molino del Rey on September 8, 1847. When the Civil War started he became colonel of the 1st New Jersey Volunteers. His appointment as brigadier general of volunteers ranked from May 1861. In June he fell from his horse while on duty at Camp Aldman, near Trenton, New Jersey, and fractured a rib. He was disabled for a few days. He was absent sick in November and December 1861 and was sick again in November 1862. Before his resignation in April 1864, he had suffered poor health for five months.[1] He returned to business in Pennsylvania. Died the night of May 31 to June 1, 1871, at Bristol, Pennsylvania, and was buried there in St. James Churchyard.

1. CSR; LR, ACP, 2043, 1886; Heitman, *Historical Register and Dictionary* 2:31.

GEORGE WEBB MORELL • *Born January 8, 1815,* in Cooperstown, New York. Graduated from the USMA in 1835. While at West Point, he was treated one time each for a sore throat, scarlet fever, calculus urinary, and nephritis. Morell resigned from the military service in 1837 and, after being involved in railroad construction, was engaged in the law. He reentered the military service as colonel of the New York militia and in August 1861 was made a brigadier general of volunteers. He served on the Peninsula, at Second Bull Run, and at Antietam. His promotion to major general ranked from July 1862. In the middle of August he developed general debility, jaundice, bilateral sciatica, painful spasmodic twitching of his muscles, and swelling of his lower limbs. According to his surgeon, all of these symptoms were the result of malarial poisoning. Morell was treated in the field by unit surgeons and continued his duties. In June 1863 he was treated for some nonspecified problem. He later reported that he had never lost a day due to sick leave. Morell's career was supposedly ruined by his testimony at Fitz John Porter's court-martial, and he was discharged in December 1864. After the war his health continued to be poor and he became more of an invalid. In 1874 Morell was very feeble and emaciated. His skin was sallow, and his nervous system was much disordered as indicated by neuralgia and nervous twitching. His condition was similar in 1880, and he continued to have edema of his lower extremities, sciatica, and other forms of nervous disease and prostration. His attending physicians stated that his symptoms were the result of chronic malarial poisoning.[1] Died February 11, 1883, at Scarborough, New York, and was buried under the chancel of St. Mary's Episcopal Church.

1. WPCHR, vols. 601, 603; RVA, Pension SC 204,042; RAGO, entry 534.

CHARLES HALE MORGAN • *Born on November 6, 1835,* at Manlius, New York. Graduated from the USMA in 1857. As a cadet he was treated for diarrhea and

catarrhus six times each, ophthalmia, odontalgia, cephalalgia, and febris intermittent tertian three times each, and vulnus incisum, eruptio, contusio, phlegmon, excoriatio, erysipelas, and colica one time each. After participating in the
1859 Mormon Expedition, he returned to the East and was assigned to an artillery battery. He served on the Peninsula; absent sick in September 1862, he rejoined the army in October. He had sick leave in August 1863 and again in December. After he passed through grades, he was made brigadier general of
volunteers in May 1865. Morgan was discharged from the volunteer service in
January 1866 and resumed his regular rank of captain. Following the war, he
had duty at various artillery garrisons. A medical examiner in February 1867
stated he was in robust health and able to perform his duties. The surgeon who
treated him from October 1874 to June 1875 reported that Morgan suffered from
frequently recurring difficulty of his brain. After any military exercise or protracted office work he suffered severely from headaches, consequent upon alterations of the blood to the brain from a diseased state of his blood vessels.
Another surgeon proposed that Morgan had a recurring hyperemia of the brain
incident to the climate. He died at Alcatraz Island, California, on December 20,
1875. First buried in the military cemetery on Angel Island, California, his remains were later moved to Golden Gate National Cemetery at San Bruno, California. According to his attending physician, the cause of his death was apoplexy, resulting from a diseased condition of his arteries.[1]

1. CSR; U.S. Army, CWS, roll 4, vol. 6, report 13, pp. 393–401; LR, ACP, 200, 1876, fiche: 000147;
RVA, Pension WC 174,454.

EDWIN DENISON MORGAN • *Born on February 8, 1811,* in Washington, Massachusetts. A rich businessman and politician in New York, he was made a major
general of volunteers in September 1861 by President Lincoln. Elected to the
U.S. Senate, he resigned his commission in January 1863. His political aspira-
tions after the war were unsuccessful, and he became better known for his phi-
lanthropy. He died in New York City on February 14, 1883, and was buried in
Cedar Hill Cemetery, Hartford, Connecticut.
DEATH CERTIFICATE: Primary, Bright's disease of the kidneys (granular form),
five-year duration and diabetes dehydration; immediate, asphyxia from cardiac weakness, forty-eight hour duration.

GEORGE WASHINGTON MORGAN • *Born on September 20, 1820,* in Washington
County, Pennsylvania. An officer in the Texas army, he entered USMA but withdrew. Morgan was wounded on August 20, 1847, at the Battle of Churubusco
and was on sick leave until the close of the Mexican War. Prior to the Civil War,
he practiced law in Ohio, was United States consul at Marseilles, France, and
minister to Portugal. In November 1861 he was commissioned brigadier general of volunteers. He was at Cumberland Gap, Chickasaw Bayou, Arkansas

Post, and Vicksburg. Morgan's health was much impaired in January 1863. In May he was judged to be disqualified for military service because of his continued poor health. He tendered his resignation, which was accepted on June 8. Morgan wanted to go to New England for medical treatment.[1] Following the war, he served in Congress three times. Died July 27, 1893, at Fort Monroe, Virginia, and was buried in Mount Vernon.

DEATH CERTIFICATE: Cause of death, pneumonia.

1. LR, ACP, 604, 1888, fiche: 000148; U.S. Army, CWS, roll 5, vol. 9, report 18, pp. 345–521; Heitman, *Historical Register and Dictionary* 2:31.

JAMES DADA MORGAN • *Born August 1, 1810,* in Boston, Massachusetts. Served in the Mexican War. A merchant and member of a local militia unit prior to the Civil War, he was made colonel of the 10th Illinois in May 1861. His promotion as brigadier general of volunteers ranked from July 1862 and he was mustered out in August 1865. He returned to Illinois and reentered business and banking. Morgan died at Quincy, Illinois, on September 12, 1896, and was buried in Woodland Cemetery in that city.

WILLIAM HOPKINS MORRIS • *Born on April 22, 1827,* in New York City. Graduated from the USMA in 1851. As a cadet he was treated for ophthalmia three times, cephalalgia twice, and subluxatio, cynanche parotitis, tonsillitis, diarrhea, rheumatism, clavus, excoriatio, catarrhus, and phlegmon one time each. While in California, he contracted a fever and resigned in 1854. After he left the Federal service, he worked with his father and invented a repeating carbine. In August 1861 he was appointed a captain of volunteers and held a staff position. He was commissioned colonel of an infantry unit in 1862 that was converted into the 6th New York Heavy Artillery. His promotion to brigadier general of volunteers ranked from November 1862. He served at Gettysburg, in the Bristol and Mine Run campaigns, and in the Wilderness. On May 9, 1864, at Spotsylvania Court House, Virginia, he received a rifle ball through the muscles below the right knee. A simple dressing was applied. The next day he was in the division hospital and then was taken to Georgetown. When able to walk on crutches, he was allowed to go to New York for further treatment and served on court-martial duty. He returned to New York after the war, took part in politics, and became a military writer. Valvular heart disease was detected in 1898, which his physician attributed to his previous rheumatism. During the last six months of his life, he suffered from severe dyspnea or cardiac asthma and paroxysms of anginoid pain. In the terminal stages of his illness, there was great venous stasis associated with cyanosis and cardiac dropsy. A marked increased amount of albumin was present in his urine. He had cerebral disturbance as evidenced by sleeplessness, vertigo, and loss of memory. Died August 26, 1900, at North Long

Branch, New Jersey, and was buried at Cold Springs, New York.[1]
DEATH CERTIFICATE: Cause of death, chronic endocarditis. Length of sickness, two years.

1. *OR*, vol. 36, pt. 1:64–65, 146, 191, 721, 724–25, pt. 2:563; WPCHR, vols. 605, 606, 607; LR, CB, roll 353, M838, 1867; RAGO, entry 534; RVA, Pension WC 653,090.

JAMES ST. CLAIR MORTON • *Born on September 24, 1829,* in Philadelphia, Pennsylvania. He graduated from the USMA in 1851, where he was treated for cephalalgia seven times, catarrhus and tonsillitis twice each, and vulnus lacerate, abscess, contusio, rheumatism, subluxatio, and dyspepsia once each. As a staff member at the military academy, he was treated for gonorrhea in November 1855 and for pleuritis in January 1857. In March 1862, while in Florida, he obtained a leave of absence on surgeon's certificate because of Chagas' fever. The next month he was placed in charge of the engineering operations at Fort Mifflin, Pennsylvania. In June 1862 he was ready for field duty and was made chief engineer of the Army of the Ohio. His promotion to brigadier general of volunteers ranked from November. He received a leave of absence for disability from July 15, 1863, into September. He was slightly wounded in the Battle of Chickamauga on September 20, 1863, but continued on duty. In November 1863 he was discharged from volunteer service and reverted to his rank of major in the Regular Army. He was killed in action in front of Petersburg on June 17, 1864.[1] He was buried in Laurel Hill Cemetery, Philadelphia.

1. CSR; *OR*, vol. 30, pt. 1:950, pt. 3:112, 701, 797; U.S. Army, CWS, roll 2, vol. 3, report 38, pp. 1145–49.

GERSHOM MOTT • *Born April 7, 1822,* in Lamberton, New Jersey. Served in the Mexican War. Engaged in business in New Jersey, he was appointed lieutenant colonel of the 5th New Jersey in 1861. Severely wounded on August 29, 1862, at Second Bull Run, he relinquished command of the regiment. He was appointed brigadier general of volunteers in September and reported back to Washington for duty in December 1862. Mott was wounded in the left hand during the Chancellorsville campaign on May 3, 1863, and rejoined his command in August. At Spotsylvania on May 19, 1864, he was slightly wounded in the side by a musket ball but was back on the field on May 23. Near Amelia Springs, Virginia, on April 6, 1865, he was seriously wounded by a musket ball passing through the upper third of his right leg. He turned over his command and was carried to the rear where a simple dressing was applied. Mott again assumed division command on May 16 and was appointed as major general of volunteers to rank from May. Following his return to civilian life, he held a number of state offices. An 1878 medical examination showed evidence of dilation of the right ventricle of the heart with marked distortion of the mitral and aortic valves. These changes gave rise to frequent attacks of palpitation of his heart.

In later years he frequently had pain from his old injuries. He died suddenly on November 29, 1884, in New York City. He was buried in Riverview Cemetery, Trenton, New Jersey. His family physician reported that the cause of Mott's death was valvular disease of the heart.[1]

1. CSR; *OR*, vol. 12, pt. 2:456; vol. 21:835, 882; vol. 25, pt. 1:179, 392, 394, 446, 462; vol. 46, pt. 1:568, 583, 682–83, 685, 783, pt. 2:740; U.S. Army, CWS, roll 1, vol. 1, report 13, pp. 187–92; ibid., roll 4, vol. 7, report 11, pp. 161–67; RAGO, entry 534; RVA, Pension WC 227,092; RG 94, Casualty Lists of Commissioned Officers: Civil War, 1861–65, entry 655, NA (hereafter cited as CLCO).

JOSEPH ANTHONY MOWER • *Born on August 22, 1827,* in Woodstock, Vermont. Served during the Mexican War, but did not get to Mexico. He was appointed a second lieutenant of the 1st U.S. Infantry in 1856. Mower was elected colonel of the 11th Missouri (Union) Infantry in May 1862. At Corinth on October 4, 1862, he was wounded in the back of the right side of his neck and was taken prisoner. Supposing the firing from his left and rear was friendly, he had ridden into a small party of the enemy. Owing to the severity of his wound, he was left on the field and later found by Federal troops in the captured Confederate field hospital. He obtained a sick leave on October 27 and returned to duty on November 13. Mower was promoted to brigadier general in March 1863 and served in the Vicksburg campaign. On July 4 he received a leave of absence on surgeon's certificate and returned in September. He was in the Red River campaign, the Atlanta campaign, and in the Carolinas. He was promoted to major general of volunteers in August 1864. He remained in the army after the war. Although an invalid for several years and nursed by members of his family, he was never totally dependent. Prior to his death he had an effusion of his lungs following congestion. Died in New Orleans on January 6, 1870, and was buried in Arlington National Cemetery. The attending physician reported that Mower died from a cerebral embolism and chronic endocarditis.[1]

1. CSR; *OR*, vol. 17, pt. 1:180, 198; LR, ACP, 3506, 1885, fiche: 000149; U.S. Army, CWS, roll 1, vol. 2, report 10, pp. 99–107; RVA, Pension WC 144,860; *Battles and Leaders* 2:752.

N

JAMES NAGLE • *Born April 5, 1822,* in Reading, Pennsylvania. Served in the Mexican War. A painter and paperhanger, he became colonel of the 6th Pennsylvania Volunteers in 1861. Although the unit was not mustered into Federal service, it did serve in the field. Nagle organized the 48th Pennsylvania, which he led at Groveton and Antietam. He was appointed brigadier general of volunteers in September 1862. In February 1863 his surgeon reported that Nagle had suffered from angina pectoris for the previous nine months. His appointment as brigadier general was not confirmed by the Senate and expired in March

1863. He was reappointed to rank from that month. For the next year and a half he was in and out of the army. The surgeon who examined him in April 1863 stated that he was suffering from cardiac hypertrophy and valvular heart disease, a diagnosis that was confirmed by a professor at Philadelphia. That month he submitted his resignation on account of disability. After his resignation was accepted, he left for home on May 21. When his health improved, he was mustered back in the service on July 4, 1863; however, on August 2 he was mustered out again. When he tried to enter the service again, there was disagreement between physicians as to whether his health had improved, and he was finally discharged in November 1864. Died August 22, 1866, in Pottsville, Pennsylvania, and was buried there in Presbyterian Cemetery. According to his attending physician, he died from valvular heart disease.[1]

1. RVA, Pension WC 196,089; U.S. Army, CWS, roll 2, vol. 3, report 8, pp. 169–79.

HENRY MORRIS NAGLEE • *Born January 15, 1815,* in Philadelphia. Graduated from the USMA in 1835. While at West Point, he was treated for a wound and a headache four times each, piles three times, a sore throat, bruise, sore feet, and a corn twice each, and diarrhea once. He resigned from the army soon after graduation and, following service in California during the Mexican War, was engaged in banking in California. At the start of the Civil War, he was appointed a lieutenant colonel in the Regular Army, but resigned to accept the rank of brigadier general of volunteers in February 1862. At Seven Pines on May 31, 1862, his horse was shot from under him and he received four contused wounds from musket balls. He was struck in the right breast, under the right shoulder blade, and had two slight marks on the right leg. Apparently he did not leave the field. In July 1862 he had typhoid fever. He required a leave and returned about the end of September. Naglee was relieved from his command in September 1863 because of a disagreement with his superiors and was finally mustered out of the service in April 1864. He returned to the banking business in California. His eldest daughter took care of him during his final sickness. After a lingering illness of six weeks, he died in the Occidental Hotel in San Francisco on March 5, 1886, while paying a visit to his doctor. The immediate cause of death was an affection of the bowels. He was buried in Laurel Hill Cemetery in San Jose.[1]

1. CSR; OR, vol. 11, pt. 1:673, 915, pt. 2:218–19, 236; vol. 51, pt. 1:647; WPCHR, vols. 601, 602, 603; U.S. Army, CWS, report of W. H. Emory, roll 1, vol. 1, report 51, p. 957; CLCO; Steiner, *Disease,* 150; *San Francisco Call,* Mar. 6, 1886.

JAMES SCOTT NEGLEY • *Born December 22, 1826,* near Pittsburgh. Served in the Mexican War. Prior to the Civil War he was involved with the local militia. After serving as brigadier general of Pennsylvania troops he was appointed brigadier general of volunteers in February 1862. From September 12–14, 1863, Negley remained on duty while his surgeon treated him for diarrhea or inflammation of the bowels. The next two days he was confined to bed with more severe symptoms. On September 17, when the command moved, he rode his horse but kept his ambulance near in case it was required. From September 18–23 he remained on duty although fatigued and with inflamed bowels. He was confined to his bed on October 8–9. On December 22, he was directed to proceed to Cincinnati, or any point outside the military division, and was to report by letter to the adjutant general for orders. Negley's military performance was criticized, and he resigned in January 1865.[1] He was elected to Congress after the war and engaged in private business. Died August 7, 1901, in Plainfield, New Jersey, and was buried in Allegheny Cemetery, Pittsburgh.

DEATH CERTIFICATE: Cause of death, diabetes (one year) and carbuncle (three weeks).

1. OR, vol. 30, pt. 1:334, 337–38, 343, 1010, 1021, pt. 3:936–37; vol. 52, pt. 1:506; RVA, Pension C 537,137.

THOMAS HEWSON NEILL • *Born on April 9, 1826*, in Philadelphia. Graduated from the USMA in 1847. While a cadet at West Point he was treated for phlegmon three times, rheumatism twice, and subluxatio, vertigo, and cephalalgia once each. After duty on the frontier he served at West Point as an instructor for three years. In February 1862 he was commissioned colonel of the 23rd Pennsylvania. In early October 1862 he sustained a severe contusion of his leg and a sprained ankle. His appointment as brigadier general of volunteers ranked from November. He was at Fredericksburg, and at Chancellorsville on May 4, 1863, his horse was shot and fell on him. Although partially disabled, he remained in command until the action was over. Neill remained sick for the first part of the month. He fought at Mine Run, the Wilderness, Spotsylvania, and Cold Harbor. In late July 1864, outside of Petersburg, he was prostrated by dysentery and malarial fever. The next month his condition was diagnosed by a different surgeon as typhomalaria. He was sent north and was treated in Philadelphia until October. On October 21, 1864, he was ordered to report to Philip Sheridan for duty as a staff officer. Neill remained in the military after the war and reverted to his grade of major of infantry in 1866. He had sick leave from August 25 to December 5, 1865, because of a fractured rib, a severe contusion of the left side and shoulder, and a lacerated wound of his forehead. How he obtained the injuries is not clear. In July 1882, while at Jefferson Barracks, Missouri, he developed septic enteritis due to malaria and went to Atlantic City for treatment. On September 28, 1882, following his return, he had a stroke. When he left Jefferson Barracks in October, according to his surgeon, he was convalescing from paralysis resulting from an embolism of one of the cerebral vessels. In late February 1883, he was on leave at Buffalo, New York, still suffering residual paralysis. The almost-constant pain in his legs deprived him of a great deal of sleep. In addition, he reported that he had for years suffered from too frequent and copious urination, which disturbed him many times during the night. He was also too deaf to hear the oral evidence before general court-martial trials. Examined by a board in March 1883, he was found to be incapacitated from his paralysis; with no prospect of recovery, he was retired. He was an invalid for the last two years of his life. Neill died suddenly in Philadelphia on March 12, 1885, and was buried at West Point. According to the attending surgeon, the immediate cause of death was paralysis.[1]

1. *OR*, vol. 25, pt. 1:601; vol. 36, pt. 1:683; vol. 43, pt. 2:437; WPCHR, vol. 605; RVA, Pension Min. C 221,515; U.S. Army, CWS, roll 4, vol. 6, report 8, pp. 269–82; LR, ACP, 2133, 1882.

WILLIAM NELSON • *Born on September 27, 1824,* near Maysville, Kentucky. Served in the navy during the Mexican War. He was made brigadier general of volunteers in September 1861 and major general in July 1862. At Richmond, Kentucky, on August 30, 1862, he received two flesh wounds. The following day he was in Lexington, Kentucky. One bullet was removed from his thigh and the wound healed rapidly. He was killed the morning of September 29, 1862, in Louisville, Kentucky, during an encounter with Gen. Jefferson C. Davis. After an argument, Nelson had slapped Davis in the face and walked off. Davis procured a pistol and followed him. They met in the hall of the hotel and Davis shot him. The ball entered Nelson's right breast, and he died shortly thereafter.[1] He was buried in Maysville.

1. CSR; *OR*, vol. 16, pt. 1:908, 923, 931–32, pt. 2:464, 557–58, 566–67, 987.

JOHN NEWTON • *Born August 24, 1823,* in Norfolk, Virginia. He graduated from USMA in 1842. After serving in the Engineer Corps, he was made a brigadier general of volunteers in September 1861. He commanded a brigade on the Peninsula and at Antietam and a division at Fredericksburg. At Salem Heights, Virginia, on May 3, 1863, he was slightly wounded.[1] Newton served with distinction at Gettysburg and in the Atlanta campaign. After the war he served in the Corps of Engineers. In March 1884 he was made chief of engineers with the rank of brigadier general. He retired from the army in 1886. Newton died in private quarters on May 1, 1895, at New York City and was buried at West Point. DEATH CERTIFICATE: Chief cause, acute articular rheumatism of six weeks' duration; contributing, endocarditis.

1. RVA, Pension, WC 429,522; CLCO.

FRANKLIN STILLMAN NICKERSON • *Born August 27, 1826,* in Swanville, Maine. A member of the U.S. Customs Service, he was elected major of the 4th Maine Infantry in June 1861 and was commended for his service at First Bull Run. In September he was made lieutenant colonel of the unit and was commissioned colonel of the 14th Maine in November. He was appointed brigadier general to rank from November 1862. While at Port Hudson, Louisiana, in July 1863, he developed rheumatism. That same month, shortly after the surrender of Port Hudson, he obtained a leave and went to New Orleans for treatment. He was home on sick leave from October to December 29, 1863. When he arrived home he walked with difficulty and used a cane. After his return to duty he was a member of a court of inquiry in New Orleans. His resignation was accepted in May 1865. After the war he returned to the practice of law. His rheumatism continued, and by 1891 he had tried Turkish baths, bandages, changes of air, and various diets, all which helped minimally. At times he was confined to his bed for days or weeks. His condition continued to deteriorate, and by 1901 he had to have almost daily attendance. The following year he had to give up his business; unable to use his right hand, he had to have his food cut. His attendants rubbed his limbs, helped him dress, and assisted him in and out of his bath. Although he could climb up stairs, he had fallen a number of times going down. Able to stand on his feet for only a short period, he had fallen frequently and could not get back up without help.[1] Died January 23, 1917, at Boston and was entombed in Forest Hills Crematory in Jamaica Plain outside of Boston. DEATH CERTIFICATE: Immediate cause of death, acute bronchitis, nine days. Chronic valvular heart, years.

1. RVA, PENSION SC 865,936.

O

RICHARD JAMES OGLESBY • *Born July 25, 1824,* in Oldham County, Kentucky. Served in the Mexican War. A practicing lawyer in Illinois and a state senator, he resigned his positions and was made colonel of the 8th Illinois Infantry in 1861. He commanded a brigade at Forts Henry and Donelson, and in March 1862 he was made brigadier general of volunteers. Oglesby was wounded by a musket ball on October 3, 1862, at Corinth. It entered his body at the lower posterior part of the left axilla and passed through the center of the lungs toward the opposite axilla. He was taken to the Tishomingo Hotel in Corinth and remained there until the Confederates almost captured the hotel. He was then transported to Sulphur Springs in an ambulance. He was moved back to Corinth when the battle was over and examined by a number of physicians who probed the wound. They could not find the ball, and all reported he would die. When Oglesby had raised the 8th Illinois in April 1861, Dr. Trowbridge, an old friend, had accepted the position as regimental surgeon and had promised to look after him. After Oglesby was promoted to brigadier general, Trowbridge had been transferred and made surgeon of Gen. John A. Logan's brigade. Oglesby requested Dr. Trowbridge to come take care of him after he was wounded, and this was approved by Gen. U. S. Grant. The surgeon arrived on the evening of October 6 and found him having to sit in a semirecumbent position in a rocking chair. Oglesby had a rapid pulse and labored respiration and expectorated small amounts of blood. His skin was covered with cold perspiration, his pupils dilated, and his kidney and bowel functions were decreased. The surgeon conjectured that the ball had passed between the costal and pulmonary pleura and lodged in the body of the fourth dorsal vertebrae. For some reason he further speculated that the ball had been dislodged by the ambulance ride and had fallen upon the diaphragm. He gave Oglesby one and a half grains of morphine to alleviate the pain and "to equalize the circulation of the blood and to reduce the respiration rate to rest the lungs." To decrease his secretions, an hour later he gave him a full portion of sulfate of magnesia as a hydrogogue cathartic. His pulse and respiration decreased, and he slept. The next morning Trowbridge met with the medical director for consideration of the case. The previous consulting surgeons had recommended that Oglesby should be given three grains of opium every three hours, fed large amounts of beef, tea, and soup, and given two bottles of Catawba wine per day. Stating the recommended amount of opium was excessive and that a stomach filled with beefsteak and heavy wine would be harmful, Trowbridge gave him no more opium, morphine, or wine and provided him a guarded diet. Oglesby became jaundiced and suffered a great deal but, with his wife and family in attendance, improved slowly. Trowbridge obtained Gen. U. S. Grant's permission to move Ogleby home, again over the protests of the medical director. Blankets on the floor of a freight car acted as a buffer, while a rocking chair provided a seat for his ride to Decatur. His promotion to major general ranked from November, and in April he reported back for duty. Because of continued pain, he tendered his resignation on June 21, 1863. He obtained leave with extensions until January 1864, when he started serving on the court-martial of Surgeon General Hammond. In May 1864, he resigned from the service to run for governor of Illinois. He served as governor for three terms and then practiced the law. Oglesby was in poor health after a severe attack of la grippe in 1895, during which he again came close to losing his life. It produced a generalized weakness from which he never fully recovered. He was subject to vertigo, and while in Chicago in October 1898 he had such an episode and fell. The first part of January 1899 he had a slight attack of la grippe. On the morning of his death, April 24, he was around the house at Elkhart, Illinois, and there was nothing to indicate his end was near. Later, Oglesby was found in the toilet room following a fall. There was blood on his face and slight discoloration on the right temple. His head was turned under his body, and a small pool of blood was found under his face from his teeth cutting his lips. The dying man was carried to the large hall on the first floor, placed on a couch, and later moved to the bed. From the time he was found until his death, he remained unconscious.[1] He was buried in the Elkhart Cemetery.

1. *OR*, vol. 17, pt. 1:155, 157, 175, 256–57, 273; vol. 24, pt. 3:165, 175, 181, 487; U.S. Army, CWS, roll 2, vol. 3, report 31, pp. 915–37; Dr. Silas T. Trowbridge, "Saving a General," *CWTI* 11, no. 4 (July 1972): 20–25; *Lincoln (Ill.) Courier*, April 25, 1899.

JOHN MORRISON OLIVER • *Born on September 6, 1828,* in Penn Yan, New York. Having spent time as a pharmacist and court recorder, in April 1861 he enlisted in Federal service as a private. By March 1862 he was colonel of the 15th Michigan and was promoted brigadier general of volunteers in January 1865. He was mustered out in August 1865 and took up practice of the law. Oliver resigned as superintendent of postal service in 1871 because of poor health. Died March 30, 1872, in Washington, D.C., and was buried in Lake View Cemetery, Penn Yan.

EMERSON OPDYCKE • *Born January 7, 1830,* in Trumbull County, Ohio. A businessman before the war, he entered Federal service as a first lieutenant of the 41st Ohio in August 1861. He was made a captain in January 1862. While carrying the colors of the 41st Ohio at Shiloh on April 7, 1862, Opdycke received two slight flesh wounds but kept possession of the flag. He was promoted through grades and in January 1863 was made colonel of the 125th Ohio. He was at Chickamauga and Chattanooga. On May 14, 1864, during the Battle of Resaca, he received a severe wound just above the left elbow. A jagged spent ball passed entirely through his arm, grazed the bone, and nearly severed the principal tendon. He fainted from loss of blood and was taken from the field. As soon as his arm was tied up to prevent further bleeding he returned to his regiment and remained with it until they were relieved. He was back in command the next month and led a brigade at Kennesaw Mountain and Franklin. In July 1865 he was made a brigadier general.[1] He returned to private life and business after the war. On April 22, 1884, he accidently shot himself; three days later, in New York City, he died of peritonitis. He was buried in Oakwood Cemetery, Warren, Ohio. DEATH CERTIFICATE (Coroner's inquest): Shock from a pistol shot wound into the abdomen one and one-half inches to the right of the naval; said pistol discharged accidently, while in the act of being cleaned on April 22, 1884, at his residence.

1. *OR*, vol. 38, pt. 1:191, 293, 295, 353, 369; vol. 42, pt. 2:295, 742; U.S. Army, CWS, roll 5, vol. 9, report 9, pp. 171–229.

EDWARD OTHO CRESAP ORD • *Born October 18, 1818,* in Cumberland, Maryland. Graduated from the USMA in 1839. Fought in Florida and was in California during the Mexican War. Promoted to captain, he took command of his company early in 1851 at Fort Independence, Boston. Within a short time he was given a five-month sick leave to go to a drier climate. After serving primarily on the frontier, he was appointed brigadier general of volunteers in September 1861. In late May 1862 he was sick for a number of days, and on May 30 he was relieved from duty. There was some question as to how real this illness was. On June 22 he was assigned to command. At the Battle of Hatchie Bridge near Corinth, on October 5, 1862, a bullet hit his ankle, and he was taken to a hospital near Pocahontas, Tennessee. An examination revealed that the ball had passed between the bones and had to be cut out from the side opposite its point of entry. On October 7 he was ordered to Carlisle, Pennsylvania, to recuperate at the home of one member of his staff. He went by rail to Jackson, Tennessee, to Columbus, Kentucky, by steamer to Cairo, by rail to Chicago, then to Carlisle. By November 10 Ord could walk using crutches, and on November 18 he reported himself fit for light duty since the wound was closed and not discharging. He served on the Buell Commission until March 1863. At Vicksburg he commanded the Thirteenth Corps. While at Vermilionville, Louisiana, he developed a fever on October 12, 1863. He had a severe respiratory infection and spent the months of November and December with his family in Louisville. His children were also sick with a similar illness during this period, and one died. He started back to duty on December 30 and arrived in New Orleans on January 8, 1864. In April he was relieved at his own request. Early in September 1864 he was bothered by piles, dyspepsia, and diarrhea. At Fort Harrison on September 29, Ord was wounded in the medial aspect of his thigh. An improvised tourniquet was used to stop the bleeding, and he tried to continue in command from an ambulance. However, the first surgeon who examined him sent him to the headquarters of the Eighteenth Corps in the rear. He took a leave and went to Baltimore before joining his family in Bellaire, Ohio. By October 27 he was still off his feet and, because of the location of his wound, unable to ride. He returned to duty in December; in February 1865 he was assigned to command the Army of the James. Ord remained in the army and retired in 1881. He became sick on July 16, 1883, aboard a steamer from Vera Cruz to New York. On his arrival at Havana on July 19, he was so sick that there was little hope for his survival. Although in a private hospital in Havana and under the care of United States sanitary inspector Dr. D. M. Burgess, Ord died of yellow fever on the twenty-second.[1] He was buried in Arlington National Cemetery.

1. CSR; *OR*, vol. 12, pt. 3:291; vol. 17, pt. 1:302–3, 306, 308, 323, pt. 2:268; vol. 26, pt. 1:339, 383, 698; vol. 33:911; vol. 34, pt. 2:104; vol. 37, pt. 2:118, 136; vol. 42, pt. 1:794–95, pt. 2:1091, 1113, 1115, 1146; vol. 46, pt. 2:421; vol. 51, pt. 1:717; vol. 52, pt. 1:259; LR, ACP, 714, 1879, fiche: 000154; U.S. Army, CWS, roll 1, vol. 2, report 49, pp. 695–99; ibid., roll 5, vol. 9, report 21, pp. 559–67; ibid., report of J. R. Kenly, roll 3, vol. 5, report 2, pp. 237–554; D. B. Birney to Gross, September 6, 1864, David Bell Birney Papers, USAMHI; Bernarr Cresap, *Appomattox Commander: The Story of General E. O. C. Ord*, 33, 91, 93, 95–96, 111–12.

WILLIAM WARD ORME • *Born February 17, 1832*, in Washington, D.C. His health before the war was good except for a furuncle on the back of his neck and an occasional bilious spell. A lawyer and friend of President Lincoln, he was elected colonel of the 94th Illinois Volunteers in August 1862. He led the regiment at Prairie Grove, and in March 1863 he was promoted brigadier general of volunteers to rank from the previous November. In late August 1863, while in camp at Carrolton, Louisiana, he had a violent attack of swamp fever. After remaining in camp very ill, he took the advice of his physicians and went north in September. Once he had partially recovered he was ordered to Washington, D.C., and sent on an inspection tour of the prison camps. He assumed command at Chicago in December 1863. Here a similar fever struck him again, and he was confined to his bed for much of the next four months. For this reason, his resignation was accepted in April. He was appointed by President Lincoln as supervising special agent of the Treasury Department at Memphis. He held this position until his resignation in November 1865. In the summer of 1866 his physician sent him to Minnesota to improve his health because of a possible tubercular condition. He obtained little benefit and died, according to his wife, from consumption in Bloomington, Illinois, on September 13, 1866.[1]

1. *OR*, vol. 26, pt. 1:709; vol. 52. pt. 1:504; RVA, Pension WC 313,340; U.S. Army, CWS, roll 2, vol. 3, report 42, pp. 1199–213; RAGO, entry 534.

THOMAS OGDEN OSBORN • *Born on August 11, 1832,* in Jersey, Ohio. He was practicing law in Chicago when the war started and was appointed lieutenant colonel of the 39th Illinois Infantry in October 1861. The following January he was made colonel of the unit. At Drewry's Bluff on May 14, 1864, a musket ball struck his right elbow and ranged downward. The wound was dressed, and the next day he was sent to the Chesapeake Hospital at Fortress Monroe, Virginia. He stayed in the hospital until the last of September with the ball apparently remaining in the arm. Osborn reported for duty in December and was assigned to command. In May 1865 he was made brigadier general and was mustered out of the military. After the war, he returned to the practice of the law, held various Federal positions, and entered business. He had ankylosis of the injured elbow.[1] Died March 27, 1904, at Washington, D.C., and was buried in Arlington National Cemetery.

DEATH CERTIFICATE: Cause of death, primary, cerebral hemorrhage, ten hours' duration; immediate, paralysis.

1. CSR; *OR*, vol. 36, pt. 2:49; vol. 42, pt. 3:888; vol. 46, pt. 2:581; RVA, Pension SC 224,604.

PETER JOSEPH OSTERHAUS • *Born on January 4, 1823,* in Coblenz, Germany. Involved in revolutionary movements in Europe, he had to flee to the United States in 1849. He entered Federal service as a major of a Missouri battalion in April 1861, became a colonel of the 12th Missouri Infantry in December and brigadier general of volunteers in June 1862. He fought at Wilson's Creek and Pea Ridge. His health was poor because of malaria and dysentery in the winter of 1861–62, and when the symptoms recurred in July 1862 he went north. He returned to Helena, Arkansas, in August. After a stay of a few days his health deteriorated again due to malaria, and on August 30 he was obliged to go back north. By September 25 his health was partially restored, and he assumed command on October 2, 1862. During the whole period he continued to take quinine. He went to St. Genevieve, Missouri, and because of repeated attacks of malaria remained in bed from October 13 to December 21. Osterhaus divided his time between St. Genevieve and St. Louis. He started for the field again on December 31. He took his medicine with his meals and was transported occasionally by ambulance. During the Vicksburg campaign on May 17, 1863, he was wounded in the inner side of his left thigh from a shell fragment. Osterhaus was able to mount his horse and made a reconnaissance of the areas. Disabled for only a short time, he recovered enough to resume command the next day. The malaria and dysentery continued in July 1864, and he turned over his command and took a sick leave. He went to Nashville and Louisville and returned on August 15. Osterhaus was mustered out of Federal service in January 1866. After the war, his left leg progressively became weaker, and he had frequent attacks of malaria and diarrhea. He served as U.S. consul in France and in Germany. In 1883 he had dysentery and chronic catarrh of the stomach and intestines, along with an enlarged liver and spleen. He was examined at Mannheim, Baden, Germany, for a pension request in May 1886. The examination revealed chronic swelling of his spleen and liver, supposedly the result of malarial poisoning, and an enlarged heart. On his left leg were two cicatrices: one on the middle of the upper thigh was the size of a pigeon's egg, and the other, a hand space above the ankle, was as large as a bean. The physician hypothesized that his occasional pain and the fatigue following even the slightest exertion were attributed to his prior wounds. Osterhaus's loss of appetite, indigestion, and frequent attacks of dysentery were supposedly due to the cardiomegaly and hepatosplenomegaly. He was retired from Federal service in 1905. Died January 2, 1917, in Diusburg, Germany. He was cremated at Crefeld and was buried in Coblenz. Report of the death of an American citizen, American Consular Service: Cause of death, inflammation of the lungs.[1]

1. *OR*, vol. 13:781; vol. 24, pt. 1:152–53, pt. 2:16–18, 26, 128, 132; vol. 38, pt. 1:103, pt. 3:42, 133–34; RVA, Pension SC 393,849; U.S. Army, CWS, roll 2, vol. 3, report 15, pp. 401–28; ibid., roll 4, vol. 7, report 14, pp. 217–71.

JOSHUA THOMAS OWEN • *Born March 29, 1821,* in Caermarthen, Wales. Before the war he was a teacher, lawyer, and politician. After serving in a ninety-day unit, he was made colonel of the 69th Pennsylvania. He obtained a sick leave in July 1862 because of chronic diarrhea and went to Philadelphia. Owen was appointed a brigadier general of volunteers in November but was not confirmed. In January 1863 he required a leave because of the chronic diarrhea and was

248 CHARLES JACKSON PAINE

ordered back to duty the next month. He had sick leave again in July. His military actions were criticized, and he was discharged in 1864, even though he had served in most of the eastern campaigns.[1] He returned to his law practice in Pennsylvania and later started a law journal. Died in Philadelphia on November 7, 1887, and was buried in Laurel Hill Cemetery.

DEATH CERTIFICATE: Cause of death, typhoid fever.

1. CSR; *OR*, vol. 25, pt. 2:109; vol. 36, pt. 1:436; U.S. Army, CWS, roll 1, vol. 2, report 38, pp. 553–65.

P

CHARLES JACKSON PAINE • *Born on August 26, 1833,* in Boston, Massachusetts. He left his Boston law practice and entered Federal service as a captain in the 22nd Massachusetts Infantry in October 1861 and colonel of the 2nd Louisiana in October 1862. He served in the Department of the Gulf and fought at Port Hudson. Paine had a sick leave in August 1863 and returned after about two months. His appointment as brigadier general of volunteers ranked from July 1864. In late September he had malaria and obtained a sick leave in October 1864. On January 18, 1865, he was assigned to command of the forces occupying the line of works facing Wilmington, North Carolina.[1] After returning to civilian life, he engaged in the development of the railroad system and later defended the America's Cup. Died August 12, 1916, in Weston, Massachusetts, and was buried in Mount Auburn Cemetery, Cambridge, Massachusetts.

DEATH CERTIFICATE: Cause of death, bronchopneumonia; contributory, edema of lungs.

1. *OR*, vol. 46, pt. 2:174; U.S. Army, CWS, roll 6, vol. 10, report 51, pp. 501–6; Sommers, *Richmond Redeemed*, 31.

ELEAZER ARTHUR PAINE • *Born September 10, 1815,* in Parkman, Ohio. Graduated from the USMA in 1839. While at West Point, he was treated for pain in his breast five times, a cold three times, wound twice, and a sick stomach, diarrhea, headache, and nausea once each. Served in the Florida wars. He resigned his commission in 1840 and practiced the law until the start of the Civil War. A friend of President Lincoln, he was made colonel of the 9th Illinois in July 1861 and brigadier general in September. He served at Paducah, New Madrid, Island No. 10, and Corinth. In January 1862 he was disabled by pains in his stomach, chest, and throat due to neuralgia of the stomach and a bronchial affection. Paine was present sick in June and August. His condition became worse, and in October, when he could be moved, he was given a sick leave. He was placed on a bed in an ambulance and was transported to a steamer, which took him to Cairo, Ohio. A couch was prepared for him in a railroad car, and he was taken with a surgeon in attendance to his home in Monmouth, Illinois. The attending physician reported he was suffering from general debility and irritation of the bowels consequent upon an attack of bilious remittent fever of a typhoid character. When Paine reported back, Gen. William S. Rosecrans determined he was still too sick for field duty and made him post commander at Gallatin, Tennessee, in January 1863. While there during the summer, he had chronic irritability of the bowels, loss of appetite, pain in the left side, and one severe spell of continued fever. In September 1864 his wife came to Paducah, Kentucky, and with a surgeon in attendance took him to their home on sick leave. His resignation dated from April 1865. Paine returned to the practice of the law after he left Federal service. The physician who took care of him the last two years of his life reported that he had general nervous and muscular debility. He was called to see Paine on December 7, 1882, and found that he had symptoms of pneumonia, which rapidly became more severe.[1] Died on December 16, 1882, at Jersey City, New Jersey, and was buried in the grounds of The Old Bergen Church in Jersey City.

DEATH CERTIFICATE: Cause of death, pneumonia of ten days' duration.

1. CSR; *OR*, vol. 17, pt. 2:193; WPCHR, vol. 604; RVA, Pension, C 242,766.

HALBERT ELEAZER PAINE · *Born on February 4, 1826*, in Chardon, Ohio. He left his law practice and was made colonel of the 4th Wisconsin Cavalry in July 1861. His promotion as brigadier general ranked from March 1863. During the attack on Port Hudson on June 14, 1863, he was wounded in three places on the left side of his body: the leg, his side, and his shoulder. He lay all day under the hot sun among the dead and wounded. A wounded private lying nearby tossed him a canteen cut from the body of a dead soldier. Paine felt this saved his life. When picked up by Federal troops, he was conveyed to the field hospital where it was found that the bones of his leg were fractured. He was taken to Hotel Dieu in New Orleans. The femoral artery had been damaged, and after three bouts of hemorrhaging, an amputation of the leg was done. Medical records differ on the date of surgery (June 23 or 24) and location (upper third of the leg or four inches below the knee). Paine was removed from the hospital on July 22, 1863, and went to Milwaukee. In September he left for Washington to serve on a military commission. Later he was able to use an artificial limb. In July 1864 he was placed on general court-martial duty and continued in this capacity until the middle of August.[1] After resigning his commission in May 1865 he was elected to Congress. Following three terms he returned to law practice and served as commissioner of patents. Died on April 14, 1905, in Washington, D.C., and was buried in Arlington National Cemetery.

DEATH CERTIFICATE: Cause of death, primary, mitral regurgitation, one year's duration; immediate, exhaustion.

1. *OR*, vol. 26, pt. 1:17, 45, 69, 148; vol. 37, pt. 2:162, 236; vol. 39, pt. 2:245, 544; *MSHW*, vol. 2, pt. 3:513, 517; RAGO, entry 623, "File D"; U.S. Army, CWS, roll 2, vol. 3, report 52, pp. 1385–464; RVA, Pension SC 72,075; *MOLLUS* 19:108.

INNIS NEWTON PALMER • *Born on March 30, 1824,* in Buffalo, New York. Graduated from the USMA in 1846. On September 13, 1847, at Chapultepec, Mexico, he was wounded. His duty before the Civil War was mainly on the western frontier, and when the war started he was a major in the Second Cavalry. Palmer's promotion as brigadier general of volunteers ranked from September 1861. He served at First Bull Run and on the Peninsula. On March 10, 1865, Palmer became ill, and on March 20 he was assigned to district command. He remained in the army following the Civil War, and in 1868 he was made colonel of the Second Cavalry and served in the area now constituting Wyoming and Nebraska. He suffered from inflammation of both the prostate gland and the neck of the urinary bladder in early August 1876. His appetite and general condition were considerably impaired. He was on continued sick leave until he retired in March 1879.[1] Died at Chevy Chase, Maryland, on September 9, 1900, and was buried in Arlington National Cemetery.

1. *OR,* vol. 47, pt. 1:935; Heitman, *Historical Register and Dictionary* 2:33; LR, ACP, 1306, 1874, fiche: 000155.

JOHN MCCAULEY PALMER • *Born September 13, 1817,* in Scott County, Kentucky. A lawyer, politician, and opponent of slavery, he was made colonel of the 14th Illinois Infantry in May 1861. In December 1861 he was promoted brigadier general of volunteers. He was at New Madrid, Island No. 10, Corinth, Stones River, Chattanooga, and the Atlanta campaign. Because of pneumonia, he was off duty starting the last of May 1862 and did not report back until the end of August. His appointment as major general ranked from November 1862. On September 26, 1863, at Redan near Chattanooga, Palmer received a severe flesh wound. Two days later he was in Chattanooga. By the last of October his wound had become greatly inflamed, so he was relieved from division command and had disability leave. On May 9, 1864, while commander of the Fourteenth Corps, he had to leave the front because of illness and go to his headquarters in the rear. In August 1864 he was relieved from command at his own request. He was elected governor of Illinois in 1868, and he continued as a politician for the rest of his life. In 1899 he reported that he had cataracts, had lost the sight in one eye, and was going blind in the other. However, he never blamed his conditions on his military service.[1] Died on September 25, 1900, in Springfield, Illinois, and was buried in Carlinville, Illinois.

1. CSR; *OR,* vol. 16, pt. 2:468; vol. 17, pt. 2:193; vol. 30, pt. 3:876, 916; vol. 31, pt. 1:81–82, 519, pt. 2:53; vol. 38, pt. 1:519; RVA, Pension C 508,886; Steiner, *Disease,* 177–79.

JOHN GRUBB PARKE • *Born September 22, 1827,* near Coatesville, Pennsylvania. Graduated from the USMA in 1849. As a cadet, he was treated for catarrhus and cephalalgia ten times each, odontalgia twice, and vertigo, constipatio, tonsillitis, pleurodynia, phlegmon, clavus, subluxatio, and excoriatio once each. He served in the corps of topographical engineers and the corps of engineers until the beginning of the war. Parke was made a brigadier general of volunteers in November 1861, and his promotion as major general ranked from July 1862. He was in the North Carolina campaign and at Antietam and Fredericksburg. In September, following Antietam, he had a sick leave but returned to duty in a short time. In August 1863, after Vicksburg, he was under his doctor's care in Cincinnati. The physician stated he should go to the seashore for the benefit of his health. In September he was ordered to proceed to Nicholasville, Kentucky, to resume command of his corps. Suffering with poor health from recent exposure, he had to remain in Knoxville in January 1864. He was absent sick in April and returned in May. He served with distinction in the Virginia campaigns in 1864–65. On July 3, 1864, he was quite ill and had three chills. He was given leave to go north and returned in August. No specific diagnosis was given for any of Parke's various illnesses.[1] He remained in the army after the war and became a colonel of engineers. From 1887 until his retirement in 1889 he was superintendent of the U.S. Military Academy. Died at his residence on December 16, 1900, in Washington, D.C., and was buried in the churchyard of St. James the Less in Philadelphia.

DEATH CERTIFICATE: Cause of death, primary, prostatitis, chronic, two years' duration; immediate, prostatic abscess, exhaustion, four weeks' duration.

1. CSR; *OR*, vol. 30, pt. 3:127, 157, 169, 656, 659; vol. 33:685; vol. 36, pt. 1:905; vol. 40, pt. 2:609; vol. 51, pt. 1:1159; WPCHR, vols. 605, 606, 607; U.S. Army, CWS, roll 1, vol. 2, report 13, pp. 141–51; Lymon, *Meade's Headquarters*, 213; Cox, *Military Reminiscences* 2:127.

LEWIS BALDWIN PARSONS • *Born April 5, 1818,* in New York state. During his youth he injured the bone in one hip. In November 1838 his health started to fail, supposedly because he studied too hard in school. On his doctor's advice he gave up school and taught for a short time. In 1840, the time of his graduation from Yale, he still suffered hip pain. He was chief executive officer of the Ohio & Mississippi Railroad when the Civil War started. After serving as a volunteer aide, he was made a captain and assistant quartermaster to rank from October 1861. Parsons played a major role in the transportation of the Union army during the war although he had an increasing number of episodes of pain in his previously injured hip, particularly when he went on long train rides. Following the Civil War, he took a disability leave and in May 1865 had some type of operation on his hip, which was apparently successful. That same month he was commissioned brigadier general of volunteers. He had a bilious attack while in St. Louis during September. In April 1866 he was discharged.[1] He returned to the railroads, business, and banking. Died in Flora, Illinois, on March 16, 1907, and was buried in Bellefontaine Cemetery, St. Louis.

DEATH CERTIFICATE: Immediate cause, acute bronchitis; contributory cause, organic heart disease.

1. *OR*, vol. 47, pt. 3:539; RVA, Pension XC 2,490,943; George Carl Schottenhamel, "Lewis Baldwin Parsons and Civil War Transportation" (diss.), 11, 14, 327, 339.

MARSENA RUDOLPH PATRICK • *Born on March 11, 1811*, near Watertown, New York. Graduated from the USMA in 1835. While a cadet, he was treated for a headache seven times, cold and diarrhea six times each, colica and pain in chest twice each, and scarlet fever, constipatio, influenza, catarrhus, fever, and sore feet once each. Served in the Florida and Mexican wars. On December 15, 1849, he had an attack of inflammatory rheumatism in his shoulder and arm and was not able to write. He had sick leave from January 1850 to June and spent most of the time at home. Patrick resigned his commission in 1850, took up farming, and developed advanced agricultural methods. He served as inspector general of the state of New York from the start of the war until March 1862, when he was made brigadier general of volunteers. On the cold night of June 22, 1864, in front of Petersburg, he fell asleep with his back against a tree. When he awoke the next morning there was some soreness in his left shoulder and arm. He kept working and remained in the saddle until the middle of July, when the pain forced him to take a few days off. His doctor prescribed palliatives. Stomach and bowel problems laid him up for a few days after he returned, but he continued to work and applied liniments to his shoulder and side. On August 1, Patrick was seen by a physician from Philadelphia who recommended electrical treatments to restore life in his shoulder and arm. He could not obtain rest except when he lay partly on his back and side, holding up the left arm and foot. Late in the month, another physician took his case, and potassium iodine was given externally and internally, along with blue pills, liniments, and rubbing. By the middle of September, his condition was regarded as "partial paralysis," and he was advised to leave the field. His symptoms were attributed to rheumatism and chronic malarial poisoning. Pain in his hip had developed to the point where he could not stand; the shoulder was more painful, and there was a feeling of numbness and a prickly sensation on his left side. Starting September 29, he used the electric battery for one half hour every night. His groom gave him dry-hand rubbing, chloroform liniments were used, and when the suffering became intense, the shoulder was cupped. Colchicine was administered, and the dry, hot, itching sensation was helped by rubbing with salt and water. From December 27 until January 8, 1865, he had an acute attack of his symptoms. After a new medicine was prescribed, he improved and about the end of January was able to travel from Fort Monroe to Washington. On February 25 the regular use of the battery was discontinued. In March he was able to do office work but could not ride a horse, and on April 11 he was ordered to Richmond. He resigned from the army in June 1865. On his return home, he tried to take an active part in farming, but his poor health limited what he could do. By 1872, he was unable to walk any distance or stand for any length of time and had to ride to take care of his farm. There was constant pain in his left shoulder and knee, and he had lumbago three to four times a year.[1] Died July 27, 1888, at Dayton, Ohio, and was buried there in the Home Cemetery.

1. WPCHR, vols. 601, 602, 603; LR, ACP, 4968, 1973, fiche: 000156; RVA, Pension C 178,850.

FRANCIS ENGLE PATTERSON · *Born May 7, 1821,* in Philadelphia. Served in the Mexican War. Promoted to first lieutenant in 1848, he remained in the Regular Army until 1857 when he resigned. After serving in a ninety-day militia unit, he was made a brigadier general of volunteers to rank from April 1862. Although very ill and unable to command, he accompanied his troops on May 31, 1862, at Seven Pines. The next day he had to relinquish his command, supposedly due to typhoid fever. He received a sick leave on June 7 and returned to duty at Harrison's Landing the first part of July. He was quite ill in November. On November 22, 1862, he was found dead in his tent, killed by the accidental discharge of his own pistol. It has also been suggested that he committed suicide because of charges preferred against him by Gen. Dan Sickles.[1] The place of death is usually fixed at "Fairfax Court House" or "near Occoquan, Virginia." He was buried in Laurel Hill Cemetery, Philadelphia.

1. CSR; *OR,* vol. 11, pt. 1:759, 819, 835–36; vol. 19, pt. 2:562; U.S. Army, CWS, report of J. B. Carr, roll 1, vol. 2, report 17, pp. 199–215; Steiner, *Disease,* 150; Edward Longacre, "Damnable Dan Sickles," *CWTI* 23 (May 1984): 16–25.

GABRIEL RENÉ PAUL · *Born on March 22, 1813,* in St. Louis. Graduated from the USMA in 1834. At West Point he was treated once each for a wound and a fever. Served in the Florida and Mexican wars. He was wounded April 18, 1847, at Cerro Gordo. He served on the frontier, and in April 1861 he was promoted major of the 8th Infantry. The following April he was promoted to lieutenant colonel. His first promotion as brigadier general was not confirmed, but he was reappointed in April 1863 and finally confirmed. He was a field commander at Fredericksburg and Chancellorsville. On July 1, 1863, at Gettysburg, he received a gunshot wound of the head. The ball entered about one and a half inches behind his right eye and emerged through the left eye socket, carrying the eye with it. Paul remained insensible in a private home in Gettysburg for several days. When he awoke he was blind with an impaired sense of smell and hearing. He remained there until about August 1, when he was removed to Baltimore, Maryland. Near the end of the month he received permission to proceed to Washington, D.C. In October, he went to Newport, Kentucky, where he remained under treatment and awaiting further orders. He was absent sick until he retired as a brigadier general of the Regular Army in February 1865. Following his wound, he had epilepsy and violent attacks of pain in his head. During the last years of his life the epilepsy attacks became more frequent and occurred up to six times a day. Died May 5, 1886, at his residence in Washington, D.C., and was buried in Arlington National Cemetery.[1]

DEATH CERTIFICATE: Cause of death, primary, epileptiform attack resulting from gunshot wound of the head. Wounded at Gettysburg. Duration, about twenty-four hours; immediate, coma. Last illness, less than two days.

1. CSR; *OR*, vol. 27, pt. 1:72, 249, 290, 705; WPCHR, vol. 602, 603; LR, ACP, 1154, 1883, fiche: 000157; RAGO, entry 534; U.S. Army, CWS, roll 1, vol. 2, report 14, pp. 153–77; Heitman, *Historical Register and Dictionary* 2:33.

JOHN JAMES PECK • *Born January 4, 1821,* in Manlius, New York. Graduated from the USMA in 1843. While at the military academy, he was treated for a headache four times, a toothache twice, and bruise, diarrhea, nausea, lameness, constipation, sprain, and sore feet one time each. Peck was wounded in Mexico. He resigned from the service in 1853 and became a successful and rich businessman. President Lincoln appointed him a brigadier general of volunteers in August 1861. His promotion as major general ranked from July 1862. He commanded a division on the Peninsula and at Suffolk. In early December 1862, Peck was close to breaking down from exhaustion, and he obtained a leave. His attending surgeon reported in July 1863 that he was suffering from a fall that he had received in April, which injured his spine and caused some hemiplegia. The injury was aggravated again in July when he had another accident. In May 1864 he was assigned to the command of the District of Saint Mary's and was granted a thirty-day leave on surgeon's certificate of disability before assuming his duties.[1] He was discharged in August 1865 and two years later organized the New York State Life Insurance Company. Peck's health was undermined by illness and the previous injuries, and on April 21, 1878, he died at Syracuse, New York. He was buried in Oakwood Cemetery, Syracuse.

DEATH CERTIFICATE: Immediate cause of death, spinal sclerosis.

1. *OR*, vol. 18:476–78; vol. 37, pt. 1:404; vol. 51, pt. 1:1161–62; WPCHR, vol. 604; RAGO, entry 534; Kearny, *Letters,* 96.

GALUSHA PENNYPACKER • *Born June 1, 1844,* in Chester County, Pennsylvania. In August 1861, at the age of seventeen, he was commissioned captain of a company in the 97th Pennsylvania. The following October he was promoted to major. In September 1863 he was prostrated by diarrhea and intermittent fever and for a time was away from active duty. However, he remained in his quarters and received the attention of his regimental surgeon and a nurse. Although still an invalid, he marched his command on September 7 in the assault on Fort Gregg. Being disqualified from active duty by his illness, he took a sick leave in late September and went north. A surgeon's certificate in October reported that he was suffering from the effects of miasma causing intermittent disease. He returned and served as a drill instructor in November. During the charge on May 20, 1864, at Green Plains, Virginia, he was wounded twice but rose each time to press forward with his men. He had been superficially wounded below the left knee and on the right side of his chest. A third wound was more serious and rendered him helpless: The ball struck him above the right elbow and injured the biceps and triceps muscles. He was carried by his men back to his tent where the regimental surgeon cared for him. On May 23 he was sent to the Chesapeake General Hospital near Fort Monroe, Virginia, for treatment. By the middle of June, the arm wound had still not healed, and flexion and extension were materially limited. There also appeared to be a potential abscess between the wound and the axilla. A circumscribed hardness suggested some foreign body. During his convalescence he returned to West Chester, Pennsylvania. Still somewhat limited in the use of his right arm, he rejoined his regiment in August. At Fort Gilmer, Virginia, on September 29, 1864, a shell fragment struck his right ankle, causing a slight but painful wound. Although suffering severely, he continued on duty and obtained what care he could. During the attack on Fort Fisher, North Carolina, on January 15, 1865, Pennypacker was seriously wounded while planting the colors of his leading regiment on the works. An enemy soldier, only a few feet away, fired his musket and wounded him through the right side and hip. The upper portion of the pelvic bone was fractured and muscles of the anus were injured. He suffered excruciating pain when any attempt to move him was made, and, under the circumstances, any movement was difficult and precarious. As soon as possible, he was moved to the Chesapeake Hospital at Fort Monroe. He was later moved to the general hospital at Norfolk, Virginia, and then back to Chesapeake Hospital. After remaining about ten months in hospitals, he returned to his home in West Chester. During the next few months he continued to experience painful relapses and was confined to his bed for several weeks at a time. His final recovery was reported to be doubtful. He was made brigadier general of volunteers to rank from February 1865. At the end of his leave, he was deemed incapable of further field service.[1] However, he remained in the army and in 1866 was appointed colonel. Pennypacker retired in 1883. Died October 1, 1916, in Philadelphia and was buried in Philadelphia National Cemetery.

1. CSR; OR, vol. 46, pt. 1:400, 416, 420, pt. 2:156, 165; U.S. Army, CWS, roll 4, vol. 6, report 30, pp. 577–668.

WILLIAM HENRY PENROSE • *Born on March 10, 1832,* at Madison Barracks, Sacket's Harbor, New York. Engaged in civil and mechanical engineering in Michigan when the Civil War started, he was appointed a second lieutenant of the 3rd U.S. Infantry. On August 31, 1862, the day after Second Bull Run, he developed camp fever and went to Washington. After being confined for three weeks to convalesce, he was detailed as an instructor of new regiments. He rejoined his regiment in November. He fought at Fredericksburg, Chancellorsville, and Gettysburg. In April 1863 he was commissioned colonel of the 15th New Jersey Volunteers. That same year his right eardrum was ruptured when an artillery piece fired too early. He had a leave of absence on September 6 because of facial neuralgia caused by carious teeth. Penrose served in the Wilderness and at Spotsylvania and was severely wounded in the arm at Cedar Creek on October 19, 1864. A minié ball, fired at a distance of twenty yards, passed through his right forearm, which was raised above his head. The ball entered from the front, passed through on the radial aspect of the arm about two inches below the elbow, and made its exit about one inch below the elbow. Three and one-half inches of the radius was badly comminuted, and the fragments were driven into the surrounding tissues. The radial nerve was divided, but the radial artery was uninjured. Eight hours afterward, he was operated on in the Sixth Corps Hospital using chloroform as an anesthetic. The wound on the radial aspect was extended to about four inches. The ends of the bone were sawed off by a chain saw and carefully smoothed. The space between the two ends of the bone was about four and a half inches long. The wound was nearly closed by a number of silk sutures. The arm was placed in temporary splints, and the next morning he was sent to the rear. Given a sick leave, he convalesced in Philadelphia and at home. The wound had to be opened three more times to remove bone fragments. In February 1865 he returned to duty. On April 2, 1865, near Petersburg, his right hip was bruised by a bullet, but he did not leave his command. His arm wound appeared to be completely healed by May. Penrose was made a brigadier general of volunteers in June. He was discharged from volunteer service in 1866 and remained in the army as a captain. Not only did his hip wound continue to bother him after the war, but also his leg was stiff, and he had to be helped on and off his horse. By 1868 his right arm was slightly bent inward, but all motions of the arm remained except for rotation. Movements of the hand and fingers were retained except for a very slight impairment of the power and mobility of the thumb and index finger. Ankylosis was present in the last joint of the index finger. However, he was able to use the thumb and finger for all functions, such as writing, and holding a pen or knife and fork. By May 1870 there was still limited rotation of the right arm, but he could draw his sword. There was a fistulous opening at the site of the resection, and at intervals pus and spicules of dead bone were spontaneously discharged. The arm wound never completely closed except for a short period of time, and over thirty pieces of bone were removed. In September 1870 he had medical care for over ten days for erythema from a poison vine. In 1873 Penrose was treated for tonsillitis in March, tertian intermittent fever in August, and a boil in December. While on duty at Camp Supply, Indian Territory, in March 1874, he fell down while drunk and was unable to reach his quarters without assistance. He was court-martialed for drunkenness. After he pledged to abstain from the use of all intoxicating drinks he was restored to duty. In June 1875 he had pain and inflammation of the right ear attended with profuse discharge of pus and complete loss of hearing. The following August he wanted to go east for treatment of his ear, which had not responded to treatment by army doctors. In September he got into a fight while drunk. He finally obtained his leave in November 1875 and went to Philadelphia, Pennsylvania, where he was under treatment through January. In late 1880 Penrose was dismissed from the service for one year because of continued drinking. Chronic eczema over the lower half of his body, which had bothered him for three years, became worse during the last half of 1884. In early 1885 the eczema affected his entire body and confined him to bed for weeks. In February 1885 he requested a leave because of sciatic pain, which his surgeon reported was due to the nerve being injured at Petersburg. In the summer of 1885 he was on sick leave at Passale, New Jersey, and under treatment by a New York specialist. After thirteen months there was little improvement in his skin disease. During July 1889 he received three days' treatment for acute diarrhea, and the following April he was treated for bronchial catarrh. His eczema again became generalized in 1890, and his surgeon hypothesized the cause for the skin disease was his injured right sciatic nerve. In October the post surgeon stated the waters of Hot Springs, Arkansas, were especially efficacious in skin disease, such as the one that afflicted Penrose. He continued on sick leave, and in September 1891 a specialist reported that Penrose's skin condition might be curable. This dermatologist theorized that it was due to toxic influences as demonstrated by the increased uric acid in his urine. All of this, he speculated, indicated an impaired "oxidation process due to faulty hepatic activity." He recommended treatment directed at Penrose's general condition rather than the localized manifestations. Penrose returned from sick leave in September 1892 and was finally made a colonel in 1893. After more sick leave, he retired on March 10, 1896. Died August 29, 1903, at Salt Lake City, Utah, and was buried in Arlington National Cemetery. He had had diarrhea for two weeks and, according to the local commanding officer, the cause of death was typhoid fever.[1]

1. CSR; *OR*, vol. 42, pt. 1:55, 131, 167; vol. 46, pt. 2:551; LR, ACP, 2104, 1874, fiche: 000158; U.S. Army, CWS, roll 6, vol. 10, report 38, pp. 317–28; *MSHW*, vol. 2, pt. 2:938, 946; RVA, Pension C 588,841.

JOHN SMITH PHELPS • *Born December 22, 1814,* in Simsbury, Connecticut. A lawyer and congressman from Missouri when the war started, he raised a six-month command and became its colonel. At Pea Ridge, Arkansas, on March 7, 1862, he had three horses shot under him and received a contusion from a shell. President Lincoln appointed him military governor of Arkansas in July 1862, and his appointment as brigadier general of volunteers ranked from that same month. For three weeks in early September 1862 he was so sick he was unable to attend to business. His appointment as general was not confirmed by the Senate and

expired in March 1863.[1] In 1864 he returned to his law practice in Missouri and for one term was governor of the state. Died in St. Louis on November 20, 1886, and was buried in Hazelwood Cemetery, Springfield, Missouri.
DEATH CERTIFICATE: Cause of death, uremic poisoning.

1. *OR*, vol. 8:260, 280; vol. 13:683.

JOHN WOLCOTT PHELPS • *Born November 13, 1813,* at Guilford, Vermont. Graduated from the USMA in 1836. He was seen at the Cadet Hospital for a cold twice and for a boil, rheumatism, and a headache once each. Served in the Florida and Mexican wars. After resigning from the military in 1859 he campaigned against slavery and the Masonic Order. He was made colonel of the 1st Vermont in May 1861, and his promotion as brigadier general of volunteers ranked from the same month. He organized the first Negro troops before receiving authorization, and his actions were disavowed by the administration. He resigned in September 1862 and continued to champion various causes until his death. Died in Guilford on February 2, 1885, and was buried there.
DEATH CERTIFICATE: Found dead in bed.

ABRAM SANDERS PIATT (First name appears as Abraham in records of the War Department) • *Born May 2, 1821,* in Cincinnati, Ohio. He left his farm and became colonel of the 13th Ohio, a three-month regiment, when the Civil War started. In September 1861 he was made colonel of the 34th Ohio and was promoted to brigadier general of volunteers in April 1862. He was at Second Bull Run and Antietam. In late March 1862 he had typhoid fever. Granted leave, he was taken to his home in Ohio where he remained until June. At Fredericksburg on December 13, 1862, his horse stumbled, and he was thrown to the ground. His back was injured so severely that he was unable to walk. He was able to return to duty the next morning, but the injury apparently led to his resignation from the service, which was accepted as of February 17, 1863. Piatt returned to civilian life and resumed farming. Died March 16, 1908, in Monroe, Ohio, and was buried in the nearby Piatt Cemetery. Record of death: Cause of death, cancer.[1]

1. *OR*, vol. 21:55, 135, 395; U.S. Army, CWS, roll 2, vol. 3, report 49, pp. 1361–71; Record of deaths, Probate Court, Logan County, Ohio.

BYRON ROOT PIERCE • *Born on September 20, 1829,* in East Bloomfield, New York. Pierce was a dentist and captain of a local militia unit that entered Federal service in June 1861 as Company K, 3rd Michigan. By January he was a colonel. He was at First Bull Run, on the Peninsula, at Second Bull Run, and at Fredericksburg. He was slightly wounded in the left hand and the right arm at Chancellorsville on May 3, 1863. After his wounds were dressed, he immediately returned to his post. At Gettysburg on July 2, 1863, he was wounded below the left knee. He was not hospitalized, and his wound was dressed by the regimental surgeon. During May 1864 he was wounded at Spotsylvania. His promotion to brigadier general of volunteers ranked from June. In front of Petersburg on June 18, 1864, he was wounded for the last time. He was sent to the hospital at City Point in late July 1864 after being sick with diarrhea for several days. In August he was on leave in Grand Rapids, Michigan, and had dysentery and general debility. He was mustered out of the service in August 1865. Pierce participated in Union veterans' groups and operated a hotel before retiring from business in 1899. In February 1921 he was completely disabled by reason of his age; he had been confined in a sanitarium since the previous November. He was unable to take care of himself and required constant attendance and assistance from a nurse.[1] Died July 10, 1924, at Grand Rapids, Michigan, and was buried in Fulton Street Cemetery, Grand Rapids.

DEATH CERTIFICATE: Cause of death, myocarditis (arteriosclerotic) and nephritis (chronic interstitial). Duration, two years.

1. CSR; OR, vol. 25, pt. 1:434, 437; vol. 27, pt. 1:521, 524; vol. 40, pt. 1:184, 368, pt. 2:166; U.S. Army, CWS, roll 5, vol. 9, report 15, pp. 335–37; RVA, Pension SC 219,956; RAGO, entry 534.

WILLIAM ANDERSON PILE • *Born on February 11, 1829,* near Indianapolis, Indiana. Pile was a minister of the Methodist Episcopal church and at the beginning of the war enlisted as a chaplain of the 1st Missouri Light Artillery. Apparently he preferred a different role in the war, and by December 1862 he was colonel of the 33rd Missouri Infantry. He was at Corinth and Vicksburg and led a brigade of black soldiers at Mobile and Fort Blakely. He was made a brigadier general of volunteers in December 1863. After being mustered out of Federal service in August 1865, he was elected the following year to Congress. Pile held Federal positions until 1876, when he became an agent of the Venezuelan government. Died July 7, 1889, at Monrovia, California, and was buried in Live Oak Cemetery. According to the attending physician, the cause of death was pneumonia.[1]

1. RVA, Pension WC 464,559.

THOMAS GAMBLE PITCHER • *Born October 23, 1824,* at Rockport, Indiana. Graduated from the USMA in 1845. Served in the Mexican War. When the Civil War started, Captain Pitcher was depot commissary at Fort Bliss, Texas. During the Battle of Cedar Mountain, August 9, 1862, he was wounded in the right knee joint. The ball lodged in the internal condyle of his femur, having struck it perpendicularly about the middle of the internal face. He was moved from Culpeper, Virginia, to Washington, where he remained confined to his room until November 19, 1862, when he proceeded to New York City for duty. His promotion to brigadier general of volunteers ranked from that month. When he was examined on February 3, 1863, it could not be determined if the ball was still present. The inflammation in his wound had left the swollen knee joint in a state of false ankylosis and subacute inflammation. He required crutches to walk, and any motion caused him pain. On examination in April, he had an unusual accumulation of fluid in the right knee joint and a general enlargement of the whole knee, and he was not able to extend the leg completely. He was ordered to Vermont in June to be assistant to the provost marshal general of the U.S. for the state of Vermont. He was still suffering from his painful knee in May 1864 and was obliged to continue using crutches. He was discharged from volunteer service in 1866 and was made colonel of the Forty-fourth Infantry. In November 1877 Pitcher was physically capable of the ordinary duties required of an officer of his rank and could ride well. However, he could not march or do the things required in a rough-and-tumble Indian campaign. A retirement board in February 1878 reported he was incapacitated due to ankylosis of his right knee joint, and he was retired in June. Died in the post hospital, Fort Bayard, New Mexico, on October 19, 1895, and was buried in Arlington National Cemetery. According to the assistant surgeon, the cause of death was exhaustion due to an abscess of the brain.[1]

1. *OR*, vol. 12, pt. 2:169; vol. 25, pt. 2:503; LR, ACP, 2721, 1877, fiche: 000160; *MSHW*, vol. 2, pt. 3:365; U.S. Army, CWS, roll 1, vol. 1, report 3, pp. 39–41; ibid., roll 4, vol. 7, report 10, pp. 157–59; RAGO, entry 534.

ALFRED PLEASONTON • *Born July 7, 1824,* in Washington, D.C. Graduated from the USMA in 1844. Served in Mexican and Florida wars. He was on sick leave and detached service from December 1846 until the following December and was with his regiment in Mexico until September 1848. He was sick at Santa Fe, New Mexico, from June 21 to December 20, 1851, and was absent sick from April 17 to July 20, 1854. Medical certificates providing authorization for the leaves are not available. In the fall of 1861 he brought his troops from Utah to Washington, D.C., and served in the city's defenses and on the Peninsula. Pleasonton's promotion to brigadier general of volunteers ranked from July 1862. Over his period of service during the Civil War he supposedly had episodes of malaria from time to time. His right ear was injured from the concussion of artillery fire at Antietam on September 17, 1862. He served at Fredericksburg, Chancellorsville, and Brandy Station. In June 1863 he was promoted to major general. Late in October 1864 he had a severe fall and on October 27 was unable to move. He requested a medical leave to go to St. Louis to obtain treatment. In late January 1865 he was in Philadelphia undergoing therapy. Not in favor with those in higher command and subordinate to those he had previously commanded, he occupied minor Federal posts until he was placed on the retired list in 1888 as a major. Pleasonton appeared broken and prematurely old when examined in March 1880 and had a number of complaints.

There was partial deafness of his previously injured ear, and he had episodes of chills and fever. He suffered from migratory neuralgia, affecting mainly the right side of his face, the right leg, and his thighs. In addition, he had pains in his stomach and back, a torpid liver, and diarrhea with hemorrhoids. His liver was slightly enlarged and the spleen was tender. The examining physician stated that Pleasonton's condition was due to chronic malaria poisoning. In October 1888 he was operated upon for an abscess of the buttocks of such a serious character that he was confined to his bed for over three months.[1] Died at his residence on February 17, 1897, in Washington, D.C., and was buried in the Congressional Cemetery.

DEATH CERTIFICATE: Cause of death, primary, Bright's disease following malaria; immediate, catarrhal pneumonia. Duration last illness, ten days.

   1. CSR; *OR*, vol. 41, pt. 1:503, 506–7, 540; vol. 48, pt. 1:746–47, 761; RVA, Pension SC 166,428.

JOSEPH BENNETT PLUMMER • *Born on November 15, 1816,* in Barre, Massachusetts. Graduated from the USMA in 1841. Cadet Plummer was treated for a cough, a pain in his side, and a headache one time each. Served in the Florida and Mexican wars. He had sick leaves from August 27, 1846, to June 27, 1847, August 21, 1851, to April 24, 1854, and from October 27, 1860, to January 30, 1861. There are no surgeon's certificates available for these leaves. Captain Plummer was on quartermaster duty on the frontier when the Civil War started. He was wounded in the hip by a rifle ball on August 10, 1861, at the Battle of Wilson's Creek. The ball was not extracted. In September he was commissioned colonel of the 11th Missouri Infantry and brigadier general of volunteers to rank from October 1861. He led a division at New Madrid and Island No. 10. Early in May 1862 he was sick, and the first of August he was seen by a physician in Baltimore. The physician stated that Plummer was suffering from his wound and hepatic and gastric derangement due to his protracted exposure to the climate and camp life. Against the advice of the army surgeon and the Baltimore physician, he reported for duty at Corinth, Mississippi. He died suddenly near Corinth on August 9, 1862, from "congestion of the brain secondary to his wounds, hepatic derangement and the fatigues and exposures of active campaigning." The Baltimore physician later theorized that the congestion of his brain resulted from his blood having been poisoned by protracted and fatiguing exposure to malaria. His liver had been so much disturbed that it could no longer function.[1] He was buried in Arlington National Cemetery.

   1. *OR*, vol. 3:72, 209–10; vol. 10, pt. 1:805; WPCHR, vol. 604; LR, ACP, 1440, 1884, fiche: 000161; RVA, Pension WC 1,253.

ORLANDO METCALFE POE • *Born on March 7, 1832,* at Navarre, Ohio. Graduated from the USMA in 1856. At West Point, he was treated for catarrhus five times, diarrhea four times, nausea three times, subluxatio and cephalalgia twice each, and rheumatism, contusio, tonsillitis, and excoriatio one time each. Graduating sixth in his class at the U.S. Military Academy, he was appointed to the engineers and spent time surveying the northern lakes. He was promoted first lieutenant in 1860 and appointed colonel of the 2nd Michigan in September 1861. In the middle of April 1862 he developed bilious remittent fever but remained on duty. At dusk on May 31, 1862, at Seven Pines, his horse was killed under him, and he received severe contusions when it fell. Because of his injury and the fever, he went home on sick leave on June 11 but returned in August for Second Bull Run. He was appointed brigadier general of volunteers in November. On December 23, 1862, he received another leave on surgeon's certificate and did not return until February. His appointment as general was not confirmed by the Senate, and in March 1863 he reverted to his rank of captain of engineers in the Regular Army. As such he served with distinction at Knoxville, in the Atlanta campaign, and in the Carolinas. After the Civil War, Poe remained in the army and in 1873 was made a staff colonel and aide-de-camp to Gen. William T. Sherman. On September 18, 1895, while on an official inspection tour at Sault St. Marie, Michigan, he slipped and struck his left tibia against a ladder. He developed traumatic erysipelas. On September 21, an area of several inches around the wound was swollen and inflamed, there was edema of the gluteus muscle, and he had constitutional symptoms. By September 24, the wound was deeper and about an inch in circumference, and the erysipelas was confined to the leg and foot. The infection had reached his face on September 28. He died at Detroit on October 2, 1895, and was buried in Arlington National Cemetery.[1]

DEATH CERTIFICATE: Cause of death, erysipelas, two weeks' duration.

1. CSR; WPCHR, vols. 608, 609; U.S. Army, CWS, roll 3, vol. 4, report 10, pp. 217–54; LR, ACP, 3757, 1883, fiche: 000162; RVA, Pension WC 419,700.

JOHN POPE • *Born on March 16, 1822*, in Louisville, Kentucky. Graduated from the USMA in 1842. Served in the Mexican and Florida wars. At Monterey, Mexico, in September 1846, two balls hit the scabbard of his saber without causing him injury. During most of the winter of 1849–50 he was confined to his bed by nervous exhaustion and stomach disorders brought on by overexertion. He was promoted to captain in 1856. His commission as brigadier general of volunteers ranked from May 1861, and he was promoted to major general in March 1862. He was successful at New Madrid, Island No. 10, and Corinth, but ruined his reputation at Second Bull Run. On June 1, 1862, Pope was ill and had to command from a number of miles behind the lines. He was able to return to full duty by June 4. A planned trip to St. Louis was delayed until February 22, 1865, because of illness. He had been commissioned a brigadier in the regular service to rank from July 1862 and was promoted major general in October 1882. Pope died on September 23, 1892, at the Soldiers' and Sailors' Home near Sandusky, Ohio, while making a visit. His remains were buried in Bellefontaine Cemetery,

St. Louis. The attending surgeon reported Pope's death was caused by a complete breaking down of his nervous system, a letting loose of all vital forces, which could very properly be styled "nervous prostration."[1]

1. *OR*, vol. 48, pt. 1:947; LR, ACP, 5013, 1883, fiche: 000281; Merlin Gwinn Cox, "John Pope: Fighting General from Illinois" (diss.), 21, 26, 133–35.

ANDREW PORTER • *Born July 10, 1820,* in Lancaster, Pennsylvania. Served in the Mexican War. He was appointed 1st Lieutenant of the Mounted Rifles on May 27, 1846. While serving on the Indian frontier, his health was impaired. In 1855, Porter had a sick leave from June 3 to December in Texas. No diagnosis was provided. In May 1861 he was made colonel of the 16th U.S. Infantry and was appointed brigadier general of volunteers in August. He served at First Bull Run and on the Peninsula but in July 1862 suffered from malarial fever and chronic dysentery. The illness confined him to his room in Philadelphia from July to September. His physician reported that his disease was particularly hard to cure because of the character imparted upon the disorder by the locality in which it was contracted and the serious exertions he had undergone. In early September Porter was assigned to duty in Pennsylvania to organize volunteers. In November 1862 he was appointed provost marshal general of the state. His chronic dysentery continued during 1863, and he developed an abscess that was present for eighteen months. Greatly debilitated, he lost physical strength. In April 1864 he was mustered out of the volunteer service and resigned his regular commission. His medical problems continued during 1865–68, and his wife was always in attendance. In July and August 1868 he was in Canada in an effort to improve his health during the summer heat. He used the medicinal waters in an attempt to arrest his disease without success. In the last week of November, Porter went to Europe for medical advice. After seeing physicians at Paris, he went to Hamburg, Germany, in the summer of 1869, again without apparent benefit. He returned to the United States in October 1869 for the healthful effects of the sea voyage. He sailed for Liverpool, England, in November. During the winter of 1869–70 he took the medical advice of a physician, who treated him using his system of electricity, and again there was no improvement. He was treated in the summer of 1870 at the Water Cure of Bellevue near Paris, France. In August he was in England under treatment at the Malvern Water Cure, again without benefit. In the winter of 1870–71 he was in Belgium for medical treatment. He went to Hamburg in August and then back to Belgium without improvement. In October 1871 he returned to Paris. His strength continued to decline until the morning of January 3, 1872, when he died in Paris, France.[1] His body was returned to the United States and he was buried in Elmwood Cemetery, Detroit. Burial records: Cause of death, consumption.

1. CSR; *OR*, vol. 19, pt. 2:214, 473; vol. 21:1003; vol. 51, pt. 1:937; LR, ACP, 3248, 1879, fiche: 000163; RVA, Pension, WC 187,382; Averell, *William Woods Averell,* 310.

FITZ JOHN PORTER • *Born on August 31, 1822,* in Portsmouth, New Hampshire. Graduated from the USMA in 1845. He received a severe contusion from a spent ball on September 13, 1847, at Chapultepec, Mexico. Before the Civil War he had duty as an instructor of artillery at the U.S. Military Academy and as Albert Sidney Johnston's adjutant in the Utah expedition. His promotion to brigadier general of volunteers ranked from May 1861. Sickness did not prevent him from going up in an observation balloon on May 3, 1862.[1] He served admirably on the Peninsula, petulantly at Second Bull Run, and ambivalently at Antietam. Loyalty to Gen. George B. McClellan and a dislike for Gen. John Pope terminated in his court-martial and dismissal from the army in January 1863. Finally in 1886, President Grover Cleveland signed a bill that restored his name upon the army rolls as colonel of infantry. Died May 21, 1901, in Morristown, New Jersey, and was buried in Green-Wood Cemetery, Brooklyn.

DEATH CERTIFICATE: Cause of death, chronic diabetes of two years' duration.

1. *OR Suppl.,* vol. 2, pt. 1:43; Heitman, *Historical Register and Dictionary* 2:34; Wilcox, *Mexican War,* 470.

EDWARD ELMER POTTER • *Born on June 21, 1823,* in New York City. A New York farmer, he was commissioned a captain in the commissary department in February 1862. He recruited the 1st North Carolina (Union) Infantry in May 1862, and his appointment as brigadier general of volunteers ranked from November 1862. On September 13, 1864, he obtained a leave on medical certificate for ill health and returned in October. On July 4, 1865, he went home sick. On July 19 he tendered his resignation, which was accepted July 24.[1] Potter returned to civilian life after the Civil War. He died in a boarding house in New York City on June 1, 1889, and was buried in Marble Cemetery in Manhattan.

DEATH CERTIFICATE: Chief cause, pneumonia of seven days' duration; contributing cause, heart failure.

1. U.S. Army, CWS, roll 6, vol. 10, report 36, pp. 287–96.

JOSEPH HAYDN POTTER • *Born October 12, 1822,* in Concord, New Hampshire. Graduated from the USMA in 1843. Potter was wounded at Monterey, Mexico, on September 21, 1846. Absent from duty on account of his wound until November, he was then on recruiting service until September 1850. Later, Samuel G. French said that Potter's old leg wound was an excellent indicator of rain. Potter participated in the Utah expedition and was stationed in New Mexico when the Civil War started. He was captured along with other regulars at San Augustine Pass on July 27, 1861, and was not exchanged for a year. In 1862 he was appointed colonel of the 12th New Hampshire Infantry. He was present sick in November and December 1862. During the Chancellorsville campaign on May 3, 1863, he was wounded in the leg and captured again. He was taken to Richmond and paroled on May 15. Potter received medical treatment in Washington from May through August. From September through December he was on court-martial duty in Washington D.C. During January and February 1864 he assumed command as assistant to the provost marshal general and superintendent of the volunteer recruiting service for Ohio. He rejoined his regiment in September 1864. He had been made a major in the regular service in 1863 and brigadier general of volunteers in May 1865. Potter remained in the army after the war and had a series of illnesses over the years: He was sick at Fort Sedgwick, Colorado Territory, in April 1867; January 21–25, 1871, catarrh; Sick at Columbus, Ohio from December 19, 1871 to March 7, 1872, acute rheumatism; April 1–7, 1873, catarrh; Sick at Fort Sanders, Wyoming, December 1873 to January 1874 and April to May 1874, acute rheumatism; December 11–15, 1874, rheumatism; Sick at Fort Brown, Texas, January 3 to February 8, rheumatism; March 6–9, cholera morbus; May 31 to June 1875, acute rheumatism; November 9 to December 3, 1875, acute rheumatism, and April 24 to May 1876, acute rheumatism. He had a sick leave on surgeon's certificate from August 1, 1876, to May 31, 1877. Potter was governor of the Soldier's Home near Washington, D.C., from July 1, 1877, to July 1, 1881. While commanding a regiment at Fort Supply, Indian Territory, he was sick at the post from January 25–28, April 18–22, 1884, and with rheumatism on May 10–16, 1885. Promoted to brigadier general in the Regular Army in April 1886, he retired the following October. Died December 1, 1892, in Columbus, Ohio, and was buried there in Greenlawn Cemetery. According to the attending physician, the cause of death was from the effects of acute rheumatism and pneumonia, the pneumonia consequent and secondary to the rheumatism.[1]

1. CSR; *OR*, vol. 25, pt. 1:391, 394, 492, 500; LR, ACP, 2514, 1877, fiche: 000164; RVA, Pension SC 373,196; Heitman, *Historical Register and Dictionary* 2:34; Samuel G. French, *Two Wars: An Autobiography of General Samuel G. French*, 130.

ROBERT BROWN POTTER • *Born on July 16, 1829,* in Schenectady, New York. He was practicing the law in New York City at the start of the Civil War and enlisted as a private in the militia. In October 1861 he was commissioned major of the 51st New York. During the fighting at Roanoke Island on February 8, 1862, he hurt his leg. On March 7 he was able to embark with his command. At the Battle of New Bern, North Carolina, on March 14, 1862, he received a gunshot wound in the hip but continued on the field. The wound was variously described as slight, severe, and a flesh wound. He was in the hospital and on leave until May 30. Potter was promoted to colonel in September after Second Bull Run. Slightly wounded twice in the Battle of Antietam on September 17, 1862, he again did not leave the field. In March 1863 he suffered with chronic diarrhea. His promotion to brigadier general of volunteers ranked from the same month. After Fredericksburg he was a division commander at Vicksburg and Knoxville and in the Virginia campaigns of 1864–65. During the attack before Fort Sedgwick, Virginia, on April 2, 1865, Potter was severely wounded and taken to a nearby house. A musket ball had transversed the pelvic cavity from a point above and slightly to the right of the symphysis pubis and went to the outer side of the left buttock. It was speculated that the axis of the wound indicated that the missile had passed near the upper curve of the great sciatic notch. Urine escaped from the shot orifices, suggesting that the bladder had been injured, but there was no evidence of a fractured pelvis. The field surgeon regarded the case as desperate. However, the flow of urine from the openings soon ceased, and in the course of a few weeks the wound appeared to heal. In September 1865 he was made major general. He was mustered out of the service in January 1866 and worked for a railroad until 1869, when he went abroad. Potter returned to the United States in 1873. An examination in January 1874 did not reveal any dysfunction of his bladder or any inconvenience consequent to the injury he had received.[1] Died February 19, 1887, at Newport, Rhode Island, and was buried in Woodlawn Cemetery, New York City.

DEATH CERTIFICATE: Cause of death, softening of the brain.

1. CSR; *OR*, vol. 9:222, 229; vol. 46, pt. 1:573, 1017, 1020, pt. 3:484, 486, 732; U.S. Army, CWS, roll 6, vol. 10, report 57, pp. 577–89; RAGO, entry 623, "File D"; *MSHW*, vol. 2, pt. 2:264, 424.

BENJAMIN FRANKLIN POTTS • *Born on January 29, 1836*, in Carroll County, Ohio. A member of the Ohio bar, Potts entered Federal service as a captain of the 32nd Ohio in August 1861 and served in West Virginia and in the Shenandoah. During the winter of 1861–62 he had a severe attack of measles, and it took him a long time to recover. He was made colonel of his regiment in December 1862. He was at Vicksburg, in the Atlanta campaign, and in the Carolinas. In August 1863 he had the onset of fever and ague, and in October he was in Carrollton, Ohio, still sick. In January 1865 he was made a brigadier general. After the war he returned to his law practice in Ohio and suffered with rheumatism.[1] Died June 17, 1887, near Helena, Montana, and was buried there.

DEATH CERTIFICATE: Died from an aneurysm of the aorta.

1. CSR; RVA, Pension WC 266,060.

WILLIAM HENRY POWELL • *Born May 10, 1825*, at Pontypool, South Wales. A well-known engineer, he was employed at various ironworks prior to the Civil War. Powell was mustered into Federal service as a company commander of the 2nd [West] Virginia Cavalry in November 1861. During March and April 1863 he was absent due to typhoid fever. At Wytheville, Virginia, on July 18, 1863, he was wounded in the back by a revolver fired by one of the Union troops. The ball entered the right side of the chest near the posterior superior angle of the right scapula and passed downward. There was no exit wound. Left on the field because it was thought he was mortally wounded, he was captured and almost hanged by the Rebel crowd. Powell was cared for in a private home until he was removed to Richmond. He was charged with having waged war contrary to the usages of war. After spending a few days in the general hospital, he was put in a coal-hole dungeon for thirty-seven days without a bed or bedding, and received only bread and water. Following his release from the dungeon, he was kept at Libby Prison until January 1864, when he was paroled. He rejoined his command in March and was made brigadier general of volunteers in October 1864. After the war he returned to his prior occupation in Ironton, Ohio, but later lived in a number of other locales. In 1867, while superintending the construction of a nail factory in Mason County, West Virginia, he was injured. In 1877 he had constant and increasing pain in his arm, occasional cough, and at times dyspnea.[1] Died at his residence on December 26, 1904, at Belleville, Illinois, and was buried in Graceland Cemetery, Chicago.

DEATH CERTIFICATE: Immediate cause, la grippe; contributory, chronic bronchitis.

1. CSR; OR, vol. 27, pt. 2:941–42, 944, 949, 1003, 1005; U.S. Army, roll 8, vol. 14, report 1, pp. 3–11; RVA, Pension C 63,245; CV 18:31; Newton Bateman, Paul Selby, A. S. Wilderman, and A. A. Wilderman, eds., Historical Encyclopedia of Illinois and History of St. Clair County 2:1094; A. W. Campbell, An Interesting Talk with General W. H. Powell, 5–6.

CALVIN EDWARD PRATT • Born January 23, 1828, in Shrewsbury, Massachusetts. A lawyer before the Civil War, he and a friend recruited and organized the 31st New York Infantry at their own expense. He was mustered in as the unit's colonel in August 1861. On June 27, 1862, he was wounded in the face during the Battle of Gaines' Mill. The ball pierced his left cheekbone about one inch below the eye, passed through the face and nose, and lodged deep in the bone of the right antrum. It had pierced the back part of the nostril near the palate. The root of the first right bicuspid tooth was fractured, and the ball was so deep in the bone that it could neither be seen nor felt. He was hospitalized for two days in a temporary hospital at Savage Station, Virginia, and then was sent to New York. In August the tissue of the right cheek was indurated and the skin red. Pressure over the area produced a ready flow of tears. Any physical jarring produced facial neuralgia. At the end of fifty days, he had sufficiently recovered from his wound to return to duty. He rejoined his regiment in August 1862, following the Second Battle of Bull Run. He still had bad neuralgia of his face, and any jarring produced severe pain. In September he was honorably discharged because of his face wound. He reentered the service the same month and was appointed brigadier general of volunteers. Pratt led a division at Fredericksburg but resigned again in April 1863 because of the suffering from his wound. The ball remained in place for the rest of Pratt's life, and he continued to suffer from its effects. Died on his farm on August 3, 1896, at Rochester, Massachusetts, and was buried in that town. According to the physician's certificate, he died of apoplexy.[1]

1. CSR; *OR*, vol. 11, pt. 2:434, 457; RVA, Pension WC 665,941; U.S. Army, CWS, roll 4, vol. 7, report 54, pp. 887–905.

BENJAMIN MAYBERRY PRENTISS • *Born on November 23, 1819,* in Belleville, Virginia. Served in the Mexican War. Prentiss was commissioned colonel of the 10th Illinois Infantry in April 1861, and his promotion to brigadier general of volunteers ranked from the next month. He distinguished himself at Shiloh, and his promotion to major general ranked from November 1862. He resigned in October 1863. He resumed his law practice and, after moving to Bethany, Missouri, he was made postmaster. When Prentiss was eighty-one years old his mind was gone, and he depended on his son for support.[1] Died at Bethany, Missouri, on February 8, 1901, and was buried in Miriam Cemetery, Bethany.

1. LR, CB, roll 49, P533, 1863.

HENRY PRINCE • *Born June 19, 1811,* in Eastport, Maine. Graduated from the USMA in 1835. At West Point he was treated for a toothache ten times, cold and influenza three times each, colica twice, and cholera, strain, cough, constipatio, and diarrhea once each. He was wounded at Camp Izard, Florida, on February 29, 1836. At Molino del Rey on September 8, 1847, Prince was so severely wounded that he was disabled for the next three years. After a period on frontier duty, he spent one year on leave of absence because of a wound. In April 1862 he was made a brigadier general of volunteers. He was captured at Cedar Mountain on August 9, 1862, and exchanged in December. On April 7, 1863, while on shipboard, he was ill and constantly retching due to a bilious sickness. The next day he awoke with a blinding headache and sickness and was unable to leave his bed or attend to his duties. He served in the Mine Run campaign and remained in the army after the war. By 1877 he held the rank of lieutenant colonel. In November 1879 it was reported that the irritable and morbid condition of his mind was such that he could not properly discharge his duties, and thus he should be retired. In December Prince sent letters from two doctors, who reported that his mind was not "irritable or morbid." Finally he was retired December 31, 1879. Prince was bathing under the attention of a physician in September 1889 at Baden, Germany, when the wound he had received at Molino del Ray reopened. Its condition became worse, so in October he went to Switzerland to undergo a surgical procedure. On August 19, 1892, he committed suicide at Morley's Hotel, London, England, by shooting himself in the head with a revolver. The bullet wound was in the right parietal bone above the temple and there was no exit wound. At autopsy the bullet was inside the base of the brain, having lacerated the brain and fracturing the skull. He had become despondent upon discovering he had Bright's disease and being told it would go to his brain and make him an imbecile. For the three months prior to his death he did everything to set his office straight, even to the point of having deposited money to pay for his funeral expenses.[1] He was buried in Hillside Cemetery, Eastport, Maine.

1. *OR*, vol. 18:224, 589; U.S. Army, CWS, roll 1, vol. 1, report 26, pp. 345–69; WPCHR, vols. 601, 602, 603; LR, ACP, 4330, 1892, fiche: 000165; Heitman, *Historical Register and Dictionary* 2:34.

Q

ISSAC FERDINAND QUINBY • *Born on January 29, 1821,* near Morristown, New Jersey. Graduated from the USMA in 1843. As a cadet he was treated for a headache twice and one time each for a boil on his forehead, a boil on his left arm, bile, sprain, and a sore throat. In 1852 he resigned from the military after teaching at the U.S. Military Academy and serving on the frontier. At the outbreak of the Civil War he was teaching at the University of Rochester. He served a short period in a three-month unit, which he led at First Bull Run. In March 1862 he accepted a commission as brigadier general of volunteers. In April 1863, when he developed an illness resembling Asiatic cholera, he went to Helena, Arkansas, and the command was given to another. He returned on May 16 and the next day resumed command of his division. He had a relapse, and in early June he left on sick leave. Quinby served in the Vicksburg campaign but resigned in December 1863 because of poor health. He returned to the academic life. Over the years he continued to have chronic diarrhea, rheumatism, weakness, and difficulty with his mental powers. During the winter of 1883 he was confined to his house most of the time because of rheumatic and bowel troubles. On the basis of an apparently enlarged spleen and his continued diarrhea, a diagnosis of chronic malarial poisoning was made in 1885. The two physicians who took care of him from 1888 until his death described a number of conditions, including athroma of the arteries, chronic catarrhal inflammation of the stomach and bowels, angina pectoris, pleural effusion, dementia, chronic diarrhea, and abdominal dropsy. Although various treatments were used, one physician felt that antimalarial medications produced the best result. Over the next couple of years he had episodes of severe dyspnea. Unable to lie down at times, he would sit gasping for breath. He raised large amounts of thick sputum that were frequently intermixed with blood. In December 1890 he was confined to bed with a mild attack of inflammatory rheumatism of the right arm. He was admitted to an asylum in July 1891 because the physician stated that he was incompetent by reasons of insanity.[1] Died September 18, 1891, in Rochester, New York, and was buried in Mount Hope Cemetery.

DEATH CERTIFICATE: Cause of death, chief cause, angina pectoris, old-age-pleurtic effusion; contributing, abdominal dropsy and general anasarca.

1. *OR*, vol. 24, pt. 1:75, 78, 85, 92, 259, pt. 2:59–60, pt. 3:259, 320; WPCHR, vol. 604; U.S. Army, CWS, roll 4, vol. 6, report 17, pp. 423–24; RVA, Pension, C 324,367.

R

GEORGE DOUGLAS RAMSAY • *Born February 21, 1802,* in Dumfries, Virginia. Graduated from the USMA in 1820. Served in the Mexican War. A captain for most of his career in the ordnance department, he was promoted to major in April 1861. In September 1864 he was made a brigadier general and chief of ordnance. On September 12, 1864, he was "retired for age." He continued to serve by special appointment until 1870. Died in Washington, D.C., on May 23, 1882, and was buried in Oak Hill Cemetery, Georgetown.

DEATH CERTIFICATE: Cause of death, primary, senile exhaustion.

THOMAS EDWARD GREENFIELD RANSOM • *Born November 29, 1834,* in Norwich, Vermont. Ransom was a civil engineer and was dealing in real estate when he recruited the 11th Illinois. The unit was mustered into Federal service for three years in July 1861. On the night of August 19, 1861, while he accompanied an expedition from Bird's Point to Charleston, Missouri, he was severely wounded in the shoulder. He received a leave of absence on August 25 but rejoined his regiment after only seven days. During the attack on Fort Donelson on February 15, 1862, he was wounded in the shoulder by a minié ball. After having his wound dressed he resumed command. At Shiloh on April 6, 1862, he was slightly wounded in the head. His wound was dressed and he returned to the field. However, during one of the subsequent attacks, his horse was killed, and the wound rendered him unfit to walk or command. He was put in the hospital at Savannah, Tennessee, from April 7–14 and then rejoined his regiment. He was on detached service and in post command until September 18, when he received a forty-day leave of absence on surgeon's certificate for disability. He reported to U. S. Grant in October. After passing through grades, he was promoted brigadier general of volunteers to rank from November 1862. He commanded a brigade at Vicksburg. In August 1863 he was assigned to the command of the post and town of Natchez, Mississippi. On April 8, 1864, at the Battle of Mansfield, he was severely wounded near the knee. He was taken from the field and went to New Orleans. He had a leave of absence from April 23 to June 11 in New York City and returned to duty in August at Atlanta, where he commanded a division and then a corps. Although quite sick, he made a reconnaissance on October 1. He was constantly in the saddle and managed his command on October 4, although suffering from dysentery. His symptoms continued and he followed the command in an ambulance. He was lying in a farmhouse on October 20, close to the point of death. On October 28, a surgeon made a diagnosis of typhoid. The next day his dysentery became worse; he was dry and feverish, his forehead cold and clammy, and the pupils of his eyes dilated. Gen. William T. Sherman ordered him to be carried to Rome, Georgia, the nearest point on a railroad. He was carried back on a litter by four men. When he grew weaker he was placed on an improvised bunk in a roadside cabin near Rome, where he died on October 29, 1864.[1] He was buried in Rosehill Cemetery, Chicago.

1. CSR; OR, vol. 3:136; vol. 7:178, 197, 199; vol. 10, pt. 1:116–17, 133, 136–37; vol. 24, pt. 3:573; vol. 34, pt. 1:244, 259, 267, pt. 3:98, 127, 580; vol. 39, pt. 3:99, 476, 493, 580; vol. 53:51; U.S. Army, CWS, roll 3, vol. 4, report 2, pp. 9–33; Hirshson, *Grenville M. Dodge*, 108; Howard, *Autobiography*, 2:66–67; *MOLLUS* 20:115–16.

GREEN BERRY RAUM • *Born December 3, 1829*, at Golconda, Illinois. He joined the 56th Illinois Infantry at the start of the Civil War and was successively the unit's major, lieutenant colonel, and colonel. He was at Corinth and Vicksburg. On November 25, 1863, at Missionary Ridge, he received a gunshot wound in the left thigh close to the bone. After being treated in a field hospital near Chattanooga, he was taken north to his home in Illinois. He returned to duty in February 1864 for the Atlanta campaign and the March to the Sea. For the remainder of his service his leg was weak, becoming painful and stiff when he rode all day. His promotion as brigadier general of volunteers ranked from February 1865. After resigning in May 1865, he practiced the law and was engaged in politics. His family physician examined him in March 1899 and found the following: On the outer and posterior surface of the left thigh, seven inches above the articulation of the femur at the knee, there was an irregular umbilicated scar about one and a quarter inches in diameter. At the median line of the inner surface of the same thigh, five inches above the articulation, there was a somewhat more irregular and umbilicated scar, one and a third inches in diameter. The first scar was evidently the entrance and the second the exit of the ball. The physician stated that the ball must have involved the great sciatic nerve with laceration of the nerves and muscles to explain the weakness, pain, and numbness in the leg below the knee, which Raum experienced most of the time.[1] Died December 18, 1909, in Chicago and was buried in Arlington National Cemetery.

DEATH CERTIFICATE: Cause of death, uremia, carcinoma of the bowel. Duration of disease, twenty-one days.

1. CSR; OR, vol. 31, pt. 2:88, 648, 650; vol. 46, pt. 3:278; vol. 47, pt. 2:62; RVA, Pension WC 696,112.

JOHN AARON RAWLINS • *Born on February 13, 1831,* at Galena, Illinois. Before the war he was a lawyer in Galena and friend of U. S. Grant. In August 1861 he became a captain and assistant adjutant general on Grant's staff. By August 1863 he was brigadier general of volunteers. After becoming wet in November 1863, he contracted bronchitis, which his physician later stated was the start of his tuberculosis. Others have said Rawlins had the disease before he entered the service. His health deteriorated, and he was given a leave of absence on August 1, 1864. Although he returned on September 29, he still had not recovered and was bothered by a cough. His promotion as brigadier general, chief of staff, U.S. Army, ranked from March 1865. His first wife died with tuberculosis, and he was diagnosed as having the disease in 1865. After the war, the recommended travel on the high plains over the proposed route of the Union Pacific Railroad failed to improve his health. Convalescing from his illness during the summer of 1867, along with Grenville M. Dodge, he explored southeastern Idaho Territory. He resigned as chief of staff to the general of the army in March 1869 to take the position of secretary of war. He died in Washington, D.C., on September 6, 1869, and was buried in Arlington National Cemetery. The attending physician who had treated him for phthisis pulmonalis stated that the cause of his death was hemorrhage from the lungs.[1]

1. RVA, Pension WC 176,018; Porter, *Campaigning with Grant,* 273, 314; Hirshson, *Grenville M. Dodge,* 3; *MOLLUS* 2:388.

HUGH THOMPSON REID • *Born October 18, 1811,* in Union County, Indiana. A lawyer and president of the Des Moines Valley Railroad, he entered Federal service as colonel of the 15th Iowa in February 1862. At Shiloh on April 6, 1862, a musket ball passed through the right trapezius muscle of his neck and knocked him from his horse. He was temporarily paralyzed but recovered in a short time, remounted his horse, and continued in command throughout the fight. He was not admitted to a hospital but was treated for about three months in his quarters and returned to duty in August. He contracted diarrhea in late September and was unable to command on October 3. The next day he rose from his sick bed and, unable to ride his horse, he accompanied his regiment, traveling in an ambulance. His promotion to brigadier general of volunteers ranked from March 1863. In October he had arrived at Cairo, Illinois, and was ordered to report by letter. Early in the next year he was ordered to assume command of the District of Cairo. He resigned April 1864 because of personal business and impaired mobility of his right shoulder and arm. Reid returned to civilian life and joined the Des Moines Valley Railroad Company. While in New York in 1869 he had a stroke. After returning home he had a second stroke, which for a time rendered him unconscious. Reid had difficulty walking, and his powers of coordination suffered, particularly when bringing his ideas into focus. He had headaches with "want of equalization in the circulatory forces of pedal capil-laries." When his simplest desires were not followed, he became irascible. Other strokes followed at intervals until they resulted in a solid right hemiplegia. In January 1870, his general health was poor, and he had occasional pain in his right foot associated with formication (sensation of small insects crawling over the skin), numbness, and muscular atrophy. His physician made a diagnosis of paresis of the right leg and malarial toxemia and visited him almost every day. He treated him with an interrupted electric current for the stimulation of the muscles and nerves, along with quinine and iron plus quinine tonics. In April 1871 Reid was treated again for malarial fever. The physician visited him on August 15, 1874, because of paroxysmal dyspnea. Examination of his lungs and heart was not remarkable. His urine contained abundant albumin, and on mi-croscopic examination it revealed tube casts and renal epithelial debris. On this basis, the physician made a diagnosis of chronic Bright's disease and visited him daily until he died. Two physicians, who both related his problem to the shock he had suffered when shot in the neck, proposed interesting speculations about his renal disease and death. The physician who had treated him and saw him when he died regarded the state of his brain as one of close similarity to the edema of the lungs, which created the dyspnea. A characteristic of edema is to alter its position in chronic albuminuria and in its turn give birth to anuria by compression. Coma supervened forty hours before his death due to brain edema, not because of phenomena of a uremic nature. The albuminuric state could be fairly attributed to shock to the cervical part of the medulla spinalis together with paludal (malaria) poison imbibed in the field, thus hindering proper sanguification (production of blood) in the liver. Another physician who, along with his father, had also treated Reid speculated that paralysis of the sphincter of the urinary bladder resulted in the retention of urine that required catherization. Later this produced morbus Bright's disease due to the draining back of urine upon the kidneys from retention. The physician had treated him frequently with the application of Moxa (a tuft of soft, combustible substance burned upon the skin) to the spine, and by alternating current from a battery. Regardless of all the treatment, Reid died August 21, 1874, at Des Moines, Iowa,[1] and was buried there in Oakland Cemetery.

1. CSR; OR, vol. 10, pt. 1:289; vol. 17, pt. 1:338, 340, 360; vol. 32, pt. 2:217; RVA, Pension WC 189,700.

JAMES WILLIAM REILLY • Born May 20, 1828, in Akron, Ohio. He was a lawyer and member of the state legislature when he was appointed colonel of the 104th Ohio in August 1862. During July and August 1863 he was present sick. He was promoted brigadier general of volunteers in July 1864. He served in the Atlanta campaign, the Battle of Franklin, and in the Carolinas. Needing time to recuperate, he was granted a short leave in December, and his resignation was accepted in April 1865.[1] He returned to his law practice after the war. Died November 6, 1905, at Wellsville, Ohio, and was buried there in St. Elizabeth's Cemetery.

1. CSR; Cox, *Military Reminiscences* 2:355.

JESSE LEE RENO • *Born June 20, 1823*, in Wheeling, [West] Virginia. Graduated from the USMA in 1846. He was wounded at Chapultepec on September 13, 1847. An ordnance officer, he taught at West Point, commanded arsenals, and served on ordnance boards before the Civil War. He surrendered the Mount Vernon, Alabama, arsenal to state forces in January 1861. In November he was commissioned brigadier general of volunteers. He commanded a brigade in the North Carolina expedition and a corps at Second Bull Run and before Antietam. He was killed by a rifle ball fired at long range on September 14, 1862, during the Battle of South Mountain.[1] His remains were first placed in a vault in Trinity Church, Boston, and then were moved to Oak Hill Cemetery, Georgetown, D.C.

1. *OR*, vol. 19, pt. 1:27, 34, 50, 177, 186, 210, 417, 423, 429, 460, 1020; vol. 25, pt. 2:140, 186; Walter Clark, ed., *Histories of the Several Regiments and Battalions from North Carolina* 2:221; Heitman, *Historical Register and Dictionary* 2:34.

JOSEPH WARREN REVERE • *Born on May 17, 1812*, in Boston. He was in the U.S. Navy for twenty-two years and resigned in 1850. He served in the Florida wars and was in California during the Mexican War. In 1850 he became an officer in the Mexican army and was wounded in May 1852. In September 1861 he entered Federal service as colonel of the 7th New Jersey Infantry. Revere was absent sick in July 1862. He was severely wounded twice at the Second Battle of Bull Run, August 30. One was a contusion from a shell and the other was by a minié ball in the right groin. He went on sick leave, first to Washington, D.C., and then to his home, and finally returned to his regiment in six weeks. He was commissioned brigadier general in October. For his actions at Chancellorsville, he was court-martialed and dismissed from the service. The president allowed him to resign, effective August 1863. After the war, he traveled abroad and wrote, although his health was poor. He continued to have problems from his old wounds, and in September 1879 he applied for a truss because of a scrotal hernia.[1] Died April 20, 1880, in a hotel in Hoboken, New Jersey, and was buried in Morristown, New Jersey.

DEATH CERTIFICATE: Cause of death, heart disease. Primary disease, rheumatism. Secondary disease, neuralgia and pericarditis.

1. CSR; U.S. Army, CWS, roll 4, vol. 6, report 18, pp. 425–28; RVA, Pension C 43,077.

JOHN FULTON REYNOLDS • *Born on September 20, 1820,* in Lancaster, Pennsylvania. He graduated from the USMA in 1841. Served in the Florida and Mexican wars. Starting in 1834 Reynolds had a preoccupation with his health; although never sick himself, he was constantly preaching about health to others. In July 1842, just a little over two weeks after arriving at St. Augustine, Florida, he developed bilious fever. He had to remain in bed for a month and was taken care of by Lt. Braxton Bragg. He did not fully recover his health until the next year. While in Mexico in April 1847 he had a chill but nevertheless performed his duty. During August and September 1853, in New Orleans, he had yellow fever but recovered by November. After returning to Fort Monroe, Virginia, from a trip to California and Oregon in December 1856, he had severe chills and fever. It was speculated that he had contracted malaria while on the return trip to the East, and he did not fully recover until the following May. When the war started he was commandant of cadets at West Point and was made lieutenant colonel of the 14th U.S. Infantry in May 1861. He was promoted brigadier general of volunteers to rank from August 1861 and major general in November 1862. He was captured on June 28, 1862, on the Peninsula and exchanged August 8. He was a corps commander at Fredericksburg and Chancellorsville. He was killed at Gettysburg on July 1, 1863, by a sharpshooter. He fell face down from his horse. There was no obvious bleeding, and at first no wound was seen. When they turned him on his back he gasped once and then smiled. He never spoke a word and must have been dead within a minute or two after he was hit. Taken under his arms, he was carried back out of the immediate range of fire. Later, when he was examined, a hole was found where a rifle ball had struck him behind the right ear and passed through his head.[1] Within three days he was buried in Lancaster, Pennsylvania.

1. *OR*, vol. 27, pt. 1:71, 114–15, 229, 245, 696; vol. 29, pt. 2:154; Steiner, *Medical-Military Portraits*, 237–54; Edward J. Nichols, *Toward Gettysburg: A Biography of General John F. Reynolds*, 6, 15, 39, 55, 72, 205–6, 253–54.

JOSEPH JONES REYNOLDS • *Born January 4, 1822,* in Flemingsburg, Kentucky. He graduated from the USMA in 1843. Served in the Mexican War. During the march from Corpus Christi to Fort Brown on the Rio Grande in March 1846 he developed a right direct inguinal hernia and had to wear a strong truss. After serving on the frontier, he resigned his commission in 1857. Until the start of the Civil War, he taught and engaged in business. Reynolds served in the Indiana militia and was made a brigadier general of volunteers to rank from May 1861. His left testicle was injured while he was in the field in West Virginia during the fall and winter of 1861–62. In March 1862 he had an abscess of the left testicle and epididymis, which nearly destroyed both organs. He led a division at Chickamauga, was a staff officer at Chattanooga, and served as a corps commander in the Mobile campaign. He commanded the Department of Arkansas from November 1864 until April 1866. In July 1866 he was made colonel of the 26th Infantry. An injury to his right testicle occurred in Texas sometime during the fall and winter of 1871–72. He continued to wear a truss, and in 1872 chronic ulcerations of his right scrotum occurred. After the summer of 1873 the intestine no longer descended into the hernia. On a physical examination in July 1876, the left testicle and epididymis were absent. In October he developed partial paralysis of his left arm, and he received leave the next month because of his disability. An examination in February 1877 revealed atrophy of his right testicle and chronic enlargement of the epididymis. No direct or indirect hernia could be detected. A suspensory bandage to retain the testicle was necessary to decrease pain in the organ. Although the paralysis of his left arm was less, it was ruled that he was incapacitated and in March was ordered to return home and to report monthly. He obtained a leave and went to Europe for over a year to improve his health. Died February 25, 1899, in Washington, D.C., and was buried in Arlington National Cemetery. According to the adjutant general's office, the cause of his death was cerebritis.[1]

1. RVA, Pension WC 495,144; LR, ACP, 1295, 1871, fiche: 000168.

AMERICUS VESPUCIUS RICE • *Born on November 18, 1835,* in Perryville, Ohio. Rice entered Federal service as a captain of the 21st Ohio, a three-month regiment. Following expiration of the unit's service, he was remustered in as captain of the 57th Ohio. He was at Shiloh, Chickasaw Bayou, and Arkansas Post. At Vicksburg on May 22, 1863, he was wounded by a sharpshooter. He was in a half-sitting position at the time he was struck. The ball entered from the front below the knee and passed through his leg. It entered a second time above the knee, ranged upwards, and lodged near his abdomen. He was sent to Memphis, then went home on sick leave and did not return to duty until February 1864. At Kennesaw Mountain on June 27, 1864, Rice received three gunshot wounds almost simultaneously. The right femur was fractured, and the knee joint was penetrated. The skin of the forehead was lacerated but there was no fracture of the skull. The remaining bullet carried away pieces of bone from near the left ankle. Because of the fracture, he underwent a primary circular amputation in the lower third of the femur twelve hours after receiving the injury. He was appointed brigadier general of volunteers in May 1865 and rejoined the army the next month.[1] Rice returned to civilian life and engaged in business and politics. Died at his residence on April 4, 1904, at Washington, D.C., and was buried in Arlington National Cemetery.

DEATH CERTIFICATE: Cause of death, cancer of kidney and exhaustion. Eighteen months' duration.

1. CSR; *OR,* vol. 24, pt. 2:270, 281; vol. 38, pt. 3:178, 188, 194, 216; RVA, Pension WC 572,902; *MSHW,* vol. 2, pt. 3:253; RAGO, entry 623, "File D."

ELLIOTT WARREN RICE • *Born on November 16, 1835,* in Allegheny City, Pennsylvania. Rice was practicing law in Iowa at the start of the Civil War and joined Company C, 7th Iowa, as a private. At the battle of Belmont, Missouri, on November 7, 1861, he was badly wounded in the leg and received a leave of absence. He was still on crutches at Fort Donelson in February 1862 but fought at Shiloh. By April 1862 he was a colonel. Supposedly he was wounded seven times during the war and carried the bullet he received at Belmont the rest of his life. He was promoted brigadier general of volunteers in June 1864.[1] He was a brigade and division commander during the Atlanta campaign, the March to the Sea, and in the Carolinas. After being mustered out of the service he returned to the practice of law. Because of poor health in 1885, he moved to the home of a sister in Sioux City, Iowa, where he died June 21, 1887. He was buried there in Floyd Cemetery.

DEATH CERTIFICATE: Cause of death, consumption of two years' duration.

1. CSR; *OR,* vol. 3:271–72, 298.

JAMES CLAY RICE • *Born December 27, 1829,* in Worthington, Massachusetts. He left his law practice and was made a lieutenant of the 39th New York in May 1861. After passing through grades, he was appointed colonel of the 44th New York in July 1862. In August he was seriously ill with typhoid and was sent home on September 4. Rice returned in late 1862, and he was made a brigadier general of volunteers in August 1863. He had served at Second Bull Run, Chancellorsville, and Gettysburg. On May 10, 1864, at Spotsylvania, he was wounded in the thigh, and his femur was fractured. Thinking the advancing line of his men could hear his voice, he had mounted the earthworks. A large artery was severed and, since it was some time before a tourniquet could be applied, he was in shock from blood loss. Under the influence of a general anesthetic he had a primary amputation in the upper third of the femur. When he regained consciousness, he asked if he was dying and was told that he was. He died that day and was buried in Rural Cemetery, Albany, New York.[1]

1. CSR; *OR,* vol. 12, pt. 2:474; vol. 36, pt. 1:191, 541, 611, 625; U.S. Army, CWS, roll 1, vol. 1, report 37, pp. 777–83; *MSHW,* vol. 2, pt 3:222; Nash, *Forty-Fourth New York,* 341.

SAMUEL ALLEN RICE • *Born January 27, 1828,* in Cattaraugus County, New York. He practiced the law and held county and state offices in Iowa prior to the Civil War. Rice was made colonel of the 33rd Iowa, which entered Federal service in October 1862. He was promoted to brigadier general of volunteers in August 1863. On April 4, 1864, at Elkin's Ferry, Arkansas, on the Little Missouri River he received a slight scalp wound from a canister shot. At Jenkins' Ferry on the Saline River, April 30, 1864, he was wounded in the right ankle. The ball entered the external malleolus, carried with it a portion of his spur and strap, and passed through the ankle joint. The injury was treated conservatively. He was in Little Rock on May 8 and then went home to Oskaloosa, Iowa, on sick leave. Rice had a number of episodes of erysipelas during May. On the first of June, he had pyaemia, and his wound was discharging unhealthy pus. He had another attack of erysipelas of the wound, and several pieces of bone were removed on June 15. In spite of all remedies, he died on July 6, 1864, at Oskaloosa.[1] He was buried there in Forest Cemetery.

1. CSR; *OR*, vol. 34, pt. 1:671, 686, 690, 698, 706, pt. 3:77; vol. 41, pt. 2:71, 282, 284; *MSHW*, vol. 2, pt. 3:585.

ISRAEL BUSH RICHARDSON • *Born December 26, 1815,* in Fairfax, Vermont. He graduated from the USMA in 1841. As a cadet he was treated for a cold twice and colica, headache, and toothache once each. Served in the Florida and Mexican wars. Richardson resigned from the army in 1855 and took up farming in Michigan. In May 1861 he entered Federal service as colonel of the 2nd Michigan Infantry and was made brigadier general of volunteers in August. He was at First Bull Run and on the Peninsula. He was hospitalized for a short period in July 1862 with a diagnosis of debility and then had a sick leave. The last of August he resumed command of his division. One of the men of the Irish Brigade accidently kicked him and injured his ribs on September 13. The two of them took a pull from the man's flask and they went back to duty. On September 17, 1862, at Antietam, while talking to Capt. William M. Graham, he was mortally wounded by a ball from a spherical case. He was taken to Gen. George B. McClellan's headquarters, the Pry House. Dr. Jonathan Letterman and one of the surgeons of his division examined Richardson soon after he had been wounded. However, they became so busy that their subsequent visits were infrequent. His sister visited him in October and after a few days felt that although he was weak and depressed, he had improved some since her arrival. The surgeons agreed that his case was hopeless, although there was disagreement about the pleuropneumonia he had developed. Most felt it was unrelated to his wound, while others thought the projectile had entered his lung. It was implied that the pneumonia was more of a factor in determining his outcome than his wound. Although many of the surgeons stated that he should be told about his bad prognosis, his attending physician felt that telling him would kill him. He died on November 3, 1862.[1] His body was taken to Pontiac, Michigan, for burial.

1. CSR; *OR*, vol. 19, pt. 1:344; vol. 51, pt. 1:738; WPCHR, vol. 604; RAGO, entry 534; Fannie to Maria, Sunday, Oct. 1862, Israel B. Richardson Papers, *CWTI* Collection, USAMHI; Conyngham, *Irish Brigade*, 293.

JAMES BREWERTON RICKETTS • *Born on June 21, 1817,* in New York City. He graduated from the USMA in 1839. Ricketts was treated for a cold and a headache twice each while at West Point. Served in the Florida and Mexican wars. At First Bull Run on July 21, 1861, Captain Ricketts was severely wounded four times and taken prisoner. Details are lacking, but one severe wound was in the leg. Gen. P. G. T. Beauregard, who had known him in his old army days, sent him his own surgeon. He was taken to the Lewis house, and on July 28 he was moved to the depot at Manassas Junction for transportation to Richmond. His wife came to Richmond, partitioned off a portion of the prison, and put in a small cot. She made daily rounds and administered to her husband and the other prisoners. In January 1862, still disabled by his wounds, he was released from prison and exchanged the next month. His promotion as brigadier general of volunteers ranked from the day he was wounded. In April 1862 he tried to mount his horse for the first time; the next month he rejoined his troops. He served at Cedar Mountain, Second Bull Run, and Antietam. Still suffering from his wounds, he was relieved from command at his own request on October 19, 1862. In November he reported to Washington, D.C., and was detailed to court-martial duty. Gen. James Garfield, also a member of the board, noted that Ricketts's forehead carried a scar that looked like a saber wound. In March 1864 he was relieved from duty as a member of a military commission and was ordered to report for assignment to duty. At the Battle of Cedar Creek on October 19, 1864, he was severely wounded and sent to Washington, D.C., for treatment. The ball had penetrated about two inches below the right clavicle and transversed the pectorals major and minor muscles. It injured the median nerve, periosteum of the scapula near the neck, and the latissimus dorsi muscle near its insertion. Although he was deprived of the use of his right arm, he resumed command in April 1865. In November 1866 he was still unable to draw his saber or mount a horse unassisted. There were paroxysms of pain in his shoulder and arm, with edema of the hand and fingers. Ricketts retired from active service in January 1867 because of disability from wounds; however, he continued on court-martial duty until 1869. Died at his residence on December 22, 1887, in Washington, D.C., and was buried in Arlington National Cemetery. The attending surgeon reported that the immediate cause of his death was exhaustion from repeated hemorrhage. Primary cause, abscess and gangrene of the right lung. It was suggested that the lung lesion was related to his wound received at Cedar Creek.[1]

1. CSR; *OR,* vol. 2:347, 403, 410, 567; vol. 12, pt. 3:117; vol. 19, pt. 2:533; vol. 33, 732; vol. 43, pt. 1:32, 55, 131, 159; vol. 46, pt. 3:747; *OR Suppl.,* vol. 1, pt. 1:161–62; WPCHR, vol. 604; U.S. Army, CWS, roll 6, vol. 10, report 48, pp. 491–94; RVA, Pension WC 237,825; LR,ACP, 4346, 1887, fiche: 000169; *Battles and Leaders* 1:213; Garfield, *Wild Life of the Army,* 187–88.

JAMES WOLFE RIPLEY • *Born on December 10, 1794,* in Windham County, Connecticut. Although in the USMA class of 1814, he graduated a year early because of the War of 1812. Served in the Florida and Mexican wars. His many years of military service prior to the Civil War were spent as an artillery officer and commander of the Springfield Armory. In April 1861 he became director of the ordnance department, and in August he was commissioned brigadier general in the Regular Army. Replaced as director in September 1863, he then served as inspector of armaments of the forts on the New England coast until 1869. His physician in Hartford, Connecticut, had detected in 1864 what he diagnosed as evidence of grave disease of the brain. The symptoms indicated to him the primary stages of general paralysis. They were, in the surgeon's opinion, "the evident and usual results of over tasking the brain. The wear and tear of the nervous system which arises from specific mental labor and from that fret and worry so naturally consequent on it."[1] Died at Hartford, Connecticut, on March 15, 1870, and was buried in Springfield, Massachusetts.

DEATH CERTIFICATE: Cause of death, debility.

1. RVA, Pension WC 157,338.

BENJAMIN STONE ROBERTS • *Born on November 18, 1810,* in Manchester, Vermont. He graduated from the USMA in 1835. At the military academy he was treated for diarrhea four times, headache three times, a wound, sprain, and cold two times each, and for influenza, cholera, syphilis, bruise, lameness, eruption, sore foot, and vomiting once each. Four years after graduation from the academy he resigned and became a civil engineer for a railroad. He reentered the army as a first lieutenant at the start of the Mexican War and served with distinction. Over the years he had the following sick leaves: October 1850 to February 1851, May to December 1851, July 1852 to June 1853, July 1854 to August 1855, and March 1856 to July 1857. Although surgeon's certificates for these absences are not available, it would appear from later records that they were due to chronic laryngitis. From the last of 1857 through the first of 1860 he was treated for chronic inflammation and ulceration of the larynx. Some of the treatment occurred while he was in Europe. In May 1861 Roberts was promoted to the rank of major and served at the engagement of Valverde. His promotion to brigadier general of volunteers ranked from July 1862. At Cedar Mountain on August 9, 1862, his left arm and breast were badly contused. In July 1864 he had a sunstroke, which disabled him for three months. During that summer he also had excessive salivation because of medications given to remove calomel from his system. The salivation, along with the hot damp weather, aggravated the disease of his larynx and ears.[1] Following the war, he was made lieutenant colonel in 1866 and retired from the army in 1870. Died at his residence in Washington, D.C., on January 29, 1875, and was buried in Oak Hill Cemetery. He was later reinterred at Manchester, Vermont.

DEATH CERTIFICATE: Cause of death, primary, pneumonia; immediate, double pneumonia. Duration of last sickness, one week.

1. WPCHR, vols. 601, 602, 603; LR, CB, roll 210, R576, 1865.

JAMES SIDNEY ROBINSON • *Born on October 14, 1827,* near Mansfield, Ohio. He was editing a newspaper in Kenton, Ohio, when the Civil War started, and initially served in a three-month state militia unit. He was made major of the 82nd Ohio in December 1861 and by August 1862 had risen to colonel. He was in the Shenandoah, at Second Bull Run, and at Chancellorsville. On July 1, 1863, as his regiment fell back into Gettysburg, he was wounded. The ball entered his left breast between the second and third ribs on a line below the junction of the middle and outer third of the clavicle and three inches below. It exited through the center of the scapula about one and a half inches below the spine. Branches of the thoracic and cervical plexus of nerves were injured. He remained under treatment on the battlefield for about two weeks. The nerve injuries produced partial paralysis of his arm, and he was absent because of his wound until December. In March 1864, Robinson returned to his brigade for the Atlanta campaign. On July 24 he asked for leave on account of sickness and the effects of his wounds, and remained in Ohio through August. From September 5–27, he was absent sick. He was appointed brigadier general of volunteers in January 1865. After the war, he returned to the railroad business, politics, and farming. Robinson had marked atrophy of the anterior and posterior walls of the chest and paralysis of the left arm and hand, with severe atrophy and loss of use of the arm. He had some disturbances of the heart, dyspnea, and at times paroxysms of pain in his precordial area. There were also marked rales in the upper lobe of the left lung over and around the area of the wound. His heart was dilated. According to the surgeon, "there was destruction of many of the pulmonary branches of the pneumogastric nerve that supplied the lung. There was also a great amount of cicatrical lung tissue, the result of the wounded lung enclosing branches of the vagus and sympathetic nerves. These being enclosed in the hardened cicatrical tissues produced reflex nervous disturbances to the heart and also to his respiratory movements producing dyspnea and at time severe paroxysm of pain in the heart and precordial region something like angina. So severe were these attacks that life was almost lost. There was marked dullness in the upper lobe of the left lung over the wound and for some distance around the area due to pleural adhesions and scarified or contracted lung tissues, evidently obliterating many of the pulmonary blood vessels. These closed blood vessels acted as a dam to the pulmonary circulation and systolic action of the heart. The heart had more labor to perform and its secondary result was dilatation of the right cavity of the organ." For some months before his death he had anasarca. Examination of his urine proved normal on a number of occasions. He died suddenly on January 14, 1892, in Kenton, Ohio. Physician's affidavit: Immediate cause of death was heart disease or heart failure, the result of the wound received at the Battle of Gettysburg.[1]

1. CSR; *OR*, vol. 27, pt. 1:744; vol. 38, pt. 2:36, 92, 107; vol. 39, pt. 1:659; RVA, Pension WC 357,783.

JOHN CLEVELAND ROBINSON • *Born April 10, 1817,* in Binghamton, New York. He entered the USMA in 1835 but was dismissed. Served in the Florida and Mexican wars. In October 1839 he was commissioned into the army as a second lieutenant of the 5th Infantry. A captain at the start of the Civil War, Robinson was commissioned colonel of the 1st Michigan Infantry in September 1861. His promotion as brigadier general of volunteers ranked from April 1862. On August 27, 1862, at Broad Run, Virginia, he was struck by a piece of shell but not injured. During the Battle of Spotsylvania Court House on May 8, 1864, he was severely wounded in the left knee joint by a musket ball. He turned his horse to the rear and had to be assisted off of the field. Gen. John Gibbon reported seeing him lying on a litter along the side of the road with a broken leg. He was admitted to the division hospital and transferred to a general hospital on May 11. On May 15 he underwent an intermediary circular amputation in the lower third of the femur because of the fracture. Three months later he notified the war department that he was ready for light duty. In September 1864 he was assigned to the command of the Military District of Northern New York with headquarters at Albany. In October 1866 an examining board reported that Robinson could perform the duties of an officer in the Veteran Reserve Corps. He was placed on the retired list in May 1869 because of disabilities arising from his wounds. He was elected lieutenant governor of New York in 1872. By 1893 he was completely deaf in his right ear and totally blind.[1] Died February 18, 1897, in Binghamton, New York, and was buried in Spring Forest Cemetery. DEATH CERTIFICATE: Cause of death, chief cause, chronic Bright's disease; contributing, old age.

1. CSR; *OR*, vol. 12, pt. 2:423; vol. 36, pt. 1:64–65, 141, 191, 549, 594, 597; U.S. Army, CWS, roll 4, vol. 7, report 38, pp. 525–31; LR, ACP, 4583, 1881, fiche: 000178; *MSHW*, vol. 2, pt. 3:295; RAGO, entry 534; Gibbon, *Personal Recollections,* 217.

ISAAC PEACE RODMAN • *Born on August 18, 1822,* in South Kingstown, Rhode Island. A prominent businessman and politician in Rhode Island prior to the Civil War, he was made captain in the 2nd Rhode Island in June 1861. In October he was commissioned colonel of the 4th Rhode Island, and his promotion to brigadier general of volunteers ranked from April 1862. The first of the year, he contracted typhoid fever and went to Rhode Island to recover. He rejoined the army as a division commander in September. At Antietam on September 17, 1862, a ball passed through his lung. He was taken to a field hospital near

Sharpsburg where he died on September 30.[1] He was buried in a family cemetery at Peace Dale, Rhode Island.

1. OR, vol. 19, pt. 1:178, 197, 203, 420, 426; RVA, Pension Min. C 490,933.

WILLIAM STARKE ROSECRANS • *Born on September 6, 1819,* in Delaware County, Ohio. Graduated from USMA in 1842. At West Point, he was treated for catarrhus twice, and sore feet, headache, cold and swollen face once each. He was sick in his teens and almost died while on a journey to Vicksburg. During the Mexican War he served in Washington, D.C., and worked so hard that his health was impaired. He resigned from the military in 1854. A lamp exploded in 1859 while he was working in a laboratory in a coal-oil production plant. In spite of being severely burned, he walked the mile and a half to his home. He remained mainly on his back for eighteen months and had just recovered when the Civil War started. The resulting scars on his forehead remained clearly visible. His appointments as colonel of the 23rd Ohio Infantry and brigadier general in the Regular Army ranked from May 1861. He served in West Virginia and then was assigned to important commands in the West. On November 29, he had recovered enough from some nonspecified illness to attend to business. His appointment as major general of volunteers ranked from March 1862. Due to indisposition, he was detained at Strasburg on April 15. After successes at Iuka and Corinth he was named commander of the Army of the Cumberland. He was in camp and on duty but was sick on January 26, 1863.[1] Rosecrans was relieved of command on October 19, 1863, and resigned his Regular Army commission on March 1867. He died March 11, 1898, on his ranch in California and was buried first in Rosedale Cemetery, Los Angeles, then reinterred in Arlington National Cemetery.
DEATH CERTIFICATE: Cause of death, pneumonia.

1. OR, vol. 5, p. 669; vol. 51, pt. 1:574; WPCHR, vol. 604; Glenn Tucker, *Chickamauga: Bloody Battle in the West,* 33–36; Garfield, *Wild Life of the Army,* 226.

LEONARD FULTON ROSS • *Born on July 18, 1823,* at Lewistown, Illinois. During the Mexican War he was left sick at Matamoros on December 24, 1846, but was back on duty in a week. Ross was a lawyer, judge, county clerk, and politician prior to the Civil War. He was appointed colonel of the 17th Illinois to rank from May 1861 and brigadier general of volunteers in April 1862. On August 19, 1862, he was quite sick and requested a few days leave to visit friends in northern Alabama. He served in Mississippi and Arkansas. His July 1863 resignation was accepted in September.[1] Died January 17, 1901, in Lewiston, Illinois, and was buried in Oakhill Cemetery in that town.

1. OR, vol. 17, pt. 2:182; vol. 22, pt. 1:475; RVA, Pension C 995,660.

LOVELL HARRISON ROUSSEAU • *Born August 4, 1818,* near Stanford, Kentucky. Served in the Mexican War. A lawyer and politician in Indiana, he was mustered into Federal service as colonel of the 3rd Kentucky (Union) Infantry in September 1861. Rousseau was an insomniac and during the war would stay up all night talking. He was promoted to brigadier general and major general in October 1862. He served at Shiloh, Perryville, Stones River, and Tullahoma. He resigned from the army in 1865 to take a seat in Congress. A political radical, he left this position and was made a brigadier general in the Regular Army in March 1867. Died January 7, 1869, in New Orleans after a three-day illness and was buried in Arlington National Cemetery. The surgeon general reported that Rousseau died of mucous engorgement and congestion of the bowels producing inflammation with probable congestion of the lungs.[1]

1. RVA, Pension WC 126,625; LR, CB, roll 201, R201, 1867; Peskin, "James A. Garfield," 266–68.

THOMAS ALGEO ROWLEY • *Born October 5, 1808,* in Pittsburgh, Pennsylvania. He served in the Mexican War. A city contractor, politician, and court clerk prior to the Civil War, he was commissioned colonel of a three-month regiment in April 1861. The unit was reenlisted as the 102nd Pennsylvania. At Seven Pines on May 31, 1862, he was struck by a ball on the back of the head and was severely stunned. The flesh was lacerated and the left side of the occipital bone was fractured. A fragment of detached bone was removed from the wound during the first dressing and additional small pieces came away at subsequent dressings. He was never a patient in a hospital but had his wound treated in a field hospital. In November 1862 he was promoted brigadier general of volunteers. After being struck several times by spent shells and shell fragments at Gettysburg on July 3, 1863, he was absent until August. In September he was sick, and the following month the surgeon diagnosed his condition as remittent fever and general disability. In October he was assigned to duty at Portland, Maine. He was court-martialed in April 1864 for drunkenness on duty and unbecoming conduct. Reinstated, he finally resigned in December 1864. After the war, he returned to his business as a contractor and practiced the law. By 1878 the sight of his left eye was seriously impaired, and he suffered severe pain in his head. He could not lie on the left side of his head because it produced pain. In late 1883, he had a slight stroke with paralysis of his left side and was confined to bed for six weeks. The surgeon who examined him in March 1884 reported that there was a cicatrix one inch to the left of the crest of the occipital bone over the inferior curved line. The cicatrix was tender with considerable thickening of the periosteum. Pain radiated from the cicatrix over the left side of his head. The partial left hemiplegia was unchanged.[1] Died May 14, 1892, in Pittsburgh and was buried in Allegheny Cemetery.

DEATH CERTIFICATE: Cause of death, primary, fatty deterioration of heart. Secondary, sudden death.

1. CSR; *OR,* vol. 11, pt. 1:890, 895; vol. 27, pt. 1:256; RVA, Pension SC 155,723.

DANIEL HENRY RUCKER • *Born April 28, 1812,* in Belleville, New Jersey. Served in the Mexican War. He entered the army as a second lieutenant in October 1837 and by the start of the Civil War was a major. He was promoted to brigadier general of volunteers May 23, 1863. He served in the quartermaster's department during the Civil War. In July 1866 he was made assistant quartermaster general with the rank of colonel. In 1882 he was appointed quartermaster general with the rank of brigadier general and was placed on the retired list. Died January 6, 1910, in Washington, D.C., and was buried in Arlington National Cemetery. According to the attending surgeon, the cause of death was uremic poisoning as the result of chronic interstitial nephritis.[1]

   1. LR, ACP, 4324, 1875, fiche: 000171.

THOMAS HOWARD RUGER • *Born on April 2, 1833,* in Lima, New York. He graduated from the USMA in 1854. While at West Point, he was treated for excoriatio fifteen times, contusio twice, and for catarrhus and phlegmon once each. Ruger resigned from the army within a year of graduation and became a lawyer. He was made lieutenant colonel of the 3rd Wisconsin in June 1861 and colonel in September. He was in the Shenandoah and at Cedar Mountain. He was wounded slightly in the head at Antietam on September 17, 1862. His commission as brigadier general of volunteers ranked from the following November. He served at Chancellorsville, Gettysburg, in the Atlanta campaign, at Franklin, and in the Carolinas. In the middle of December 1864 he was disabled by illness. Following the Civil War, he remained in the army and was appointed a colonel. On April 27, 1869, he was treated for tonsillitis. He was commissioned brigadier general in 1886 and major general in 1895. On the night of May 30, 1907, he suddenly became ill with marked cardiac asthma, faintness, a small feeble pulse, and extreme prostration. For the next thirty-six hours his condition improved, but then he began to grow weaker and became unconscious.[1] Died June 3, 1907, at Stamford, Connecticut, and was buried at West Point.
DEATH CERTIFICATE: Primary cause of death, dilatation of heart. Secondary, endocarditis.

   1. *OR,* vol. 19, pt. 1:478; vol. 45, pt. 2:311; WPCHR, vols. 608, 609; RVA, Pension C 675,542; RAGO, entry 534.

DAVID ALLEN RUSSELL • *Born December 10, 1820,* in Salem, New York. He graduated from the USMA in 1845. Served in the Mexican War. He was ill while stationed on the west coast during the spring of 1858. After serving on the frontier and on garrison duty, he had risen to the rank of captain by the time the Civil War started. In January 1862 he was made colonel of the 7th Massachusetts Volunteer Infantry and brigadier general in November. He was on the Peninsula and at Antietam, Fredericksburg, Chancellorsville, and Gettysburg. Russell was slightly wounded in the foot at Rappahannock Station, Virginia, on November 7, 1863. He remained on the field on his horse but later was able to leave on foot. He had a sick leave on November 20 but returned in three days. However, the wound was more serious than first thought, and he later required over two months of hospitalization. He was slightly wounded in the arm at Cold Harbor on June 1, 1864, but remained on the field. Struck by a ball at Winchester on September 19, 1864, he fell forward upon his horse. He straightened up and continued on the field. Soon afterward he was killed when a piece of shell passed through his heart. An officer who was there reported that the shell had been fired from a Federal gun. The next day Russell's body was taken to Harpers Ferry and after being embalmed was forwarded to New York.[1] He was buried in Evergreen Cemetery, Salem, New York.

1. CSR; *OR*, vol. 43, pt. 1:25, 54, 112, 164, pt. 2:110, 124; Will to Dave, June 13, 1864, David A. Russell Papers; Civil War Papers Generals, USAMHI; *Battles and Leaders* 4:87–88, 215; A. D. Slade, *That Sterling Soldier,* 70, 147, 153.

FRIEDRICH (FREDERICK) SALOMON • *Born April 7, 1826,* in Strobeck, Saxony. He had served as a lieutenant in the Prussian army before he emigrated to Wisconsin in 1848. Salomon volunteered in May 1861 as a captain of the 5th Missouri, a three-month unit, and fought at Wilson's Creek. In November he was appointed colonel of the 9th Wisconsin and was made brigadier general to rank from July 1862. Salomon had a sick leave starting December 21 and reported back on January 9, 1863. He commanded a division at Helena and Jenkins' Ferry. During the Yazoo Pass expedition in March and April 1863, he contracted malaria. He was assigned to the Command of the District of East Arkansas on August 2, 1863. However, because of impaired health due to malaria, he obtained a leave on surgeon's certificate on August 9. While on sick leave in Wisconsin he developed jaundice. Supposedly his liver was affected; although he suffered from its effects for some time he was able to report for duty on September 27. In July 1864 he had an attack of malaria that required another sick leave, and he went to Wisconsin. This episode was followed by dysentery and chronic diarrhea. He returned to duty in September. He was mustered out of service in August 1865 and served as surveyor general of Missouri and of the Territory of Utah. In 1883 he continued to suffer from his liver problem.[1] Died March 8, 1897, at Salt Lake City and was buried there in Mt. Olivet Cemetery.

DEATH CERTIFICATE: Immediate cause of death, atheroma, coronary artery. Three weeks' duration.

1. *OR*, vol. 22, pt. 1:475, pt. 2:575; vol. 41, pt. 2:384; vol. 53:547; U.S. Army, CWS, roll 2, vol. 3, report 11, pp. 233–49; RVA, Pension WC 462,529.

JOHN BENJAMIN SANBORN • *Born December 5, 1826,* in Epsom, New Hampshire. At the start of the Civil War he was appointed quartermaster general and adjutant general of Minnesota. He was made colonel of the 4th Minnesota in late 1861 and commissioned brigadier general in August 1863. Sanborn served at Iuka, Corinth, Vicksburg, and in Missouri against Sterling Price. During 1865–66 he dealt with the Indian tribes in the West. After the war he returned to Minnesota and became a politician. He died in St. Paul, Minnesota, on May 16, 1904, and was buried in Oakland Cemetery.

DEATH CERTIFICATE: Cause of death, arteriosclerosis, cerebral thrombosis, gangrene of foot. Duration, two months.

WILLIAM PRICE SANDERS • *Born August 12, 1833,* probably in Frankfort, Kentucky. Graduated from the USMA in 1856. While a cadet he was treated for catarrhus nine times, phlegmon four times, contusio and clavus three times each, and vulnus incisum, odontalgia, excoriatio, and cephalalgia one time each. After graduation he had duty on the frontier and was a captain serving in the Washington defenses during the first part of the Civil War. His promotion to colonel of the 5th Kentucky (Union) Cavalry ranked from March 1863. He was commissioned brigadier general of volunteers in October. During the Battle of Knoxville on November 18, 1863, his horse was shot from under him, and he was shot in the area of the spleen and mortally wounded. He was taken to Knoxville and died the next day in the Lamar House. Initially he was interred in the yard of the Second Presbyterian Church at Knoxville, but later his remains were removed to the National Cemetery at Chattanooga.[1]

1. *OR,* vol. 31, pt. 1:269, 275, 292, 296; WPCHR, vols. 608, 609; RAGO, entry 534; "Daily Journal 1863," August Valentine Kautz Papers, USAMHI.

RUFUS SAXTON • *Born on October 19, 1824,* in Greenfield, Massachusetts. Graduated from the USMA in 1849. He was treated while at West Point for odontalgia seven times, vulnus twice, and rheumatism, contusio, catarrhus, fatigue, cephalalgia, and dyspepsia once each. Served in the Florida wars. An artillery officer, he was in command of a unit at the St. Louis arsenal in 1861 and helped disperse the Missouri State Guard at Camp Jackson. First a chief quartermaster for Gen. Nathaniel Lyon, he was then a member of Gen. George McClellan's staff in West Virginia until appointed brigadier general of volunteers as of April 1862. Saxon commanded at Harpers Ferry in May and June 1862. He was absent from the army for one month that year while recovering from an unspecified serious illness. On July 9, 1864, he was admitted to the USA hospital steamer, *Cosmopolitan,* but returned to duty the next day. In 1866 he reverted to major in the quartermaster's department and served there until he retired in October 1888. In September 1881 he had been sick for at least six months with malarial cachexia, dyspepsia, and debility and required a sick leave. He applied for a transfer from the Military Division of the Pacific in June 1882 at the surgeon's suggestion because the high winds from the water were causing acute rheumatism.[1] Died at Washington, D.C., on February 23, 1908, and was buried in Arlington National Cemetery.

DEATH CERTIFICATE: Cause of death, primary, old age, general debility; immediate, syncope.

1. WPCHR, vols. 605, 606; U.S. Army, CWS, roll 1, vol. 1, report 16, pp. 251–61; RAGO, entry 534; LR, ACP, 1302, 1879, fiche: 000172.

ELIAKIM PARKER SCAMMON • *Born December 27, 1816,* in Whitefield, Maine. He attended the USMA as E. Parker Scammon and graduated in 1837. While at the military academy he was treated for a cold three times and for a pain in the side, a boil, a swollen face, diarrhea, a bruise, and a sore throat once each. Served in the Florida and Mexican wars. He was an officer in the topographical engineers in various parts of the country before being dismissed from the service in 1856 because of disobedience of orders and poor conduct. In June 1861 he was commissioned colonel of the 23rd Ohio Volunteers and served in West Virginia. He was promoted to brigadier general to rank from October 1862. Scammon was captured by Confederate guerrillas in February 1864 and was not released until August. In October and November his health was impaired by his imprisonment and the weather. It was recommended that he be transferred, and by the middle of November he was placed in command of the District of Florida, Department of the South. In February and March 1865 he was seriously ill and unfit for duty. He left the district on April 7 on sick leave and was mustered out of the service in August.[1] He was United States consul on Prince Edward Island from 1866 until 1870, and then became a teacher. Died at his residence in New York City on December 7, 1894, and was buried in Calvary Cemetery, Long Island City.

DEATH CERTIFICATE: Chief cause, cancer of rectum; contributing cause, exhaustion.

1. CSR; OR, vol. 35, pt. 1:28, pt. 2:317, 325; vol. 46, pt. 2:864; vol. 47, pt. 2:392, 452–53, 857; WPCHR, vols. 602, 603.

ROBERT CUMMING SCHENCK • *Born October 4, 1809,* in Franklin, Ohio. A lawyer, congressman from Ohio, and minister to Brazil, Schenck was made a brigadier general of volunteers to rank from May 1861. He went home in November 1861 dangerously ill and returned the first part of 1862. At the Battle of Second Bull Run, August 30, 1862, he was wounded in the right wrist joint. The ball entered the palmar side of the wrist, passed between the radius and ulna, fractured the radius, and exited from the dorsum of the arm. The radial nerve was injured and produced paralysis of the thumb and index finger. He was carried to a nearby hospital tent, conveyed to Alexandria that night, and then was admitted to a hospital in Washington, D.C. After treatment for about seven weeks, he was transferred to Baltimore for further therapy. On June 13, 1863, he was in Baltimore, too sick for active work. In late August he had an accident and was prevented from attending the Court of Inquiry on the Gettysburg campaign. He was temporarily absent and returned on October 10. Schenck resigned in December 1863 to enter Congress. When he was not reelected in 1870, he was sent as minister to London. By 1876 he had complete ankylosis of the right wrist, and the grip of the hand was weak. After slowly recovering from a long illness he was able to walk around Washington, D.C., in late November 1880.[1] Died March 23, 1890, at his residence in Washington, D.C., and was buried in Woodland Cemetery, Dayton, Ohio.

DEATH CERTIFICATE: Cause of death, primary, bronchopneumonia and diphtheria, six days' duration; immediate, pulmonary edema. Duration of last sickness, about two weeks.

1. *OR*, vol. 5:258–59, 657; vol. 12, pt. 2:48, 269, 282–83, 342, pt. 3:582; vol. 27, pt. 2:151, pt. 3:95; vol. 29, pt. 2:27, 116, 224, 290; RVA, Pension SC 142,349; RAGO, entry 534; Hayes, *Diary,* 299.

ALEXANDER SCHIMMELFENNIG • *Born July 20, 1824,* in Lithauen, Prussia. At age sixteen he entered the Prussian service as an ensign. He attended the military academy of Berlin and by 1842 had risen to the rank of lieutenant. He joined the revolutionary army of Bavarian Palatinate and, when they lost, had to flee to Switzerland. He came to the United States in 1853 and settled in Philadelphia. When the Civil War started, Schimmelfennig was engaged in engineering in Washington, D.C., and in September 1861 was made colonel of the 74th Pennsylvania Volunteers. He was en route to Washington, passing through Philadelphia with his regiment in 1861, when his horse fell, causing Schimmelfennig to injure his ankle. While remaining behind for treatment he contracted smallpox and was hospitalized for several weeks. He rejoined his regiment, but the active camp life aggravated his ankle and he had to take sick leave for another seven months. He rejoined his regiment in time to participate in the campaign that ended in the Second Battle of Bull Run in August 1862. He served at Chancellorsville, and on July 1, 1863, at Gettysburg, he became separated from his men and was surrounded by Confederate troops. While climbing over a fence, he was knocked on the head with the butt of a rifle. He dropped on the opposite side of the fence and acted as if he were dead. He crawled into a nearby pigsty and remained there until the morning of the fourth, when the Confederates retreated. In November 1863 he contracted dysentery and was forced to take a two-month sick leave. Still weak from dysentery, he reportedly contracted tuberculosis in August 1864, and on September 1 went north by steamer on a leave of absence. In February 1865 he accepted the surrender of Charleston. He remained there until April 8 when he left South Carolina on a leave of absence on surgeon's certificate. He went to Dr. Aaron Smith's Living Springs Water Cure Establishment at Cushing Hill Springs, near Wernersville, Pennsylvania, in the summer of 1865. On September 5, he was visited by his wife. In the midst of their conversation he reached for a glass of water and took a drink. As he returned the glass to its place on the table, he suddenly collapsed in his chair and died. A postmortem examination revealed that his lungs were almost entirely destroyed.[1]

1. CSR; *OR*, vol. 28, pt. 2:138; vol. 35, pt. 1:28, 39, pt. 2:264; vol. 47, pt. 3:577; Pula, *For Liberty and Justice*, 60; Alfred C. Raphelson, "General Alexander Schimmelfennig's Burial in Reading, Pennsylvania" (typewritten copy), Historical Society of Berks County, Reading, Penn.

ALBIN FRANCISCO SCHOEPF • *Born March 1, 1822*, in Podgorz, Poland. A captain in the Austrian army, he came to the United States in 1851. Schoepf was employed first as a clerk in the patent office and then in the war department. He was commissioned a brigadier general of volunteers in September 1861. On June 1, 1862, he was given a sick leave on surgeon's certificate. He was hospitalized in October because he was disabled by chronic enlargement and irritability of a testicle, and deafness due to neuralgia in his head. On March 13, 1863, he was relieved from service on a military commission and was ordered to report for duty. Schoepf applied for a certificate on which to base his resignation, and the medical director's office reported the following about his examination in March 1863: He had a large varicocele on the left side, which subjected him to considerable pain and inconvenience when in the saddle. Also, he had pain in the right upper abdomen that was accompanied by a cough, particularly when he rode on horseback. His general health was good. He was in command of Fort Delaware from April 1863 to January 1866, when he was mustered out of service. Schoepf returned to the United States patent office after the war. He was unfit for work for at least the last year of his life and was almost constantly in bed from January 1886 until his death in May. The attending physician who took care of him reported that he died from cancer of the stomach. He stated that Schoepf had obscure symptoms, which the physician theorized were due to gastric catarrh that led to an ulcer of the stomach that finally developed a malignant cancerous condition. Another physician who had taken care of him violently disagreed with the diagnosis of cancer because of the long period of Schoepf's symptoms. In 1869, Schoepf had complained to this physician of a burning sensation in his stomach, heartburn, and of pains in his side that had been present ever since the Kentucky campaign. The physician had written prescriptions for him in 1870 for pyrosis and attributed his condition to exposure and improper foods. He had treated him by having him avoid coarse food, such as hardtack, oatmeal, pork, beans, and peas to protect the gastric region. Over the last sixteen years of Schoepf's life the physician had treated him frequently; at first his complaints would temporarily respond to treatment, but over time they became worse. [1] Died May 10, 1886, at Hyattsville, Maryland, and was buried in the Congressional Cemetery in Washington, D.C.

1. CSR; *OR*, vol. 16, pt. 2:625, 676–77; vol. 25, pt. 2:211; RVA, Pension WC 267,008.

JOHN MCALLISTER SCHOFIELD • *Born September 29, 1831,* in Gerry, New York. Graduated from the USMA in 1853. During the summer encampment at West Point, he caught a cold and his eyes became inflamed, requiring him to stay in the hospital for the rest of the encampment. In addition, while a cadet he was treated for catarrhus five times, subluxatio and excoriatio four times each, phlegmon and odontalgia three times each, diarrhea twice, and febris ephemeral, obstipatio, luxatio, colica, and fever intermitt. one time each. In Florida in 1855 he had a fever that was variously recorded as yellow fever or typhoid fever. On leaving Florida he had a relapse and was cared for by A. P. Hill. He became so ill that the surgeon used chloroform on him. When he was well enough, he was taken to A. P. Hill's home at Culpeper Court House where he was kept in bed and every morning given a brandy mint julep before he got up. Schofield served as an instructor at the U.S. Military Academy and was treated there in October 1857 for catarrhus. He was on leave from the army, teaching physics at Washington University in St. Louis, when the Civil War began. Initially, he held a number of positions, including a staff appointment at Wilson's Creek, until he was made a brigadier general of volunteers in November 1861 and was given command of the Union militia of the state of Missouri. On November 11, 1862, he was sick at Springfield with typhoid and had to turn over his command on November 20. He went to St. Louis, Missouri, to recover. He took command of the Army of the Frontier in December 1862. In the Atlanta campaign he commanded the Army of Ohio. While finding his way in the forest near Cassville on the night of May 25, 1864, he was injured when his horse fell. Disabled, he had to give up his command for two days but returned on May 28 partially recovered. He was made a brigadier in the Regular Army to rank from November 1864. He did notable service as a corps commander at Franklin and Nashville. After the war, he was secretary of war for a short time, superintendent at West Point, commander of various departments, and, in 1888, general in chief of the army. In the summer of 1871 he had a cold that developed into pneumonia, which bothered him for some months. He was promoted to lieutenant general in February 1895 and retired the following September. He died from a stroke at St. Augustine, Florida, on March 4, 1906, and was buried in Arlington National Cemetery.[1]

1. *OR*, vol. 13, 787; vol. 22, pt. 1:789, 853; vol. 38, pt. 2:512, 681; WPCHR, vols. 607, 608; Schofield, *Forty-Six Years in the Army*, 4, 24–28, 429–31; *Battles and Leaders* 3:453, 4:307; Howard, *Autobiography* 1:547; James L. McDonough, "John McAllister Schofield," *CWTI* 13 (Aug. 1974): 10–17; *MOLLUS* 12:28.

CARL SCHURZ • *Born March 2, 1829,* in Liblar, Prussia. A revolutionary in Germany, he fought at Ubstatt on June 23, 1849, and Bruchsal on June 24, 1849. In one of the battles he received a slight flesh wound when a bullet grazed his shin bone, but it did not disable him. Throughout his life he had a number of undefined illnesses for short periods of time. Because of his activities as a revolutionary, he had to flee to Switzerland and was sick in a small inn in Dornachbruck for a few days late in 1849. He slipped in a public bath in Berlin in August 1850 and sustained a severe contusion that confined him for over two weeks. In July 1852, soon after he was married in England, Schurz developed a high fever and could not swallow or speak. He went to Malvern to take the water and, nursed by his wife, recovered by the end of the month. They came to the United States in September 1852 and settled in Philadelphia, where he entered politics and joined the antislavery cause. During the fall of 1855, while Schurz was on the way to his new farm at Watertown, Wisconsin, his horse stumbled and fell on Schurz' left leg, making him unable to walk for several days. Schurz took an active part in Wisconsin and national politics. On his arrival at Philadelphia in March 1858 he became ill. When he finally arrived back at Watertown he contracted chicken pox. Continuing his political activism, he took part in the antislavery movement. Headaches and general malaise kept him in bed in Philadelphia for a few days during March 1862. Although he had little military experience, his political views and ability to attract the German-American population gained him a commission as brigadier general of volunteers to rank from April. At Sperryville, Virginia, he was sick for several days in August 1862 but participated in the Second Bull Run campaign. He had jaundice in March 1863 and returned first to Washington and then to Philadelphia to recuperate. He was at Chancellorsville and Gettysburg. Early in September he had "camp fever" and went on sick leave. During the first of 1864 he was sick with fever while camped near Lookout Mountain. Toward the end of February 1864, Schurz had diarrhea and went to New York on leave. He returned to civilian life after the war and continued his interests in politics and various other causes. In March 1869 he was sworn in as senator from Missouri. During 1874 he had a fever, intermittent headaches, and could not attend the senate sessions or spend time on his reelection. After the adjournment of Congress, he went to Narragansett for the sea bathing. While in his office on March 25, 1878, he had an attack of heart trouble and was prostrated. He was carried home and, after medical treatment, rallied. He sprained both feet in 1885 when he stumbled over a rock in the street. In 1887, he fell at the corner of 42nd street and 6th Avenue in Washington, D.C., and fractured his thigh. Apparently his recovery was complete. In the summer of 1887 he was afflicted with rheumatism. During the summer of 1892 he had symptoms suggesting gallbladder disease and could not be very active. In 1899 he ate fish while on a river steamer and contracted what was diagnosed as ptomaine poisoning. With proper medical attention he recovered. Over his remaining years, Schurz had attacks of bronchial infections and gallbladder disease. In November 1905 he slipped and fell while getting off a trolley car and had a concussion of his head. Early in 1906 he became ill and continued to be so until his death.[1] Died May 14, 1906, at New York City and was buried in Sleepy Hollow Cemetery, Tarrytown, New York. DEATH CERTIFICATE: Bilateral septic pneumonia, lower lobes, resulting from chronic suppurative pericholangitis.

1. U.S. Army, CWS, roll 1, vol. 1, report 29, pp. 383–84; Hans L. Trefousse, *Carl Schurz: A Biography,* 23, 28–29, 31, 42, 55, 69, 114, 116, 120, 129, 139, 143–44, 199, 222, 270, 272, 274, 294; Hayes, *Diary,* 133.

ROBERT KINGSTON SCOTT · *Born July 8, 1826,* in Armstrong County, Pennsylvania. He was practicing medicine and was engaged in real estate investments when the Civil War began. He was mustered into Federal service as major of the 68th Ohio and had risen to colonel by July 1862. Being a physician, he treated himself during the war. He served at Vicksburg and in the Atlanta campaign. At Atlanta on July 22, 1864, a shell exploded near him, and he was wounded in the left side of the neck and stunned. He was taken prisoner, was marched to East Point, Georgia, and then was taken to Jonesboro. On July 25 he was placed on a railcar for transfer to a Confederate prison. That evening, near Macon, he attempted to escape by jumping from the moving train in the dark. He fell down the embankment and injured his back, chest, right knee, and leg. Nine weeks after his capture he was exchanged and in October was back with his troops. Scott's promotion to brigadier general ranked from January 1865. Following the war, he could not resume his medical practice or be a merchant because of continued trouble from his previous back, knee, and leg injuries. He could not ride a horse or remain standing very long. He was made head of the South Carolina branch of the Freedman's Bureau and retained his military rank until 1868, when he was elected governor of that state. Scott became a part of the state corruption and finally went back to Ohio in 1877. Christmas Day in 1880 he shot a druggist whom he accused of making his son an alcoholic. On a plea of accidental homicide, he was acquitted. He had a stroke sixteen months before his death and was confined in his home for most of the period. Died August 12, 1900, in Henry County, Ohio, and was buried in Glenwood Cemetery, Napoleon, Ohio.[1]
DEATH CERTIFICATE: Cause of death, paralysis.

1. *OR,* vol. 38, pt. 1:109; RVA, Pension C 964,002; *(Napoleon, Ohio) Democratic Northwest,* Dec. 30, 1880, Aug. 16, 1900; "Grave Matters" 5, no. 2 (1995): 8.

WINFIELD SCOTT · *Born on June 13, 1786,* near Petersburg, Virginia. During the War of 1812, Scott was taken prisoner at Queenston Heights, Canada, on October 13 and paroled November 20. During the capture of Fort George, Canada, on May 27, 1814, one of the magazines blew up. Splinters of the stoneway struck Scott; hurled from his horse to the ground, he suffered a fracture of his left collarbone. He continued on the field, and later the bone was set and his arm strapped to his side. At Lundy's Lane on July 25, 1814, Scott was bruised on the side by a rebounding spent cannonball but continued to encourage his troops. Later, while he was trying to get cartridges, his left shoulder joint was fractured by a musket ball. He was carried unconscious to the rear and propped against a tree, then taken by ambulance to the camp on the Chippewa. The next morning he was ferried across the Niagara with other wounded men. He stayed at Batavia until the August heat became unbearable, and he had to be moved to Geneva. Placed on a litter, he was carried the seventy miles by citizens. A mattress was placed in a carriage, and he was moved to Albany. It was recommended that he go to Philadelphia, where the best surgeon was located. Scott was taken from Albany to New York by river steamboat and from there to Philadelphia in a carriage. On the way he stopped off at Princeton to receive an honorary Master of Arts degree. In October he was able, with help, to mount a horse, and he took command of the defenses of the Chesapeake. In December his shoulder wound was still draining. In 1833, Scott spent a few days in Charleston with a sprained ankle. He was made commander in chief of the army in 1841 and breveted lieutenant general in 1847. While in Mexico during May 1848, he had the vomito. Almost seventy-five years of age at the start of the Civil War, he had been the most prominent American military figure for decades. During December 28–30, 1860, he was very sick from protracted diarrhea and could not answer his correspondence or go to church. He weighed 350 pounds and was given to dozing during meetings. He could take only a few steps at a time and required a hoist to mount a horse. Adding to his other problems were vertigo, gout, and dropsy. On November 1, 1861, the president announced Scott's retirement from active command.[1] Died at West Point on May 29, 1866, and was buried there.

1. *OR*, vol. 1:112–14, 579; vol. 5:639; Heitman, *Historical Register and Dictionary* 2:36; RAGO, entry 623, "File D"; Arthur D. Howden Smith, *Old Fuss and Feathers*, 56, 71–73, 130, 135–41, 186, 345.

JOHN SEDGWICK • *Born September 13, 1813,* at Cornwall Hollow, Connecticut. Graduated from the USMA in 1837. Served in the Florida and Mexican wars. He was major of the 1st Cavalry and became its colonel when the senior officers left to join the Confederacy at the start of the Civil War. In the spring of 1861 he was ill in Washington, D.C., with possible cholera, making him unable to take the field with his troops. Sedgwick was commissioned brigadier general of volunteers to rank from August 1861. Ill with camp fever, he was unable to sit in his saddle on June 27, 1862. On June 29, although still sick, he mounted his horse and rode with his men. At Glendale on June 30 Sedgwick was slightly wounded twice. The first ball struck his arm; a short time later, his leg was grazed by a bullet. He was promoted to major general to rank from July. On September 17, 1862, he was severely wounded at Antietam. First, a bullet went through his leg, then another fractured his wrist. He remained on his horse, and the surgeon who examined his wounds recommended he go to the rear. He refused and mounted another horse, but he could not control it due to his broken wrist. A third wound, located in his shoulder, compelled him to leave the field, and he was carried to a little hut alongside a road in the rear. After remaining in a field hospital near Kedysville for a few days, he was carried by ambulance into Hagerstown, Pennsylvania. Later he went home where he was treated by his sister for about three months. When he reported back, his wounds were not healed, and he spent two weeks in Washington before returning to field duty in the middle of December. He is quoted as saying, "If I am ever hit again, I hope it will settle me at once. I want no more wounds." He served at Fredericksburg, Chancellorsville, and in reserve at Gettysburg. In late March and early April 1863 he had trouble with his eyes. At Spotsylvania on May 8, 1864, a spent ball hit him in the stomach, but he was uninjured. The next day Sedgwick was killed by a ball that entered just below his left eye and transversed the base of the brain. When warned about his exposed position, Sedgwick supposedly made the often-quoted statement that "they couldn't hit an elephant at this distance."[1] He was buried in Cornwall Hollow.

1. CSR; OR, vol. 19, pt. 1:30, 57, 173, 192, 276, 306; vol. 21:882; vol. 36, pt. 1:15, 19, 64–65, 144, 191, 228, 356, 541; U.S. Army, CWS, roll 1, vol. 1, report 20, pp. 293–96; Richard Elliott Winslow III, *General John Sedgwick*, 3, 22–23, 26–27, 47–48, 50, 52, 59, 60, 170; *Battles and Leaders* 4:175; Clark, *North Carolina Regiments*, 4:195; *SHSP* 27:37–8; *MOLLUS* 21:163.

WILLIAM HENRY SEWARD, JR. • *Born on June 18, 1839*, at Auburn, New York. Prior to the Civil War, he was his father's private secretary and engaged in banking. He recruited troops in early 1862 and in August was made lieutenant colonel of the 138th New York. Seward was absent on sick leave from October 6, 1863, to February 24, 1864. In June he was promoted to colonel. On July 9, 1864, at Monocacy, he was wounded in the right leg. He went on sick leave on July 12 and did not assume command again until December. His promotion as brigadier general ranked from the previous September. In June 1865, he resigned from the army and returned to the banking business and charitable interests. An examination in February 1908 revealed a large scar above his right knee.[1] Died at Auburn on April 26, 1920, and was buried there in Fox Hill Cemetery. DEATH CERTIFICATE: Cause of death, chief cause, lobar pneumonia; contributory, *Strep. viridans* infection of throat.

1. CSR; OR, vol. 36, pt. 1:93; vol. 37, pt. 2:145, 190; vol. 43, pt. 2:594, 754; RVA, Pension C 2,479,276.

TRUMAN SEYMOUR • *Born September 24, 1824*, in Burlington, Vermont. He graduated from the USMA in 1846. Served in Florida and Mexican wars. At Fort Moultrie, South Carolina, on November 23, 1860, his health was poor, and he was not able to undergo much exercise. After participating in the defense of

Fort Sumter at the start of the Civil War, he was on duty recruiting and in the defenses around Washington. Seymour was made a brigadier general of volunteers in April 1862. He served on the Peninsula and at Second Bull Run and Antietam. In April 1863 he was granted a leave of absence on medical certificate, and he was a member of a board in Washington until early June. During the assault on Battery Wagner, South Carolina, on July 18, 1863, he was wounded by grapeshot. He was temporarily assigned to command of troops on Morris Island in October. Seymour was captured in the Wilderness in May 1864 and not released until August, after which he served in the Shenandoah and at Petersburg and Appomattox. He had a sick leave from May to July 1865. In 1866 he was promoted to major of the 5th Artillery and held this position until he retired in 1876. From February 4–22, 1872, he was treated for pleuritis. Over the last six years of his life, he had chronic bronchial asthma and degenerative heart disease. He died October 30, 1891, in Florence, Italy, and was interred there in the Cimitero degli Allori. According to the attending physician, he died from heart disease.[1]

1. CSR; *OR*, vol. 1:75; vol. 14:451; vol. 28, pt. 1:348, pt. 2:110; RVA, Pension WC 400,123.

JAMES MURRELL SHACKELFORD • *Born July 7, 1827*, in Lincoln County, Kentucky. Served in the Mexican War. He left his law practice in Louisville and in January 1862 was commissioned colonel of the 25th Kentucky (Union) Infantry, which he led at Fort Donelson. In February he was ill for a short period. Shackelford resigned his original commission and was made colonel of the 8th Kentucky Cavalry in September 1862. He was severely wounded in the foot on September 3, during an engagement at Geiger's Lake, Kentucky, and bled profusely. The ball struck him on the outside of the left foot at the articulation of the fifth metatarsal bone and the cuboid bone and emerged on the inner side of the foot just below the scaphoid bone. He was taken to Henderson, Kentucky, and treated by the surgeon for two weeks. After being moved to Evansville, Indiana, he was treated for a month. A number of small pieces of bone were discharged from the wound before it healed. He was never in a hospital and, after eight weeks of confinement, went on recruiting duty, using a crutch and traveling in a buggy. His promotion to brigadier general ranked from January 1863. He resigned from the service in January 1864. Shackelford returned to the law, was made United States judge for the Indian Territory in 1889, and practiced law in Muskogee in what is now Oklahoma. Ever since he had been wounded, he was slightly lame, and the foot was painful whenever he stood for very long. The scars were contracted, adherent, and tender when pressure was applied. The physician who attended him the last two months of his life diagnosed his case as a general breakdown in consequence of his advanced years. There was a failure of assimilation along with urine retention. Toward the end there was congestion of the lungs due largely to the effects of gravity, since Shackelford was obliged to lie much of the time in one position. Edema of the lungs was a terminal event.[1] Died September 7, 1909, at Port Huron, Michigan, and was buried in Cave Hill Cemetery, Louisville, Kentucky.

DEATH CERTIFICATE: Cause of death, complications arising from old age.

1. CSR; RVA, Pension C 701,391.

ALEXANDER SHALER • *Born on March 19, 1827,* in Haddam, Connecticut. Before the war he was a dealer in bluestone and building material. In April 1861 he was mustered into Federal service as a major of the 7th New York Volunteers, and in June 1861 he was commissioned lieutenant colonel of the 65th New York Volunteers. By May 1863 he had been promoted to brigadier general. He served on the Peninsula and at Antietam, Fredericksburg, and Chancellorsville. He was captured in the Wilderness on May 6, 1864, exchanged in August, and given an extended medical leave. In October Shaler reported to New Orleans for duty and was discharged in August 1865.[1] After returning to civilian life, he dealt in real estate. He died December 28, 1911, in New York City and was buried in Ridgefield, New Jersey.

DEATH CERTIFICATE: Cause of death, general arteriosclerosis, senility and exhaustion.

1. CSR; *OR*, vol. 36, pt. 1:2, 64, 126, 190, 660; vol. 41, pt. 4:177, 268; U.S. Army, CWS, roll 7, vol. 11, report 3, pp. 491–517; LR, ACP, 763, 1875, fiche: 000174.

ISAAC FITZGERALD SHEPARD • *Born on July 7, 1816,* in Natick, Massachusetts. He graduated from Harvard in 1842 and was a principal in the Boston school system, editor of a Boston newspaper, and member of the Massachusetts legislature. After going to St. Louis in 1861, he served as a major on Gen. Nathaniel Lyon's staff at Wilson's Creek. In January 1862 he was made colonel of the 3rd Missouri. After serving at Arkansas Post, he was commissioned colonel of the 51st U.S. Colored Infantry in May 1863 and was promoted brigadier general of volunteers to rank from October 1863. His nomination as general was not approved by the Senate and his commission expired. Following the war he held a number of political positions. He died in Ashland, Massachusetts, on August 25, 1889, and was buried in Ashland Cemetery, Middlesex County, Massachusetts.

DEATH CERTIFICATE: Immediate cause, chronic dysentery.

GEORGE FOSTER SHEPLEY • *Born January 1, 1819,* in Saco, Maine. A graduate of Dartmouth, he studied the law and went into practice in Maine. Except for a four-year period, he was United States district attorney for Maine from 1848 until the start of the Civil War. In November 1861 he was commissioned colonel of the 12th Maine Infantry. He was made post commander at New Orleans after its capture and military governor of Louisiana the following month, June 1862. His promotion as brigadier general of volunteers ranked from July 1862. He held his position in Louisiana until early 1864. After Richmond was occupied, Shepley was made military governor of the city and remained in this position until resigning from the army in July 1865. He returned to his law practice in Maine. Died July 20, 1878, in Portland, Maine, reportedly of Asiatic cholera. He was buried there in Evergreen Cemetery.

PHILIP HENRY SHERIDAN • *Born on March 6, 1831,* in Albany, New York, according to his own later account. He graduated from the USMA in 1853. While at West Point, he was treated for obstipatio and cephalalgia twice each, and clavus, nausea, excoriatio, and subluxatio once each. Before the war, he served on the frontier and on expeditions against the Indians. On March 28, 1857, in a fight with the Yakima Indians at Middle Cascade, Oregon, a bullet grazed the bridge of his nose. He was made captain of the 13th Infantry in May 1861, colonel of the 2nd Michigan in May 1862, and was appointed brigadier general of volunteers in September 1862. He served notably at Corinth, Perryville, Stones River, Chickamauga, and Chattanooga. Afterward he became commander of cavalry in the Army of the Potomac. The night of July 29, 1864, prior to the Petersburg mine explosion, he was sick. In November 1864 he was made a major general. He remained in the army and was promoted to lieutenant general in March 1869 and general of the army in June 1888. He was sick in November 1869. In January 1880 he was given permission to travel for the benefit of his health, and was in Europe from July 1880 to May 1881. In September 1883, following a trip to Yellowstone Park with the president, he was exhausted and in poor health. As he aged, Sheridan put on weight, his face became more flushed and his rapid pulse more noticeable. He began to tire easily and had trouble digesting food. In November 1887 his physician diagnosed disease of his mitral and aortic heart valves. On May 22, 1888, he collapsed with a heart attack and continued to have similar episodes with increasing severity. During one attack his heart ceased functioning, and he was revived with stimulants. Frail, emaciated, and wasted, he was taken to his seaside home at Nonquitt, Massachusetts, hoping that the cooler weather would help his condition. He died at Nonquitt on August 5, 1888, and was buried in Arlington National Cemetery. The attending physician reported that he died due to disease of the mitral and aortic valves, originating in the line of duty.[1]

1. *OR,* vol. 40, pt. 1:52, pt. 3:638; WPCHR, vols. 606, 607, 608; RVA, Pension XC 2,662,504; LR, ACP, 5904, 1885, fiche: 000054; Paul Andrew Hutton, *Phil Sheridan and His Army,* 9, 359, 370–72.

FRANCIS TROWBRIDGE SHERMAN • *Born December 31, 1825,* in Newtown, Connecticut. Before the war he was a hotelier. He entered Federal service in November 1861 as lieutenant colonel of the 56th Illinois Volunteers. When this three-month unit was mustered out, he was made major of the 12th Illinois Cavalry in March 1862. The following September he was appointed colonel of the 88th Illinois. He fought at Stones River and Chattanooga. In September 1863 he was suffering from spasmodic asthma and requested sick leave. On October 17 he was assigned to command of troops. He was captured in July 1864 near Atlanta and was not exchanged until October. In the middle of that month, he had the onset of intermittent fever of a congestive form, which occurred at irregular intervals. The paroxysms were accompanied by a prolonged cold stage, delirium, and prostration. In November he was at home in Chicago as a paroled prisoner of war to recover his health. In January 1865 he was ordered to report for temporary duty and in July was made brigadier general. He was mustered out of the army in February 1866 and after a short and unsuccessful period in Louisiana moved back to Chicago. Here he had a business and entered politics. In October 1904 he filed for an invalid pension on the basis of his age. His wife helped nurse him during his final illness. Died November 9, 1905, in Waukegan, Illinois, and was buried in Graceland Cemetery, Chicago. According to his wife, the cause of death was mitral regurgitation with degeneration of heart muscle and pneumonia due to asthma.[1]

1. CSR; RVA, Pension WC 624,088.

THOMAS WEST SHERMAN • *Born March 26, 1813,* in Newport, Rhode Island. Graduated from the USMA in 1836. At West Point he was treated one time each for eruptions, tonsillitis, and fever. Served in the Florida and Mexican wars. Appointed brigadier general of volunteers to rank from May 1861. During the battle before Port Hudson on May 27, 1863, he was wounded in the right leg by a musket ball. The tibia and fibula were fractured at the upper third. The wound was extensive and the tissue greatly lacerated. Along with other wounded, Sherman was sent that night in a tugboat to New Orleans. Three or four days after he reached New Orleans, the examining surgeon found the wound had been very tightly sewn up with one continuous suture. When the suture was cut, there was a large discharge of decomposing coagula, pus, and bone splinters. His constitutional symptoms had assumed a most aggravated character, and he remained in very poor condition for nearly two weeks. Fragments of bone were discharged from day to day. It was decided that surgery was his only hope for recovery, and an amputation at the middle third of the thigh was performed by Dr. Warren Stone. Sherman left New Orleans on sick leave in July 1863. He was in Washington in August, where his improvement was slow. He planned to start using his artificial limb in October, but a surgeon advised a delay. Using the limb in late November, he required a crutch because of the comparatively small amount of leverage from the short stump. The next month, after extensive practice, he was able to walk with the assistance of one crutch. Because of the lack of elasticity of the artificial leg, he was unable to get the foot into a stirrup and required slight elevation to mount a horse. Using just a cane, he rejoined his command in February 1864. In May 1864 he had two problems: First, his stump had shrunk and impaired the fit of his artificial leg. Second, he had to be confined to his bed because of a large, painful abscess upon the stump induced by the artificial leg while riding. Although his surgeon stated the climate was bad for his health, he remained on duty, and in June he took over command of New Orleans. Sherman was mustered out of the volunteer service in April 1866. From 1866 until 1879, he commanded his regiment at various stations on the Atlantic Coast. On August 8, 1870, he was confined to his bed in the Metropolitan Hotel in Washington, and the retirement board had to visit him in his room. They determined he was not fit for active duty, and he was retired on December 31, 1870, with the rank of major general. He died at his residence in Newport on March 16, 1879, and was buried there in Island Cemetery. According to the assistant adjutant general, the cause of death was pneumonia.[1]

1. *OR*, vol. 26, pt. 1:17, 58, 124, 510–11, 518, 522; vol. 34, pt. 3:437, pt. 4:406; WPCHR, vols. 602, 603; *MSHW*, vol. 2, pt. 3:279; LR, ACP, 1382, 1879, fiche: 000175; U.S. Army, CWS, roll 3, vol. 4, report 3, pp. 35–68; ibid., roll 4, vol. 7, report 5, pp. 93–119.

WILLIAM TECUMSEH SHERMAN • *Born February 8, 1820,* in Lancaster, Ohio. Graduated from the USMA in 1840. At six years of age he was thrown from a horse, which resulted in a residual scar on his right cheek. He was treated at the military academy one time each for a sore foot, a headache, a sprain, an inflamed eye, dizziness, fever intermittent and a cold. In the autumn of 1845 he dislocated his shoulder when he fell while hunting deer and received a three-month leave. He developed asthma in 1846. He served in California during the Mexican War. During March and April 1850 he had severe diarrhea. There was a recurrence of his asthma in October 1850, March 1851, and May 1852. Sherman resigned from the army in 1853 and engaged unsuccessfully in the banking business in California. Over the next few years he continued to have episodes of asthma. For particularly bad attacks he would breath the vapors of burning niter papers and, on at least one occasion, had cupping of his back. At Fort Riley, Kansas, in September 1858, he had an attack of chills and fever. His law practice in Kansas failed, and on January 2, 1860, he was superintendent of the new Louisiana Military School when it opened. In March 1861, after Louisiana issued an ordinance of secession, he left New Orleans for St. Louis to work for the railroad. In May he was appointed colonel of the 13th U.S. Infantry. At First Bull Run on July 21, 1861, balls grazed one knee and his shoulder without causing injury. He was made brigadier general of volunteers in August. His physical and mental system was so broken down in November, according to Gen. Henry W. Halleck, that he was unfit for duty and required a rest. The newspapers reported he was insane. However, the only physician who reportedly saw him diagnosed his condition as "one of such nervousness that he was unfit for command." Sherman, however, appeared in better spirits and health after visiting his family. He suffered bouts of rheumatism during January 1862 and had diarrhea in March. He was severely wounded in the right hand at the battle of Shiloh, Tennessee, on April 6, 1862, and a spent ball bruised his shoulder. His promotion as major general of volunteers ranked from May. In June 1862 he had an attack of malaria that lasted for a month and required that he ride in an ambulance for two days. Sherman commanded a corps at Chickasaw Bluffs, Arkansas Post, and Vicksburg. He also led a corps at Chattanooga and then assumed overall command in the West. He had a respiratory infection in the middle of January 1864. His health had improved by the last of April, and he was almost ready for duty. On August 2 he was ill again. During November he had neuralgia in his right arm and shoulder and had trouble writing. His servant continued to rub his shoulder. Sherman was made brigadier general and major general in the Regular Army during the war. Appointed lieutenant general in 1866, he became full general and general-in-chief of the army in 1869. Asthma continued to bother him in 1869, and he was confined to bed with rheumatism on one occasion. He retired in February 1884. On February 5, 1891, he had a cold; the next day, because of a sore throat, he cancelled a dinner appointment. On the seventh he developed erysipelas of the face and nose along with a fever. The infection spread the following day and he had trouble talking. His face was painted with iodine. The asthma returned, and chloroform plasters applied to his chest did not help. The only nourishment he could take was whiskey and milk. Died February 14, 1891, in New York City and was buried in Calvary Cemetery, St. Louis. According to the surgeon, the cause of death was facial erysipelas.[1]

1. *OR*, vol. 3, 570; vol. 8:374, 441; vol. 10, pt. 1:103, 110; vol. 17, pt. 2:11, 13, 19; vol. 24, pt. 3:541; vol. 32, pt. 2:75; vol. 33:1019; vol. 38, pt. 5:330; vol. 43, pt. 2:552; vol. 44:528; vol. 52, pt. 1:198, 200; WPCHR, vol. 604; LR, ACP, 610, 1884, fiche: 000176; Steiner, *Military-Medical Portraits*, 54–118; Sherman, *Memoirs* 1:132–33, 217, 256; John F. Marszalek, *Sherman: A Soldier's Passion for Order*, 5, 80, 164, 168, 175, 485–86; 491–92; *Battles and Leaders* 4:663.

JAMES SHIELDS • *Born May 10, 1810*, in County Tyrone, Ireland. He came to the United States in 1826 and settled in Illinois. He practiced law and entered politics, serving as a member of the Illinois legislature, a senator from Illinois, and a senator from Minnesota. On April 18, 1847, in storming a battery at Cerro Gordo, Mexico, a grapeshot hit him below the right nipple and passed out through his back on the same side. The American surgeons gave up on him, but a Mexican surgeon drew a silk handkerchief through the wound and removed the extravasated blood. Shields was back on the field in August 1847 and wounded during the storming of Chapultepec on September 13. The ball struck the posterior aspect of the left arm on the ulnar side, a little above the wrist. By 1859, the chest wound had diminished the breathing capacity of his right lung, making him less capable of active exercise or prolonged exertion. He had lost strength in his left arm, and the power of extending the fingers was somewhat impaired. He was commissioned a brigadier general of volunteers in August 1861. During a skirmish outside of Winchester on March 22, 1862, a shell fractured his left arm above the elbow, bruised his shoulder, and injured his side. He was taken into Winchester where he remained in bed. However, he was never in a hospital. Having recovered sufficiently, he returned to duty on April 30 and rode in a buggy. His resignation from the army was accepted in March 1863.[1] He returned to politics in Missouri. Died in Ottumwa, Iowa, on June 1, 1879, and was buried in St. Mary's Cemetery, Carrollton, Missouri.

1. OR, vol. 12, pt. 1:336, 339, 354, pt. 3:12; U.S. Army, CWS, roll 2, vol. 3, report 30, pp. 859–911; James Shields, Civil War Miscellaneous Collection, USAMHI; B. Huger to wife, Aug. 23, 1847, Benjamin Huger Papers, UV; RVA, Pension C 280,224; Conyngham, Irish Brigade, 98–100.

HENRY HASTINGS SIBLEY • Born February 29, 1811, in Detroit, Michigan. He engaged in the fur business for years and in 1858 was elected the first governor of Minnesota. In 1862 he was placed in command of the state's forces sent against the Sioux. Late in September 1862 he was ill. His commission as brigadier general of volunteers was not confirmed, but the following March he was reappointed and finally confirmed. His service during the Civil War was against the Sioux rather than Confederate forces. He was mustered out in April 1866.[1] Following the war, he led an active life as an author, businessman, and politician. Died February 18, 1891, in St. Paul, Minnesota, and was buried there in Oakland Cemetery.

DEATH CERTIFICATE: Cause of death, granular kidney.

1. OR, vol. 13:687, 694.

DANIEL EDGAR SICKLES • Born on October 20, 1819, in New York City. He later reported he was born on October 20, 1825. During a political meeting in the early 1840s he was thrown down a stairwell. He seized the railing; though stunned and bleeding, he was not seriously injured. A lawyer, he was a New York state senator and a representative in Congress from 1857 to 1861. In February 1859, he shot and killed his young wife's lover, Philip B. Key, in Washington, D.C. In April he was acquitted on grounds of temporary insanity and in later years was condemned more for taking his wife back than for killing Key. He was made brigadier general of volunteers to rank from September 1861 and major general to rank from November 1862. Sickles served on the Peninsula and at Antietam, Fredericksburg, and Chancellorsville. He required treatment for diarrhea with some enteritis in June 1863. The evening of July 2 at Gettysburg, his right leg was shattered by a solid shot. He was moved back, where a saddle strap was fastened about the thigh as a tourniquet. While being carried off the field on a stretcher, he smoked a cigar. Placed in an ambulance, he was given brandy and taken to the Third Corps field hospital, which consisted of tents near Taneytown Road. Using candles for light, chloroform was administered and the injured leg was amputated in the lower third of the thigh. The limb was wrapped up, placed in a small coffin, and later sent to the Army Medical Museum, where Sickles would visit it after the war. Sickles was borne to the rear on a stretcher with his cap over his eyes, his hands folded on his chest, and a cigar in his mouth. He was taken the twelve miles to the nearest Union-controlled rail point at Littlestown. Given a few opium pills for pain, he was accompanied by a surgeon, a medical aide, and twelve men to carry the stretcher. They traveled four miles the first day, and the next morning he shaved himself. They reached Washington on July 5, and he was placed in a lodging on F Street, still attended by his surgeon. Not allowed to be lifted, he was placed on the stretcher on the floor and the stump was kept moist with water. He had occasional attacks of anxiety, which he blamed on the chloroform. He started to use crutches, and on July 22 he used them to visit President Lincoln at the White House. The next month the stump was painful, and he was unable to ride in a carriage at more than a slow walk. By December his stump had shrunk enough so that he could be fitted for an artificial limb. He started a tour in April 1864 of the Union-held Southern territory for the government. Sickles retired from Federal service in April 1869 with the rank of major general in the Regular Army. He returned to politics and held a number of federal and state positions, including serving in Congress from New York. In later years he preferred the crutches more than his artificial leg. When Gen. Philip Kearny's body was reinterred in April 1912, Sickles was there on crutches. On April 27, 1914, he had a cerebral stroke and remained unconscious until he expired. Died May 3, 1914, at his residence in New York, and was buried in Arlington National Cemetery. The adjutant general's office reported he died of paralysis.[1]

1. CSR; *OR*, vol. 27, pt. 1:72, 116, 133, 370, 483, 533; *MSHW*, vol. 2, pt. 3:242, 254; RVA, Pension WC 785,655; RAGO, entry 534; Davis, *David Bell Birney*, 184–85; W. A. Swanberg, *Sickles the Incredible*, 54–55, 82, 216–22, 224–25, 227, 243, 269; Kearny, *Letters of Philip Kearny*, 228.

FRANZ SIGEL • *Born November 18, 1824,* at Sinsheim, Germany. He graduated in 1843 from the military academy at Kalsruhe. In early 1847 he took part in a duel where, in addition to fatally wounding another officer, he suffered a wound himself. Imprisoned because of the affair, he resigned his commission in the fall. He was with the revolutionary elements during the 1848 and 1849 insurrections in Germany. He was wounded in the head during one of the engagements toward the end of May 1849. Forced to leave Germany, he finally arrived in New York in 1852. He was director of schools in St. Louis in 1861 and was made a brigadier general of volunteers to rank from May. On leaving the U.S. arsenal at St. Louis on May 10, he was injured and had to be taken to Camp Jackson in a carriage. Later in the day, Sigel obtained a horse, which slipped and fell on the paved street, injuring Sigel's leg. A doctor ran forward, and Sigel was able to join his regiment in a carriage after being treated. Following his arrival at Rolla he had a severe case of the flu, and on November 27, 1861, he had a sick leave and returned to St. Louis. He went back to Rolla in late December. On December 29 he still complained of being ill but appeared able for duty. During the night of February 13, 1862, while advancing to Little York over icy roads, his feet were frozen. In March he was promoted to major general. Seriously ill with influenza after the Battle of Pea Ridge, he was given a sick leave on April 4 to go to St. Louis. Following an extension of his leave, he was ordered to Washington, D.C., about the end of May and then to Harpers Ferry to take command. At Second Bull Run on August 30, 1862, Sigel received several wounds, the most serious to his left hand. He was in poor health in the middle of November, and in February 1863 he was given sick leave. Again in March 1864 he was afflicted with influenza. His military performance on the field during the rest of the war was considered marginal, and he finally resigned his commission as major general in May 1865.[1] Following the war he returned to politics and served as United States pension agent at New York. He died in his residence in New York City on August 21, 1902, and was buried in Woodlawn Cemetery.

1. *OR*, vol. 8:438, 472; vol. 19, pt. 2:574; U.S. Army, CWS, roll 5, vol. 8, report 7, pp. 501–87; ibid., report of Julius Stahel, roll 7, vol. 11, report 1, pp. 1–135; Stephen D. Engle, *Yankee Dutchman: The Life of Franz Sigel*, 4–7, 15–16, 32, 58–59, 89–90, 119, 145, 156–57, 171; Monaghan, *Western Border*, 131–32; *Battles and Leaders* 1:315, 317.

JOSHUA WOODROW SILL • *Born on December 6, 1831,* in Chillicothe, Ohio. He graduated from the USMA in 1853. As a cadet he was treated for excoriatio thirteen times, febris intermittent three times, phlegmon, rheumatism, and catarrhus each twice, and vulnus incisum and phlegmon one time each. Brevetted an ordnance subaltern, he served at various arsenals and as an instructor at West Point for three years. In January 1861 he resigned his commission to become a professor at Brooklyn Polytechnic Institute, but at the start of the Civil War he offered his services to the governor of Ohio. He was made colonel of the 33rd Ohio in August 1861 and brigadier general of volunteers in July 1862. Sick and exhausted, he arrived at Huntsville, Alabama, on July 2, 1862. The surgeon reported he had jaundice and should remain there in the general hospital for a few days. At the Battle of Stones River, Tennessee, on December 31, 1862, he died almost instantly when struck below the cheekbone by a musket ball. His body was taken to a nearby hospital.[1] He was buried in Grand View Cemetery near Chillicothe, Ohio.

1. CSR; *OR*, vol. 20, pt. 1:193, 209, 348, 356–57, 666, 846, 857, 862, 888, 948; WPCHR, vols. 607, 608; *CV* 16:452.

JAMES RICHARD SLACK • *Born September 28, 1818,* in Bucks County, Pennsylvania. Prior to the war he taught school and became a lawyer in Indiana. He was county auditor for nine years and served seven terms in the state senate. In December 1861 he was commissioned colonel of the 47th Indiana Infantry. He was a brigade commander at New Madrid, Island No. 10, Vicksburg, and Mobile. His regimental surgeon treated him for sciatic rheumatism, supraorbital neuralgia, and vertigo at different times during the war. While he was at Dauphin Island, Alabama, he suffered from supraorbital neuralgia accompanied with vertigo and numbness of óne of his limbs. In Louisiana in 1864, Slack had dengue fever. He was promoted to brigadier general of volunteers in November. In the spring of 1865 he had an urticarial eruption over his body, which was accompanied by redness of his joints resembling ordinary rheumatism. On his return home after the war, he suffered from debility and prostration, resulting from his recent attack of "break bone fever," and walked with a cane. In the spring of 1866 he had severe and painful rheumatism in his legs and could get around only with difficulty. Afterward he had such attacks of rheumatism at irregular intervals over the years. In the summer of 1875, he was confined to his house for a long time with erysipelas. Slack served on the Twenty-Eighth Judicial Circuit and was reelected to this position in 1878. He had shortness of breath, especially when walking up hills, and frequent attacks of fainting after exertion compelled him to lie down. He had at least three episodes of a sudden sensation of numbness and paralysis in his arm and leg. After these attacks he dragged his foot when he walked. He died July 28, 1881, in the Alexian Brothers' Hospital at Chicago and was buried in Mount Hope Cemetery, Huntington, Indiana. Hospital Records: Cause of death, apoplexy.[1]

1. RVA, Pension WC 424,300.

ADAM JACOBY SLEMMER • *Born January 24, 1829,* in Montgomery County, Pennsylvania. He graduated from the USMA in 1850. While at West Point he was treated for catarrhus four times, excoriatio and diarrhea twice each, and for obstructio and contusio once each. Served in the Florida wars. When the Civil War started he was a first lieutenant, 1st Artillery. He commanded Fort Barrancas, Florida, and the barracks on Pensacola Bay. In May 1861 he was promoted to major of the 16th Infantry. While inspecting troops at Huttonville, Virginia, on October 25, 1861, he became seriously ill with typhoid fever. In late November he was near death. He was confined to a bed in a private house five miles from Beverly, Virginia, and his wife was with him. On December 11 he received a leave of absence and did not return to duty until March 1862. However, he was still too ill for service and required another sick leave. He returned to command of his regiment in May. Slemmer was severely wounded just below the left knee at the Battle of Stones River on December 31, 1862. On January 1, while being carried from the battlefield, he was captured by Confederate cavalry. Too badly wounded to be transported, he was given a parole and left behind. He remained in Nashville in a hospital from January 2 until March 11, 1863, when he received a leave. His promotion to brigadier general of volunteers in April ranked from the previous November. He proceeded to Norristown, Pennsylvania, where he remained until July 3, 1863, when he was ordered to Columbus, Ohio. He arrived still on crutches. For the rest of the war he served there as presiding officer of a board for examination of sick officers. He remained in the army and served on garrison duty and on examination boards. After his arrival at Fort Laramie, Dakota Territory, in 1867, he had a tendency to dyspnea upon the slightest exertion and occasional dropsical changes of his legs. On October 6, 1868, he went about eight miles from the post in an open wagon to inspect a detachment of men cutting wood on Deer Creek. The day was extremely cold and his breathing was very labored when any walking was required. He returned to the post, dined very heartily, and was drowsy all that evening. He went to bed; shortly after midnight his wife awakened to find him sitting up in bed vomiting. Immediately afterward he fell back upon his pillow and remained motionless. The doctor arrived in a few minutes and found Slemmer without a pulse or respiration. No heart sounds could be heard on auscultation. The surgeon rubbed Slemmer vigorously with brandy, dashed cold water on his face, and applied a mustard mixture to his extremities. He sent for a galvanic battery and applied the poles to the nape of Slemmer's neck, the insertion of his diaphragm, and to his precordium. He resorted to artificial respiration for a short time but to no purpose. Slemmer died October 7, 1868, at Fort Laramie, Dakota Territory. A postmortem examination was made thirty-two hours after death. His lower extremities were edematous. The left lung was deeply congested throughout and had evidently become pneumonic. Two ounces of serous fluid was present in the pericardium. The heart was covered with adipose tissue and its right side was largely dilated. The walls of the right ventricle were thin and softened while the walls of the left ventricle were somewhat thickened. The cavities of the heart contained between ten and eleven fluid ounces of blood and clots. Dense fibrinous deposits were present on the mitral valve. Fluid was found in both pleural cavities. The liver was enlarged and weighed about six pounds. Both kidneys were contracted and granular. Some effusion was evident in the abdomen. The mucous membranes of the stomach were slightly congested on the posterior side. The dura mater of the brain was adherent to the skull posteriorly and there was about two fluid ounces of serous fluid in the membrane. Other organs were normal.[1] He was buried in Montgomery Cemetery, Norristown, Pennsylvania.

1. *OR,* vol. 5:251, 670; vol. 20, pt. 1:380, 395, 398, 401; WPCHR, vols. 605, 606, 607; RVA, Pension WC 125,031; U.S. Army, CWS, roll 1, vol. 1, report 4, pp. 43–46.

HENRY WARNER SLOCUM • *Born September 24, 1827,* at Delphi, New York. He graduated from the USMA in 1852. While at the military academy he was treated once each for febris ephemeral, catarrhus, odontalgia, colica, and excoriatio. Served in the Florida wars. He resigned from the U.S. Army in 1856 and started a law practice. Slocum held county and state positions and was a colonel in the New York state militia before the Civil War. In May 1861 he was made colonel of the 27th New York. At the first battle of Bull Run, July 21, 1861, he was wounded in the right thigh by a musket ball. He remained in the infirmary on Fifth Street in Washington with his estranged wife in attendance until August 20, when he went home on sick leave. He was promoted to brigadier general in August and in September was back on duty. His promotion to major general ranked from July 1862. He served on the Peninsula, at Second Bull Run, Antietam, Chancellorsville, Gettysburg, and Chattanooga, in the March to the Sea, and in the Carolinas. Slocum resigned his commission in September 1865[1] and returned to the practice of the law and politics. He died April 14, 1894, in Brooklyn and was buried there in Green-Wood Cemetery.

DEATH CERTIFICATE: Primary cause, pneumonia, cirrhosis of liver. Secondary, ascites.

1. CSR; *OR,* vol. 2:386, 389; WPCHR, vols. 607, 608; U.S. Army, CWS, roll 1, vol. 1, report 17, pp. 263–75.

JOHN POTTS SLOUGH • *Born February 1, 1829,* in Cincinnati, Ohio. After being expelled from the Ohio legislature for having struck another member, he moved first to the Kansas Territory and then to Denver in 1860. Made colonel of the 1st Colorado Infantry in 1862, he was made brigadier general of volunteers in August of that same year. The rest of the war he served as military governor of Alexandria. After he was mustered out of service in August 1865, he was appointed chief justice of the New Mexico Territory. On December 15, 1867, Slough was shot in the billiard room of the La Fonda Hotel in Santa Fe by a member of the territorial legislature. The politician had introduced a resolution censuring him for unprofessional conduct. Slough died on the seventeenth from his wound. The man who killed him was acquitted on a plea of self defense. Initially buried in Santa Fe, Slough's remains were later removed to Spring Grove Cemetery in Cincinnati.[1]

1. *New Mexico (Santa Fe, N.M.),* Dec. 17, 1867; William A. Keleher, *Turmoil in New Mexico, 1846–1868,* 204.

ANDREW JACKSON SMITH • *Born April 28, 1815*, in Bucks County, Pennsylvania. He graduated from the USMA in 1838. He was treated one time each for sore eyes and a sore throat while at West Point.[1] Served in the Mexican War. Smith had duty at various posts in the West prior to the Civil War and was commissioned colonel of the 2nd California Cavalry in October 1861. He resigned this position and was made chief of cavalry under Gen. Henry W. Halleck. Appointed a brigadier general of volunteers in March 1862, he was promoted to major general in May 1864. Following the war he was made colonel of the 7th Regular Cavalry in March 1866, a position he resigned from in 1869 to become postmaster of St. Louis. He was reappointed colonel of cavalry in January 1889 and retired with that rank the same day. Died at his home in St. Louis on January 30, 1897, and was buried in Bellefontaine Cemetery.

DEATH CERTIFICATE: Cause of death, cerebral apoplexy.

1. WPCHR, vols, 603, 604.

CHARLES FERGUSON SMITH • *Born on April 24, 1807*, in Philadelphia. He graduated from the USMA in 1825. During the Mexican War he had diarrhea, which was later stated to be a contributing factor in his death. After an active service, mainly on the frontier, he was in command of the Department of Utah from February 1860 until the following February. He was appointed brigadier general of volunteers in August 1861. His wife later reported that he was wounded at Fort Donelson, but this could not be confirmed. On March 7, 1862, he was assigned to command the expedition that was to move up the Tennessee River. While making a personal inspection, Smith missed a step getting into a small boat and abraded his shin. Soon infection set in and he was confined, sick, on board the *Hiawatha* at Pittsburg Landing. As senior officer, he was appointed to the command of the post at Pittsburgh on March 26. A cripple, he was upstairs in a brick house at Shiloh on April 6. The injury became so aggravated he had to turn over his command and go to Savannah, Tennessee. He died April 25, 1862, at Grant's headquarters at Savannah. The cause of death was reported by the surgeon to be from the infection of his leg and the chronic dysentery contracted during the Mexican War.[1] He was buried in Laurel Hill Cemetery, Philadelphia.

1. *OR*, vol. 2:17, 130; vol. 10, pt. 1:153, 181, 331, pt. 2:53, 67, 100–101, 130; vol. 52, pt. 1:236, 243; LR, ACP, 1850, 1885, box 957; RVA, Pension Min. C 99,888; Sherman, *Memoirs* 1:227.

GILES ALEXANDER SMITH • *Born on September 29, 1829*, in Jefferson County, New York. He was a proprietor of a hotel in Bloomington, Illinois, when the Civil War started. In June 1861 he was made a company captain in the 8th Missouri Infantry. He was granted a seven-day leave of absence on November 23 for the benefit of his health. In June 1862 he was made colonel of his unit. In Memphis in December 1862, he was sick, could perform little duty, and was confined in his quarters. During the assault on Vicksburg on May 19, 1863, he was slightly wounded in the right hip by a musket ball. Although not considered severe, it incapacitated him during the assault on May 22 and the siege that followed. His promotion to brigadier general of volunteers ranked from August 1863. In the attack on the north end of Missionary Ridge on November 24, 1863, Smith received a wound to the right superior area of his chest, and a conical ball hit his right arm. The ball was cut out of the arm. In the winter of 1863–64 he had a cough, weak voice, and hemorrhages from the lungs, and he remained indoors as much as possible. He was absent on account of his wounds until February. While stationed at Brownsville, Texas, during July through September 1865, he again had episodes of hemorrhage from his lungs and was unable to command much of the time. In November 1865 he was promoted to major general of volunteers and mustered out in 1866. In 1872 Smith had to resign from his position as second assistant postmaster because of deteriorating health. He went to California in 1874 to try and improve his condition; however, when he came home in the fall of 1876 he was in the last stages of consumption. He said he returned to die. Died November 5, 1876, in Bloomington, Illinois, and was buried in Bloomington Cemetery. According to the attending physician's statement, he died of consumption.[1]

1. CSR; *OR*, vol. 8:259, 263; vol. 24, pt. 2:259; vol. 31, pt. 2:573; RVA, Pension WC 224,194; U.S. Army, CWS, roll 2, vol. 3, report 6, pp. 139–66; RAGO, entry 534.

GREEN CLAY SMITH • *Born July 4, 1826*, in Richmond, Kentucky. He served during the Mexican War as a second lieutenant. Smith was left with the other sick men at Louisville on August 31, 1846, and was back in command of his company on October 15. On December 31 he was absent sick in Camargo, Mexico. A practicing lawyer, he was a member of the Kentucky legislature in 1860. He was made colonel of the 4th Kentucky (Union) Cavalry in March 1862 and brigadier general of volunteers to rank from June. During the battle of Lebanon on May 5, 1862, he was wounded in the right leg, and the kneecap was fractured. After being confined for about three or four weeks in Lebanon and Wartrace, Tennessee, he went home on leave. In July he was sent to Henderson, Kentucky, and took command. On September 7 he was sick. While at Murfreesboro in late April 1863, he became ill and could not command. Smith had been elected to Congress in 1862 and resigned his army commission in December 1863. In October 1864 he was made commandant of the camp of rendezvous at Covington, Kentucky, for a regiment he was raising. Smith remained in Congress until 1866 when he took the post of territorial governor of Montana. In 1869 he was ordained a minister. From the end of the war until 1875 he was treated for bleeding piles; he often lost considerable quantities of blood, which at times debilitated him. He took frequent baths to obtain relief.

By 1885 he could use his leg without his knee joint becoming stiff; however, he still had pain and weakness in the whole leg and required care and frequent rubbing of the limb.[1] He died June 29, 1895, at his residence in Washington, D.C., and was buried in Arlington National Cemetery.

DEATH CERTIFICATE: Cause of death, carbuncle, septic poisoning, one month's duration.

1. CSR; *OR*, vol. 10, pt. 1:884; vol. 16, pt. 2:493; vol. 23, pt. 2:288; RVA, Pension WC 427,547; U.S. Army, CWS, roll 8, vol. 13, report 2, pp. 211–25.

GUSTAVUS ADOLPHUS SMITH • *Born on December 26, 1820,* in Philadelphia. Before the war he was an affluent manufacturer of carriages in Illinois. In September 1861 he was made colonel of the 35th Illinois Infantry. Because of an attack of remittent fever and camp colic, he left Rolla without official permission and arrived at his home in Decatur, Illinois, on December 3, 1861. He suffered day and night with fever and was taken care of by his family physician. By December 18 his fever had broken, but he had paroxysms of diarrhea. At Pea Ridge, Arkansas, on March 7, 1862, he was wounded twice, and his horse was killed at about the same time. First, a ball entered the lower part of the left deltoid muscle near its insertion into the shaft of the humerus and then passed out at the axilla. At the same time, the right side of his head was struck by a shell fragment. The skull was fractured near the junction of the right parietal and occipital bones. On March 12 he went home on sick leave. During May and June, bone fragments discharged from his skull wound. Smith's promotion to brigadier general of volunteers ranked from September. Because of his physical state, the Senate did not act on his nomination, and when it expired in March 1863, he reverted to his previous rank of colonel. In late April he was not sufficiently recovered from his wounds to take an active command but was qualified to command a convalescent camp. Smith asked for a leave of absence from command on August 29. He still had discharge from his head wound, which his surgeon reported was due to caries of the bone. He left the service in September 1863. In January 1865, he reentered the service, accepted regimental command, and reported at Nashville for duty. However, on account of his wounds and the state of his health, he was refused duty and was detailed on court-martial duty. He was mustered out of service in December 1865. In February 1866 his head wound was still discharging bone fragments but had apparently healed two years later. President U. S. Grant appointed him collector of internal revenue for the District of New Mexico in 1870. By November 1876 he had partial paralysis of his left shoulder and arm, which were also at times quite painful. According to his wife, he died in Santa Fe on December 7, 1885, of kidney and stomach trouble.[1] Smith was initially buried in Fairview Cemetery in Santa Fe and was later reinterred in the U.S. National Cemetery in the same city.

1. CSR; *OR*, vol. 8:259, 263; vol. 53:36; RVA, Pension WC 399,843.

JOHN EUGENE SMITH · *Born August 3, 1816,* in Berne, Switzerland. A jeweler and goldsmith, he was elected county treasurer in Galena, Illinois, in 1860. In July 1861 he was commissioned colonel of the 45th Illinois and was made a brigadier general of volunteers in November 1862. After the war, he was appointed colonel of the 27th Infantry in July 1866. Smith served on the frontier until his retirement in May 1881. Died January 29, 1897, in Chicago and was buried in Greenwood Cemetery, Galena.

MORGAN LEWIS SMITH · *Born March 8, 1821,* in Mexico, New York. After a varied career, including five years in the Regular Army, Smith was a river boatman when the Civil War started. He recruited the 8th Missouri Infantry and was made the unit's colonel. In July 1862 he was commissioned brigadier general of volunteers. While reconnoitering in the morning fog at Vicksburg on December 28, 1862, he was hit in the hip by a chance bullet. The ball penetrated the left ilium of the pelvis and passed toward the sacrum. The ball was wedged tight, and the surgeon did not think it could be removed safely. Disabled, he was sent by boat to Memphis. An examination in August 1863 revealed a cicatrix three inches long over the posterior part of the left ilium near its crest. In its center was a suppurating canal the size of an ordinary quill and about an inch in depth. Its discharge was small in quantity and consisted of "healthy" pus. The surgeon did not feel it communicated with bone. When Smith returned to duty in December, he still suffered from his wound and had developed bronchial catarrh and a cough. During the Atlanta campaign in August 1864, he was compelled to go on sick leave because of disabilities arising from his old wound. The leg was becoming partially paralyzed; the foot and ankle were nearly useless and extremely painful. On November 9 Smith reported for duty and was ordered to assume command of the post and defenses of Vicksburg. He resigned from the service in July 1865. Smith was appointed U.S. consul general in Honolulu by President Johnson and afterward became a businessman in Washington, D.C. During the winter of 1871–72 his lungs were particularly sensitive to exposure of any kind, and night air caused him to cough.[1] Died December 29, 1874, at Jersey City, New Jersey, and was buried in Arlington National Cemetery.

DEATH CERTIFICATE: (Postmortem performed.) Congestion of the lungs.

1. *OR,* vol. 17, pt. 1:607, 635, 654; vol. 38, pt. 3:42, 106, pt. 5:352; vol. 39, pt. 3:726; LR, ACP, 5317, 1882, fiche: 000179; RVA, Pension Min. C 267,238; RAGO, entry 534; RAGO, entry 623, "File D."

THOMAS CHURCH HASKELL SMITH · *Born March 24, 1819,* in Acushnet, Massachusetts. He practiced law in Cincinnati until 1848, when he undertook construction of telegraph lines connecting the North and South. He was made lieutenant colonel of the 1st Ohio Cavalry in September 1861 and in July 1862 was appointed aide-de-camp to Gen. John Pope. Smith was promoted to brigadier general of volunteers in March 1863 and was mustered out of the service in 1866. He raised livestock but lost his sources of income in the Chicago fire of 1871. In early 1872 he was in very poor health. He was made a paymaster in the Regular Army with the rank of major in 1878. While serving at Santa Fe, New Mexico, in the summer of 1879, and for a year afterward, his health was impaired by the service and exposure. In the winter of 1882–83 he went by stage from Winnemucca, Nevada, to Fort McDermitt, Nevada. The temperature fell to about twenty degrees below zero. Smith contracted a severe cold and was never again completely well. In 1883 he was retired from the army because of his age. He had paralysis in May 1885. For several years before his death he could not walk and used an invalid chair because he had lost the use of his lower extremities due to rheumatism and paralysis. There was progress of his disease, and he had increasing constipation and urine retention. He died on April 8, 1897, at Nordhoff, California. An affidavit by the physician stated that Smith was not afflicted with la grippe and his death was not due to heart failure; however, it implied that his secondary constipation and urinary retention were factors.[1] He was buried in Santa Barbara Cemetery in Santa Barbara, California.

1. U.S. Army CWS, roll 4, vol. 7, report 6, p. 121; RVA, Pension WC 508,752.

THOMAS KILBY SMITH · *Born September 23, 1820,* in Dorchester, Massachusetts. He held various minor Federal positions before the Civil War. Smith entered the U.S. Army as lieutenant colonel of the 54th Ohio in September 1861 and was made colonel the following month. On December 13, 1862, he was unable to perform any duty due to dysenteric diarrhea. Because of the dampness of the interior of his tent, Smith was urged by his surgeon to seek shelter in a comfortable house, which would give him relief. In August 1863 he was promoted brigadier general of volunteers. His health improved in early 1864; however, in the summer he developed malarial fever and had to remain in Tennessee. On June 2 he obtained a leave because of disability. He went to Yellow Springs, Ohio, and remained an invalid because of the malarial fever and chronic diarrhea. Although not completely recovered, he was summoned in January 1865 as a witness before the Joint Committee of Congress on the Conduct of the War. Although still afflicted with diarrhea, he was assigned as military commander of the District of Florida and Southern Alabama in March. He remained at this post until August 1865, when he was granted leave because of chronic diarrhea and debility. His diarrhea continued, and he was discharged from the army in January 1866. In 1867 he was appointed consul at Panama, but the change in climate did not improve his health as proposed. He returned to the United

States in 1869 and remained an unemployed invalid at his residence due to his diarrhea and general physical condition. From 1875 to 1880, his physician treated him for sleeplessness, diuresis, and chronic diarrhea, using homeopathic methods. Throughout the 1880s he continued to have diarrhea and malarial poisoning.[1] He died December 14, 1887, in St. Luke's Hospital at New York City and was buried in Torresdale Cemetery in Philadelphia, Pennsylvania.

DEATH CERTIFICATE: Cause of death, acute gastritis, fatty degeneration and dilatation of heart.

1. CSR; RVA, Pension WC 241,435; U.S. Army, CWS, roll 2, vol. 3, report 32, pp. 939–1012.

WILLIAM FARRAR SMITH • *Born February 17, 1824,* in St. Albans, Vermont. He graduated from the USMA in 1845. Served in the Florida wars. In 1855 he contracted malaria, which precipitated attacks of chills and fever the rest of his life. During the same year he also had insolation (sunstroke). He was made colonel of the 3rd Vermont to rank from July 1861 and was promoted to brigadier general of volunteers in August. He had typhoid fever in October 1861 and did not resume command until December. On April 16, 1862, at Lee's Mill, his horse was going full speed and stepped into a hole. Smith was thrown to the ground and was dazed for the rest of the day. He went on sick leave in July. On January 23, 1863, there was an order stating that Smith could give no further service to the army; Smith was temporarily relieved from duty but no reason was given. He had irritability of the urinary bladder in April, which his surgeon attributed to sitting in the saddle. During May his surgeon stated he had a tendency to congestion of the brain when subjected to hot summer weather. In June he reported for duty at Hagerston, Maryland. He had a boil on his arm in July. Smith was relieved at his own request in August and returned in October. In June 1864 he had fever and weakness, which he attributed to sleeping on low, wet ground and drinking the swamp water at Cold Harbor. By the fifteenth he had such bad dysentery that he could hardly stay on his horse. On July 1 he was in such poor health that he had to ask for a short leave of absence. The trouble was with his head, which, during the heat of the day, caused him to feel quite helpless, and he was unable to go out even to visit his lines. Similar problems had driven him from the southern climate three times before. Initially, U. S. Grant refused the leave, but later, after a repeat request, the leave was granted. Smith left on July 9 and returned in ten days. During December 1865 he had a painful knee. He resigned his volunteer commission in 1865 and his regular commission in 1867. After the war he was president of a cable company, civilian engineer for the government, and a prolific author. From 1871 through 1879 he was treated in Europe and New York for recurring attacks of chills and fever considered to be due to chronic malaria. He had chronic enlargement of the spleen accompanied with congestion of the liver.[1] Died February 28, 1903, in Philadelphia and was buried in Arlington National Cemetery.

DEATH CERTIFICATE: Cause of death, nephritis.

1. *OR,* vol. 21:999; vol. 27, pt. 3:240, 771; vol. 29, pt. 2:102; vol. 30, pt. 4:62; vol. 40, pt. 2:594–96, pt.3:119, 334; vol. 51, pt. 1:989; RVA, Pension C 163,387; *Battles and Leaders* 4:106; William F. Smith, *Autobiography of Major General William F. Smith, 1861–1864,* 35, 50, 71, 99, 102, 114–15.

WILLIAM SOOY SMITH • *Born on July 22, 1830,* in Tarlton, Ohio. He graduated from the USMA in 1853. While at West Point he was treated once each for subluxatio, catarrhus, cephalalgia, diarrhea, and excoriatio. A year after graduation he resigned his commission and established an engineering firm. He was made colonel of the 13th Ohio Infantry in June 1861 and brigadier general of volunteers in April 1862. Following the Battle of Shiloh in April he had a short sick leave. He moved with his division to the vicinity of Nashville where he was sick in the hospital during the last of December 1862. Shortly afterward he was assigned to command. In June 1863 he was hospitalized in Nashville for a week but the diagnosis was not recorded. On July 17 he was quite ill and required a leave to go home for the benefit of his health. In early 1864 he was prostrated by a severe attack of inflammatory rheumatism, and on February 20, 1864, he was very sick. He resigned July 15, 1864, because of continued poor health due to inflammatory rheumatism.[1] He returned to civilian life and over the years made major contributions to the engineering of bridges and tall buildings, particularly in Chicago. Died in Medford, Oregon, on March 4, 1916, and was buried in Forest Home Cemetery, Riverside, Illinois.

DEATH CERTIFICATE: Cause of death, pneumonia and senility.

1. *OR,* vol. 24, pt. 2:528–29, pt. 3:537, 544; vol. 32, pt. 2:440; WPCHR, vols. 607, 608; U.S. Army, CWS, roll 5, vol. 9, report 12, pp. 273–303; RVA, Pension C 814,506; RAGO, entry 534.

THOMAS ALFRED SMYTH • *Born on December 25, 1832,* in the parish of Ballyhooley, County Cork, Ireland. Smyth came to the United States in 1854 and participated in William Walker's expedition to Nicaragua. He was a coach maker when the Civil War started and entered a three-month unit. After he was mustered out he was made major of the 1st Delaware Infantry. In September 1862 he was sick and ordered to report to the medical director in Baltimore. He returned the next month. By February 1863 he had risen to colonel of his regiment. Ill in May, he was excused from duty. On July 3 at Gettysburg he was wounded in the head and face by a shell. However, he was able to return to duty the next day. After a week of suffering from bilious remittent fever and extreme disability, he was confined to bed on August 10. On the sixteenth he was given a fifteen-day sick leave. The next year in October he was promoted to brigadier general of volunteers. Near Farmville on April 7, 1865, he was mortally wounded in the face by a Confederate sharpshooter. He was taken to a nearby residence used as a field hospital and then moved to a general hospital. Smyth lived for two days and finally died on the ninth at Burkesville, Virginia. He was the last Federal general killed during the war.[1] Smyth was buried in the Wilmington and Brandywine Cemetery in Wilmington, Delaware.

1. CSR; *OR*, vol. 27, pt. 1:454, 465; vol. 46, pt. 1:76, 567, 583, 674, 683, 759, 768; LR, ACP, 1227, 1874, fiche: 000182; RAGO, entry 534; *MOLLUS* 4:158.

JAMES GALLANT SPEARS • *Born on March 29, 1816,* in Bledsoe County, Tennessee. A lawyer in Tennessee, he was also a land and slave owner before the Civil War. Because of his strong Unionist feelings, he was almost arrested by the Confederate government and had to go to Kentucky. He was made lieutenant colonel of the 1st Tennessee (Union) Infantry in September 1861 and brigadier general in March 1862. Upset by the Emancipation Proclamation, he came into conflict with Federal authorities and in August 1864 was court-martialed and dismissed because of disloyal language and conduct prejudicial to good order. Died at Branden's Knob, Bledsoe County, Tennessee, on July 22, 1869, and was buried in Pikeville, Tennessee.

FRANCIS BARRETTO SPINOLA • *Born on March 19, 1821,* at Stony Brook, New York. After being admitted to the New York bar in 1844 he entered politics. In October 1862 he was appointed a brigadier general of volunteers. Following the Battle of Gettysburg on July 23, 1863, near Manassas Gap, Virginia, he was wounded twice—once in the right foot and then in the right side of his abdomen. Neither wound was considered serious and he was not hospitalized. He was first treated at the Metropolitan Hotel in Washington, D.C., and then was sent to his home in Brooklyn, where his own physician continued his treatment. In August and September he was convalescing in Brooklyn. From the middle of October to the middle of January 1864 he was on recruiting duty in New York, although the foot continued to be tender and painful. Spinola resigned from the service in June 1865. Shortly afterward, he developed rheumatism, which affected him the rest of his life. A physical examination in October 1886 revealed that the entrance scar on the right foot was one inch below the right internal malleolus and a quarter of an inch in diameter and circular. It was depressed, somewhat retracted, and painful. From that point, the cicatrix extended in a linear shape about to the posterior portion of the os calcis, where the missile exited. In addition, there was a scar on the right side of his body, on a level with the crest of the ilium, one and a half inches long and a quarter-inch wide. There was no retraction or adherence, but it was painful. He also had a curvature of the spine, which was stated to be due to rheumatism. The pelvis was elevated on the right side because of the curvature, such that the left leg appeared one to one and one-half inches longer than the right. To compensate, he wore a thick sole on the right boot. The right knee joint had an inward curvature from alteration of the structure of the joint. He walked slowly with apparent difficulty and pain from rigidity of the tendons. A left hydrocele was present. There were bilateral varicose veins of the legs, the right leg more than the left. In July 1888 he filed an additional claim for disability because of an injury to his right shoulder. He reported this was the result of a fall from his horse while in service near New Bern, North Carolina. There was crepitus in both shoulder joints. Motion of the right shoulder joint was restricted and the arm could not be raised to more than forty-five degrees without associated movement of the scapula. With all the movement the scapula would permit, the arm could not be raised to a right angle. On the outer aspect of the right arm just below the shoulder was a cystic tumor half the size of a hen's egg, which had first appeared after the fall. It was reported that there had been a partial dislocation of the shoulder joint at the time of the injury.[1] Died in Washington on April 14, 1891, at the Arlington Hotel and was buried in Green-Wood Cemetery, Brooklyn.

DEATH CERTIFICATE: Primary, perirectal abscess of nearly one year duration; immediate, asthenia. Duration of last illness, five weeks.

1. CSR; *OR*, vol. 27, pt. 1:99, 490, 496, 539; RVA, Pension SC 166,389.

JOHN WILSON SPRAGUE · *Born on April 4, 1817,* in White Creek, New York. An Ohio businessman, he entered the 7th Ohio Infantry when the war started. He was made colonel of the 63rd Ohio in January 1862 and brigadier general in July 1864. After the war he entered the railroad business. Died December 24, 1893, in Tacoma, Washington, and was buried in Tacoma Cemetery.

DEATH CERTIFICATE: Cause of death, chronic cystitis and enlargement of heart; immediate cause, heart failure.

JULIUS STAHEL · *Born November 5, 1825,* in Szeged, Hungary. He served in the Austrian army as a lieutenant and lived in London and Berlin before he came to America in 1859. He was working for a German-language weekly in New York City at the start of the Civil War and was made lieutenant colonel of the 8th New York in 1861. He was promoted to colonel in August 1861 and to brigadier general in November. On July 7, 1862, he had sick leave and returned on August 13 because he knew his command would be receiving their marching orders. Stahel was wounded in the shoulder at Piedmont on June 5, 1864, and left his command only for the time required to allow his surgeon to dress the injury. Relieved from field duty on the ninth because of the painful wound, he was ordered to Martinsburg and Harpers Ferry to collect and organize troops. He was given a leave of absence on surgeon's certificate of disability on July 16. Having recovered from his wound in August, he was ordered to report back to duty. He was mustered out in 1865. Following the war Stahel was in consular

service in Japan and China for several years; on his return to the United States
he entered the insurance business. It is of interest that when he was examined
in July 1892, no scar or evidence that he had been wounded was reported. However, he did have large internal and external hemorrhoids.[1] Died December 4,
1912, in New York City and was buried in Arlington National Cemetery.
DEATH CERTIFICATE: Chronic interstitial nephritis and cardiosclerosis.

1. *OR*, vol. 37, pt. 1:595, 613; vol. 43, pt. 1:686; vol. 46, pt. 2:356; RVA, Pension C 852,3344; U.S.
Army, CWS, roll 7, vol. 11, report 1, pp. 1–135.

DAVID SLOANE STANLEY • *Born June 1, 1828,* in Cedar Valley, Ohio. He graduated
from the USMA in 1852. As a cadet he was treated for cephalalgia five times,
excoriatio three times, diarrhea, contusio, and phlegmon each twice, and pyrosis, odontalgia and pleurodynia one time each. In May 1855 he was in Hot
Springs, Arkansas, with a squamous inflammation of his skin. His skin disease
continued into December while he was at New Port Barracks, Kentucky. The
condition baffled every mode of treatment, and the continued use of sulphur
vapor baths were recommended. In 1856 he was on sick leave conducting recruits to Fort Pierre in the Dakotas. During a fight with Indians on July 27,
1857, his gun jammed, and one of the Indians prepared to shoot him. J. E. B.
Stuart dashed up to the Indian and took the ball himself. Stanley was convinced that Stuart had saved his life. Later, south of the Wichita River in August, during another fight with Indians, his horse slipped, and Stanley's leg
was badly bruised. When the Civil War started, Stanley was at Fort Washita,
Indian Territory, and took his troops back to Fort Leavenworth, Kansas. In
September 1861 he was appointed a brigadier general of volunteers. In the first
week of November at Syracuse, Missouri, his horse jumped as he was getting
into the saddle, and when his foot struck the ground he broke his ankle. He
had a Pott's fracture, was laid up for six weeks, and needed a crutch for three
months. Part of the time was spent in the hospital in St. Louis. He was able to
return in January 1862 and was detailed as president of a military commission
on February 1. The commission was dissolved on March 30, and he was assigned to command on April 10. His promotion as major general dated from
November. On September 10, 1863, he was sick with dysentery and confined to
his bed. Unable to stay in the saddle and having to be transported in an ambulance, he was compelled to turn over his command on September 15. The next
day he was taken to Nashville by rail and did not return until October. At
Jonesborough on September 1, 1864, Stanley sustained a slight but very painful
contusion in his left groin. Although he was sick, he was on the field at Franklin
on November 30 when his horse was killed. He had no sooner returned to his
feet after being thrown to the ground when he received a musket ball in the
back of his neck. The ball passed transversely through the skin and the

integuments of the posterior and inferior part of his neck and emerged about three inches from the point of entrance. He obtained a remount and remained on the field and in command. After arriving at Nashville, he turned over the command on December 2 and took a sick leave. Although his general health was good, by late December there was localized inflammation and suppuration of the wound. Stanley took command of the Fourth Army Corps on January 31, 1865. In July 1866, following the war, he was commissioned colonel of the 22nd Infantry. At Fort Clark, Texas, in May 1882, he was treated in his quarters for inflammation of the stomach and returned to duty in six days. After serving on the western frontier, Stanley was retired for age in 1892. Died March 13, 1902, in Washington, D.C., and was buried in the Soldiers' Home cemetery in that city. According to the attending surgeon, he died from chronic interstitial nephritis.[1]

1. CSR; OR, vol. 30, pt. 1:35, 126, 150, 152, 343, 349, 353, 889, 892, pt. 3:589, 605, 637, 653, 689; vol. 45, pt. 1:112–18, 152, 353; vol. 49, pt. 1:19; U.S. Army, CWS, roll 2, vol. 3, report 13, pp. 255–59; West-Stanley-Wright Family Papers, David S. Stanley folder, USAMHI; WPCHR, vols. 606, 607, 608; LR, ACP, 6571, 1880, fiche: 000183; David S. Stanley, Personal Memoirs of Major-General D. S. Stanley, 45, 52, 79–80, 84, 183; RAGO, entry 534.

GEORGE JERRISON STANNARD • Born October 20, 1820, in Georgia, Vermont. He worked at a St. Albans foundry in Vermont and was colonel of a militia regiment in 1860. In June 1861 he was made lieutenant colonel of the 2nd Vermont, and in July 1862 he was made colonel of the 9th Vermont. While in the field in 1862 he developed piles. In March 1863 he was promoted to brigadier general of volunteers. Near the end of the fight at Gettysburg on July 3 he was wounded in his right thigh by a shell fragment. He did not leave the field until nightfall. The next day his wound became so painful that he had to retire. He proceeded to Washington, D.C., where he remained for a short time, then was granted a leave to return to Vermont. Stannard reported back in September for duty that would not require him to ride a horse. He commanded troops in New York City harbor and New York City from September 9 to May 1864. At Cold Harbor on June 3 he received two slight wounds in the left thigh but did not leave the field. In July at Petersburg he received a gunshot wound of the second finger of his left hand. He spent August in the U.S. general hospital in Burlington, Vermont, and returned to duty on September 15. At Fort Harrison on September 30, 1864, a musket ball shattered the bone of his right arm above the elbow. The arm was amputated that evening in a field hospital. After a sick leave, he was ordered in January 1865 to report for such duties as could be assigned to him during his convalescence. He continued to serve in the Department of the East until the close of the war. Following his resignation from the army in 1867, Stannard was appointed collector of customs for the District of Vermont. The piles that had developed during the war continued to bother him, and in 1884 he had an attack of severe rheumatic pain with the loss of flesh, strength, and the ability to sleep. For the last four years of his life he was doorkeeper of the House of Representatives.[1] Died June 1, 1886, in Washington, D.C., and was buried in Lake View Cemetery, Burlington.

1. *OR*, vol. 27, pt. 1:262, 353; vol. 29, pt. 2:164; vol. 36, pt. 1:88; vol. 42, pt. 1:134, 801, pt. 2:1137, 1143, pt. 3:984; vol. 46, pt. 2:159; vol. 51, pt.1:1255–62; *MSHW*, vol. 2, pt. 2:712; RVA, Pension WC 225,375; U.S. Army, CWS, roll 2, vol. 3, report 45, pp. 1287–98; RAGO, entry 534.

JOHN CONVERSE STARKWEATHER • *Born on May 11, 1830,* in Cooperstown, New York. Starting in 1858, he had annual attacks of rheumatism that on some occasions would render him totally unfit for periods of three or four months. He had a law practice at Milwaukee, and in May 1861 he was made colonel of the 1st Wisconsin Infantry, a three-month regiment. In October the unit was mustered back in service for three years. While being transported by steamboat from Jeffersonville, Indiana, to the mouth of the Salt River on November 16, 1861, Starkweather was exposed to a bad storm. He contracted a cold that resulted in bronchitis and acute rheumatism. Following this illness, he developed chronic lung disease and had episodes of pulmonary hemorrhage. In January 1862 he had a similar attack of rheumatism and was so incapacitated that he had to leave his regiment for about six weeks. Again in January 1863 he suffered from rheumatism and neuralgia. He continued to perform his duties, but on March 5 his surgeon advised him to leave his command to recover his health. A surgeon's certificate in June, to be used either for a leave of absence or for a resignation, stated that for months he had suffered from rheumatism, neuralgia, and diarrhea. The exposure during two years' service had reduced his condition to "barely a life sustaining point," according to his surgeon. Starkweather did not enjoy food and lacked an appetite. His rest was disordered and night sweats prostrated him. He did not respond to ordinary remedies prescribed by the surgeon; they even seemed to make his depression worse. Only by the use of stimulants was he able to discharge the lightest camp duties. In July he was promoted to brigadier general of volunteers. On the morning of September 20, 1863, at the Battle of Chickamauga, he was slightly wounded in the left leg. He remained on the field in full command until the next day, when the army returned to Chattanooga and he went on leave. Supposedly from overexertion of his voice during the battle he had hemorrhage from his lungs. On October 9 he was back in command. Because of his poor health he was placed on court-martial duty in July 1864, and he resigned in May 1865. Following a short period practicing law in Milwaukee, he moved to Washington, D.C. He continued to suffer with his lung disease and rheumatism. Died November 15, 1890, at his residence in Washington, D.C., and was buried in Forest Home Cemetery, Milwaukee, Wisconsin.[1]

DEATH CERTIFICATE: Cause of death, primary, phthisis pulmonalis and vesica urinaria (urinary bladder); immediate, exhaustion. Duration of last illness, three weeks.

1. CSR; *OR*, vol. 30, pt. 1:280, pt. 4:337; LR, ACP, 1950, 1875, fiche: 000184; U.S. Army, CWS, roll 2, vol. 3, report 1, pp. 27–84; ibid., roll 5, vol. 8, report 12, pp. 619–29; RVA, Pension WC 287,153.

JAMES BLAIR STEEDMAN • *Born July 29, 1817,* in Northumberland County, Pennsylvania. He served in the Texas army during the Mexican War. Prior to the Civil War he was a printer, Ohio legislator, and owner of a newspaper. He was made colonel of the 14th Ohio in the summer of 1861 and brigadier general in July 1862. At Chickamauga on September 20, 1863, he was severely bruised when his horse was killed. However, he was able to remain on the field during the day. He was promoted to major general in April 1864 and resigned in August 1866.[1] He was collector of internal revenue at New Orleans, and after moving to Toledo, he was a newspaper editor and politician. At the time of his death he was a captain of police. Died October 18, 1883, at his residence in Toledo, Ohio, and was buried in Woodlawn Cemetery.

DEATH CERTIFICATE: Cause of death, immediate, pneumonia of two weeks' duration.

1. *OR,* vol. 30, pt. 1:855.

FREDERICK STEELE • *Born January 14, 1819,* in Delhi, New York. He graduated from the USMA in 1843. Served in the Mexican War. He had duty on the frontier and had risen to major by 1861. Appointed colonel of the 8th Iowa Volunteers in September, he was promoted to brigadier general in January 1862. After the war he was appointed colonel of the 20th Infantry, and in 1867 was mustered out of volunteer service. He died on January 12, 1868, at San Mateo, California. His death was caused by a sudden attack of apoplexy; he had been in good health the day before.[1] He was buried in Woodlawn Memorial Park, Colma, California.

1. *San Francisco Alta California,* Jan. 13, 1868.

ISAAC INGALLS STEVENS • *Born on March 25, 1818,* at Andover, Massachusetts. He graduated from the USMA in 1839. He was wounded September 13, 1847, at Chapultepec, Mexico. In 1853 he resigned his army commission and became governor of the Washington Territory. He was elected territorial delegate to Congress in 1856 but was defeated for reelection in 1860 when he joined the proslavery national ticket. In spite of his political orientation he was appointed colonel of the 79th New York regiment in July 1861 and brigadier general of volunteers in September 1861. He had a severe attack of bilious fever from which he recovered slowly. At the battle of Chantilly on September 1, 1862, after passing by his wounded son, Stevens took the flag and ran in front of his troops. He was killed by a bullet through his brain and died still holding the colors.[1] His remains were buried in the Island Cemetery, Newport, Rhode Island.

1. *OR,* vol. 12, pt. 2:48, 86, 261; pt. 3:588, 797, 805; Heitman, *Historical Register and Dictionary* 2:37; Steiner, *Disease,* 74; Henry Steele Commanger, ed., *The Blue and the Gray* 2:191.

JOHN DUNLAP STEVENSON • *Born June 8, 1821,* in Staunton, Virginia. Served in the Mexican War. He participated in Stephen W. Kearny's invasion of New Mexico in August 1846. A practicing lawyer in St. Louis and a politician, he was appointed colonel of the 7th Missouri (Union) in June 1861. His promotion to brigadier general ranked from November 1862. He served at Shiloh, Corinth, and Vicksburg. Made colonel of the 38th Infantry in 1869, he was discharged from the army in December 1870 and returned to his law practice. He died on January 22, 1897, at St. Louis and was buried there in the Bellefontaine Cemetery. Burial certificate: Cause of death, chronic nephritis.

THOMAS GREELY STEVENSON • *Born February 3, 1836,* in Boston, Massachusetts. He was involved with local militia affairs from an early age, and in the spring of 1861 he was orderly sergeant of the New England Guards. Upon the organization of the 4th Battalion of Massachusetts Infantry he was elected a company captain. In December 1861 he became colonel of the 24th Massachusetts. His promotion to brigadier general of volunteers ranked from March 1863. Stevenson had two leaves on surgeon's certificates of disability. The first, from September 15 to October 19, 1863, was due to malarial fever. The second was an extended leave from January through March 1864 because of chronic diarrhea. On the morning of May 10, 1864, in front of Spotsylvania Court House, he was instantly killed when a sharpshooter's bullet hit him in the head.[1] He was buried in Mount Auburn Cemetery, Cambridge, Massachusetts.

1. *OR,* vol. 36, pt. 1:147, 191, 325, 916, 941, 944; U.S. Army, CWS, roll 1, vol. 2, report 33, pp. 483–89; RAGO, entry 534.

JAMES HUGHES STOKES • *Born June 1815,* in Hagerstown, Maryland. There is some question concerning both the date and location of his birth. He graduated from the USMA in 1835. At the military academy he was treated for nausea and headaches twice each, and one time each for a sore throat, bruise, wound, fever, boil, and tonsillitis. Served in the Florida wars. While Stokes was in Florida, he had a sick leave because of gastroenteritis and severe dysentery and went north from July to September 9, 1841. Markedly emaciated and broken down, he recovered slowly. Following his leave, he was on duty at Buffalo, New York, from September 1841 to April 1843, when his dysentery returned and he developed inflammation of the prostate. The severe intestinal problem, according to his physician brother, led to the inflammation of his prostate. When he was ordered to return to Florida in 1843, he resigned his commission because of ill health. He moved to New York in 1844, but as a result of his continued illness he was compelled by the physician to dispose of his business. The doctors stated that he had been poorly treated in Florida by having been given excessive amounts of arsenic for the ague and fever. Unable to support his family without an occupation, and trying to recover his health, Stokes moved to Connecticut and finally to Illinois. From 1858 until 1861 he was an executive of the Illinois Central Railroad. He volunteered for the army in 1862, although in ill health, and was mustered in as a captain of the "Chicago Board of Trade Battery" in July. During the war he had at least two attacks of inflammation of the prostate, once while at Nashville and once later at New Orleans. He was in the major battles in the west from Perryville to Chattanooga. After being in the saddle day and night pursuing Wheeler's cavalry, he developed a right inguinal hernia. Appointed brigadier general of volunteers in July 1865, he was mustered out of Federal service in August. After the war, the sight in his right eye was destroyed, and there was inflammation of the optic nerve of the left eye with an associated decreased vision. Until 1880 he was engaged in the real estate business in Chicago. His hernia was aggravated by having to strain to pass his urine. By 1887, because of the loss of his eyesight and his continued poor health, he was unable to work.[1] Died in a boarding house in New York on December 27, 1890, and was buried in Washington Street Cemetery, Geneva, New York.

DEATH CERTIFICATE: Cause of death, pneumonia.

1. WPCHR, vols. 601, 602, 603; RVA, Pension WO 501,260.

CHARLES JOHN STOLBRAND • *Born on May 11, 1821,* near Kristianstad, Sweden. During the Schleswig-Holstein campaign of 1848–50 he took part in the defense of Denmark against the Prussian intervention. In the early 1850s he came to the United States and settled in Chicago. Stolbrand organized an artillery company and was promoted from captain to major in December 1861. On March 31, 1862, near Union City, Missouri, he was unable to ride because of a contusion received when he fell from his horse. However, he was still able to follow the artillery advance. In 1865 he was promoted to brigadier general of volunteers and was mustered out in January 1866.[1] After the war he moved to South Carolina, where he entered politics and held various state and federal positions. Died February 3, 1894, at Charleston, South Carolina, and was buried in Arlington National Cemetery.

DEATH CERTIFICATE: Cause of death, primary, influenza (grippe); immediate, passive congestion of right lung.

1. *OR,* vol. 8:117.

CHARLES POMEROY STONE • *Born September 30, 1824,* in Greenfield, Massachusetts. Graduated from the USMA in 1845. Served in the Mexican War. During a climb of the volcano Popocatepelt in Mexico, he, along with other officers, developed snow blindness and had to be taken down the mountain with his eyes bandaged. In July 1847, Stone was not completely well but had nearly recovered from some nonspecified illness. He resigned from the army in 1856 and surveyed the state of Sonora for the Mexican government. He was appointed colonel of the 14th Regular Infantry and brigadier general of volunteers in May 1861. Blamed for the disaster at Ball's Bluff, he was arrested in February 1862 and imprisoned without a trial. He was confined at Fort Lafayette where his limited cell space prevented him from obtaining adequate exercise. Finally released in August, Stone was not assigned back to duty until 1863. He resigned in September 1864.[1] After the war he served in the Army of the Khedive of Egypt for thirteen years. Died January 24, 1887, while on a visit to New York City and was buried at West Point.

DEATH CERTIFICATE: Chief cause, pneumonia, five days' duration; contributing, asthenia.

1. *OR*, vol. 42, pt. 2:143, 370; vol. 48, pt. 1:1102; ser. 2, vol. 3:373, 380; Henry Heath, *The Memoirs of Henry Heath*, 64–65; B. Huger to wife, July 19, Aug. 3, 1847, UV.

GEORGE STONEMAN • *Born on August 22, 1822,* in Busti, New York. Graduated from the USMA in 1846. Served in the Mexican War. In the 1850s he developed hemorrhoids and had an unsuccessful operation while serving in Texas. At the start of the Civil War he was promoted from captain to major. After duty on Gen. George B. McClellan's staff, Stoneman was made chief of cavalry of the Army of the Potomac and promoted to brigadier general of volunteers to rank from August 1861. In May 1862 he remained in the saddle although ill. The following month he took a sick leave and returned on July 5. He was made major general to rank from November 1862. By June 1863 he was having a copious loss of blood from his hemorrhoids and was being treated by a surgeon at West Point. An anesthetic process and applications of some type appeared to provide some relief. He stated that part of the poor performance on his raid in 1864 was due to his prostration from blood loss. Following arduous horseback riding in March and April 1865, he developed a prolapsed anus. When he walked or stood much, he assumed a bent posture to prevent the anal tissue from protruding. Some type of appliance was used to help prevent its protrusion. Following the war he was appointed colonel of the 21st Infantry. In September 1868 in Richmond, Virginia, he had surgery by former Confederate surgeon Dr. Hunter McGuire, who was assisted by two army surgeons. After it became obvious that the operation had not been successful, the surgeons stated that it was not possible to produce a permanent cure. Relief could only be obtained by a life of rest and quiet in a cool climate, and remaining in a reclining posture as much as possible. In 1871, when he was retired for disability, the examining board had an interesting discussion of his disability and whether it qualified as a wound. The medical board expressed the opinion that his hemorrhoids and anal prolapse were frequently wounded by the saddle in the line of duty, thus meeting the definition of the law. Others did not agree.[1] Died

September 5, 1894, at Buffalo, New York, and was buried in Lakewood, New York.

DEATH CERTIFICATE: Cause, paresis; contributing, exposure and hardships of army life.

1. *OR*, vol. 51, pt. 1:725; LR, ACP, 3414, 1871, fiche: 000185; *Battles and Leaders* 2:430, 433.

EDWIN HENRY STOUGHTON • *Born June 23, 1838*, in Chester, Vermont. He graduated from the USMA in 1859. While a cadet he was treated for catarrhus seven times, neuralgia five times, odontalgia and diarrhea each four times, colica three times, cephalalgia twice, and phlegmon, tonsillitis, and clavus each once. In March 1861 he resigned his commission and in September was appointed colonel of the 4th Vermont. During July and August 1862 he was absent sick. He was promoted brigadier general of volunteers in November 1862. However, Confederate John S. Mosby captured him in March 1863; as a result, his appointment as general was not confirmed by the Senate. He saw no more duty after he was exchanged in May.[1] He moved to New York City and practiced the law. Died in New York on December 25, 1868, and was buried in Immanuel Cemetery, Rockingham, Vermont.

1. CSR; WPCHR, vol. 609.

GEORGE CROCKETT STRONG • *Born October 16, 1832*, in Stockbridge, Vermont. He graduated from the USMA in 1857. While at the military academy, Strong was treated for odontalgia six times, clavus, cephalalgia, catarrhus, excoriatio, and hemorrhoids three times each, nausea twice, and colica and vulnus incisum one time each. Breveted a second lieutenant of ordnance, he had duty at a number of arsenals before the Civil War. He served as an ordnance officer for Gens. Irvin McDowell and George B. McClellan and in September 1861 was assigned to Gen. Benjamin F. Butler's staff as a major of volunteers. During the summer of 1862 he was in poor health, and in October Gen. Benjamin F. Butler reported that Strong was still not fully recovered. His promotion to brigadier general of volunteers ranked from November 1862. In the attack on Battery Wagner on July 18, 1863, he was wounded in the right thigh by a shell. Asked by Gen. Quincy A. Gillmore if it was a bad wound, Strong replied that it was only a severe flesh wound near the hip. He was admitted to the USA hospital steamer, *Cosmopolitan,* and was taken to the general hospital at Beaufort, South Carolina, where he was well attended. However, he wanted to go home and without permission took a steamer for the North. He developed lockjaw and died soon after reaching New York City on July 30, 1863.[1] He was buried in Green-Wood Cemetery in Brooklyn.

1. CSR; *OR*, vol. 15:160; vol. 28, pt. 1:16, 77, pt. 2:31; WPCHR, vol. 609; RVA, Pension WC 49,289; RAGO, entry 534; *Battles and Leaders* 4:59–60.

WILLIAM KERLEY STRONG • *Born April 30, 1805,* in Duanesburg, New York. He retired at an early age after becoming rich as a wool merchant. When the Civil War started, Strong went to France to purchase weapons for the Union. In September 1861, President Lincoln commissioned him a brigadier general. During the war he held various district commands and had duty on commissions. In late 1863, while driving in New York City's Central Park, he was thrown from his carriage and was so severely injured that he was paralyzed for the remainder of his life. On October 10, 1863, he was given sick leave.[1] He had an attack of apoplexy on February 28 and died March 16, 1867, in New York City. He was buried in Green-Wood Cemetery, Brooklyn.

DEATH CERTIFICATE: Cause of death, sanguineous apoplexy. Secondary, inanition.

1. U.S. Army, CWS, roll 1, vol. 2, report 8, pp. 87–92; Warner, *Generals in Blue,* 484.

DAVID STUART • *Born March 12, 1816,* in Brooklyn, New York. A lawyer, he served one term in Congress from Michigan. When the Civil War started he lived in Chicago and was solicitor for the Illinois Central Railroad. In July 1861 he was commissioned lieutenant colonel of the 42nd Illinois Infantry, and the following October was made colonel of the 55th Illinois. At Shiloh on April 6, 1862, Stuart was wounded in the shoulder. He turned over his command and went to the landing to have his injury examined. He returned to the field the next day, but compelled to leave because of the wound, he gave up his command. Although appointed brigadier general in November 1862, his promotion was rejected by the Senate in March 1863. He resigned the following April.[1] Returning to civilian life, he practiced law in Detroit and New Orleans. Died September 11, 1868, in Detroit, Michigan, and was buried in Elmwood Cemetery, Detroit. Burial records: Cause of death, paralysis.

1. *OR,* vol. 10, pt. 1:104, 251–53, 259, 305.

FREDERICK SHEARER STUMBAUGH • *Born on April 14, 1817,* near Shippensburg, Pennsylvania. He developed rheumatism in 1852, which continued to affect him over the years. In 1854 he became a lawyer and took part in local militia affairs. After entering Federal service in a three-month regiment, Stumbaugh was appointed colonel of the 77th Pennsylvania in October 1861. He was treated in camp for an episode of diarrhea in January 1862. In August during the march from Battle Creek, Tennessee, he had a violent attack of diarrhea that prostrated him so that he had to be put in an ambulance. After a few days' rest at Nashville, he returned to his command. However, the diarrhea continued, and in October, following the onset of severe rheumatism, his health deteriorated further. He received treatment for one night at a Louisville hospital and the next day requested to continue his treatment in the Louisville Hotel. Finally, in

November he managed to return to his home in Pennsylvania. Stumbaugh was appointed brigadier general of volunteers to rank from November 1862 but his appointment was revoked by the Senate. His medical problems continued and he became debilitated. In May 1863 he was discharged from the service and returned to his legal practice in Pennsylvania. He had some relief from his rheumatism in the summer of 1867 he stated, because he had drunk the water of the Gettysburg springs. By 1889 he had almost constant episodes of diarrhea and rheumatism and received various medications from his local druggist and from his physician's office. He found that abstinence from drinking fluids relieved his diarrhea. For several years Stumbaugh was often so weak and debilitated that he was unable to stand up longer than fifteen to twenty minutes at a time, and he could not practice the law. He died in Topeka, Kansas, on February 25, 1897, while playing chess in his office just after being checkmated. He was buried in Topeka Cemetery. Burial record: Cause of death, paralysis.[1]

1. CSR; RVA, Pension SC 463,919; *Topeka Daily Capital,* Feb. 26, 1897; Topeka City Clerk.

SAMUEL DAVIS STURGIS • *Born June 11, 1822,* in Shippensburg, Pennsylvania. He graduated from the USMA in 1846. Served in the Mexican War and was a prisoner during February 1847. He had duty on the frontier; when the Civil War started, he was in command at Fort Smith, Arkansas. After taking his troops to Fort Leavenworth, he was promoted to major. His promotion to brigadier general of volunteers ranked from August 1861. Although too sick to give testimony during an inquiry on July 1, 1864, he appeared at the inquiry the next day. Mustered out of the volunteers in August 1865, Sturgis reverted to his rank of lieutenant colonel of the 6th Cavalry. He was sick in Austin, Texas, from February 1 to March 3, 1867. He developed an acute and continuous pain in his right side in October 1872, reported to be due to torpidity of the liver. From October 29, 1877, to February 28, 1878, he had sick leave and went to Hot Springs, Arkansas, for the waters. In addition, in December 1877 he developed sciatic trouble that his surgeon stated would increase if he returned North. He had an ulcerated throat and general prostration and required a sick leave from March 17 to April 10, 1886. The surgeon who saw him in the spring of 1886 went into his past history and speculated that he had a nephritic disorder that had developed during the Indian campaign in 1876–77. He was retired for age in 1886. Died September 28, 1889, in St. Paul, Minnesota, and was buried in Arlington National Cemetery. According to the attending physician, he died from diabetes.[1]

1. *OR,* vol. 39, pt. 1:155; LR, ACP, 1398, 1881, fiche: 000186; RVA, Pension C 315,785.

JEREMIAH CUTLER SULLIVAN • *Born on October 1, 1830,* at Madison, Indiana. He graduated from the U.S. Naval Academy in 1841 and served in the U.S. Navy until he resigned in April 1854. After duty as a captain of a three-month regiment, he was made colonel of the 13th Indiana in the summer of 1861. His promotion to brigadier general of volunteers ranked from April 1862. Seriously contused by a shell splinter on October 3, 1862, at Corinth, he gave up his command. When the fighting became general the next day he got out of his bed and took command. On June 5, 1864, near Piedmont, West Virginia, his horse was killed and he was violently thrown to the ground. His right hand was broken by his sword hilt, his head injured, and he was badly ruptured. The rupture was sustained when he was thrown forward on the metal ornament of his Mexican saddle. His hand was bandaged on the field and required a bandage for a month. The next day he was carried by ambulance into Staunton and was unable to perform his duties. Not able to ride on horseback for any length of time, he had to be transported by ambulance. His resignation was accepted in May 1865. After the war he was unemployed or held minor clerical jobs. Died October 21, 1890, in Oakland, California, and was buried there in Mountain View Cemetery. Burial records: Cause of death, apoplexy.[1]

   1. *OR*, vol. 17, pt. 1:207, 227, 230, 232; vol. 37, pt. 1:613; RVA, Pension WC 306,730.

ALFRED SULLY • *Born May 22, 1820,* in Philadelphia. He graduated from the USMA in 1841. While at West Point he was treated for headache four times, cold three times, wound and toothache twice each, and swollen face, sore fingers, cholera morbus, catarrhus, bruise, hemorrhoids, nausea, and swollen feet one time each. Served in the Florida and Mexican wars. Before the Civil War he served on the frontier and was sick with varying medical problems: November 20 to December 8, 1843, catarrhal fever; February 13–18, 1845, diagnosis not stated; July 26–31, 1846, morbi. varii. After making the trip around Cape Horn from the East and arriving in Monterey, California, Sully had a fever in early 1849. In the middle of the year he was unable to go with a hunting detail from Benicia, California, because infected flea bites on his legs made walking too painful. During the summer of 1853, after a trip up the Sacramento River, he developed fever and chills like most of his men. His surgeon told him that "none who pass through the valley of the Sacramento ever escape it," yet cured him in a few days with quinine. In September 1856 Sully was treated for hemorrhoids. During September and in November 1857 he was sick again, but the diagnosis was not available. After he reported with his company to the commander of the City Guard in Washington in November 1861, he stated he was unable to do field duty because of rheumatism. He was appointed colonel of the 1st Minnesota in March 1862. A bullet grazed his ear on June 1 at Fair Oaks but did little damage. On the night of June 29 during the Seven Days' battles he was unwell and remained behind. He sent his staff orders to send for him if they became engaged. Soon afterward the battle opened on the field, and he tried to rally the men who were retreating. He was commissioned brigadier general of volunteers in September 1862. Sick, he quartered himself with a Virginia family for a few days in early

November. At the Battle of Fredericksburg on December 12, 1862, he was grazed on the leg, but it was so minor he did not consider it a wound. The last of January 1863, he obtained a leave to go to Philadelphia for surgical treatment because of prolapsus ani produced by excessive exertion. Apparently, he had some type of procedure and returned about the first week in March. Ordered to the Department of the Northwest in Milwaukee in May, he continued to suffer poor health. For the rest of the war he primarily fought against the Indians in Minnesota and the Dakotas. Sick with rheumatism and dysentery, he was unable to mount his horse and had to ride in a wagon during the Indian expedition of August 1864. From August 22 to December 1864 he was absent on sick leave. He remained in the army and reverted to his rank of major of infantry. During his pursuit of the Indians in 1869, he still had to travel in an ambulance. From March 14–29, 1873, he had inflammation of his bowels, and from April 2–23, 1873, he had chronic diarrhea. On May 10 he wrote from Baton Rouge and requested six months' leave on surgeon's certificate. He was debilitated from chronic malarial poisoning attended by diarrhea. From June to December 11, 1873, he was given a sick leave. In February 1874, while en route to Fort Vancouver, Washington, he became ill with remittent fever, diarrhea, and debility. Although not on sick report and able to attend to his duties, Sully was not in good enough health to travel across the Plains, and he did not report to his regiment until May. While at Vancouver Barracks he was given sick leave starting April 21, 1879. Ill with quotidian intermittent fever, he died suddenly from arterial hemorrhage resulting in cardiac paralysis on April 27, 1879, at Fort Vancouver. The first hemorrhage was slight and had occurred on the twenty-fourth. It was followed by others of increased severity, although the intervals between hemorrhages decreased. An autopsy revealed the hemorrhage was due to a perforation of the descending aorta by a chronic ulcer of the esophagus. The ulcer involved all of the esophageal coats, causing infiltration of its tissues an inch above and below, including nearly the whole of its circumference. The condition had evidently existed for some time though no symptoms sufficient to lead to a correct diagnosis were apparent. The dissection of the ulcer was from the esophagus downward so that its aortic orifice (quarter of an inch in diameter) was half an inch below the esophageal opening, which was larger and irregularly defined. Owing to the greater obstruction by infiltration of the esophageal tissues above, the hemorrhages from the mouth were never very large and most of the blood passed by way of the intestines. All the thoracic and abdominal organs were healthy. No microscopic findings were reported but the degree of gross infiltration reported is suspicious of a malignancy.[1] He was finally buried in Laurel Hill Cemetery, Philadelphia.

1. *OR*, vol. 11, pt. 2:87; vol. 21:264, 268; vol. 22, pt. 2:277, 288; WPCHR, vol. 604; LR, ACP, 727, 1874, fiche: 000187; U.S. Army, CWS, roll 1, vol. 1, report 23, pp. 311–30; RVA, Pension WC 946,506; Langdon Sully, *No Tears for the General*, 34, 50, 101, 137, 149, 158, 190, 217–19, 231.

EDWIN VOSE SUMNER · *Born January 30, 1797,* in Boston, Massachusetts. He was wounded April 17, 1847, at Cerro Gordo, Mexico, but was only disabled for a few days. While on garrison duty on the frontier he had a severe attack of indigestion from drinking alkaline water. To the surprise of his troops, he showed up for reveille the next day. Sumner had a distinguished record before the war. He was made colonel of the 1st Cavalry in 1855 and in 1861 was appointed a brigadier general in the Regular Army. In late December 1861, outside of Alexandria, Virginia, his horse stepped into a blind posthole and threw him forward to the ground when it fell. His shoulder and lungs were injured, but he remounted the horse and rode back to camp. In December and January 1862 he was absent sick in Washington, D.C. When he returned in March he slept in a nearby house and not in his Sibley tent. At Glendale on June 30, 1862, he was struck twice by spent balls—once on the arm and once on the hand—but did not leave the field. In October 1862, Gen. George B. McClellan reported that because of Sumner's age, his state of health, and the many exposures he had undergone, it was doubtful if he could stand the fatigues of another campaign. Sumner was assigned to the Department of Missouri at St. Louis, but he had to stop at Syracuse, New York, because he became ill. A physician saw him on March 16, 1863, and he was laboring under an active state of fever and congestion of the lungs. The disease continued without abatement until his death.[1] Died March 21, 1863, at Syracuse and was buried there in Oakwood Cemetery.

1. CSR; *OR,* vol. 19, pt. 2:483–84; vol. 22, pt. 2:167; vol. 25, pt. 2:568; *OR Suppl.,* vol. 2:87; RVA, Pension C 37,248; Heitman, *Historical Register and Dictionary* 2:38; Howard, *Autobiography* 1:181–83, 190–91, 194; Wilcox, *Mexican War,* 284, 618.

WAGER SWAYNE · *Born November 10, 1834,* in Columbus, Ohio. Practicing law in Ohio when the war started, he was made major of the 43rd Ohio in August 1861. In late May 1862 he was absent sick and returned in June. He was promoted to lieutenant colonel in December 1861 and colonel in October 1862. At River's Bridge, South Carolina, on February 2, 1865, a piece of shell struck him on the right knee. Gen. O. O. Howard saw him being carried back on a stretcher and in great pain. He found a large pinecone and used it to support the fractured leg. Swayne was taken to an old barn on the bluff where, with the wind blowing through and lighted by two tallow candles, he was laid upon a carpenter's bench to undergo amputation. A primary flap amputation in the lower third of the femur was performed. On the thirteenth there was hemorrhage from the face of the stump, and he underwent an operation that day during which a small artery was ligated. Swayne's promotion as brigadier general ranked from March 1865, and toward the end of the year he was selected to direct the Freedmen's Bureau in Alabama. In 1866 he was commissioned colonel of the 45th Regular Infantry. He was retired from active service July 1, 1870, because of his amputated leg. After returning to civilian life he practiced law in Toledo and New

York. Died December 18, 1902, in New York City and was buried in Arlington National Cemetery. The assistant general's office reported he died from diabetic coma.[1]

1. CSR; *OR*, vol. 47, pt. 1;49, 194, 376, 387, 398; RVA, Pension WC 610,283; *MSHW*, vol. 2, pt. 3:255, 800; Howard, *Autobiography* 2:107; *MOLLUS* 22:164–65.

THOMAS WILLIAM SWEENY • *Born on December 25, 1820,* in County Cork, Ireland. He came to the United States at the age of twelve with his widowed mother. He joined the United States Army in 1846 and was wounded on the forehead at Contreras, Mexico, during a hand-to-hand fight with a Mexican lancer. At Churubusco on August 20, 1847, he was struck in the groin by a spent ball but remained on the field. Soon afterward he was wounded by a musket ball in the right arm above the elbow. Again he continued to lead his men until he had to be assisted off of the field because of exhaustion and loss of blood. An amputation of the arm was performed in the middle third. Sweeny returned to New York City in 1848 and was commissioned into the Regular Army as a lieutenant. During January through April he was on recruiting duty. He was sent to California in April 1849. In May 1852 he was severely wounded in the neck by an arrow during an engagement with the Yuma Indians in Cocopa County. At Wilson's Creek, August 10, 1861, he received a ball in his right thigh that remained there the rest of his life. The wound did not appear to heal, and about the first of September he received a leave and returned in a month. In January 1862 he was made colonel of the 52nd Illinois Infantry. At Shiloh on April 6, 1862, he was wounded, once in the fleshy part of his remaining left arm and once in the foot. His horse received eight balls, and Sweeny had to have assistance to mount another horse. On June 26, 1862, he received a sick leave because of his wounds; after two months he resumed brigade command. A spent ball struck him on the right leg without doing any harm at Corinth in October 1862. His promotion to brigadier general of volunteers ranked from November. He had a sick leave starting July 11, 1863, because of his wounds and did not return until September. After a fistfight with Gen. Grenville M. Dodge on July 25, 1864, Sweeny was relieved from duty but was later acquitted of the charges. He was dismissed from the service in December 1865 for being absent without leave, but he was restored with the rank of major in November 1866.[1] Following the war, he left Federal service to be involved with the Irish Fenian movement and their invasion into Canada. Restored to his former position in the army, he was placed on the retired list in May 1870 with the rank of brigadier general. Died April 10, 1892, in Astoria, New York, and was buried in Green-Wood Cemetery, Brooklyn.

DEATH CERTIFICATE: Cause of death, chief cause, Bright's disease; contributing, uremic convulsions. Duration, two years.

1. CSR; *OR,* vol. 3:70; vol. 10, pt. 1:101; vol. 17, pt. 1:276; U.S. Army, CWS, roll 5, vol. 9, report 31, pp. 861–944; William M. Sweeny, "Brigadier-General Thomas W. Sweeny, United States Army," *Journal of the American Irish Historical Society* 27 (1928): 257–69; Leslie Anders, "Fisticuffs at Headquarters: Sweeny vs. Dodge," *CWTI* 15 (Feb. 1977): 8–15.

GEORGE SYKES • *Born on October 9, 1822,* at Dover, Delaware. Graduated from the USMA in 1842. He was treated twice for a headache while at West Point. Fought in the Florida and Mexican wars. After duty on the frontier he was made major of the 14th Infantry in 1861 and brigadier general of volunteers in September 1861. Sykes was relieved in December 1863 because Gen. George G. Meade reported he acted too slowly during the Mine Run campaigns. On August 25, 1864, Sykes was to relieve Gen. Thomas J. McKean if his health would permit. He was unable to take the field on September 22. On the first of December 1864 he wrote that he had been at Fort Leavenworth since October 10 awaiting orders. His command had been given to another because Sykes's health was not considered equal to undertaking a campaign. He remained in the army and reverted to his rank of lieutenant colonel, 5th Infantry, in 1866. In 1868 he was made colonel, 20th Infantry. In late July of the same year, he had a short illness due to intermittent fever. Died February 8, 1880, at Fort Brown (Brownsville), Texas, and was buried at West Point. According to the assistant surgeon, the cause of death was cancer of the left side of his face.[1]

1. *OR,* vol. 41, pt. 2:862, pt. 3:315, pt. 4:741–42; LR, ACP, 4242, 1880, fiche: 000188; RAGO, entry 534.

T

GEORGE WILLIAM TAYLOR • *Born November 22, 1808,* in Hunterdon County, New Jersey. Served in the Mexican War. When the Civil War started, he was engaged in mining and the manufacture of iron. He was made colonel of the 3rd New Jersey, and his promotion to brigadier general ranked from May 1862. At Bull Run bridge on August 27, 1862, he was wounded in the left leg and taken from the field on a litter. He was next moved on a handcar, then taken to Alexandria. He was admitted to the Mansion House Hospital, Alexandria, thirteen hours after the injury. The ball had entered at the inner edge of the tibia, about six inches above the internal malleolus, passed directly through, and comminuted the bone very badly for about six inches above and below. It made two exit openings on the anterior and outer aspect of the leg about five inches above the external malleolus. Twenty-six hours after he was injured, the surgeon, using chloroform, amputated the lower limb at the middle third by the double flap method. Taylor lost considerable blood, and all the vessels required ligation.

His blood appeared to be very much "vitiated by the morbific influence of malaria." After the amputation it was determined that the fibula was not broken by the force of the ball but by the weight of the patient coming upon it suddenly when the support from the tibia was destroyed by its fracture. Taylor's arterial system did not fully react; his pulse, which was feeble, tremulous, and very irregular at times, evidently denoted a weakened condition of his system. He refused to take stimulants except sparingly. This condition continued until September 1, 1862, when he died at 4 A.M. The amputated parts were contributed to the Armed Forces Museum (Specimen 313, surgery, A.M.M.). The cause of death was exhaustion.[1] He was buried in Rock Church Cemetery, Hunterdon County.

1. CSR; OR, vol. 12, pt. 2:406, 408, pt. 3:698–99; MSHW, vol. 3, pt. 3:480, 491.

JOSEPH PANNELL TAYLOR • *Born May 4, 1796,* near Louisville, Kentucky. He was a second lieutenant of the 28th Infantry in 1813 during the war with Great Britain. He was appointed a second lieutenant in the artillery corps in May 1816. Served in the Mexican War. From November 1841 until September 1861 he was assistant commissary general of subsistence, with the rank of lieutenant colonel. He was made commissary general and in February 1863 was commissioned staff brigadier general. Died June 29, 1864, in Washington, D.C., and was buried in Oak Hill Cemetery, Georgetown, D.C. According to the attending surgeon, the cause of death was diarrhea and partial paralysis resulting from cerebral and general physical disability.[1]

1. CSR; RVA, Pension WC 43,774.

NELSON TAYLOR • *Born June 8, 1821,* in Norwalk, Connecticut. Served in California during the Mexican War. He remained in California after the war with Mexico and held various county and state positions until he returned to New York in the late 1850s to study law. When the Civil War started he entered Federal service as colonel of the 72nd New York and in September 1862 was made a brigadier general. Having been in bad health for some months and told that medicine would do him no good while in the field, he tendered his resignation, which was accepted January 19, 1863.[1] He returned to his law practice and took part in local and state politics. Died January 16, 1894, at South Norwalk, Connecticut, and was buried there in Riverside Cemetery. Interment record: Cause of death, pneumonia.

1. U.S. Army, CWS, roll 4, vol. 7, report 1, pp. 1–23.

WILLIAM RUFUS TERRILL • *Born April 21, 1834,* in Covington, Virginia. Graduated from the USMA in 1853. Terrill was on the sick list while at West Point with tonsillitis four times, catarrhus and diarrhea each three times, excoratio and contusion each twice, and clavus, colica, and cephalalgia each once. Served in the Florida wars. He had garrison and recruiting duty and was an instructor at the U.S. Military Academy before the Civil War. In May 1861 he was commissioned a captain in the 5th Regular Artillery. He served at Shiloh, Corinth, and Richmond, Kentucky. There was some question about his health in late August 1862. His promotion to brigadier general of volunteers ranked from September. At Perryville on October 8, 1862, he was struck in the side by a shell fragment that carried away a portion of his left lung. He died that night in a field hospital.[1] He was buried at West Point.

1. OR, vol. 16, pt. 1:1023, 1026, 1031, 1034, 1040–41, 1061, 1065, pt. 2:449; WPCHR, vols. 607, 608; P. E. Steiner. "Medical-Military Studies on the Civil War. 11, Brigadier General William R. Terrill, U.S.A., and Brigadier General James B. Terrill, C.S.A." Military Medicine 131 (1966): 178–82.

ALFRED HOWE TERRY · Born on November 10, 1827, in Hartford, Connecticut. He enlisted as a private in a militia organization known as the New Haven Grays and served with this unit from 1849 to 1856. From 1854 to 1860 he was a clerk of the New Haven County superior court. He was made a colonel of a three-month regiment at the start of the Civil War. On June 14, 1861, he not able to go with his troops because erysipelas, involving one foot, confined him to his quarters. He rejoined his regiment in Virginia on June 25, although still forced to prop his infected foot in a chair. Terry was at First Bull Run, and in August he was appointed colonel of the 7th Connecticut Regiment. On April 25, 1862, he was promoted to brigadier general of volunteers. For some reason while at Pulaski, Georgia, in May 1862, Terry did not eat, so he lost weight and was weak. By July he was so thin that his uniform hung on him. In November he was weakened by overexertion and looked ill. His sister came, took care of him, and fed him so that by December his health had improved. He was given a leave on surgeon's certificate on May 10, 1863, because for some months he had become debilitated and enervated from exposure to the malarious influences of the area. He went home to New Haven on sick leave and returned in June. In July he assumed command of U.S. forces at Morris Island, South Carolina. He had a bilious attack late in 1863, which continued into the next year. In May 1864 he was assigned to the command of the Tenth Corps. Early in June he had malaria and was unfit for duty. The next August he developed a large painful "Jobs" comforter (boil). In February 1865 he had a rapid succession of huge boils and carbuncles and was unable to stand or sit down because of the pain. He was commissioned a brigadier general in the Regular Army in January 1865. By mid-March he was in better health and had markedly improved by April. After the war he commanded the Department of Dakota. Terry was confined to the house with illness at St. Paul, Minnesota, in late August 1877. A sharp attack of sciatica detained him at Fort Snelling on March 31, 1884. Starting in May 1885, he was treated for Bright's disease by diet and reduced exposure to the elements. His general condition improved; although weak, he was able to perform all his duties at headquarters. Over the next year and a half he was nervous, could not eat, and had palpitations of his heart. An examination of his urine revealed large amounts of albumin and casts. In 1886 he was promoted to major general. From December 23, 1887, to January 20, 1888, Terry was under treatment in New York City by a physician and his brother, who was also a physician. The diagnosis was chronic interstitial nephritis and a gouty diathesis with pleural adhesions. He had considerable dyspnea, some enlargement of his heart, nervousness, sleeplessness, painful dyspepsia, and a cough. Urine albumin varied from a trace to 10 percent. According to his brother, using treatment of some unspecified type, the pleural adhesions were supposedly, in great measure, removed with marked relief of the dyspnea, cough, and dyspepsia and with some diminution of the cardiac enlargement. He applied for discharge on disability in 1888. According to the inspector general he died at a residence on December 16, 1890, in New Haven, Connecticut, from heart failure.[1] He was buried there in Grove Street Cemetery.

1. CSR; *OR*, vol. 36, pt. 2:348, pt. 3:743, 757; Carl William Marino, "General Alfred Howe Terry: Soldier from Connecticut" (diss.), 30, 40, 54, 57, 84, 159, 169, 195, 199, 262, 312, 314, 493, 525; U.S. Army, CWS, roll 1, vol. 2, report 29, pp. 449–55; LR, ACP, 567, 1876, fiche: 000061.

HENRY DWIGHT TERRY • *Born March 16, 1812,* in Hartford, Connecticut. Practicing law in Detroit when the Civil War started, he was commissioned colonel of the 5th Michigan Infantry in June 1861. During late 1861 he developed rheumatism from exposure to the elements, and the following year he was more or less disabled from pain in his limbs and body. From January through April he had diarrhea. At the Battle of Williamsburg, Virginia, on May 5, 1862, he received a slight wound from a spent ball and left the field for only ten minutes. He was in poor health during May, gave up regimental command early in June, and occupied an ambulance. His promotion as brigadier general ranked from July. In April and May 1863 he temporarily relinquished command of a division in the Sixth Corps because he could not undergo the fatigue of a long march during the extremely hot weather. Terry was at Gettysburg and in the Overland campaign and then commandant of the prison at Johnson's Island, Ohio. He resigned from the service in February 1865[1] and returned to his law practice. Died in Washington, D.C., on June 23, 1869, and was buried in Clinton Grove Cemetery, Mt. Clemens, Michigan, near Detroit.

DEATH CERTIFICATE: Cause of death, Bright's disease of the kidneys, four months' duration.

1. *OR*, vol. 11, pt. 1:505, 508; RVA, Pension WC 259,725.

JOHN MILTON THAYER • *Born January 24, 1820,* in Bellingham, Massachusetts. After practicing law in Massachusetts, Thayer moved to the Nebraska Territory in 1854. He was made the first brigadier general of the territorial militia when the Pawnee Indians became a problem to the white settlers. At the start of the Civil War he was appointed colonel of the 1st Nebraska. In October 1862 he was promoted to brigadier general but not confirmed by the Senate. He was reappointed to rank from March 1863 and confirmed. Thayer served at Forts Henry and Donelson, Vicksburg, and in Arkansas. In July 1865 his resignation was accepted. After the war Thayer was governor of Nebraska from 1886 until 1892. At Lincoln, Nebraska, in early March 1906 he became ill. He rallied in a few days and was able to go to town but became weaker and was confined to his bed. On March 18 he was dangerously ill, suffering from no specific disorder; rather, he seemed to be ill from the effects of old age. The next day he became unconscious and died. He was buried in the Wyuka Cemetery, Lincoln.[1] DEATH CERTIFICATE: Cause of death, old age.

1. *(Omaha) Morning World Herald,* March 19, 20, 1906.

GEORGE HENRY THOMAS • *Born on July 31, 1816,* in Southampton County, Virginia. Graduated from the USMA in 1840. While at West Point, Thomas was treated one time each for toothache, cold, inflamed eye, earache, diarrhea, and cholera morbus. Served in the Florida and Mexican wars. After fifteen years' duty with the artillery he was made a major in the 2nd Cavalry in 1855. While serving in the cavalry at Clear Fork on the Brazos River, Texas, on August 26, 1860, an Indian arrow hit his chin and went into his chest. Although in pain, he was able to withdraw the shaft. He had the wound dressed and continued on the field. On his way home in November 1860, Thomas was on the train from Richmond to Washington by way of Norfolk. When the train stopped to take on water, he stepped out on what he thought in the moonlight was the roadbed but was in fact a deep depression. He fell twenty feet or more and injured his back. In pain, he continued on to Norfolk where he remained for six weeks with his wife in attendance. He went to his home for further rest; although never fully recovered from his injury, he returned in January. In May 1861 he was promoted to lieutenant colonel and colonel. The following August he was made a brigadier general of volunteers, and his promotion to major general ranked from April 1862. Thomas served in the Shenandoah and at Mill Springs, Corinth, Perryville, and Stones River. Because of his actions at the Battle of Chickamauga, Thomas was made a brigadier general in the Regular Army in October 1863. He was at Chattanooga and commanded the Army of the Cumberland in the Atlanta campaign and at Franklin and Nashville. On

February 18, 1864, he reported that he could not take the field because the cold and damp weather had brought on an attack of neuralgia. His promotion to major general in the Regular Army ranked from December 1864. Weighing 175 pounds in 1850, he weighed 246 pounds at the end of the Civil War. He was ordered to take command of the Fifth Military District in August 1867, but his physician wired that he had a liver disorder and could not withstand the trip to New Orleans. In 1869 he was assigned to the command of the Division of the Pacific. Died in his office in San Francisco on March 28, 1870, and was buried in Oakwood Cemetery at Troy, New York. According to his wife and an attending physician, he died of apoplexy.[1]

1. *OR*, vol. 32, pt. 2:421; WPCHR, vol. 604; RVA, Pension WC 183,243; Heitman, *Historical Register and Dictionary* 2:38; Freeman Cleaves, *Rock of Chickamauga: The Life of General George H. Thomas*, 62–63, 66, 304–5; Frank A. Palumbo, *George Henry Thomas: The Dependable General*, 55–56; Jordan, *Winfield Scott Hancock*, 201; *MOLLUS* 10:398, 20:293.

HENRY GODDARD THOMAS • *Born April 4, 1837*, in Portland, Maine. A lawyer, he enlisted as a private in the 5th Maine in April 1861. The following June he was commissioned a captain. A surgeon's certificate from New Orleans reported that on the way across the gulf, Thomas had been sick while on shipboard. At the camp near Brashear City, Louisiana, in the summer of 1863, he developed malarial fever that became gastric and then typhoid. He was sent north in the latter part of June and was on sick leave in Portland, Maine, in July. That month his surgeon reported that Thomas was weak and exhausted from malarial fever, which had been followed by gastroenteritis and chronic diarrhea. He rejoined his regiment in September 1863. When he was ordered to return to Louisiana, he resigned his volunteer position. After recruiting and organizing Negro troops, he was commissioned colonel of the 79th U.S. Colored Infantry in March 1863 and colonel of the 19th Colored Infantry in January 1864. He served in the Overland campaign and at the Battle of the Crater. In November 1864 he was made a brigadier general of volunteers. After the war Thomas was mustered out of the volunteer service. Made a captain in the 11th Infantry in January 1866, he was appointed major of the 4th Infantry in 1876. In 1878 he transferred to the paymaster's department. He was assigned to Colorado, but he tolerated the weather there poorly. He had chronic eczema from 1880–82, and in 1882 he had neurasthenia. In January 1883 Thomas was under treatment for loss of "nervous force" and had frequent attacks of mental depression, which for several hours totally incapacitated him for duty. The physician attributed his condition to the mental stress of his position. Another physician made a report the next month in regard to his dental decay. He stated that the extensive decay—thirteen teeth already having been filled—was due to a systemic cause. Many other teeth required attention, and there was marked lithic diathesis.

"The excessive loss of phosphate which uniformly accompanied it was very apparent." He suggested rest and a change in climate—specifically, to the seashore. He told Thomas, "[This] will accomplish more than all the physicians, dentists or drugs in the state for the preservation of your teeth." A year later in February 1884, his surgeon stated that Thomas was suffering from serious derangement of his nervous system manifest by insomnia, confusion of thought, and impairment of memory and general vigor. The impaired nervous force was especially noted in his lack of efficiency and sexual appetite. He could not concentrate on any subject requiring close attention. The surgeon reported that his present condition was "clearly that of neurasthenia with defective assimilation and faulty elimination induced by too protracted residence in the altitude" at Denver, Colorado. Rest, along with no duty for six months and either a voyage or a visit to the seashore, was again recommended. Dr. William A. Hammond in May 1884 reported that Thomas was suffering from cerebral congestion of the passive type and required brain rest. In November 1884 he went to Paris, France, where Dr. C. E. Brown Sequard made a similar diagnosis. That same month he had a chronic dry nasal catarrh and an aggravated form of eczema of his entire face, neck, and lower extremities. There was an associated inflammation of one eye. The physician suggested rest and no duty for at least six months. In April 1885 he was back in Colorado and had eczema and cellulitis of his face, associated with edema of his eyelids and iritis. He was on sick leave in Portland, Maine, in 1889, and in December the physician reported a diagnosis of diabetes mellitus for the first time. His surgeon in November 1890 stated his neurasthenia, cerebritis, and diabetes were progressive and did not respond to treatment. He retired in July 1891. Died January 23, 1897, in Oklahoma City and was buried in Portland, Maine. According to a local retired army officer, the cause of death was a carbuncle.[1]

1. LR, ACP, 3426, 1871, fiche: 000190; U.S. Army, CWS, roll 6, vol. 10, report 35, pp. 279–85.

LORENZO THOMAS • *Born October 26, 1804,* in New Castle, Delaware. Graduated from the USMA in 1823. Served in the Florida and Mexican wars. From 1853 until 1861 he was chief of staff to the commander in chief, Gen. Winfield Scott, with the staff rank of lieutenant colonel. In August 1861 he was made adjutant general with the rank of brigadier general. Having had bad relations with the secretary of war, Thomas was sent to the military division of the Mississippi in 1863 to organize colored regiments. At Milliken's Bend, Louisiana, on April 12, 1863, he had diarrhea.[1] He retired from the army in 1869. Died in Washington, D.C., on March 2, 1875, and was buried in Oak Hill Cemetery, Georgetown.

DEATH CERTIFICATE: Cause of death, primary, debility. Immediate, congestion of the lungs, half hour duration.

1. *OR,* vol. 24, pt. 1:74.

STEPHEN THOMAS • *Born December 6, 1809,* in Bethel, Vermont. He was a well-known politician in Vermont before the war, having served in the legislature, as a state senator, as registrar, and as judge of the probate court of Orange County. In February 1862 he entered Federal service as a colonel of the 8th Vermont. The summer of 1862 he had diarrhea that continued more or less until the next summer, when he became very sick. In May, during the march to Port Hudson, Thomas had a bad throat; the physician made a diagnosis of diphtheria. While involved in the early siege of Port Hudson he had diarrhea, which took on a typhoid type causing great exhaustion. The surgeon tried to get him to go to the hospital but he refused until June 1863, when his condition became worse and he entered the regimental hospital. When he heard firing he got up and went back to duty. He returned to the hospital for a few days after the action was over. During this period he had almost constant nausea and no appetite. His weight, which had been 160 to 165 pounds, was reduced to 117 pounds. After the surrender of Port Hudson in July, Thomas marched with his brigade to a steamer, although he was emaciated and had diarrhea of a typhoid-malarious character. His pulse was intermittently irregular. When they arrived at Donalsonville, Louisiana, he helped his men off the boat until he became so weak that the physician had to assist him back on board. He went to New Orleans and was hospitalized at Hotel Dieu Hospital. From November 1863 until January 1, 1864, he was on recruiting duty in Vermont. He was better by February but still had diarrhea and a miasmatic condition of his system. By July he had become so deaf that he had to have his adjutant nearby to relay him orders. He developed rheumatism in the fall of 1864. Appointed brigadier general of volunteers in February 1865, he was discharged in August 1865. Thomas was lieutenant governor of Vermont during 1867–68 and United States pension agent from 1870 until 1877, when he took up farming. Supposedly he never recovered from the effects of his malaria, but he lived to the age of ninety-four years. The last year of his life he required the constant attention of a nurse or attendant.[1] Died in Montpelier, Vermont, on December 18, 1903, and was buried there in Green Mount Cemetery.

DEATH CERTIFICATE: Cause of death, senile decay.

1. RVA, Pension SC 277,638.

CHARLES MYNN THRUSTON • *Born February 22, 1798,* in Lexington, Kentucky. Graduated from the USMA in 1813. Served in the Florida wars. In August 1836 he resigned from the army and took up farming. He later became president of a bank. He was appointed a brigadier general of volunteers in September 1861. He resigned in April 1862 and returned to his farm. Died in February 18, 1873, on his farm near Cumberland, Maryland, and was buried in Rose Hill Cemetery.

WILLIAM BADGER TIBBITS · *Born March 31, 1837,* in Hoosick Falls, New York. He was commissioned captain in the 2nd New York Infantry in May 1861. At New Market Bridge on June 8, 1861, he was stunned and for a few minutes rendered insensible by the concussion from a nearby Confederate field piece. He was promoted to major in October 1862. Tibbits served on the Peninsula and at Second Bull Run and Fredericksburg. At Chancellorsville, May 4, 1863, he was slightly injured when he was hit in the groin by a ball. He left the service when his unit's two years of service ended in August and reentered in February as colonel of the 21st New York Cavalry. At Piedmont, Virginia, on June 5, 1864, he used a pistol because his wrist was weak and gave out soon after the fight commenced. Near Winchester on March 7, 1865, his horse fell with him; when thrown to the ground, he struck his head. He was delirious and depressed, but by the next morning, reason had partially returned. When convalescent, he was given leave and started for home on March 14. However, he returned and reported to duty on March 23. Outside of Millwood on April 18, his horse reared violently several times, and Tibbits threw himself off just as the horse fell over backwards. He fractured his wrist, which the surgeon set with such conveniences as he could procure. Tibbits turned over the command on April 19, and on April 23 he applied for and received a leave of absence. He returned May 4 to Washington, D.C. In October 1865 he was commissioned brigadier general and was mustered out in 1866.[1] Died February 10, 1880, in Troy, New York, and was buried in Oakwood Cemetery. Burial records: Cause of death, pneumonia.

1. CSR; *OR,* vol. 46, pt. 3:911; U.S. Army, CWS, roll 5, vol. 8, report 4, pp. 53–195; RAGO, entry 534.

DAVIS TILLSON · *Born April 14, 1830,* in Rockland, Maine. He entered the USMA in July 1849 but in 1850 had to have one of his legs amputated. Cadet Tillson was seen on sick report at West Point for a puncture wound on July 9 and subluxation on September 2, 1849, sites not specified. He was treated again for subluxation from October 14–19 and October 24–November 1, 1849. On December 14, 1849, he was on sick report for pain in his foot, although he later stated his foot had given him some trouble earlier while he was in camp. On December 18 he returned to duty but was again on sick report on December 24 for a subluxation. He was finally admitted into the hospital on January 2, 1850, where he remained under treatment until March 21, when he was removed to New York City. Later he was moved to the U.S. Hospital at Governors Island, and on March 23 the diseased portion of the limb was removed. It is not clear what initially happened to his leg or the indications for amputation. Tillson remained at the hospital on Governors Island, attended by the surgeon of that post, until April 28, when he was sufficiently improved to be brought back to the academy. He was in the hospital to convalesce until he was able to walk with the aid of crutches. After his resignation from the academy, he held state positions in Maine and entered Federal service in November 1861 as a captain of the 2nd Maine Battery. He was promoted to major in May 1862. At the end of August he was granted a leave on account of illness and to allow him an opportunity to have his artificial limb repaired. In October he returned to duty. He was promoted to lieutenant colonel in December 1862, and his appointment to brigadier general in March 1863 ranked from November 1862. Tillson served at Cedar Mountain, Second Bull Run, and in East Tennessee. After the war he remained in the army directing branches of the Freedmen's Bureau in Tennessee and Georgia until December 1866.[1] In 1868 he returned to Maine and engaged in the lime and granite business. Died in Rockland, Maine, on April 30, 1895, and was buried there in the Achorn Cemetery.

DEATH CERTIFICATE: Cause of death, angina pectoris.

1. WPCHR, vol. 607; Captain Henry Brewerton to Brig. Gen. Joseph G. Totten, May 30, 1850, Transcript, U.S. Military Academy, West Point, N.Y., vol. 2, p. 883, July 2, 1849–Feb. 15, 1853; Letters Sent, 1838–40 and 1845–1902; Records of the United States Military Academy, Record Group 404; National Archives at USMA Archives, West Point, N.Y.; U.S. Army, CWS, roll 1, vol. 2, report 44, pp. 625–29.

JOHN BLAIR SMITH TODD • *Born April 4, 1814,* in Lexington, Kentucky. Graduated from the USMA in 1837. As a cadet, he was treated for a toothache three times, headache and pain in the chest twice each, and lameness, fever, a sore throat, a sore hand, and a wound one time each.[1] Served in the Florida and Mexican wars. Following garrison and frontier duty, Todd resigned from the army in September 1856 and became a sutler at Fort Randall, South Dakota. After studying the law, he was admitted to the bar in 1861 and commissioned a brigadier general of volunteers in September. In July 24, 1862, he was relieved at his own request. Todd was a delegate to Congress from the Territory of Dakota until March 1863 and again from June 1864 until March 1865. He held state positions until 1868. Died January 5, 1872, in Yankton County and was buried in Yankton City, South Dakota.

1. WPCHR, vols. 602, 603.

ALFRED THOMAS ARCHIMEDES TORBERT • *Born July 1, 1833,* in Georgetown, Delaware. He graduated from the USMA in 1855. While at the military academy, he was treated for excoriatio seven times, catarrhus four times, odontalgia five times, phlegmon three times, cephalalgia, contusio, subluxatio, and colica each twice, and vulnus incip., abscesses, and clavus one time each. Served during the Florida wars. He was absent sick for four months in early 1857 while in Florida. In February 1861 he was promoted to first lieutenant. Unknown to him at the time, he was nominated and confirmed as a first lieutenant of artillery by the Confederate Congress! After being on recruiting duty, in September 1861 Torbert became colonel of the 1st New Jersey. During the Union advance to Centreville and Manassas, Virginia, in March 1862 he was unable to ride on horseback because of rheumatism. However, he remained on the field. On June 27, 1862, during the engagement on the left bank of the Chickahominy River, he was confined to his bed with "Chickahominy fever" (remittent fever). When informed his regiment was going into action, he started for the battlefield at once. Soon he was physically unable to remain in command and had to take a sick leave. At Crampton's Pass, Maryland, on September 14, 1862, he was slightly wounded but remained on the field. In November he was made a brigadier general of volunteers. He was absent sick with malaria starting in April 1863 and rejoined his brigade at Dranesville in June. At Chancellorsville on May 5, 1863, he had to give up his brigade command because he had an abscess (pilonidal cyst) near the end of his spine. He underwent an operation using chloroform at Fredericksburg on May 9. He was sent to Washington, D.C., where he remained until May 16, when he returned to his command for Gettysburg and the Shenandoah campaigns of 1864. During the spring of 1865 he had another attack of malaria. In January 1866 he was mustered out of volunteer service and reverted back to his rank of captain. The surgeon who examined him in March reported that Torbert had been suffering for several years with an extensive and suppurating cyst in contact with and over the base of the coccyx. Suppurating tracts extended on both side of the cyst under the fasciae and its covering. The surgeon performed extirpation of the cyst and its covering, leaving a large wound that would take several months to heal. Torbert resigned from regular service in October 1866 and held a number of diplomatic posts. He was intermittently sick with malaria during the period from 1873 through 1875. En route to Mexico on business, he lost his life on August 29, 1880, when the steamer *Vera Cruz* was wrecked off Cape Canaveral by a hurricane. Wearing a life jacket, he was swept off of the ship and climbed into a raft, only to be washed off again. His body was recovered on August 31, and he was buried in the Methodist Episcopal Cemetery in Milford, Delaware.[1]

1. CSR; *OR*, vol. 5:538; vol. 11, pt. 2:438, 440; vol. 36, pt. 1:128, 803; WPCHR, vols. 608, 609; LR, ACP, 5383, 1880, fiche: 000192; A. D. Slade, *A. T. A. Torbert: Southern Gentleman in Union Blue*, 22, 39, 41, 46, 61, 66, 95–96, 98, 185, 187, 202, 204, 206, 213–14; *(Tallahassee) Semi-Weekly Floridian*, Sept. 7, 1880.

JOSEPH GILBERT TOTTEN • *Born April 17, 1788*, in New Haven, Connecticut. Graduated from the USMA in 1805. Served in the War of 1812 and the Mexican War. A distinguished engineer, he was chief engineer of the army when the Civil War started and was commissioned brigadier general in the Regular Army in 1863. He died suddenly from pneumonia in Washington on April 22, 1864, and was buried in the Congressional Cemetery.

ZEALOUS BATES TOWER • *Born on January 12, 1819,* in Cohasset, Massachusetts. Graduated from the USMA in 1841. While at the military academy, he was treated for a headache twice and for a cold, sore throat, and nausea one time each. He was wounded in the head on September 13, 1847, during the storming of Chapultepec. In 1861, Tower was chief engineer for the defenses of Fort Pickens, Florida. His promotion to brigadier general of volunteers ranked from November. He was severely wounded in the left knee on August 30, 1862, at the Second Battle of Bull Run, and was taken with the other wounded to Washington, D.C. In the middle of March 1863 the ball was still in the bone, and the surgeon reported he needed a new type of probe to extract it. On May 20, 1863, he was given leave to go north. Not sufficiently recovered to be useful, he reported his progress monthly by letter to the adjutant general's office. After several relapses, his wound appeared to be adequately healed by January 1864. However, that same month his condition was complicated by erysipelas and fever. As a consequence, he did not return until June when he was ordered to West Point as superintendent. Unable to take the field again because of his wound, he was sent to Nashville in September 1864 to examine the fortifications. After the war he was promoted to lieutenant colonel of engineers in November 1865 and colonel in January 1874. He retired in 1883. Died in Cohasset on March 19, 1900, and was buried in Central Cemetery. Physician's certificate: Cause of death, cystirrhagia (hemorrhage from the urinary bladder). Duration, six years.[1]

1. CSR; *OR,* vol. 12, pt. 2:48, 255, 342, 345, 384; vol. 39, pt. 2:377; WPCHR, vol. 604, LR, ACP, 1537, 1882, fiche: 000193; Heitman, *Historical Register and Dictionary,* 2:39; B. Huger to wife, Sept. 16, 1847, Benjamin Huger Papers UV; U.S. Army, CWS, roll 1, vol. 1, report 22, pp. 305–10; ibid., roll 3, vol. 5, report 10, pp. 859–61; *OR Suppl.,* pt. 1, reports, vol. 4, 455.

JOHN BASIL TURCHIN (IVAN VASILOVITCH TURCHINOFF) • *Born January 30, 1822,* in the Province of the Don, Russia. He graduated from the Russian military academy, became a colonel of the Imperial Guard, and fought in the Crimean War. In 1856 he received a leave of absence for one year with permission to go abroad on account of sickness. He emigrated to the United States in the summer of that year. He was an employee in the engineering department of the Illinois Central Railroad when he was commissioned colonel of the 19th Illinois Infantry in June 1861. Because he encouraged his troops to pillage and plunder Confederate civilian property in Athens, Alabama, in April 1862, Turchin was court-martialed. During his trial in July he had a fever, which gave him a severe headache. Through the efforts of his wife and President Lincoln, his verdict was set aside and his commission as brigadier general of volunteers ranked from July 1862. He served creditably at Chickamauga, Chattanooga, and in the Atlanta campaign. After the war, a committee reported such conduct as that shown by his troops was almost standard by the end of the war and was called "foraging." On July 14, 1864, he had a sunstroke. His examining surgeon reported that he was peculiarly susceptible to solar influences that produced violent pain in his head, approaching coup-de-soleil (sunstroke). A change of climate was recommended, and the next day he went north on sick leave. In October 1864 he resigned because of his poor health. On his return to civilian life he became a solicitor of patents in Chicago. In later life he had severe mental problems and died on June 19, 1901, in the Southern Illinois Hospital for the Insane at Anna, Illinois. He was buried in the National Cemetery at Mound City. The cause of death was listed in the hospital records as senile dementia.[1]

1. *OR*, vol. 38, pt. 1:96, 742, 755, 761; RVA, Pension WC 532,314; Garfield, *Wild Life of the Army*, 123.

JOHN WESLEY TURNER • *Born July 19, 1833*, near Saratoga, New York. Graduated from the USMA in 1855. According to the medical records between the period of July 7, 1851, and September 29, 1864, he was treated at intervals for catarrhous, diarrhoea, tonsillitis, excoriates, cephalalgia, influenza, subluxatio, intermittent fever, quotidian fever, and phlegmon. In the summer of 1861 he was appointed captain and became chief commissary in Kansas for Gen. David Hunter. Turner was made chief of staff and chief of artillery in the Department of the South in 1863 and his promotion to brigadier general ranked from September of that year. In August 1864 he was ill and not expected to live due to some unspecified disease. By the next month he had recovered enough to go on sick leave, not returning until late November, when he was appointed chief of staff of the Department of Virginia and North Carolina.[1] In 1866 he was mustered out of volunteer service and reverted to his regular staff rank of colonel. Until his resignation from the army in September 1871, Turner served as depot commissary at St. Louis. Died in St. Louis on April 8, 1899, and was buried there in Calvary Cemetery.

DEATH CERTIFICATE: Double pneumonia (la grippe).

1. CSR; *OR*, vol. 40, pt. 1:123; WPCHR, vols. 608, 609; RVA, Pension WC 784,853; U.S. Army CWS, roll 6, vol. 10, report 32, pp. 213–17; RAGO, entry 534; John Wesley Turner Papers (Folder: Official Correspondence, 1864), USAMHI.

JAMES MADISON TUTTLE • *Born September 24, 1823*, in Summerfield, Ohio. He held local county offices in Van Buren County, Iowa, before the war, and in May 1861 joined Federal service as lieutenant colonel of the 2nd Iowa. The following September he was made the unit's colonel. At Fort Donelson on February 15, 1862, he was standing on a log when it was struck by a cannonball. He fell backwards, and his lower back hit a branch. When he got up he was in great pain and had difficulty walking but did not require hospitalization. The fall produced a left inguinal hernia, and he was later furnished with a truss. After Shiloh he was absent on sick leave and returned in May. Tuttle was made brigadier general of volunteers in June 1862 and commanded a division at Vicksburg. In

June 1864 he resigned from the army, probably because he faced a charge of misconduct. He returned to Iowa and engaged in business and politics until 1877, when he became involved in mining in the Southwest. He continued to have difficulty walking and became more feeble over the years. On Sunday, October 23, 1892, he suffered a stroke while visiting the Jack Rabbit Mine, of which he was principal owner, located south of Casa Grande, Arizona. Medical aid was summoned from Casa Grande and Florence, but he never regained consciousness and died on October 25. He was buried in Woodland Cemetery, Des Moines, Iowa.[1]

1. *OR*, vol. 7:230; vol. 39, pt. 2:186; RVA, Pension WC 366,717; *(Florence) Arizona Enterprise*, Oct. 27, 1892.

DANIEL TYLER • *Born January 7, 1799*, in Brooklyn, Connecticut. Graduated from the USMA in 1819. After resigning from Federal service in 1834, he was successfully engaged with railroad and canal companies until the Civil War. He was made colonel of a ninety-day regiment, brigadier general of Connecticut Volunteers, and led a division at First Bull Run. Mustered out in August 1861, he was appointed a brigadier general of volunteers in March 1862. In June 1862 he received a leave of absence because of a severe case of dysentery and reported back to duty in August. He resigned in April 1864.[1] Tyler founded the town of Anniston, Alabama, which became an industrial center. While on a visit to New York City, he died after a very brief illness in a hotel on November 30, 1882, and was buried in Hillside Cemetery, Anniston.

DEATH CERTIFICATE: Chief cause, pneumonia, seven days' duration. Contributing, senile anemia and atheroma.

1. CSR; LR, ACP, 6736, 1882, fiche: 000195; U.S. Army, CWS, roll 1, vol. 1, report 11, pp. 167–77.

ERASTUS BARNARD TYLER • *Born April 24, 1822*, in West Bloomfield, New York. A fur dealer, he helped organize the 7th Ohio Volunteers and in 1861 was elected its colonel. In May 1862 he was commissioned brigadier general of volunteers. He was absent sick with acute enteritis in January 1863. Since he did not have an official leave, he was placed under arrest on February 12 but was released the next month. Near Fredericksburg on December 13, 1862, a shell burst near Tyler, and spent fragments struck him on the left side of his body and head. Although injured, he did not leave the field. The head wound left a hard, bony prominence as large as half a walnut, although Tyler always felt the side injury had been worse. In August 1865 he was discharged from the army. He married a woman from Baltimore, where he remained after the war. The time sequence is uncertain, but Tyler developed pain in his right arm and occasional numbness in his right leg in later years. A gradual paralysis developed, first noticed in the right leg and then extending to the right arm, which increased in severity. In

1891, two physicians, one who had known him during the war and another who had treated him for twelve years, stated his paralysis was due to his old head injury. On January 9, 1891, he died in Calverton, now a part of Baltimore, Maryland, and was buried in Green Mount Cemetery. The attending physician listed the cause of death as obstruction of the intestines.[1]

1. CSR; RVA, Pension WC 288,115; RAGO, entry 534.

ROBERT OGDEN TYLER · *Born December 22, 1831,* in Hunter, New York. Graduated from the USMA in 1853. While at West Point, he was treated for catarrhus four times, cephalalgia three times, febris intermittent and diarrhea each twice, and phlegmon, nausea, excoriatio, and subluxatio once each. Served in the Florida wars. Before the Civil War Tyler had duty at various posts throughout the country, and in May 1861 he was transferred to the staff of the Quartermaster's Department. In September 1861 he was commissioned colonel of the 4th Connecticut Infantry, which was designated the 1st Connecticut Heavy Artillery the following January. In November he was made brigadier general of volunteers. On July 3, 1863, at Gettysburg, he supervised movement of the artillery back into a less exposed position. From the extreme heat and overexertion, Tyler had a sunstroke which prostrated him so that he had to turn over his command. At dusk he had sufficiently recovered to resume his position. At Cold Harbor on June 3, 1864, the bones of his foot were fractured by a gunshot, and it was feared that he might lose his foot. He was admitted to a hospital and apparently had some type of surgical procedure. Although he could proceed by the usual modes of travel, his lameness and inability to mount a horse prevented him from being of much service in the field. In January 1865 Tyler wanted to be assigned to temporary duty near Philadelphia. His civilian surgeon recommended another operation, which he stated would help restore Tyler's foot. It is not clear whether he had the surgery. The next month, although still physically unfit, he was ordered to New York City for duty.[1] He remained in the army after the war and in 1866 was made deputy quartermaster with the rank of lieutenant colonel. Most of his service was interrupted by trips abroad in an effort to improve his declining health. Died at the Coolidge House in Boston, Massachusetts, on December 1, 1874, and was buried in Cedar Hill Cemetery, Hartford, Connecticut.
DEATH CERTIFICATE: Immediate cause of death, neuralgia of heart.

1. *OR,* vol. 27, pt. 1:1021; vol. 36, pt. 1:88, 168, 345, 434, 460; vol. 46, pt. 2:66–67, 76; vol. 49, pt. 1:716; WPCHR, vols. 607, 608; RAGO, entry 534.

GEORGE HECTOR TYNDALE · *Born on March 24, 1821,* in Philadelphia. Before the war he was an importer of glass and china. He was commissioned major of the 28th Pennsylvania in June 1861 and lieutenant colonel the following April. In the summer of 1862 he developed diarrhea. He was at Cedar Mountain and

Second Bull Run. A musket ball struck him on the back of his head at Antietam on September 17, 1862. Unconscious, he was dragged by one of his lieutenants at least fifty yards back behind a haystack. Tyndale had a compound fracture of the skull. The ball had struck him over the occipital protuberance and had passed to the right side of the neck under the deep muscles. The surgeon removed the ball from a position between the jaw and sternum. Tyndale was ordered to his home in Philadelphia and remained there suffering from his wound and diarrhea until the end of March 1863. In April he was commissioned a brigadier general of volunteers. There was numbness in his hand while pains and numbness extended to his right leg, at times to the point of paralysis. When he reported back he was still too weak to resume his duties and was sent home in September to recuperate. He finally rejoined his command on October 19 and commanded a brigade at Chattanooga. Because of the continued diarrhea and residual from his wound, Tyndale had sick leave starting in May 1864. On the advice of his surgeon, he resigned the following August. After returning to Philadelphia, he continued to engage in business and civic affairs. Died in Philadelphia on March 19, 1880, and was buried there in Laurel Hill Cemetery. A postmortem examination revealed the ball had entered at the occipital protuberance and the wound of exit was in the right carotid region. The skull was depressed where it had been struck and the bone thickened. On the inside of the skull the surface of this portion of the bone was rough and corresponded to the position of a large venous sinus of the dura mater. The attending physician stated the wound and enlargement of the venous sinus accounted for Tyndale's nervous symptoms following the war.[1]

DEATH CERTIFICATE: Cause of death, angina pectoris.

1. CSR; *OR*, vol. 19, pt. 1:179, 199, 478, 505, 507; vol. 30, pt. 4:324; vol. 38, pt. 2:84–85; vol. 43, pt. 1:969; U.S. Army, CWS, roll 2, vol. 3, report 23, pp. 623–57; ibid., roll 4, vol. 7, report 26, pp. 397–435; RVA, Pension WC 198,392.

U

DANIEL ULLMANN · *Born April 28, 1810,* in Wilmington, Delaware. He was engaged in politics and his law practice in New York City before the war. In April 1862 he was made colonel of the 78th New York. In July 1862, following constant exposure to the rain and not having any rest, he was barely able to sit erect on his horse. However, he remained in command, and when he was finally examined by his regimental surgeon, a diagnosis of typhoid fever was made. Ullman was taken by ambulance to Little Washington, Virginia, and, too sick to be moved farther, was left in private quarters under the supervision of a local physician. Following a relapse in the middle of August, he was captured on August 22 when Confederate troops took the town. Still too ill to be moved, he remained in private quarters until early October, when he was taken to Libby Prison in

Richmond. In December he was exchanged and went to Washington, D.C., and then to New York City to recover his health. In January 1863 he was made a brigadier general of volunteers and was sent to New Orleans to organize Negro troops. Ill in February 1865, he finally went back to New York in April in an attempt to recover. The following August he was mustered out of the army and went back to New York. The last few years of his life his eyes were so impaired that he could not see to read or write. His whole left side was affected with paralysis, and he was permanently lame in his left leg.[1] Died near Nyack, New York, on September 20, 1892, and was buried in Oakhill Cemetery, Nyack.

DEATH CERTIFICATE: Cause of death, chief cause, old age, a general loss of the vital force with malarial complications.

1. *OR*, vol. 48, pt. 1:984–85; U.S. Army, CWS, roll 8, vol. 14, report 4, pp. 25–167; RVA, Pension SC 552,367.

ADIN BALLOU UNDERWOOD • *Born May 19, 1828,* in Milford, Massachusetts. He was admitted to the Massachusetts bar in 1853 and went to Boston two years later. In May 1861 he was made captain of the 2nd Massachusetts Infantry. The first year of the war he contracted malaria and was hospitalized for a few days. In August 1862 he was promoted to lieutenant colonel of the 33rd Massachusetts and to colonel the following April. He served at Chancellorsville and Gettysburg. On October 29, 1863, at the foot of Lookout Mountain at Wauhatchie, Tennessee, Underwood was wounded two or three times in the right thigh by minié balls. One ball had entered a few inches below the greater trochanter, passed horizontally through the soft parts, fractured the upper third of the femur, and passed out and into the dorsum of the penis. The ball, along with a piece of bone the size of half of a pea, was extracted by the surgeon. After staying in a log cabin near the battlefield for two weeks, he was removed to Nashville, Tennessee. Here his wife joined him, and they remained in private quarters for five months, with his care supervised by three physicians. His treatment consisted of perfect rest, a good diet, and immobilization of the wounded extremity. His appointment as brigadier general ranked from November 1863. Transported by rail and steamboat, he returned home. He was confined to his bed for six months and remained in the house for almost an additional year. In May 1865 he reported himself as fit for light duty and was detailed on court-martial duty that month. The femur had united, the wound had closed, and his general health was good, except that the injured leg was four to five inches shorter than before. The following August Underwood was mustered out of the army. After he returned to Boston, he was made surveyor of the port. There was prominent stiffness of the left knee. From time to time the wound would break down and he would be confined to his bed for weeks. He had subsequent surgical operations and protracted healing of the wound, which was complicated by malaria and nervous strain. Died January 14, 1888, at his residence in Boston and was buried in the Newton Cemetery, Newton, Massachusetts.[1]

DEATH CERTIFICATE: Immediate cause of death, pneumonia, due to cardiac failure.

1. CSR; *OR*, vol. 31, pt. 1:95, 98, 101, 104; U.S. Army, CWS, roll 4, vol. 7, report 3, pp. 49–79; RVA, Pension WC 247,166.

EMORY UPTON • *Born August 27, 1839*, on a farm near Batavia, New York. Graduated from the USMA in 1861. While at West Point, Upton fought with one of the other students and received a slight cut on his cheek. In addition, while a cadet he was treated for phlegmon twelve times, odontalgia six times, catarrhus four times, diarrhea and excoriatio twice each, and morbus cutis, contusio, nausea, morbi. varii., and fracture one time each. Upton was made colonel of the 121st New York in October 1862 and brigadier general to rank from May 1864. Near Blackburn's Ford on Bull Run on July 21, 1861, he was wounded in the left side and arm by a minié ball. He remained on the field and delivered messages for Gen. Daniel Tyler. Following his recovery he joined an artillery battery in the defenses of Washington in August 1861. On July 5, 1864, he had some type of unspecified slight surgery. He was wounded by a shell near the close of the battle at Winchester on September 19, 1864. It tore his thigh muscles open and laid bare the femoral artery. His staff surgeon stopped the bleeding with a tourniquet, and Upton was carried about the field on a stretcher giving orders. Soon afterwards he went home on sick leave to Batavia. On December 13, 1864, when he was assigned to command of a division, he was still limping but took part in the Selma raid in 1865. He remained in the army after the war and in 1866 was made lieutenant colonel of the 25th Infantry. While commandant of cadets at West Point in 1870–75, he went to the academy dentist. During one of his early visits, the dentist heard a distinct and regular throbbing in Upton's head that was not beating in unison with the temporal artery. When the finding was mentioned to Upton, he was surprised and said that he had noticed the sound occasionally for some time. Over further visits, the dentist noticed the sound became more distinct, and it annoyed Upton to the point where it interfered with his sleep. The dentist considered an aneurysm as a possibility. He saw him at intervals over the next few years after he left West Point, the last time in early 1880, and could still hear the sound. In 1880 Upton stated that he had been having headaches for some time, which he attributed to malaria, and he had treated himself with thirty to forty grains of quinine in a thirty-six hour period with success. In March 1880 a Philadelphia physician diagnosed him with chronic nasal catarrh and treated him daily for six weeks with electrical cauterization of the mucous membrane of the nasal passage utilizing a fine-coiled wire. This was supposed to restore circulation of the membranes and "renew the proper vital action." He noted that Upton on occasion had an unusual symptom: bloody, chocolate-colored phlegm. The physician last treated him in November 1880 and stated that in his opinion there was no correlation between the nasal condition and his headaches since the nasal condition improved but the headaches did not. This physician later speculated that he may have had a brain tumor. In spite of the fact that Upton was supposed to have more electric treatments, he joined his regiment in California in late 1880. His headaches became more frequent and severe. Although in pain and confused, Upton continued to work. The pain made sleep impossible, and he was not able to think rationally. Despondent, he felt the military tactics he was working on were a failure and believed he had lost the respect of the other officers. He displayed signs of memory loss on March 13 and wrote a letter stating he should not continue with a system of military tactics that may cause the loss of life. On March 15, 1881, he killed himself in his quarters at the Presidio. He wrote and signed his resignation and then shot himself with his Colt .45 pistol. The ball entered his mouth and exited near the occipital protuberance.[1] He was buried in Fort Hill Cemetery, Auburn, New York.

1. CSR; *OR*, vol. 2:351; vol. 43, pt. 1:164; vol. 45, pt. 2:171; WPCHR, vol. 609; U.S. Army, CWS, roll 5, vol. 9, report 10, pp. 231–35; LR, ACP, 2666, 1881, fiche: 000196; Stephen Edward Ambrose, "Upton and the Army" (diss.), 13–14, 23–24, 58–61, 210–11, 214–15, 218; Peter S. Michie, *The Life and Letters of Emory Upton*, 478, 481–83, 484–95; James M. Greiner, Janet L. Coryell, and James R. Smither, eds., *A Surgeon's Civil War*, 215.

V

JAMES HENRY VAN ALEN • *Born on August 17, 1819,* at Kinderhook, New York. When the war started he recruited and equipped at his own expense the 3rd New York Cavalry. He entered the Federal service in August 1861 as colonel of the unit. In April 1862 he was promoted to brigadier general of volunteers and served on the Peninsula. The last of August 1862 he had a twenty-day sick leave. After having a series of disabling fevers, Van Alen resigned in July 1863. Wealthy, he traveled after the war. He was returning from a trip to England with his grandchildren when he fell overboard from the Cunard liner *Umbria* in the early morning of July 22, 1886. The sea was rough and there is no evidence to support the theory that he committed suicide. His body was never recovered.[1]

1. CSR; U.S. Army, CWS, roll 6, vol. 10, report 34, pp. 275–77; *New York Herald*, July 26, 1886; *Newport (R.I.) Herald*, July 25, 1886.

HORATIO PHILLIPS VAN CLEVE • *Born November 23, 1809,* in Princeton, New Jersey. Graduated from USMA in 1831. After serving on garrison duty he resigned from the army in 1836. Van Cleve was a farmer, engineer, and teacher in Michigan, Minnesota, and Ohio before the war. He was commissioned colonel of the 2nd Minnesota Infantry in July 1861 and brigadier general in March

1862. He served at Mill Springs and Corinth. He was wounded in the popliteal space of the right leg by a musket ball at Stones River on December 31, 1862, and was sent back to Nashville the next day. The internal and external popliteal nerves were injured, but the artery was missed. Disabled, he was furloughed on January 9, 1863. He reported for duty on March 12 and resumed command of his division. On September 27, 1863, other officers stated that Van Cleve should be relieved on account of his age, the confusion of his mind, and the incapacity he had displayed during the battle of Chickamauga. In August 1865 he was mustered out of service. After the war, the pain in his right hip, leg, and back prostrated him for days at a time and therapy provided only temporary relief.[1] He was adjutant general of the state of Minnesota from 1866 to 1870 and from 1876 to 1882, and postmaster at St. Anthony from 1871 to 1873. He was commissioned a second lieutenant of infantry on July 1, 1890, and placed on the retired list with that rank on the same day. Died April 24, 1891, in his residence in Minneapolis and was buried there in Lakewood Cemetery.

DEATH CERTIFICATE: Cause of death, pneumonia, four days' duration.

1. CSR; OR, vol. 20, pt. 1:608; vol. 30, pt. 1:203; U.S. Army, CWS, roll 1, vol. 2, report 51, pp. 711–18; RVA, Pension, WC 438,435.

FERDINAND VAN DERVEER • *Born February 27, 1823,* in Middletown, Ohio. Served in the Mexican War. Prior to the Civil War he practiced law and was county sheriff of Butler County, Ohio. He was made colonel of the 35th Ohio in September 1861. He served at Corinth, Perryville, Stones River, Chattanooga, and in the Atlanta campaign. After being ill for a long time Van Derveer was compelled to give up his command and go on sick leave on June 27, 1864. He was mustered out the following July but was reappointed with the rank of brigadier general of volunteers in October. He resigned again in 1865.[1] He returned to his law practice and became judge of the court of common pleas in Butler County. Died in Hamilton, Ohio, on November 5, 1892, and was buried in Greenwood Cemetery. Burial records: cause of death, paralysis.

1. OR, vol. 38, pt. 1:96, 739, 789.

WILLIAM VANDEVER • *Born March 31, 1817,* in Baltimore, Maryland. A lawyer, he was elected to Congress from Iowa in 1858 and reelected in 1860. In September 1861 he entered Federal service as colonel of the 9th Iowa Volunteers and in November 1862 was promoted to brigadier general. He was at Pea Ridge, Arkansas Post, Vicksburg, in the Atlanta campaign, and in the Carolinas. In August 1865 he was mustered out of service and returned to his law practice. He later moved to California and served in Congress from 1886 until 1891. Died in the Flor del Mar Hospital in Ventura, California, on July 23, 1893, and was buried in Ventura Cemetery. According to the attending physician, he died from fatty degeneration of the heart. His remains were transferred by his surviving daughter in 1932 to Ivy Lawn Cemetery, Ventura.[1]

1. RVA, Pension SC 388,501; "Grave Matters" 5, no. 2 (1995): 7.

STEWART VAN VLIET • *Born July 21, 1815,* in Ferrisburg, Vermont. Graduated from the USMA in 1840. At the military academy he was treated for contusio and catarrhus twice each, and excoriatio, fatigue, cephalalgia, and subluxatio one time each. Served in the Florida and Mexican wars. He served in the artillery and had duty in the Quartermaster's Department. When the Civil War started, he was stationed at Fort Leavenworth, Kansas. In August 1861 he was promoted to major and made chief quartermaster of the Army of the Potomac. His appointment as brigadier general of volunteers on September 1861 expired in July 1862. Van Vliet was relieved from duty that month but was later appointed brigadier general to rank from March 1865. In 1866 he was appointed deputy quartermaster general with the rank of lieutenant colonel. He was made a colonel in 1872 and retired due to age in 1881. Died in Washington, D.C., on March 28, 1901, and was buried in Arlington National Cemetery.[1]

DEATH CERTIFICATE: Cause of death, primary, aortic and mitral valvular disease of the heart. Immediate, hemorrhage of stomach of 36 hours.

1. WPCHR, vol. 604; LR, ACP, 4017, 1872, fiche: 000197.

CHARLES HENRY VAN WYCK • *Born May 10, 1824,* in Poughkeepsie, New York. A practicing lawyer, he was elected to Congress from New York in 1858 and served in this capacity until March 1863. In September 1861 he was commissioned colonel of the 56th New York Infantry. Van Wyck was slightly wounded in the left knee by a bursting shell on May 31, 1862, at Fair Oaks, Virginia, and was treated by the regimental surgeon. During December and through the middle of February 1864 he was ill with miasmatic fever and spent most of the time in the hospital. In March he was sent north both for the benefit of his health and to recruit. He was appointed brigadier general of volunteers in September 1865. After the war Van Wyck continued to have pain in his injured knee, which affected his walking. He was again elected to Congress from New York but in 1874 moved to Nebraska, where he continued to engage in politics. When he was examined in September 1894, very slight atrophy of the leg and a floating piece of cartilage on the inner aspect of the knee were present. There was also crepitation of the knee on palpation. Although he required a cane, there was no limitation of motion.[1] Died in Washington, D.C., on October 24, 1895, and was buried in Milford, Pennsylvania.

DEATH CERTIFICATE: Cause of death, atheroma of the cerebral vessels associated with hemorrhage, compression, encephalitis, coma.

1. CSR; RVA, Pension SC 883,644.

JAMES CLIFFORD VEATCH • *Born December 19, 1819,* in Elizabethtown, Indiana. He practiced law in Indiana and was a member of the state legislature during the 1861–62 term. However, he was appointed colonel of the 25th Indiana Infantry in August 1861. In the fall of the year, Veatch had a severe attack of typhoid fever, diarrhea, rheumatism, and heart trouble. He had to remain behind with an aide near Warrensburg, Missouri. There was a return of his rheumatic heart trouble and diarrhea in February 1862 while he was at Fort Donelson. In April he was commissioned a brigadier general of volunteers and served at Shiloh. Similar episodes of diarrhea and heart difficulty occurred in May and the fall of 1862. These episodes were accompanied by neuralgia and incapacitated him for duty. At Corinth (Battle of the Hatchie) on October 5, 1862, his side was badly contused by a grapeshot, and he was compelled to leave the field. In January 1863, Veatch was assigned to the command of the District of Memphis. He was sick in January 1864. He had a twenty-day sick leave in July and then was on court-martial duty until October. In August 1865 he was mustered out of the service at New Orleans. He returned to Indiana and was state adjutant general in 1869. From 1870 until 1883 he was U.S. collector of internal revenue for his district. According to the physician who examined him in 1887, Veatch still had diarrhea, piles, rheumatism, and heart disease. There was a precordial friction rub and loud murmurs over the apical area of the heart, which probably were of rheumatic origin. The joints of the lower extremities were stiffened with some enlargement and tenderness and motion was limited by half. There were five to six internal, ulcerated hemorrhoids. He appeared emaciated and was incapacitated for any form of physical work. He died in Rockport, Indiana, on December 21, 1895, and was buried there in Sun Set Hill Cemetery.[1]

DEATH CERTIFICATE: Cause of death, rheumatic heart disease complicated by bronchitis.

1. *OR*, vol. 17, pt. 1:302, 324; vol. 32, pt. 2:75; vol. 38, pt. 1:108, pt. 3:486; RVA, Pension WC 425,692; William A. Veitch to author, Lexington, Ky., June 9, 1980.

EGBERT LUDOVICUS VIELE • *Born June 17, 1825,* in Waterford, New York. Graduated from the USMA in 1847. While a cadet, he was treated twice each for contusio and catarrhus and once each for excoriatio, fatigue, cephalalgia, and subluxatio.[1] He was stationed in Mexico City during the occupation. In 1853 Viele resigned his commission and engaged in engineering in New Jersey and New York. He served as a captain of engineers in the 7th New York Militia for the first part of the war and in August 1861 was appointed brigadier general of volunteers. He resigned in October 1863 and returned to his engineering practice in New York. Died in a private house in New York on April 22, 1902, and was buried at West Point.

DEATH CERTIFICATE: Myocarditis.

1. WPCHR, vol. 605.

STRONG VINCENT • *Born on June 17, 1837,* in Waterford, Pennsylvania. He had just started practicing the law in Pennsylvania when the Civil War started. After serving in a three-month regiment, Vincent was commissioned lieutenant colonel of the 83rd Pennsylvania in September 1861. In May 1862 he had malaria, and after a leave, he rejoined the army in December. He was made colonel of the regiment in June 1862. Vincent served at Fredericksburg and Chancellorsville, and on July 2, 1863, on Little Round Top at Gettysburg, he was mortally wounded by a minié ball. Placed on a stretcher, he was carried to a farmhouse about four miles southeast of Gettysburg. The ball had passed clear through the left groin and lodged in the other. The thigh bone was fractured. The next day he wanted to go home, but the brigade surgeon stated his condition was too critical for him to be moved. Although constantly attended by the surgeon and visited by friends, his condition became worse and he died on July 7. He was commissioned brigadier general of volunteers to rank from July 3, 1863. Vincent's remains were buried in Erie Cemetery at Erie, Pennsylvania.[1]

1. *OR,* vol. 27, pt. 1:192, 593, 603–4, 617, 620; RVA, Pension C 19,397; O. W. Norton, *The Attack and Defense of Little Round Top: Gettysburg, July 2, 1863,* 210, 244; Amos M. Judson, *History of the Eighty-Third Regiment Pennsylvania Volunteers,* 64, 96, 128, 138–40.

FRANCIS LAURENS VINTON • *Born June 1, 1835,* at Fort Preble, Maine. He graduated from the USMA in 1856. At West Point he was treated for rheumatism four times, excoriatio and catarrhus three times each, contusio, colica, and phlegmon twice each, and diarrhea, vulnus incisum, cholera morbus, and dyspepsia one time each. Immediately after graduation he resigned to study engineering. When the Civil War started, Vinton was mustered back into the Regular Army as a captain, and in October 1861 he was commissioned colonel of the 43rd New York Infantry. At Fredericksburg on December 13, 1862, he was badly wounded when a minié ball passed into his abdomen just above the crest of the ilium and came out near the spine. The wound appeared healed by February but the entrance wound broke down and drained the next month. His appointment as brigadier general in September 1862 had not been acted on by the Senate and expired in March 1863. Vinton was reappointed brigadier general to rank from that month but resigned the following May because of poor health. On returning to civilian life he engaged in mine engineering. Died of erysipelas in Leadville, Colorado, on October 6, 1879, and was buried there in Evergreen Cemetery.[1] At a later date, his remains were moved to Providence, Rhode Island, where he was reinterred in Swan Point Cemetery.

1. CSR; *OR,* vol. 21:60, 141, 524, 529–30, 533; WPCHR, vols. 608, 609; RAGO, entry 534; RAGO, entry 623, "File D"; Warner, *Generals in Blue,* 528–29.

ISRAEL VOGDES • *Born on August 4, 1816,* in Willistown, Pennsylvania. Graduated from the USMA in 1837. While a cadet he was treated for a headache and diarrhea three times each, toothache and influenza twice each, and sprain, catarrhus, cough, colica, vomiting, nausea, and fever one time each. Served in the Florida wars. Vogdes taught mathematics for twelve years at the U.S. Military Academy and had duty as an artillery officer prior to the Civil War. He was advanced from captain to major in May 1861. He was captured on October 9, 1861, at Santa Rosa Island. While a prisoner at Richmond in May 1862, his health was undermined, and there was a question of him surviving if he remained in captivity. Vogdes was exchanged in August and was made a brigadier general of volunteers in November 1862. After the war he remained in the army with the rank of colonel before retiring in 1881. Died in the New York Hotel in New York City on December 7, 1889, and was buried at West Point.[1]

DEATH CERTIFICATE: Chief cause, gastric ulcer. Contributing, hemorrhage from stomach.

1. *OR,* ser. 2, vol. 3:557; WPCHR, vols. 602, 603; LR, ACP, 7229, 1889, fiche: 000198.

ADOLPH WILHELM AUGUST FRIEDRICH, BARON VON STEINWEHR • *Born on September 25, 1822,* at Blankenburg in the Duchy of Brunswick. He attended a Prussian military academy. Married in 1847 while on leave in the United States, he took his wife back to Brunswick. They returned to the United States in 1854 and settled on a farm in Connecticut. At the start of the Civil War he was made colonel of the 29th New York, and his commission as brigadier general of volunteers ranked from October 1861. He served at First and Second Bull Run, Chancellorsville, and Gettysburg. Throughout the war he was bothered by hemorrhoids. From January 15 to February 15, 1863, he had acute and chronic dysentery and was on leave. He was left sick at Graysville, Georgia, on November 27, 1863, and from December 26, 1863, to March 3, 1864, he was on sick leave in Connecticut for the same complaint. Again in May and June 1864 he had chronic diarrhea "caused by ulceration of the bowel" but reported he was ready for duty in September. His resignation was accepted to take effect in July 1865. After the war he became a noted geographer and cartographer. Died suddenly in his hotel in Buffalo, New York, on February 25, 1877, and was buried in Albany Rural Cemetery, Albany, New York. His wife reported that he died from dysentery.[1]

1. *OR,* vol. 31, pt. 2:350; U.S. Army, CWS, roll 1, vol. 2, report 54, pp. 759–61; ibid., roll 6, vol. 10, report 26, pp. 121–22; RVA, Pension, WC 537,358; LR, CB, roll 228, V73, 1865.

W

MELANCTHON SMITH WADE • *Born December 2, 1802,* in Cincinnati, Ohio. He had risen to the rank of brigadier general in the Ohio militia before the Civil War. He retired from his drygoods business; after helping recruit and organize men from Ohio, he was appointed a brigadier general of volunteers in October 1861. Wade's age and poor health prevented him from having much of an active role during the war. In March 1862 his resignation was accepted and he returned home, where he developed an interest in the cultivation of fruit. Died at his estate in Avondale, now a part of Cincinnati, on August 11, 1868, and was buried in Spring Grove Cemetery, Cincinnati.

JAMES SAMUEL WADSWORTH • *Born October 30, 1807,* in Geneseo, New York. After being engaged in politics, he was made a volunteer aide to Gen. Irvin McDowell at the start of the war. On McDowell's recommendation he was appointed brigadier general of volunteers in August 1861. In March 1862 Wadsworth was made military governor of the District of Columbia. He was treated for a perineal abscess in November 1862 and assigned to field command in December. He led a division at Gettysburg and in the Overland campaign. At the Wilderness on May 6, 1864, he was shot off his horse. A bullet had entered his forehead and he was captured. John Haskell saw him along the road and had two of his men set up muskets and spread a blanket over them as an awning. He obtained a surgeon to examine him; he did not think Wadsworth was conscious, so he gave him morphine and tried to give him water. He was taken to a Confederate field hospital and placed alone in an officer's tent that had been erected for his benefit. A wounded Union surgeon who examined him found that his eyes did not react upon lifting his eyelids. The ball had entered the top of his head a little to the left of the median line, had passed forward, and was lodged in the anterior lobe of the left side of the brain. His pulse was regular and his breathing a little labored. There was no expression of pain, and his mouth was drawn down on the left side. His right arm appeared to be paralyzed. A Confederate surgeon who examined him the night after he had been wounded removed a piece of bone and probed the wound. Wadsworth was unable to swallow, and when more than a teaspoonful of water was placed between his lips it ran out the corners of his mouth. He died on May 8 without regaining consciousness. His body was later recovered and was buried in Temple Hill Cemetery, Geneseo.[1]

1. *OR*, vol. 21:876; vol. 36, pt. 1:2, 64, 67, 124, 190, 325–26, 540, 549, 1028, 1091; RAGO, entry 534; John Haskell, *The Haskell Memoirs: The Personal Narrative of a Confederate Officer,* 64; *MOLLUS* 53:373–99.

GEORGE DAY WAGNER • *Born September 22, 1829,* in Ross County, Ohio. An active worker for Abraham Lincoln's election, he had served in the Indiana legislature and senate before the Civil War. In June 1861 he was commissioned colonel of the 15th Indiana. His promotion to brigadier general of volunteers ranked from November 1862. He served at Shiloh, Stones River, Chattanooga, in the Atlanta campaign, and at Franklin. Wagner was on sick leave from January 19 to February 19, 1864, and from July 10–24 because of dysentery. In August 1865 he was mustered out of Federal service and started a law practice in Indiana. Died in the Bates House at Indianapolis on February 13, 1869, and was buried near Greenhill, Warren County, Indiana. He had been sick for four or five days. The immediate cause of his death was an overdose of a prescription medication left by his physician to alleviate his nervous suffering.[1]

1. CSR; *OR*, vol. 38, pt. 1:91, 338; RAGO, entry 534; *Indianapolis Journal*, Feb. 15, 1869.

CHARLES CARROLL WALCUTT • *Born February 12, 1838,* in Columbus, Ohio. He left his position as a county surveyor in Ohio and initially joined a state unit when the Civil War started. In October 1861 he was appointed a major of the 46th Ohio. Already sick with dysentery and debility, Walcutt was wounded in the left arm near the shoulder at Shiloh on April 6, 1862. The regimental surgeon treated him in his tent every day until he went north on April 27. His treatment was continued on the steamboat until he reached Cincinnati. Healing was complicated by repeated abscesses in the area of the wound. He was promoted to brigadier general of volunteers in July 1864. On November 22, 1864, at Duncan's Farm near Griswoldville, Georgia, he was severely wounded by a shell fragment in the lower part of the calf of the right leg and left the field. The bones escaped injury, but the soft parts, including the tendons of some of the principal muscles, were extensively lacerated. A simple dressing was used. The wound was complicated by gangrene and abscess. After being treated daily in his tent, he was taken on the USA hospital steamer, *Cosmopolitan,* to a general hospital at Beaufort, South Carolina. Walcutt arrived at the hospital in the middle of December and remained there for two weeks before being sent north. In April 1865, although not fully recovered, he returned and assumed command. He was on recruiting duty in October and was mustered out of service in January 1866. Except for a four-month period when he reentered the Regular Army, he was warden of the Ohio Penitentiary until 1869. Medical examinations in 1882 and 1891 showed similar findings: It was reported that the ball had struck his left arm in front of the anatomical head of the humerus and probably still remained in the area of the axilla. At times he had numbness and temporary paralysis of the arm. On the anterior aspect of his arm, four inches below the tip of the acromion process, there was a circular cicatrix ⅝ inches in diameter that was deeply depressed and adherent to the deeper structures. There was considerable impairment in strength of the arm with atrophy. Besides the muscles, it was reported that probably the median and radialis nerves were injured and that there were adhesions, since elevation of the arm above ninety degrees or retrotraction caused pain. He had a feeling of formication (sensation of small insects crawling over the skin) and numbness of the arm and hand, particularly the palmar aspect. There was also a large scar from a shell wound in the inner side of the lower third of his right leg. He was slightly lame and complained of stiffness and weakness of the leg associated with twitching of the muscles. Examination of the heart and lungs was normal but he complained of considerable dyspnea on exertion. Died while on a visit to Omaha, Nebraska, on May 2, 1898, and was buried in Greenlawn Cemetery, Columbus, Ohio. Cause of death, uremia.[1]

1. CSR; *OR*, vol. 10, pt. 1:252; vol. 44:19, 67, 83, 98; vol. 47, pt. 3:90; RVA, Pension SC 233,758; RAGO, entry 534; Douglas County, Neb., Death Register, vol. 3, roll 4.

LEWIS "LEW" WALLACE • *Born April 10, 1827,* in Brookville, Indiana. Served in the Mexican War. In 1832, his brother died of scarlet fever, but Wallace recovered from the disease, supposedly because he was dosed with boiling saffron tea. A prolific and well-known author, he was also a lawyer and politician in Indiana before the Civil War. In July 1861 he was made colonel of a three-month regiment, the 11th Indiana, which was mustered back into service in August for three years. He was promoted to brigadier general of volunteers in September and major general to rank from March 1862. Wallace served at Fort Donelson, Shiloh, and in the Shenandoah in 1864. In June 1862 he took a leave to attend to business and see a dentist. In early 1866 he had a brief episode of ague, which recurred at intervals throughout his life. After the war he continued his writing but also served as governor of the New Mexico Territory and United States minister to Turkey. While at Constantinople in early 1885, Wallace had a recurrence of the intermittent fever. He had minor surgery on a malignant ulcer in his nose in 1895. His health began to decline in 1901, and he required further surgeries on his nose in 1901 and 1902. During the summer of 1904 he had trouble assimilating food, and his nutritional status continued to decline. By autumn he stopped all work and had difficulty walking.[1] Died in Crawfordsville, Indiana, on February 15, 1905, and was buried there in Oak Hill Cemetery.
DEATH CERTIFICATE: Primary cause of death: atrophy of stomach.

1. Irving McKee, *Ben-Hur Wallace*, 2, 52, 103, 168, 214, 264–66.

WILLIAM HARVEY LAMB WALLACE • *Born July 8, 1821,* in Urbana, Ohio. Served in the Mexican War. A practicing lawyer and politician before the Civil War, he was made colonel of the 11th Illinois, which reenlisted for three years. He was at Fort Donelson, and in March 1862 he was appointed brigadier general of volunteers. At Shiloh on April 6, 1862, he was mortally wounded while taking his men to the rear. He died at Gen. U. S. Grant's headquarters in Savannah, Tennessee, on April 10 and was buried in a private cemetery near Ottawa, Illinois.[1]

1. *OR*, vol. 10, pt. 1:101, 110, 149, 158, 279; Heitman, *Historical Register and Dictionary* 1:999.

JOHN HENRY HOBART WARD • *Born June 17, 1823,* in New York City. He was
wounded at Cerro Gordo, Mexico. After the Mexican War he was assistant to
the New York commissary general and then commissary general. When the
Civil War started he was commissioned colonel of the 38th New York. He was at
First Bull Run, on the Peninsula, at Second Bull Run, Fredericksburg, and
Chancellorsville. In October 1862 he was made a brigadier general of volunteers. On July 2, 1863, Ward was slightly wounded at Gettysburg. The next day
he resumed command and participated in the battle. He had twenty days' sick
leave and returned January 19, 1864. He was wounded on the side of the head by
a piece of shell at Spotsylvania on May 10, 1864, but did not leave the field. He
was mustered out of service in July. After the war Ward served as clerk of the
superior and supreme courts of New York. On July 24, 1903, while vacationing
in Monroe, New York, he was run over by a train on the Erie Railroad and
killed.[1] He was buried in Monroe, New York, in Community Cemetery.
DEATH CERTIFICATE: Chief cause, shock. Contributing cause, injury received
on railroad and old age.

1. *OR,* vol. 36, pt. 1:470–71; U.S. Army, CWS, roll 1, vol. 1, report 33, pp. 513–47; *New York Times,*
July 25, 1903.

WILLIAM THOMAS WARD • *Born August 9, 1808,* in Amelia County, Virginia. Served
in the Mexican War. He practiced law in Kentucky and served in the Kentucky
legislature and Congress prior to the Civil War. In September 1861 he was commissioned a brigadier general of volunteers. His major service was in the Atlanta campaign and the Carolinas. On May 15, 1864, at Resaca, Georgia, Ward
was wounded. With the aid of two of his soldiers, he returned to the works on
the hill and found a surgeon who dressed his wound. The ball had struck his
left arm, partially severed the insertion of the deltoid muscle, passed backwards
and inward, grazed the bone, and injured the musculospiral muscle. It came
out on the under surface of the arm and contused his chest just below the nipple.
The surgeon advised him to go to the hospital, but Ward thought the hospital
air would injure him, and he preferred remaining with his command. He kept
his arm bandaged and in a sling until September. After Gen. Joseph E. Johnston's
surrender in 1865, he marched with his troops through Richmond to Washington, D.C. Sick for ten days in May, he was mustered out in September 1865.
When Ward returned to civilian life he practiced law in Louisville. A physical
examination in January 1874 revealed slight distal atrophy of the left arm. When
the limb was elevated and stimulated, it was painful at the point of entry of the
ball. The fingers of the left hand could not be approximated nearer than two
inches from the palm. Prior to his death Ward was affected with some type of
brain disease; delirious for a number of days, speechless, he finally sank into
complete stupor.[1] Died in Louisville, Kentucky, on October 12, 1878, and was
buried there in Cave Hill Cemetery.

1. CSR; *OR,* vol. 38, pt. 2:321–30, 339–42; U.S. Army, CWS, roll 5, vol. 9, report 7, pp. 117–66; RVA,
Pension C 270,956.

JAMES MEECH WARNER • *Born January 29, 1836,* in Middlebury, Vermont. Graduated from the USMA in 1860. Warner was treated at the Cadet Hospital for diarrhea six times, catarrhus five times, and neuralgia, nausea, and contusio one time each. After serving on the frontier, he was made colonel of the 11th Vermont Infantry to rank from September 1862. At Spotsylvania Court House on May 18, 1864, while walking up and down on the earthworks, Warner was wounded. The ball entered the back of his neck, passed upward to the base of his skull, and came out under the right ear. Within a few weeks there was exfoliation of the base of the os occipitus. Disabled by this wound for two months, he went home on leave and returned in July to participate in the defense of Washington against Confederate general Jubal Early. His promotion as brigadier general of volunteers ranked from May 1865.[1] He resigned early in 1866 and entered business in Albany. Died on March 16, 1897, while attending the Daley's theater in New York City, and was buried in Middlebury, Vermont.
DEATH CERTIFICATE: Cerebral apoplexy.

1. CSR; *OR,* vol. 36, pt. 1:705, 717; WPCHR, vol. 609; U.S. Army, CWS, roll 6, vol. 10, report 39, pp. 331–55; *MOLLUS* 11:131.

FITZ-HENRY WARREN • *Born January 11, 1816,* in Brimfield, Massachusetts. Before the war he lived in Iowa and was a politician and assistant postmaster general. Commissioned colonel of the 1st Iowa Cavalry in June 1861, he was made a brigadier general of volunteers in July 1862. During the first part of January 1863 he was incapacitated for field duty by poor health. Seemingly he continued to have ill health, since on September 30, 1864, he was ordered to report to the commanding general of Department of the East for assignment to such duty as he may be able to perform.[1] He was mustered out in August 1865 and returned to Iowa, where he held state and Federal positions. Died June 21, 1878, in Brimfield, where he was also buried.
DEATH CERTIFICATE: Cause of death was not recorded.

1. *OR,* vol. 22, pt. 1:189; vol. 43, pt. 2:225.

GOUVERNEUR KEMBLE WARREN • *Born January 8, 1830,* in Cold Spring, New York. Graduated from the USMA in 1850. At West Point he was treated for diarrhea five times, cephalalgia and colica twice each, and catarrhus, contusio, rheumatism, nausea and morbi. varii. one time each. For the next decade after graduation Warren served in the topographical engineers and as an instructor of mathematics at the U.S. Military Academy. In May 1861 he was made a lieutenant colonel of the 5th New York. He had a very bad headache on May 26, 1862, which made writing difficult. At the battle of Gaines' Mill on June 27, 1862, he was bruised on the knee by a spent shell but remained on the field. He served at Second Bull Run and Antietam, and in September he was promoted to brigadier general of volunteers. Warren was sick for a week in December and was slightly wounded by a musket ball in the throat on July 2, 1863, at Gettysburg. He stopped the hemorrhage with a handkerchief and remained on duty. In spite of the wound he attended a staff conference that night. On August 12, 1863, he was temporarily assigned to corps command. He felt quite sick on February 6, 1864, and was unable to leave his quarters for a couple of days. Warren participated in the siege of Petersburg and later at Five Forks, but difficulties with Gen. Philip Sheridan and Gen. U. S. Grant caused him to be relieved. He resigned as a general of volunteers on May 20, 1865, and requested a leave of absence since he was exhausted and felt unable to properly continue on duty in the hot and debilitating climate. Although his career was ruined, he still remained in the army as a major and served in the Engineer Corps. In later years a court of inquiry was convened and cleared his record. He was promoted to lieutenant colonel in March 1879. In late 1881 he took a cruise for his health.[1] Died in Newport, Rhode Island, on August 8, 1882, and was buried there in Island Cemetery.

DEATH CERTIFICATE: Cause of death, diabetes mellitus.

1. CSR; OR, vol. 11, pt. 1:678, pt. 2:379; vol. 27, pt. 1:72; vol. 33:119–20, 524; vol. 48, pt. 2:520; vol. 51, pt. 1:1084; WPCHR, vols. 606, 607; Norton, Little Round Top, 311; Steiner, Medical-Military Portraits, 248; Battles and Leaders 3:313; Emerson Gifford Taylor, Gouverneur Kemble Warren, 101, 243.

CADWALLADER COLDEN WASHBURN • Born April 22, 1818, in Livermore, Maine. A lawyer in Wisconsin, he became rich through speculation and a variety of businesses. He served four terms in Congress. Possibly because of family connections, he rose from colonel in February 1862 to brigadier general of volunteers in July and to major general to rank from November. In early November 1862 Washburn was sick, but he improved when cooler weather arrived. His major service was in the Vicksburg campaign. He resigned from the army in May 1865. After the war he again served in Congress and was governor of Wisconsin. During 1880 he had a stroke and suffered from Bright's disease of the kidneys. He went to Europe to see physicians, and on his return was taken care of by a prominent physician in Philadelphia. In February 1882 Washburn went to Eureka Springs for the benefit of the waters. On May 5 he became suddenly worse and was delirious. The next night he had an apoplectic seizure, followed by another attack of apoplexy on the ninth, and his condition became hopeless.[1] Died at Eureka Springs, Arkansas, on May 14, 1882, and was buried in Oak Grove Cemetery, La Crosse, Wisconsin.

1. OR, vol. 13:781; (Madison) Wisconsin State Journal, May 12, 15, 1882.

LOUIS DOUGLASS WATKINS • Born probably on November 29, 1833, near Tallahassee, Florida. In May 1861 he was commissioned first lieutenant in the Regular Army and served in the 5th Cavalry. He was severely wounded at Gaines' Mill on June 27, 1862, near the Woodbury's bridge on the Chickahominy. At the same time he was trampled by several horses of the regiment. Watkins was made colonel of the 6th Kentucky (Union) Cavalry in February 1863 and brigadier general of volunteers in September 1865. He served at Chickamauga, Chattanooga, and in the Atlanta campaign. He remained in the army after the war and was appointed lieutenant colonel of the 20th Infantry in 1866. He was on court-martial duty in New Orleans and died there on March 29, 1868. He was initially buried in the old Girod Street Cemetery and later was reinterred in Arlington National Cemetery. The local commanding officer reported he died from paralysis and congestion of the brain.[1]

1. OR, vol. 11, pt. 2:46–47; LR, CB, roll 311, W1467, 1866.

ALEXANDER STEWART WEBB • *Born February 15, 1835,* in New York City. Graduated from the USMA in 1855. At West Point he was treated for phlegmon thirteen times, excoriatio ten times, catarrhus five times, diarrhea twice, and an abscess, cephalalgia, ophthalmia, odontalgia, neuralgia, and subluxatio once each. Served in the Florida wars. In 1857 Webb was made an instructor at the U.S. Military Academy. From July 1861 to April 1862 he was assistant to William F. Barry, chief of artillery of the Army of the Potomac. In June 1863 he was promoted to brigadier general of volunteers and took command of the Second Brigade of John Gibbon's division. At Gettysburg, close to the point of the deepest Confederate penetration of his lines, he was wounded near his groin by a bullet on July 3, 1863. At Spotsylvania on May 12, 1864, Webb was severely wounded in the head. The bullet passed through the corner of his right eye, came out behind his ear, and exposed the temple bone. While falling from his horse, he recalled a conversation about head wounds he had previously had with Gen. James S. Wadsworth; after he hit the ground, he made an effort to raise his head. Realizing he could move his head, he decided that he was not going to die and promptly fainted. This wound apparently did not impair his mental abilities. He returned to duty as superintendent of recruiting for the Second Army Corps and served on court-martial duty in New York City to January 1865. In 1866 Webb was appointed lieutenant colonel of the 44th Infantry. He was again an instructor at the U.S. Military Academy until 1870, when he was discharged from the army. He then served as president of the College of the City of New York for thirty-three years but periodically was bothered by his wounds.[1] Died in Riverdale, New York, on February 12, 1911, and was buried at West Point.

1. CSR; OR, vol. 36, pt. 1:68, 138, 192, 339, 431, 437, 440; vol. 42, pt. 2:93–94, 178, 886; vol. 46, pt. 2:93–94, 178; WPCHR, vols. 608, 609; RAGO, entry 534; *Battles and Leaders* 4:160; New York Commission, *Final Report* 3:978–86.

MAX WEBER • *Born August 27, 1824,* in Achern in the Grand Duchy of Baden. Weber graduated from the military school at Karlsruhe in 1843 and came to the

United States in the late 1840s. He ran the Hotel Konstanz in New York City until the start of the Civil War. In May 1861 Weber entered the army in the 29th New York Infantry and in April 1862 was made brigadier general of volunteers. At the battle of Antietam on September 17, 1862, his right arm was fractured and he had to be carried off the field. The ball entered the outer condyle of the humerus and emerged about midway at the inner surface of the forearm, carrying away about three inches of the radius. That same day, on the field, he underwent a primary excision of three inches of the radius, including the head. He was treated at the Sixth Corps hospital until December 20, when he was transferred to the Gerhardts Hotel in Washington D.C. At that time there was necrosis of the bones and some pieces were removed. In the summer of 1863, Weber returned to limited duty in Washington, D.C., and served on court-martial duty. He was assigned to command the defenses of Harpers Ferry in April 1864. His wound reopened in August, and he was on leave until late September. Still unfit for field duty upon his return from sick leave, he was sent to Hagerstown, Maryland, where he remained until he resigned in May 1865. After the war Weber held state and federal positions. When he was examined in 1890 the right forearm was permanently semi-flexed at 45 degrees and was associated with atrophy of the muscles of the forearm and paralysis agitans of the entire arm. He was incapable of feeding himself. The examining surgeon stated that the limb was good for nothing and expressed the opinion that the arm should have been amputated at the time Weber was wounded.[1] Died at his residence in Brooklyn on June 15, 1901, and was buried there in Evergreen Cemetery.

DEATH CERTIFICATE: Pneumonia, edema of lungs.

1. CSR; *OR*, vol. 19, pt. 1:173, 193, 276, 324, 336; vol. 33:833; vol. 46, pt. 2:357; vol. 51, pt. 1:1178–79; *MSHW*, vol. 2, pt. 2:848, 859; U.S. Army, CWS, roll 4, vol. 7, report 39, pp. 533–35; RVA, Pension SC 55,839.

JOSEPH DANA WEBSTER • *Born August 25, 1811,* in Hampton, New Hampshire. Served in the Mexican War. In 1838 he was commissioned in the Regular Army's topographical engineers. He resigned in 1854 and moved to Chicago. In July 1861 Webster reentered the army as a staff paymaster. He was made a colonel in February 1862 and served as Gen. U. S. Grant's chief of staff. His commission as brigadier general of volunteers ranked from November 1862. He later was chief of staff for Gen. William T. Sherman, and then served in this position for Gen. George H. Thomas. After the war he returned to Chicago and held city and Federal positions. He died at the Palmer House in Chicago on March 12, 1876, and was buried in Rosehill Cemetery.

STEPHEN HINSDALE WEED • *Born November 17, 1831,* in Potsdam, New York. Graduated from the USMA in 1854. While a cadet, he was treated for phlegmon three times, contusio twice, and odontalgia, catarrhus, excoriatio, influenza, and cephalalgia one time each. Served in the Florida wars. An officer of artillery, Weed had duty on the frontier prior to the Civil War. In May 1861 he was promoted to captain of the 5th Artillery and was stationed in Pennsylvania. At Gaines' Mill on June 27, 1862, he was slightly wounded in the face by a piece of shell. He served at Second Bull Run, Antietam, Fredericksburg, and Chancellorsville and was promoted to brigadier general of volunteers in June 1863. At Gettysburg, July 2, 1863, while directing the fire of his guns, he was mortally wounded by a bullet and paralyzed below the shoulders. Carried first behind some rocks, he was then moved to a hospital where he died within a few hours.[1] He was buried in the Moravian Cemetery at New Dorp, Staten Island, New York.

1. *OR*, vol. 11, pt. 2:239, 353; vol. 27, pt. 1:593, 652; vol. 29, pt. 2:148, 154; WPCHR, vols. 607, 608, 609; *MOLLUS* 42:35–46.

GODFREY WEITZEL • *Born November 1, 1835,* in Cincinnati, Ohio. Graduated from the USMA in 1855. At the military academy he was treated for excoriatio, diarrhea, catarrhus, ophthalmia, and subluxatio once each. He was commissioned in the Engineer Corps and served in this capacity at New Orleans and at West Point until 1861. The following year he was made chief engineer of Gen. Benjamin F. Butler's expedition against New Orleans. In August 1862 Wietzel was promoted to brigadier general of volunteers. On May 17, 1863, he temporarily turned over his command, having had dysentery for four days. After serving in the campaign against Port Hudson, he reported to New Orleans in March 1864 and, sick and unable to take the field, was assigned to duty there. In the middle of July he was sick again; when the illness continued into the next month he took a sick leave. He was assigned to duty on September 30, 1864, and was made a major general in November. He served at Fort Fisher and in the Appomattox campaign. Weitzel remained in the army and reverted to his regular rank of captain of engineers. He was promoted to major in August 1866 and to lieutenant colonel in 1882. In 1882, poor health from chronic catarrh, both nasopharyngeal and bronchial, prompted his assignment to lighter duties in Philadelphia. Soon after he arrived there, a large carbuncle developed on his thigh, which confined him to his house for almost two months, and he recovered slowly. His health improved; although at work most of the time in 1883, he had catarrh and contracted colds with changes in the weather. Late in the year he had a severe cold, and early in January 1884 he developed jaundice with loss of appetite, impaired digestion, and great debility. Although under treatment, the jaundice intensified, and he became more debilitated. The surgeon speculated that exposure to great variations of temperature incident to his profession brought about the diseases that ultimately resulted in his death. He gradually passed into a typhoid condition and, after being in bed for less than two weeks, died on March 19, 1884, in Philadelphia.[1] Buried in Spring Grove Cemetery, Cincinnati.

DEATH CERTIFICATE: Cause of death, congestive liver.

1. *OR,* vol. 40, pt. 3:246, 711; vol. 42, pt. 1:657, pt. 2:1146; WPCHR, vols. 607, 608, 609; U.S. Army, CWS, roll 2, vol. 3, report 27, pp. 741–801; LR, ACP, 1639, 1884, fiche: 000201; RVA, Pension C 207,962.

WILLIAM WELLS • *Born December 14, 1837,* in Waterbury, Vermont. A merchant in Burlington, Vermont, before the war, he enlisted as a private in the 1st Vermont Cavalry. By the summer of 1863 he had risen to major with service at Second Bull Run and Gettysburg. He was temporarily disabled during a skirmish at Culpeper Court House on September 13, 1863, by a bursting shell. He turned over the command for only a short time. In May 1865 Wells was appointed brigadier general of volunteers and was discharged in 1866.[1] After the war, he was adjutant general of Vermont, collector of internal revenue, and a member of the state senate. Died in New York City on April 29, 1892, and was buried in Lake View Cemetery, Burlington.

DEATH CERTIFICATE: Exhaustion from angina pectoris.

1. *OR,* vol. 29, pt. 1:129.

THOMAS WELSH • *Born May 5, 1824,* in Columbia, Pennsylvania. He was severely wounded at Buena Vista on February 23, 1847, and was treated in the general hospital in Saltillo. Welsh was a well-to-do merchant, canal boat owner, and justice of the peace at Columbia, Pennsylvania, before the war. In April 1861 he recruited a three-month regiment and, after it was mustered out of service, became colonel of the 45th Pennsylvania in October 1861. He was at South Mountain, Antietam, and Fredericksburg. In November 1862 he was promoted to brigadier general of volunteers. The day after leaving Snyder's Bluff, on or about August 6, 1863, he became sick on the boat with chills and fever. Upon arrival at Cairo, Illinois, he was too sick to travel in a common railroad car and remained there until a sleeping car could be found. He arrived at Cincinnati on August 14, 1863, and was taken to a private home, where he died the same day. The attending surgeon reported he died from congestive chills.[1] Buried in Mount Bethel Cemetery, Columbia, Pennsylvania.

1. CSR Mexican Service; *OR,* vol. 30, pt. 3:17, 30, 45; RVA, Pension C 19,444.

HENRY WALTON WESSELLS • *Born February 20, 1809,* in Litchfield, Connecticut. Graduated from the USMA in 1833. Cadet Wessells was treated for a headache four times, and for a toothache and a wound once each. Served in the Florida and Mexican wars. He was dangerously wounded on August 20, 1847, at Churubusco. From October to November 1847 he was sick in Mexico City. He was ill at Benicia, California, in January and February 1850. After service on the frontier, Wessells became a major of the 6th Infantry in June 1861. In September he was made colonel of the 8th Kansas Infantry and in April 1862 was promoted to brigadier general of volunteers. He had a severe contusion of his shoulder from a spent musket ball at Seven Pines on May 31, 1862, but did not leave the field. He was ill in November 1862. He was captured at Plymouth, North Carolina, in April 1864, and was a prisoner of war for four months. After his release he went to Connecticut to restore his health, then returned to duty in September. In 1865 he became lieutenant colonel of the 18th U.S. Infantry and remained in the army. In October 1869 he was treated for varoloid. Wessells's health, until he retired from the service in January 1871, was good except for the usual colds, toothaches, and bilious attacks. His health started to fail during the last two years of his life. The immediate cause of his death was listed by the adjutant general's office as heart failure. However, he was reported to have felt unusually well and had a warning of only fifteen to twenty minutes before his death, which does not sound correct for a diagnosis of heart failure.[1] Died in Dover, Delaware, on January 12, 1889, and was buried in the cemetery at Litchfield, where he had his residence.

1. OR, vol. 11, pt. 1:915, 927; vol. 18:20; WPCHR, vol. 601; U.S. Army, CWS, roll 4, vol. 7, report 29, pp. 449-55; LR, ACP, 545, 1889, fiche: 000203; RVA, Pension, WC 407,823; RAGO, entry 534; Heitman, *Historical Register and Dictionary* 2:41.

JOSEPH RODMAN WEST · *Born September 19, 1822,* in New Orleans, Louisiana. Served during the Mexican War. A newspaperman in California when the Civil War started, he was commissioned lieutenant colonel of the 1st California Volunteers. He was made colonel of the regiment in June 1862 and was promoted to brigadier general in October. West served in the Red River campaign and in Arkansas and Missouri. He was discharged in January 1866 and returned to New Orleans where he was deputy U.S. marshal, auditor for customs, and U.S. senator. He then moved to Washington and was a member of the board of commissioners of the District of Columbia from 1882 to 1885. By 1894 he was disabled by paralysis agitans and senile debility.[1] After being hospitalized in the Garfield Hospital he died on October 31, 1898, in Washington, D.C., and was buried in Arlington National Cemetery.

DEATH CERTIFICATE: Cause of death, primary, paralysis agitans. Immediate, asthenia, four months.

1. RVA, Pension SC 879,932.

FRANK WHEATON · *Born May 8, 1833,* at Providence, Rhode Island. He was commissioned into the 1st U.S. Cavalry as a first lieutenant in 1855. After service on the frontier, Wheaton became lieutenant colonel and then colonel of the 2nd Rhode Island Infantry in July 1861. He was at First Bull Run, on the Peninsula, and was promoted brigadier general of volunteers in November 1862. He served as a brigade and division commander at Fredericksburg, Chancellorsville, in the Wilderness, and in the Petersburg campaign. In March 1865 he suffered with piles and was uncertain if he would be able to do cavalry service. He was mustered out of volunteer service in 1866 and was made lieutenant colonel of the 39th Infantry. He developed yellow fever on September 13, 1867, in New Orleans and, on recommendation of the medical officer, went north to recuperate. Wheaton was made colonel in 1874, brigadier general, U.S. Army, in 1892, and major general in 1897. During the spring of 1899, while in Berlin, Germany, he had an acute attack of glaucoma in his right eye. There was continued deterioration in the vision in the eye and, on January 17, 1900, he had the eye removed to preserve the other eye. Died at his residence in Washington, D.C., on June 18, 1903, and was buried in Arlington National Cemetery. According to his attending surgeon, the cause of death was cerebral hemorrhage from arteriosclerosis. He was also suffering with acute bladder trouble at the time of his death.[1]

1. *OR*, vol. 46, pt. 3:29; RVA, Pension WC 648,469; LR, ACP, 2392, 1887.

AMIEL WEEKS WHIPPLE • *Born October 15, 1816*, in Greenwich, Massachusetts. He graduated from the USMA in 1841. During his time at West Point he was treated for a cough seven times, nausea and headache four times each, hemorrhoids twice, and a sore throat, pain in side, cold, earache, and fever one time each. He joined the topographical engineers and spent his years before the Civil War surveying boundaries, railroad routes, and clearing waterways in the Great Lakes. In April 1862 he was commissioned brigadier general of volunteers. At Chancellorsville on May 4, 1863, he was sitting on his horse, writing an order, when he was mortally wounded. He died in Washington on May 7, 1863, and was buried in South Cemetery, Portsmouth, New Hampshire.

1. CSR; *OR*, vol. 25, pt. 1:174–85, 302, 393, pt. 2:569; vol. 51, pt. 1:1040; WPCHR, vol. 604; LR, ACP, 6069, 1885, fiche: 000206.

WILLIAM DENISON WHIPPLE • *Born August 2, 1826*, in Nelson, New York. He graduated from the USMA in 1851. Whipple was treated at the military academy for phlegmon three times, diarrhea and catarrhus twice each, and fatigue, odontalgia, tonsillitis, dysentery, subluxatio, febris ephemeral, cephalalgia, and pleurodynia one time each. Prior to the Civil War, Whipple had frontier duties and in 1861 was captured by Southern troops at Indianola, Texas. During the war he served as a staff officer and, after passing through grades, was promoted to brigadier general of volunteers in July 1863. In October 1863 there was a question of whether his health was adequate for him to be assigned to duty. In January 1864 he complained that frequently after he ate he had neurologic pains in his jaw, which he blamed on the poor job his dentist, or "butcher," as he called him, in Cincinnati had done. After the war Whipple served on Gen. George H. Thomas's and Gen. William T. Sherman's staffs. He was adjutant general of different divisions and departments from 1878 until his retirement in 1890. On

January 26, 1888, he slipped on the icy deck of a boat while returning to Governors Island and fractured his left patella. The fracture was transverse and there were no complications. He died April 1, 1902, in New York City and was buried in Arlington National Cemetery. According to his son, he died from bronchial pneumonia.[1]

1. *OR*, vol. 30, pt. 4:59; WPCHR, vols. 606, 607; LR, ACP, 4566, 1890, fiche: 000207; W. (Whipple) to Caso, Jan. 22, 1864 (Maj. General William D. Whipple, Letters to and from friends, family); Lewis Leigh Collection, USAMHI.

WALTER CHILES WHITAKER • *Born August 8, 1823,* in Shelbyville, Kentucky. Served in the Mexican War. Whitaker was a landowner, lawyer, and politician in Kentucky before the Civil War. He was made colonel of the 6th Kentucky (Union) Infantry in December 1861. That same month he was sick at Louisville with diarrhea, which continued to bother him even after the war. He supposedly had contracted the gastrointestinal complaint from drinking pond and surface water. Whitaker served at Shiloh and Perryville. At Stones River, Tennessee, on December 31, 1862, he was wounded by a gunshot just above the left elbow. The bone was scaled, and later the arm was greatly weakened and reduced in size. During March 1863 he had recurring attacks of illness and in April was seriously ill in Louisville, Kentucky. In June he was made a brigadier general of volunteers. At the battle of Chickamauga on September 20, 1863, he was wounded in the right side of his abdomen and was on sick leave until the following April. At Resaca, Georgia, on May 15, 1864, a shell burst near his head, and the resulting concussion produced total deafness of his left ear. In June he was compelled to obtain a leave of absence because his health was seriously impaired by two months of exposure and subacute dysentery. Whitaker was at Franklin and Nashville; after his discharge in 1865 he returned to his law practice. In the winter of 1865–66 he was treated for an exacerbation of his chronic diarrhea, and for the rest of his life he intermittently required treatment for the condition. He had no further acute serious illness until he had bilious and intermittent fever in May, September, and October 1878, and a similar but milder attack in July 1879. Died in Lyndon, Kentucky, on July 9, 1887, and was buried in Grove Hill Cemetery, Shelbyville. According to his wife he died from chronic diarrhea.[1]

1. CSR; *OR*, vol. 30, pt. 1:855; vol. 38, pt. 1:90, 226, 245, 247; RVA, Pension WC 240,185.

JULIUS WHITE • *Born September 23, 1816,* in Cazenovia, New York. He conducted various businesses in Illinois and Wisconsin over the years and in 1861 was appointed collector of customs in Chicago. Soon after accepting this position, White resigned to become colonel of the 37th Illinois Volunteers. His leg was fractured in March 1862, and he left on sick leave the last of the month. He went north and, in addition to the fracture, his recovery was complicated by some

nonspecified illness during December. In June 1862 he was promoted to brigadier general. At the time of the explosion at the Crater on August 21, 1864, he
had typhoid fever; when the fighting was over he obtained a sick leave. Initially
treated at Norfolk, he was then sent home by order of the Medical Director.
White was confined to his bed for nearly two months. Although he had recovered enough to leave the house, he was still too enfeebled to return to the field
for several months. As a consequence, he resigned his commission, which was
accepted in November 1864.[1] Died in Evanston, Illinois, on May 12, 1890, and
buried in Rosehill Cemetery, Chicago.

1. *OR*, vol. 42, pt. 1:72, pt. 2:684; U.S. Army, CWS, roll 2, vol. 3, report 28, pp. 805–53; ibid., roll 3,
vol. 5, report 8, pp. 825–41.

EDWARD AUGUSTUS WILD • *Born November 25, 1825,* in Brookline, Massachusetts. After he graduated from Jefferson Medical College in 1847, he served as a
surgeon during the Crimean War. Wild practiced medicine until the start of
the Civil War when he became a company captain in the 1st Massachusetts
Infantry in May 1861. He was at First Bull Run and was wounded twice near
Fair Oaks on June 25, 1862. One of his knees was slightly injured by a minié ball.
The other projectile was a small rifle ball that passed through his right hand
between the first and second knuckle joints and made its exit in the palm. The
thumb and metacarpal bones of the first and second fingers were injured. On
June 26 he went to Philadelphia and remained there until July 19, when he went
to Boston. He had permanent disability of the first and second fingers and
stiffness of his whole right hand. On July 24 he was placed in command of the
camp of recruits at Camp Stanton, Lynnfield, Massachusetts. In August Wild
was made colonel of the 35th Massachusetts and returned to the field with his
right arm in a sling. His left arm was shattered by an explosive bullet on September 14, 1862, at the Battle of South Mountain, Maryland, and he had to walk
two or three miles to the rear for help. Two days later his arm was amputated
(exarticulation) at the shoulder joint. After remaining at Middletown, Maryland, for two weeks, he was transported to Philadelphia. On December 1 he was
moved to Boston. Healing was delayed by the repeated formation of abscesses
on the stump. When he returned to duty the wound still suppurated at times.
He recruited black troops during February through April 1863. In April the stump
had almost healed, and he was commissioned brigadier general of volunteers.
Wild was at Cold Harbor and Appomattox. He had a six-day leave to go to
Philadelphia for dental work in February 1865. Wild was mustered out in January 1866 and became engaged in mining. In later years he had no power or
grasp in his remaining injured hand, and with his other arm missing, he was
unable to return to the practice of medicine. His diarrhea, which had started
during the war, continued for the rest of his life, and his wife stated that it was
the cause of his death. He usually treated himself for the condition and never

discussed it with anyone, so nothing was recorded about his self treatment.[1] Died August 28, 1891, in Medellin, Colombia, and was buried there in the Cementerio de San Pedro.

1. CSR; *OR*, vol. 19, pt. 1:448; *MSHW*, vol. 2, pt. 2:629; U.S. Army, CWS, roll 1, vol. 2, report 59, pp. 817–30; ibid., roll 6, vol. 10, report 42, pp. 379–98; RVA, Pension WC 579,214; Military Life of Edward A. Wild, Brig. Gen. Vol., Norfolk, Va., Mar. 12, 1864, Edward Augustus Wild Papers, File 2149, USAMHI.

ORLANDO BOLIVAR WILLCOX • *Born April 16, 1823,* in Detroit, Michigan. Graduated from the USMA in 1847. At the military academy, he was treated for cephalalgia five times, catarrhus twice, and phlegmon and odontalgia one time each. Served in the Florida wars. Following the Mexican War he had garrison duty there. In 1857, Willcox resigned from the army and practiced the law in Detroit. He was appointed colonel of the 1st Michigan Infantry in 1861. At First Bull Run on July 21, 1861, a shell wounded his right forearm, which was bound up on the field. He was captured and, after being confined in a Confederate hospital at the Lewis house on the battlefield for two weeks, he was sent to the depot at Manassas Junction. After a few days he was transported by train to Richmond and was placed in the St. Marks Hospital (Alms House Hospital) where he remained for six weeks. Over the next year Willcox was transferred to prisons at both Charleston and Columbia, South Carolina, Libby Prison, and Salisbury, North Carolina, until he was paroled in August 1862. He was commissioned a brigadier general of volunteers the same month to rank from April 1861. Willcox served at Antietam, Fredericksburg, Knoxville, in the Overland campaign, and at Petersburg. In 1866 he was mustered out of the service. In July when the Regular Army was enlarged he was reappointed colonel of the 29th Infantry. He served at San Francisco until 1878, when he took command of the Department of Arizona. In August 1885 he was treated for a carbuncle on his neck. He was promoted brigadier general in 1886 and retired the next year. Died in Coburg, Ontario, on May 10, 1907, and was buried in Arlington National Cemetery. According to the adjutant general's office, he died of acute bronchitis.[1]

1. *OR*, vol. 2:315, 323, 413, 550; *OR Suppl.*, vol. 1, pt. 1:161–62; WPCHR, vol. 605; U.S. Army, CWS, roll 5, vol. 9, report 11, pp. 237–71; RVA, Pension WC 648,468; LR, ACP, 4009, 1874.

ALPHEUS STARKEY WILLIAMS • *Born September 20, 1810,* in Saybrook, Connecticut. Served in the Mexican War. He started a law practice in 1836 in Detroit, Michigan, and at the beginning of the Civil War was a brigadier general of state troops. His commission as brigadier general of volunteers ranked from May 1861. On April 29, 1862, after having been exposed to the rain all day, he had a terrible cold and was sick for the first time since he had been in the service. On May 26, 1864, the day after the fight at New Hope Church, Georgia, Williams went to sleep against a tree. A sudden sharp stinging sensation on his elbow joint woke him up. A ball had struck a tree and then hit him. Although the skin was not broken, he sustained a lump on the elbow, and since it had struck near the "funny bone" it paralyzed his forearm for awhile. He had it rubbed with spirits. Near Atlanta on July 26, 1864, he was feeling unwell and was taking quinine to build him up. Following the grand review of troops in May 1865 he had a sore stomach and was not able to ride until May 28, 1865.[1] He was in the Shenandoah, at Cedar Mountain, Second Bull Run, Antietam, Chancellorsville, Gettysburg, and in the Atlanta campaign, the March to the Sea, and in the Carolinas. Following the Civil War, he was appointed minister resident to the Republic of Salvador in 1866 and was later elected to Congress for two terms. Died in a hotel in Washington, D.C., on December 21, 1878, and was buried in Elmwood Cemetery, Detroit.

DEATH CERTIFICATE: Cause of death, primary, nausea and vomiting from food. Immediate, apoplexy. Duration of last sickness, since December 16.

1. Alpheus S. Williams, *From the Cannon's Mouth*, 72, 314, 336, 389.

DAVID HENRY WILLIAMS • *Born March 19, 1819*, on a farm in Otsego County, New York. Served in the Mexican War. He was a civil engineer and railroad surveyor at the start of the Civil War when he entered the army as colonel of the 82nd Pennsylvania (32nd Pennsylvania). He was on the Peninsula and at Antietam and Fredericksburg. In March 1863 his appointment as brigadier general of volunteers, which had not been acted on by the Senate, expired. Williams left the army in 1863 and became a professor of engineering in Pittsburgh. In poor health, he was an invalid for many years. He died in Allegheny (now Pittsburgh) on June 1, 1891, and was buried in Allegheny Cemetery. Burial records: Cause of death, apoplexy.

NELSON GROSVENOR WILLIAMS • *Born May 4, 1823*, in Bainbridge, New York. He entered the USMA in 1839 but withdrew because of his poor performance in mathematics. Following a career in business, he settled on a farm in Iowa. In June 1861 he was commissioned colonel of the 3rd Iowa Infantry. At Shiloh on April 6, 1862, Williams was severely injured when his horse was shot and fell on him. He immediately had pain in both ears, and the sight in his right eye was diminished. He was paralyzed for a number of weeks, reportedly as a result of injury to his spine. After being treated on a hospital boat at Pittsburg Landing for two days, he was sent to a private house at Memphis, Tennessee. During the period he was at Pittsburg Landing he had contracted diarrhea, which remained with him during the rest of his service. In July, having partially recovered from the injury, he developed jaundice and had a severe attack of dysentery that was complicated by a marked prolapse ani. During September and October 1862 he was absent sick in Iowa. Williams resigned his commission on November 27, 1862. He had been made brigadier general of volunteers the same month, but since he was no longer in the service, his appointment was not confirmed by the Senate. He returned to his farm in Iowa, and in 1869 President U. S. Grant appointed him a deputy collector of customs in New York City. Williams continued to have episodes of frequent pain in his ears, sometimes lasting for months. For the rest of his life he had decreased vision in his eye, problems with his rectal prolapse, and almost continuous suffering from rheumatism.[1] Died at his residence in Brooklyn on November 30, 1897, and was buried in Green-Wood Cemetery.

DEATH CERTIFICATE: Cause of death, disease of the heart, hypertrophic chronic bronchitis and cirrhosis of the liver. Associated with edema of the limbs.

1. CSR; *OR*, vol. 10, pt. 1:206, 211, 217; RVA, Pension WC 840,456.

SETH WILLIAMS • *Born March 22, 1822,* in Augusta, Maine. Graduated from the USMA in 1842. Served in the Mexican War. Early in his military career he was transferred to the adjutant general's department. He was made a major in August 1861 and a brigadier general of volunteers in September. In March 1864, Gen. U. S. Grant appointed him as his inspector general. He was ill the last of February 1866 and went to his sister's home in Boston, where he died on March 24. His remains were taken to Augusta and buried in Forest Grove Cemetery.[1]

DEATH CERTIFICATE: Immediate cause of death, inflammation of brain, five weeks' duration.

1. LR, CB, G108, 1866; LR, CB, roll 240, B263, 1866.

THOMAS WILLIAMS • *Born January 10, 1815,* in Albany, New York. He graduated from the USMA in 1837. As a cadet, he was treated for a toothache twice and nausea, cold, fever, and catarrhus one time each. Served in the Black Hawk, Florida, and Mexican wars. Following garrison duty on the frontier, Williams was at the Artillery School for Practice at Fort Monroe when the Civil War started. In May 1861 he was made major of the Fifth Artillery and in September was appointed brigadier general of volunteers. He was killed by a rifle ball, which hit him in the chest on August 5, 1862, at Baton Rouge. The transport carrying his body collided with a gunboat and sank. The following day his coffin was found and sent to his family.[1] He was buried in the family plot in Elmwood Cemetery, Detroit.

1. *OR*, vol. 15:40–41, 52, 54, 57; vol. 25, pt. 2:569; WPCHR, vols. 602, 603; Norman C. Delaney, "General Thomas Williams," *CWTI* 14 (July 1975): 4–9, 36–47.

JAMES ALEXANDER WILLIAMSON • *Born February 8, 1829,* in Adair County, Kentucky. A lawyer and politician in Iowa, he had become colonel of the 4th Iowa by July 1862. He was wounded at Elkhorn, Arkansas, on March 7, 1862. Near the

Chickasaw Bayou on December 29, 1862, he was struck by three balls; not seriously injured, he stayed on the field. He served at Vicksburg, Chattanooga, and in the Atlanta campaign and the March to the Sea. On September 1, 1864, he was slightly wounded in the hand.[1] His appointment as brigadier general of volunteers ranked from April 1865, and Williamson was mustered out the following November. After returning to civilian life, he dealt with land and railroads in the West. Died at his summer home in Jamestown, Rhode Island, on September 7, 1902, and was buried in Rock Creek Cemetery, Georgetown, D.C. Burial records: Cause of death, cancer of the liver.

1. Major General G. M. Dodge, "General James A. Williamson," *Annals of Iowa* 6, no. 3 (1903): 161–84; LR, CB, roll 451, W28, 1869.

AUGUST (VON) WILLICH • *Born November 19, 1810,* in the Prussian city of Braunsberg. He served as a lieutenant and captain in the Prussian army and, after becoming a follower of Karl Marx's work, came to the United States in 1853. He found employment as a carpenter in the Brooklyn Navy Yard and was editor of a German-language labor newspaper in Cincinnati. Willich entered Federal service as first lieutenant adjutant of the 9th Ohio Infantry in May 1861. He rose rapidly through ranks and was made brigadier general of volunteers in July 1862. In September, while in Louisville, Kentucky, he was sick with typhoid fever. After he recovered he took command near Nashville, Tennessee, in November. He served at Shiloh and Perryville. On December 31, 1862, at Stones River he was wounded and captured. He was exchanged in May 1863 and returned to command to lead a brigade at Chickamauga. Willich was wounded at Resaca on May 15, 1864. A rifle ball entered his right arm about five inches below the head of the humerus, passed internally to the bone and out through the lower part of the scapula. The projectile severely injured the axillary plexus of nerves. He returned to duty in May 1865 and was mustered out in January 1866. After returning to civilian life he settled in Cincinnati. By 1867 there was considerable atrophy and loss of strength in his right arm and hand, and he could not grasp objects. Over the years the paralysis of the arm and hand increased.[1] Died January 22, 1878, in St. Mary's, Ohio, and was buried there in Elmwood Cemetery.

1. CSR; *OR*, vol. 20, pt. 1:208, 255, 296, 912; vol. 23, pt. 2:317, 368; vol. 38, pt. 1:91, 375, 385, 391, 431; vol. 49, pt. 2:923; CLCO; U.S. Army, CWS, roll 1, vol. 1, report 48, pp. 909–19; RVA, Pension SC 77,658.

JAMES HARRISON WILSON • *Born September 2, 1837,* on a farm near Shawneetown, Illinois. Graduated from the USMA in 1860. While at the military academy he was treated once each for contusio, odontalgia, phlegmon, diarrhea, nausea, a boil, and neuralgia. On the way from New York to Washington he contracted "cholera morbus" and stopped at Wilmington, Delaware, for treatment on August 24, 1861. Within a few days he was able to continue the trip. Wilson was a member of the topographical engineers and, during the winter of 1861–62, served in this capacity. A spent bullet was deflected by his boot-top on Wilmington Island, Georgia, on April 18, 1862. Following a tour of the Department of Tennessee, and after recovering from a bout of malaria and a fall from his horse, he went to Vicksburg on September 21, 1863. In October 1863 he was made brigadier general of volunteers. He was a major cavalry commander on the Virginia campaigns in 1864 and at Franklin and Nashville. At Selma, Alabama, on April 2, 1865, he was thrown to the ground when his horse was shot. He was stunned but not seriously injured. His promotion to major general of volunteers ranked from May 1865. Wilson remained in the army, was made lieutenant colonel of the 35th Infantry in 1866, and resigned in1870. He served as a major general of volunteers in the war with Spain in 1898 and took part in the Boxer Rebellion in China. In 1901 he was placed on the retired list. Died in Wilmington, Delaware, on February 23, 1925, and was buried in Old Swedes Churchyard.[1]

DEATH CERTIFICATE: Cause of death, acute dilatation of heart. Duration, one half hour. Contributing, myocarditis.

1. WPCHR, vol. 609; Edward G. Longacre, *From Union Stars to Top Hat*, 41–42, 52, 86, 208, 289.

ISAAC JONES WISTAR • *Born November 14, 1827*, in Philadelphia. On April 5, 1849, he left Philadelphia on the way to the California gold mines. While going from St. Louis by boat on the Missouri, he had a severe but short episode of "cholera." Crossing the plains, and while traveling along the Little Blue River in late May 1849, Wistar was confined to his wagon with "Missouri River cholera" or diarrhea. He had a headache and symptoms of a severe bilious attack when they left Salt Lake in July 1849. After he arrived in California he was a miner, trapper, mountain man, and farmer, and he also hauled goods for the miners. At one point he had mountain fever, "probably one of the protean forms of bilious intermittents." Wistar was put in a small canvas lodging-house, where he lay ill for a few days. Taken to San Francisco, he recovered. During a night fight with Indians one summer, he had an arrow break off in the front part of his upper thigh. The arrow entered on one side, passed an inch below the skin, and the point projected slightly on the other side. There was considerable laceration and bleeding and, because of the barb, it was impossible to draw the arrow back. After getting rid of the broken end, with difficulty he pushed it through in the original direction and tied up the wound as best he could. Because of nearby Indians, he had to remain hiding in the cold water of an arroyo for an hour or two. It took him two days to get back to a miners' camp. Seeking a better life, Wistar studied the law, passed his examination for the bar in California in 1854, and set up a practice. He left San Francisco in September 1857 by boat and arrived at New York Harbor the next month. In the spring of 1859, following the discovery of gold at Pike's Peak, he started for Colorado. At Bloomfield, Indiana, that summer he had a bad case of ague. There was no doctor or quinine available, and he took any quack medicine available. He never got to Colorado but ended up taking cattle from Burlington to Chicago to sell. Wistar was practicing the law in Philadelphia when the war started. In 1861 he entered Federal service as a captain and by November was a colonel. Early in the fight at Ball's Bluff on October 21, 1861, he was struck in the jaw by a bullet or small stone. Although not severe, it caused pain, and a considerable amount of blood dripped down and matted in his beard. Later a bullet passed through his thigh, close to the old arrow wound. Only a flesh wound, it filled his boot with blood, and he had to cut a hole in the boot to let the blood out. Before dark a ball struck his right elbow, shattered the external condyle of the humerus and the head of the radius, and chipped the olecranon as it passed out. Years later, Wistar wrote Captain Rogers and thanked him for putting a tourniquet on his arm, which he attributed to saving his life. He had to be carried from the field to the river and was placed in a rowboat. The boat took him to a nearby island where he was taken care of by a surgeon in a farmyard. He was administered stimulants and the arm was tied up. When he could be moved, he was taken across the Maryland branch of the river, placed on a stretcher, and carried two miles to a small house near the regimental camp. The wound had little reaction during the first two weeks but had to be opened about three weeks after the injury because of inflammation and to extract loose pieces of bone and lead. Despite the surgery, his condition became worse and amputation was seriously considered. Maggots appeared in the wound and were occasionally removed in large numbers. When it became apparent he was going to have ankylosis of the principal joints, his arm was fixed in the position and at the angle where it would remain for the rest of his life. He stayed near the regimental camp for weeks without the bedsheets being changed. One of the surgeons and a small detail of men took him to his home in Philadelphia in time to enjoy Christmas. He learned to write with his right hand; since the fingers were in a fixed position and could not be closed, he had to use a thick-handled pen. In April 1862 at Yorktown, he developed typhoid fever and was carried unconscious to a hospital steamer in the York River. When he could be transported, he was sent home where he had a relapse. Once he was able to get out of the house, he was married on July 9 and rejoined the army in August. At Antietam on September 17, 1862, he was severely wounded in his good left arm near the elbow, but the bones were not injured. One of the men used Wistar's handkerchief and his bayonet for a tourniquet and left him on the field. Union and Confederate forces passed back and forth over the area, and at one point a Confederate rearranged the tourniquet and gave him a drink of water. (After the war, he discovered the man was supposedly John S. Mosby.) That night, two wounded Union men carried him to the regimental field hospital in the rear. Before long an ambulance took him to the general hospital at Keedysville. He lay there for three weeks before it was determined that the condition of the injured artery made it safe for him to travel, and he was taken by ambulance to Hagerstown. Along with his wife, who had joined him, they were moved in a boxcar to Philadelphia. His promotion as brigadier general ranked from November 1862. His right arm was already useless and the left was now paralyzed. He had some return of nerve function in the left arm; although able to use it to some extent, it was still much impaired. The fingers were so devoid of sensation that their use was limited to times they could be guided by sight. Wistar was discharged from the service because of his wounds in December 1862 and was reinstated in February 1863. When he had recovered from his wound to some extent, he was assigned to command in May. During the fall of 1863 he had "every variety of fever and diarrhea," and quinine was served daily at reveille. He entered the campaign before Petersburg in poor health, and the fever and diarrhea became worse with the exposure. Stimulating drugs were required to keep him in the saddle. Finally, he was put on a steamer and sent to the general hospital at Fortress Monroe. From there he went to the general hospital in Philadelphia, where the nearly constant pain in his left elbow required hypodermic injections. Because of the disability of both his arms and chronic malarial diarrhea, Wistar was discharged in September 1864 and returned to his legal practice. Following the war and up to 1873, because of the pain from his old wounds, he required for many weeks and even months subcutaneous injections of morphia and other strong remedies. By 1875, the entrance and exit wounds of the right elbow were united by a broad cicatrix. The elbow was firmly ankylosed at a right angle. The hand was in a good position and its functions were excellent except for minor limitations in handling small objects. Pain, neuralgic in character, was occasionally present in the right elbow and would extend over the whole arm and forearm. The left elbow was in good condition. There was an adherent cicatrix on the inner side of the left arm at about the middle with some numbness of the little, ring, and middle fingers. The hand's functions were perfect except for some limitation in handling small objects. He engaged in business and helped fund the Wistar Institute of Anatomy and Biology in Philadelphia. In 1903 he had a severe attack of intestinal complaints but recovered. His health was bad in September 1905, and he was in bed when his sister arrived at his home in Claymont, Delaware, on the sixteenth. He extended his hand to welcome her and seemed pleased but said nothing. A physician came down from Philadelphia to see him and, finding him quite ill, stayed all night. Later when Wistar's sister visited him he listened to her but said nothing and moaned a good deal; however, when asked if he was in pain he said no. He slept some that night but was given medication to ensure rest. The next morning he appeared better, took his bath, and shaved but went back to bed rather than go downstairs. Thinking the trouble was with his bowels, as it had been two years before, the doctor gave him calomel followed by two or three heavy doses of castor oil at intervals, with little effect. The pain became very severe, at times almost un-bearable, and the doctor was called again. On his arrival, he appeared disap-pointed that Wistar had not improved and gave him a hypodermic of mor-phine. Another physician, who was called because his family physician was not available, remarked that the trouble was not in the bowels but was uremia. Other physicians arrived, four of whom worked with hot water applications and seemed to have some success. But there was no response, and the last thing they did was to bleed him, which relieved his head. Prior to that his face was dark purple. He was kept under the influence of hypodermics, which kept him quiet since he had been very restless most of the time. He became par-tially unconscious and did not appear to know or to notice the doctors or their efforts. Three of the doctors remained with him all night. The family was at breakfast when they heard a knock from above and all went upstairs. He died just past eight o'clock on September 18. Wistar had extracted a promise from the doctor that he would, as soon as convenient after death, remove the brain and take the wounded right arm for scientific purposes for the benefit of the Wistar Institute. At the request of one of the physicians, his sister also agreed to an examination of the abdominal organs. Later that afternoon the procedures were performed. The liver and kidneys were heavily diseased. The heart and lungs were in good condition. The arteries of the intestines were diseased and the walls of the arteries covered with many little pustules from which there had been several hemorrhages. There is some confusion as to whether he was buried at Laurel Hill Cemetery, Philadelphia, and then trans-ferred to the Wistar Institute or sent to the institute immediately. The bones of his wounded arm and his brain are at the institute while his ashes are in the atrium area of the main entrance.[1]

1. CSR; *OR*, vol. 5:321–22, 326, 329; vol. 18:686; vol. 19, pt. 1:307; *OR Suppl.*, vol. 1, pt. 1:401; RVA, Pension SC 36,244; *MSHW*, vol. 2, pt 2:831; U.S. Army, CWS, roll 1, vol. 1, report 52, pp. 975–83; ibid., roll 4, vol. 7, report 8, pp. 137–51; Wistar, *Autobiography*, 43, 64, 99, 146–47, 204, 266, 302, 337, 346, 376, 380–81, 385–86, 409–12, 444, 458–60; Mother (Wistar's sister) to Cappy, September 24, 1905, Wistar, "Last will and testament," Archives of the Wistar Institute of Anatomy and Biology, Philadelphia, Pa.

THOMAS JOHN WOOD · *Born September 25, 1823,* in Munfordville, Kentucky. He graduated from the USMA in 1845. During the time he was at West Point he was treated for dysentery twice and one time each for diarrhea, ophthalmia, sprain, and cough with fever. Served in the Mexican War. Having transferred to the cavalry the year after graduation, Wood served on the frontier. From May 2 to 14, 1857, he was treated for parotitis. He was commissioned brigadier general of volunteers in October 1861. In March 1862 he was given a sick leave for twenty days. In mid-December he was afflicted with quotidian intermittent fever. Although wounded in the left foot at Stones River on December 31, 1862, he remained on his horse throughout the day. The minié ball had struck the inner side of the left heel at an oblique angle and injured the os calcus. His boot was torn open and the foot lacerated and severely contused. Taken to Murfreesboro that night, he was transported by ambulance to Nashville, Tennessee, the next day. After a forty-day absence because of the wound and intermittent fever, Wood rejoined the division in February 1863. In April he obtained another twenty-day leave on surgeon's certificate because of his poor health. In late September he developed diarrhea, which lasted for the next three months. In January 1864 he took a thirty-day leave for the benefit of his health and rejoined his division the next month. At Lovejoy's Station, Georgia, on September 2, 1864, Wood was wounded in the left foot again, and the os calcus was fractured. He did not leave the field. For six months he used crutches and had to be transported in an ambulance with his command. His promotion to major general ranked from January 1865. The next month he was given a medical leave of absence and returned in March. He joined his regiment at Fort McPherson, Nebraska, on December 17, 1867. Because of the cold weather and necrosis of the bones of his foot from his last wound, he applied to be placed on the retired list. In January 1868 he was treated for catarrh. He was retired from active service in June for disability from wounds.[1] Died on February 25, 1906, in Dayton, Ohio, and was buried at West Point.

1. CSR; *OR*, vol. 20, pt. 1:202, 211, 451, 463–64; vol. 32, pt. 1:23; vol. 38, pt. 1:91, 216, 384, 429, 452; vol. 39, pt. 1:603–4; vol. 49, pt. 1:607, 648; U.S. Army, CWS, roll 1, vol. 2, report 11, pp. 111–35; ibid., roll 4, vol. 7, report 17, pp. 287–99; RVA, Pension, C 661,291.

DANIEL PHINEAS WOODBURY • *Born December 16, 1812,* in New London, New Hampshire. He graduated from the USMA in 1836. As a cadet, he was treated for an ulcer and a bruise twice each, and measles, fever and diarrhea one time each. Before the Civil War he engaged in a number of engineering projects and had been promoted to a captaincy. He served at First Bull Run, on the Peninsula, and at Fredericksburg. Woodbury's commission to brigadier general of volunteers ranked from March 1862, and he assumed command at Key West, Florida, in April 1863. He developed yellow fever on August 5, 1864, which appeared to be responding to treatment until he had a sudden loss of vital force and died on August 15.[1] His remains were first buried at Key West, but later were removed to Fort Barrancas National Cemetery, Pensacola, Florida.

1. CSR; *OR*, vol. 41, pt. 3:198; WPCHR, vols. 602, 603; LR, CB, roll 73, B1268, 1864; RVA, Pension C 56,787.

CHARLES ROBERT WOODS • *Born February 19, 1827,* at Newark, Ohio. He graduated from the USMA in 1852. While at West Point, he was treated for catarrhus
ten times, cephalalgia nine times, diarrhea five times, febris ephemeral, nausea,
clavus, and nausea twice each, and subluxatio, contusio, gonorrhea, vulnus
incisum, ophthalmia, luxatio, and debilitos one time each. Woods performed
the regular duties of an infantry officer prior to the Civil War. In December 1861
he was made colonel of the 76th Ohio and served in West Virginia, at Fort
Donelson, Shiloh, Corinth, Chickasaw Bluffs, and Arkansas Post. While on duty
in the trenches during the siege of Vicksburg in 1863, he had an attack of rheumatism. He was made brigadier general of volunteers in August 1863. He was
on the Atlanta campaign, the March to the Sea, and in the Carolinas. He reported that he was absent because of sickness for only ten days during the Civil
War. Woods remained in the army and was made lieutenant colonel of the 33rd
Infantry in July 1866. On December 31, 1868, he was admitted to the post hospital at Newport Barracks, Kentucky, because of rheumatism, and returned to
duty the middle of the next month. From 1869 to 1874 he had as many as six
attacks of rheumatism per year; each lasted from three to five weeks. The intervals between episodes became shorter and each attack more aggressive. Woods
had sick leaves from February 20 to July 15, 1871, March 1872 to March 5, 1873,
and from March 28, 1873, until the time he retired in 1874. A surgeon in October
1874 at Hot Springs, Arkansas, stated that Woods suffered with chronic muscular and articular rheumatism. On physical examination there was effusion of
the right knee beneath the insertion of the tendons of the muscles of extension
and plastic deposits in the connective tissue on each elbow near the ulnar extremity. The surgeon reported he had the signs of a rheumatic diathesis. Died
near Newark, Ohio, on February 26, 1885, and was buried there in Cedar Hill
Cemetery. According to the adjutant general's office, the cause of his death was
paralysis of the heart.[1]

1. WPCHR, vols. 606, 607, 608; U.S. Army, CWS, roll 1, vol. 2, report 23, pp. 295–339; RVA,
Pension WC 216,236; RAGO, entry 534.

WILLIAM BURNHAM WOODS • *Born August 3, 1824,* on the family farm at Newark, Ohio. In 1847 he was admitted to the Ohio bar and entered state politics.
He was made lieutenant colonel of the 76th Ohio in February 1862 and colonel
of the unit the following September. After service at Corinth and Chickasaw
Bluffs, Woods was wounded during the Battle of Arkansas Post, Arkansas, on
January 11, 1863. He served in the Atlanta campaign, the March to the Sea, and
in the Carolinas, and in May 1865 he was commissioned a brigadier general of
volunteers.[1] President Ulysses S. Grant appointed him U.S. circuit court judge
for the area of Georgia and the gulf states in 1869. Woods held this position
until he was appointed associate justice of the U.S. Supreme Court in 1880.

Died in Washington on May 14, 1887, and was buried in Cedar Hill Cemetery, Newark, Ohio.

DEATH CERTIFICATE: Cause of death, primary, nephritis. Immediate, edema of lungs.

1. *OR*, vol. 17, pt. 1:769.

JOHN ELLIS WOOL • *Born February 29, 1784*, at Newburgh, New York. Served in the War of 1812 and the Mexican War. On October 13, 1812, at Queenston Heights, Canada, a bullet passed through both his thighs. Remaining in the army after the War of 1812, Wool was made a full brigadier general in 1841. He distinguished himself in the Mexican War. His promotion as major general in the Regular Army ranked from May 1862. He retired in August 1863 because of his advanced age and infirmities. Wool died in Troy, New York, on November 10, 1869, and was buried in Oakwood Cemetery. He had tripped and fallen, hurting himself severely. After a short time he regained consciousness, but then slowly deteriorated.[1]

1. *OR*, vol. 27, pt. 2:917; U.S. Army, CWS, roll 1, vol. 1, report 60, p. 1067; Heitman, *Historical Register and Dictionary* 2:42.

GEORGE WRIGHT • *Born October 21, 1801 or 1803*, in Norwich, Vermont. He graduated from the USMA in 1822. Served in the Florida and Mexican wars. In Florida during April 1841, he became sick and went north on leave. He did not return to Fort Brooke, Florida, until the end of October 1841. He was so ill he could not sit up in the canoe while scouting in the Everglades the last of January 1842. Early the next month, rheumatism in his knees prevented him from marching. He was wounded at Molino del Rey on September 8, 1847. His wound was not serious, and he was in command of troops for most of the time until February 1848. Wright spent a month of detached service in Mexico City and then obtained a three-month leave for health reasons. In 1855 he was made colonel of the 9th Infantry. From September 1861 until June 1864 he was in command of the Department of the Pacific. He had an attack of asthma while in San Francisco in November 1862. In June 1865 he was placed in command of the Department of the Columbia, which was headquartered at Fort Vancouver, Washington Territory. On July 28 Wright left San Francisco with his wife on the overloaded steamship, *Brother Jonathan*, for his new station. The steamship was old, had been repaired a number of times, and on July 20 had had hull damage that had only been patched. After some of its freight had been unloaded at Crescent City, the steamship went up the coast until the captain decided to turn back because of a severe storm. It hit a reef on the thirtieth and sank with only nineteen surviving. Wright's body was found in October at Bay Flat near

Shelter Cove, 150 miles from the scene of the wreck. His remains were interred in the City Cemetery at Sacramento.[1]

1. Heitman, *Historical Register and Dictionary* 2:42; Carl P. Schlicke, *General George Wright: Guardian of the Pacific Coast,* 56, 58, 79–80, 83, 263, 300, 323, 327, 329–30, 332, 342; "Steamship Brother Jonathan" (typed copy), California State Library, Sacramento, California.

HORATIO GOUVERNEUR WRIGHT • *Born March 6, 1820,* in Clinton, Connecticut. He graduated from the USMA in 1841. While a cadet he was treated for a headache twice and once each for diarrhea, bruise, cough, colica, nausea, and sore feet. Served in the Florida wars. Before the Civil War Wright had duty in the corps of engineers and was made brigadier general of volunteers in September 1861. He was at Cincinnati on November 6, 1862, after having been sick at Lexington, Kentucky. Wright was at First Bull Run, Gettysburg, and the Mine Run campaign. Near the captured salient at Spotsylvania on May 12, 1864, a shell exploded among the officers. Wright was hit in the thigh by a shell fragment and was knocked for a distance of several feet. Although injured, he remained at his post. His first appointment as major general was rejected by the Senate, but he was reappointed in May 1864 and confirmed. At the Battle of Cedar Creek on October 19, 1864, he was wounded in the chin by a musket ball. The wound bled profusely. The first of January 1865 he had an accident and was hardly able to move, even when in bed. The surgeon reported he may have broken a rib or two. He was given a leave of absence to Washington, D.C., on January 16.[1] Wright remained in the army and rose from lieutenant colonel of engineers to brigadier general and chief engineer of the army. He was retired for age in 1884. Died in his residence in Washington, D.C., on July 2, 1899, and was buried in Arlington National Cemetery.

DEATH CERTIFICATE: Cause of death, primary, cirrhotic (interstitial) nephritis. Immediate, cardiac thrombosis. Duration last illness, since March 29, 1899.

1. *OR,* vol. 20, pt. 2:24; vol. 36, pt. 1:359, pt. 2:657; vol. 43, pt. 1:32, 55; vol. 46, pt. 2:34–35, 42, 147, 300, 329; WPCHR, vol. 604; LR, ACP, 1245, 1884, fiche: 000213; U.S. Army, CWS, roll 4, vol. 6, report 22, pp. 473–77; ibid., report of W. Dwight, roll 7, vol. 12, report 1, pp. 1–416.

SAMUEL KOSCIUSZKO ZOOK • *Born March 27, 1821,* in Chester County, Pennsylvania. Employed by the Washington and New York Telegraph Company, he was lieutenant colonel of the 6th New York Militia at the start of the Civil War. After the enlistment period of his first regiment expired, he was commissioned colonel of the 57th New York in October 1861. He was on the Peninsula, at Fredericksburg, and at Chancellorsville. His promotion to brigadier general ranked from November 1862. At Gettysburg on July 2, 1863, he was fatally wounded in the abdomen and died the next day in a field hospital on the Baltimore Pike.[1] Buried in Norristown, Pennsylvania, in Montgomery Cemetery.

1. CSR; *OR,* vol. 27, pt. 1:72, 133, 369, 380, 396; vol. 29, pt. 2:159; Heitman, *Historical Register and Dictionary* 2:173; New York Commission, *Final Report* 3:1358.

Sequence of Events during the Civil War

KEY:
Accident (A)   Died (D)   Mortally wounded (MW)
Bruise (B)   Grazed (G)   Wounded (W)
Contusion (C)   Killed in action (KIA)

DATE	PLACE	NAME
1861		
May 10	Lindell Grove, Mo.	N. Lyon (A)
	St. Louis, Mo.	F. Sigel (A)
June 3	Phillippi, W.Va.	B. F. Kelly (W)
June 6	New York Armory	O. O. Howard (A)
June 8	New Market, Va.	W. B. Tibbits (C)
June 10	Big Bethel, Va.	H. J. Kilpatrick (W)
	Caseyville, Ill.	J. McArthur (A)
July 21	First Bull Run, Va.	A. Ames (W)
		J. S. Brisbin (W)
		M. Corcoran (W)
		S. P. Heintzelman (W)
		D. Hunter (W)
		G. Marston (W)
		T. F. Meagher (C)
		J. B. Ricketts (W)
		W. T. Sherman (G)
		H. W. Slocum (W)
		E. Upton (W)
		O. B. Willcox (W)
August 10	Wilson's Creek, Mo.	G. W. Deitzler (W)
		C. C. Gilbert (W)
		N. Lyon (KIA)
		R. B. Mitchell (W)
		J. B. Plummer (W)
		T. W. Sweeny (W)
August 19	Charleston, Mo.	T. E. G. Ransom (W)

DATE	PLACE	NAME
September 10	Carnifex Ferry, W.Va.	W. H. Lytle (W)
September 21	New Albany, Ind.	M. D. Manson (A)
October 1	Edwards Ferry, Md.	S. Miller (A)
October 16	Bolivar Heights, W.Va.	J. W. Geary (W)
October 21	Ball's Bluff, Va.	E. D. Baker (KIA)
		I. J. Wistar (W)
October 22	Edwards Ferry, Md.	F. W. Lander (W)
November 7	Belmont, Mo.	J. G. Lauman (W)
		J. A. McClernand (G)
		E. W. Rice (W)
December 20	Dranesville, Va.	T. L. Kane (W)
December 27	Rolla, Mo.	G. M. Dodge (W)

1862

DATE	PLACE	NAME
January 19	Logan's Cross Roads, Ky.	S. S. Fry (W)
		R. L. McCook (W)
February 8	Roanoke Island, N.C.	R. B. Potter (A)
February 15	Ft. Donelson, Tenn.	C. Cruft (W)
		M. K. Lawler (W)
		J. A. Logan (W)
		J. A. Maltaby (W)
		T. E. G. Ransom (W)
		J. M. Tuttle (A)
March 2	Camp Chase, Va.	F. W. Lander (D)
March 7	Pea Ridge, Ark.	A. S. Asboth (W)
		E. A. Carr (W)
		G. M. Dodge (W)
		F. J. Herron (W)
		J. L. Kiernan (W)
		J. S. Phelps (W)
		Gus. A. Smith (W)
		J. A. Williamson (W)
March 14	New Berne, N.C.	R. B. Potter (W)
March 22	Kernstown, Va.	J. Shields (W)
March 31	Near Union City, Mo.	C. J. Stolbrand (A)

DATE	PLACE	NAME
April 4	Near Shiloh, Tenn.	U. S. Grant (A)
April 6	Warrenton, Va.	L. Blenker (A)
April 6	Shiloh, Tenn.	W. W. Belknap (W)
		A. Chambers (W)
		A. L. Chetlain (A)
		C. C. Cruft (W)
		I. N. Haynie (W)
		J. McArthur (W)
		T. E. G. Ransom (W)
		H. T. Reid (W)
		W. T. Sherman (W)
		D. Stuart (W)
		T. W. Sweeny (W)
		C. C. Walcutt (W)
		W. H. L. Wallace (MW)
		N. G. Williams (A)
April 7	Shiloh, Tenn.	F. Fessenden (W)
		W. Grose (W)
		E. N. Kirk (W)
		E. Opdycke (W)
April 10	Savannah, Tenn.	W. H. L. Wallace (D)
April 16	Lee's Mill, Va.	W. F. Smith (A)
April 18	Wilmington Island, Ga.	J. H. Wilson (B)
April 19	Fredericksburg, Va.	H. J. Kilpatrick (W)
April 24	Yorktown, Va.	W. F. Bartlett (W)
April 25	Savannah, Tenn.	C. F. Smith (D)
April 27	Siege of Yorktown, Va.	J. D. Davidson (A)
May 4	Williamsburg, Va.	G. A. Custer (A)
May 5	Williamsburg, Va.	W. Dwight (W)
		H. D. Terry (W)
	Lebanon, Tenn.	G. C. Smith (W)
May 7	West Point, Va.	N. M. Curtis (W)
May 9	Farmington, Miss.	Ed. Hatch (W)
May 10	Giles Court House, Va.	R. B. Hayes (W)
May 18	Harrisburg, Pa.	W. H. Keim (D)
May 23	Lewisburg, Va.	G. Crook (C)

DATE	PLACE	NAME
May 23	Near Winchester, Va.	J. R. Kenly (W)
May 25	Winchester, Va.	J. F. Knipe (W)
May 27	Hanover Court House, Va.	E. P. Chapin (W)
May 30	Corinth, Miss.	W. Grose (C)
May 31	Fair Oaks, Va.	J. J. Abercrombie (W)
		H. S. Briggs (W)
		C. T. Campbell (W)
		S. G. Champlin (W)
		C. Devens (W)
		L. C. Hunt (W)
		C. D. Jameson (A)
		H. M. Naglee (C)
		O. M. Poe (C)
		T. A. Rowley (W)
		C. H. Van Wyck (W)
		H. W. Wessells (W)
June 1	Fair Oaks, Va.	J. R. Brooke (W)
		T. W. Egan (W)
		O. O. Howard (W)
		N. P. Miles (W)
		A. Sully (G)
June 6	Harrisonburg, Va.	T. L. Kane (W)
June 8	Port Republic, Va.	I. H. Duval (W)
June 18	Manassas, Va.	I. McDowell (A)
June 25	Near Fair Oaks, Va.	E. A. Wild (W)
June 27	Gaines' Mill, Va.	N. J. Jackson (W)
		C. E. Pratt (W)
		G. K. Warren (W)
		L. D. Watkins (W)
		S. H. Weed (W)
June 29	Savage's Station, Va.	W. T. H. Brooks (W)
		W. W. Burns (W)
June 30	Glendale, Va.	W. W. Burns (A)
		S. P. Heintzelman (C)
		E. W. Hincks (W)
		J. Sedgwick (W)
		E. V. Sumner (W)
	New Market, Va.	G. A. McCall (W)
		G. G. Meade (W)

DATE	PLACE	NAME
June 30	Charles City Cross Roads, Va.	P. Kearny (B)
July 1	Malvern Hill, Va.	H. A. Barnum (W) H. G. Berry (W)
July 4	Livermore, Me.	O. O. Howard (A)
July 7	Cache Bayou, Ark.	C. E. Hovey (W)
August 5	Malvern Hill, Va.	W. Gamble (W)
	Near New Market, Ala.	R. L. McCook (MW)
	Baton Rouge, La.	T. Williams (KIA)
August 6	Roadside, Ala. to Tenn.	R. L. McCook (D)
August 9	Cedar Mountain, Va.	C. C. Augur (W) N. P. Banks (A) I. H. Duval (A) J. W. Geary (W) J. F. Knipe (W) T. G. Pitcher (W) B. J. Roberts (W)
	Near Corinth, Miss.	J. B. Plummer (D)
August 14	On Rapidan, Va.	S. S. Carroll (W)
August 22	Freeman's Ford, Va.	H. Bohlen (KIA)
August 27	Second Bull Run Camp	J. C. Robinson (W) G. W. Taylor (MW)
August 28	Bull Run Camp	L. Cutler (W) S. A. Meredith (W)
August 29	Second Bull Run, Va.	A. Hays (W) R. S. Mackenzie (W) S. Meredith (A) G. Mott (W)
August 30	Second Bull Run, Va.	A. Duryee (W) W. L. Elliott (W) M. D. Hardin (W) J. P. Hatch (W) W. Krzyzanowski (I) J. W. Revere (W) R. C. Schenck (W) F. Sigel (W) Z. B. Tower (W)
	Richmond, Ky.	C. Cruft (W)

DATE	PLACE	NAME
August 30	Richmond, Ky.	M. S. Manson (AW) W. Nelson (W)
September 1	Chantilly, Va.	P. Kearny (KIA) I. I. Stevens (KIA)
	Alexandria, Va.	G. W. Taylor (D)
September 3	Geiger's Lake, Ky.	J. Shackelford (W)
September 6	Olive Branch, Miss.	B. H. Grierson (B)
September 13	Fredericksburg, Va.	W. Birney (C)
	Near South Mt., Md.	I. B. Richardson (A)
September 14	South Mountain, Md.	J. P. Hatch (W) R. B. Hayes (W) J. L. Reno (KIA) E. A. Wild (W)
	Crampton Gap, Md.	N. J. Jackson (W) A. T. A. Torbert (W)
September 17	Antietam, Md.	F. C. Barlow (W) H. Baxter (W) G. L. Beal (W) E. S. Bragg (W) W. T. H. Brooks (W) R. F. Catterson (W) S. W. Crawford (W) N. J. T. Dana (W) A. Doubleday (A) A. Duryee (W) G. L. Hartsuff (W) E. W. Hincks (W) J. Hooker (W) J. K. F. Mansfield (MW) T. F. Meagher (A) A. Pleasonton (C) R. B. Potter (W) I. B. Richardson (MW) I. P. Rodman (MW) T. H. Ruger (W) J. Sedgwick (W) H. Tyndale (W) M. Weber (W) I. J. Wister (W)
September 18	Confederate Hospital	J. K. F. Mansfield (D)

DATE	PLACE	NAME
September 19	Iuka, Miss.	A. Chambers (W)
September 29	Louisville, Ky.	W. Nelson (D [shot])
September 30	Field Hospital	I. P. Rodman (D)
October 3	Corinth, Miss.	P. A. Hackleman (KIA) R. J. Oglesby (W) J. C. Sullivan (C)
October 4	Corinth, Miss.	J. A. Mower (W)
October 5	Corinth, Miss.	E. O. C. Ord (W) J. C. Veatch (C)
October 7	Perryville, Ky.	D. C. Buell (A)
October 8	Perryville, Ky.	J. S. Jackson (KIA) W. H. Lytle (W) W. R. Terrill (KIA)
October 30	Beaufort, S.C.	O. M. Mitchel (D)
November 3	Antietam, Md.	I. B. Richardson (D)
November 6	Old Town, Me.	C. D. Jameson (D)
November 22	Fairfax Court House, Va.	F. E. Patterson (A, D)
December 11	Fredericksburg, Va.	H. Baxter (W)
December 12	Fredericksburg, Va.	A. Sully (G)
December 13	Fredericksburg, Va.	G. Bayard (MW) J. Caldwell (W) C. T. Campbell (W) J. L. Chamberlain (W) J. Gibbon (W) W. S. Hancock (G) C. F. Jackson (KIA) N. Kimball (W) N. P. Miles (W) A. S. Piatt (A) E. B. Tyler (W) F. L. Vinton (W)
December 14	Fredericksburg, Va.	G. Bayard (D)
December 25	Hartwood Church, Va.	J. B. McIntosh (I)
December 28	Vicksburg, Miss.	M. L. Smith (W)
December 29	Chickasaw Bayou, Miss.	J. A. Williamson (W)
December 31	Stones River, Tenn.	W. Grose (C)

DATE	PLACE	NAME
December 31	Stones River, Tenn.	W. B. Hazen (B)
		J. H. King (W)
		E. N. Kirk (MW)
		E. Long (W)
		J. F. Miller (W)
		J. W. Sill (KIA)
		A. J. Slemmer (W)
		H. P. Van Cleve (W)
		W. C. Whitaker (W)
		A. Willich (W)
		T. J. Wood (W)

1863

DATE	PLACE	NAME
January 8	Springfield, Mo.	E. B. Brown (W)
January 11	Arkansas Post, Ark.	C. E. Hovey (W)
		W. B. Woods (W)
March 17	Kelly's Ford, Va.	A. N. A. Duffie (W)
March 21	Syracuse, N.Y.	E. V. Sumner (D)
March 28	Columbus, Ohio	J. Cooper (D)
April 17	Chancellorsville, Va.	N. J. Jackson (W)
April 18	Vicksburg, Miss.	T. J. Lucas (W)
April 28	Fredericksburg, Va.	H. W. Benham (A)
May 1	Port Gibson, Miss.	R. A. Cameron (W)
May 2	Chancellorsville, Va.	C. Devens (W)
		O. O. Howard (A)
		P. H. Jones (W)
May 3	Chancellorsville, Va.	H. G. Berry (KIA)
		D. N. Couch (W)
		J. W. Geary (W)
		W. S. Hancock (B)
		W. Hays (W)
		J. Hooker (C)
		E. Kirby (MW)
		N. P. Miles (W)
		G. Mott (W)
		B. R. Pierce (W)
		J. H. Potter (W)

DATE	PLACE	NAME
May 4	Chancellorsville, Va.	T. H. Neill (A)
		W. B. Tibbits (B)
		A. W. Whipple (MW)
	Fredericksburg, Va.	S. Conner (W)
May 6	Near Port Gibson, Miss.	J. L. Kiernan (W)
May 7	Washington, D.C.	A. W. Whipple (D)
May 17	Big Black River, Miss.	P. J. Osterhaus (W)
May 19	Vicksburg, Miss.	C. Ewing (W)
		Giles A. Smith (W)
	Champion's Hill, Miss.	A. L. Lee (W)
May 22	Vicksburg, Miss.	T. J. Lucas (W)
		A. V. Rice (W)
May 27	Port Hudson, La.	W. F. Bartlett (W)
		E. P. Chapin (KIA)
		N. Dow (W)
		T. W. Sherman (W)
May 28	Washington, D.C.	E. Kirby (D)
May 29	White Oak Church, Va.	E. S. Bragg (A)
June 9	Brandy Station, Va.	W. Merritt (W)
June 10	Baton Rouge, La.	J. W. McMillan (W)
June 14	Port Hudson, La.	H. E. Paine (W)
June 15	Winchester, Va.	R. H. Milroy (A)
June 25	Vicksburg, Miss.	M. D. Leggett (W)
		J. A. Maltaby (W)
	Liberty Gap, Tenn.	J. F. Miller (W)
July 1	Gettysburg, Pa.	F. C. Barlow (W)
		L. Fairchild (W)
		W. Krzyzanowski (A)
		Solomon Meredith (A)
		G. R. Paul (W)
		J. F. Reynolds (KIA)
		J. S. Robinson (W)
		A. Schimmelfennig (B)
July 2	Gettysburg, Pa.	J. Barnes (W)
		D. B. Birney (B)
		J. R. Brooke (W)
		J. L. Chamberlain (W)

DATE	PLACE	NAME
July 2	Gettysburg, Pa.	C. K. Graham (W)
		J. Hayes (A)
		B. R. Pierce (W)
		D. E. Sickles (W)
		S. Vincent (MW)
		J. H. H. Ward (W)
		G. K. Warren (W)
		S. H. Weed (KIA)
		S. K. Zook (MW)
July 3	Gettysburg, Pa.	D. Butterfield (W)
		A. Doubleday (C)
		E. J. Farnsworth (KIA)
		J. Gibbon (W)
		W. S. Hancock (W)
		H. J. Hunt (A)
		T. A. Rowley (W)
		T. A. Smyth (W)
		G. J. Stannard (W)
		A. S. Webb (W)
		S. K. Zook (D)
July 7	Gettysburg, Pa.	S. Vincent (D)
July 18	Battery Wagner, S.C.	T. Seymour (W)
		G. C. Strong (MW)
	Wytheville, Va.	W. H. Powell (W)
July 20	Vicksburg, Miss.	B. H. Grierson (A)
July 21	Chicago, Ill.	E. N. Kirk (D)
July 23	Near Manassas, Va.	F. B. Spinola (W)
July 26	Greenbrier, Va.	J. S. Brisbin (W)
July 30	New York City, N.Y.	G. C. Strong (D)
August 14	Cincinnati, Ohio	T. Welsh (D)
August 16	Battery Wagner, S.C.	J. B. Howell (C)
September 1	Jonesboro, Ga.	D. S. Stanley (C)
September 4	Near Carrollton, La.	U. S. Grant (A)
September 13	Raccoon Ford, Va.	G. A. Custer (W)
	Culpeper Court House, Va.	W. Wells (W)

DATE	PLACE	NAME
September 19	Chickamauga, Ga.	S. Beatty (A) L. P. Bradley (W) W. P. Carlin (W)
September 20	Chickamauga, Ga.	J. T. Croxton (W) W. Grose (W) W. H. Lytle (KIA) J. St. Clair Morton (W) J. C. Starkweather (W) J. B. Steedman (B) W. C. Whitaker (W)
September 24	Near Culpeper, Va.	J. Hayes (A)
September 25	Near Vicksburg, Miss.	R. P. Buckland (A)
September 26	Redan, Tenn.	J. M. Palmer (W)
October 1	Catlett's Station, Va.	J. B. McIntosh (A)
October 7	Farmington, Tenn.	E. Long (W)
October 10	Near Chattanooga, Tenn.	U. S. Grant (A)
October 14	Bristoe Station, Va.	S. S. Carroll (W)
October 29	Wauhatchie, Tenn.	G. S. Greene (W) A. B. Underwood (W)
October 31	Rockland County, N.Y.	L. Blenker (D)
November 7	Rappahannock River, Va.	D. A. Russell (W)
November 18	Knoxville, Tenn.	W. P. Sanders (MW)
November 19	Knoxville, Tenn.	W. P. Sanders (D)
November 24	Lookout Mt., Tenn.	H. A. Barnum (W)
	Missionary Ridge, Tenn.	Giles A. Smith (W)
November 25	Missionary Ridge, Tenn.	J. T. Croxton (B) C. L. Matthies (W)
	Tunnel Hill, Tenn.	J. M. Corse (W)
	Chattanooga, Tenn.	G. B. Raum (W)
December 4	Moscow, Tenn.	E. Hatch (W)
December 14	Catlett's Station, Va.	M. D. Hardin (W)
December 16	Washington, D.C.	J. Buford (D)
December 22	Fairfax Court House, Va.	M. Corcoran (D)
December 23	Blain's Cross Roads, Tenn.	J. G. Foster (A)

DATE	PLACE	NAME

1864

January 24	Grand Rapids, Mich.	S. G. Champlin (D)
April 4	Elkin's Ferry, Ark.	S. A. Rice (W)
April 8	Mansfield, La.	J. Bailey (W)
April 8	Mansfield, La.	W. B. Franklin (W)
		T. E. G. Ransom (W)
	Sabine Cross Roads, La.	J. S. Brisbin (A)
April 9	Pleasant Grove, La.	J. I. Gilbert (W)
April 22	Washington, D.C.	J. G. Totten (D)
April 23	Monett's Crossing, La.	F. Fessenden (W)
April 30	Jenkins' Ferry, Ark.	S. A. Rice (W)
May 5	Wilderness, Va.	S. S. Carroll (W)
		J. Hayes (W)
		A. Hays (KIA)
May 6	Wilderness, Va.	W. F. Bartlett (W)
		H. Baxter (W)
		S. Connor (W)
		G. W. Getty (W)
		J. S. Wadsworth (MW)
May 8	Spotsylvania, Va.	S. W. Crawford (I)
		J. C. Robinson (W)
		J. Sedgwick (G)
	Mill Creek Gap, Ga.	P. H. Jones (A)
	Confederate Hospital	J. W. Wadsworth (D)
May 9	Spotsylvania, Va.	W. H. Morris (W)
		J. Sedgwick (KIA)
May 10	Cove Mountain, Va.	W. W. Averell (G)
	Wilderness, Va.	S. S. Carroll (W)
	Spotsylvania, Va.	J. C. Rice (D)
		T. G. Stevenson (KIA)
		J. H. H. Ward (W)
May 12	Spotsylvania, Va.	D. B. Birney (C)
		A. S. Webb (W)
		H. G. Wright (W)
May 13	Spotsylvania, Va.	S. S. Carroll (W)
	Resaca, Ga.	H. J. Kilpatrick (W)

DATE	PLACE	NAME
May 14	Resaca, Ga.	C. G. Harker (W) M. D. Manson (W) E. Opdycke (W)
	Drewry's Bluff, Va.	T. O. Osborn (W)
May 15	Resaca, Ga.	J. F. Knipe (W) W. T. Ward (W) W. C. Whitaker (C) A. Willich (W)
May 18	Spotsylvania, Va.	J. M. Warner (W)
May 19	Spotsylvania, Va.	G. Mott (W)
May 20	Atlanta Campaign	J. A. Logan (B)
	Green Plain, Va.	G. Pennypacker (W)
May 23	North Anna River, Va.	M. D. Hardin (W)
May 25	Mobile, Ala.	C. C. Andrews (A)
	Near Cassville, Ga.	J. M. Schofield (A)
May 26	New Hope Church, Ga.	A. S. Williams (B)
May 27	Pickett's Mill, Ga.	O. O. Howard (B)
May 28	New Hope Church, Ga.	Rich. W. Johnson (W)
May 30	Dallas, Ga.	J. A. Logan (W)
June 1	Cold Harbor, Va.	D. A. Russell (W)
June 3	Cold Harbor, Va.	J. R. Brooke (W) G. J. Stannard (W) R. O. Tyler (W)
June 5	Piedmont, Va.	J. Stahel (W) J. C. Sullivan (A)
June 16	Petersburg, Va.	T. W. Egan (W)
June 17	Petersburg, Va.	J. St. Clair Morton (KIA)
June 18	Petersburg, Va.	J. L. Chamberlain (W) B. R. Pierce (W)
June 19	Petersburg, Va.	R. B. Ayres (W)
June 22	Petersburg, Va.	R. S. Mackenzie (W)
June 27	Kennesaw Mt., Ga.	C. G. Harker (KIA) D. McCook, Jr. (MW) A. V. Rice (W)
June 29	Washington, D.C.	J. P. Taylor (D)

DATE	PLACE	NAME
July 6	Oskaloosa, Iowa	S. A. Rice (D)
July 9	Vining Station, Ga.	G. P. Estey (B)
	Monocacy, Md.	W. H. Seward (W)
July 13	Offutt's Cross Roads, Md.	Q. A. Gillmore (A)
July 17	Steubenville, Ohio	D. McCook, Jr. (D)
July 20	Near Atlanta, Ga.	W. Q. Gresham (W)
July 22	Atlanta, Ga.	M. F. Force (W)
		J. B. McPherson (KIA)
July 24	Winchester, Va.	R. B. Hayes (W)
July 28	Morgan's Ferry, La.	M. H. Chrysler (W)
July 30	Crater, Va.	J. H. Ledlie (B)
August 15	Key West, Fla.	D. P. Woodbury (D)
August 16	Front Royal, Va.	T. C. Devin (W)
August 18	Weldon Road, Va.	S. W. Crawford (W)
August 19	Atlanta, Ga.	G. M. Dodge (W)
		J. A. J. Lightburn (W)
August 20	Lovejoy's Station, Ga.	E. Long (W)
August 21	City Point, Va.	L. Cutler (W)
September 1	Jonesboro, Ga.	D. S. Stanley (C)
September 2	Lovejoy, Ga.	T. J. Wood (W)
September 12	Petersburg, Va.	J. B. Howell (A)
September 14	Petersburg, Va.	J. B. Howell (D)
September 19	Winchester, Va.	G. H. Chapman (W)
		I. H. Duval (W)
		J. B. McIntosh (W)
		R. S. Mackenzie (W)
		D. A. Russell (KIA)
		E. Upton (W)
September 27	Marianna, Fla.	A. S. Asboth (W)
September 29	Ft. Harrison, Va.	H. Burnham (KIA)
		E. O. C. Ord (W)
	Fort Gilmer, Va.	G. Pennypacker (W)
September 30	Fort Harrison, Va.	G. J. Stannard (W)
October 5	Allatoona Pass, Ga.	J. M. Corse (W)

DATE	PLACE	NAME
October 18	Philadelphia, Pa.	D. B. Birney (D)
October 19	Cedar Creek, Va.	D. D. Bidwell (KIA)
		C. Grover (W)
		J. E. Hamblin (W)
		R. B. Hayes (A,W)
		C. R. Lowell (MW)
		R. S. Mackenzie (W)
		W. H. Penrose (W)
		J. B. Ricketts (W)
		H. G. Wright (W)
October 20	Cedar Creek, Va.	C. R. Lowell (D)
October 29	Near Rome, Ga.	T. E. G. Ransom (D)
November 6	Prairie Landing, Ark.	E. R. S. Canby (W)
November 14	Petersburg, Va.	T. W. Egan (W)
November 22	Griswoldville, Ga.	C. C. Walcutt (W)
November 29	Spring Hill, Tenn.	L. P. Bradley (W)
November 30	Franklin, Tenn.	D. S. Stanley (W)
December 21	Savannah Campaign, Ga.	J. H. Ketcham (W)

1865

DATE	PLACE	NAME
January 15	Fort Fisher, N.C.	N. M. Curtis (W)
		G. Pennypacker (W)
February 2	Salkehatchie River, S.C.	W. Swayne (W)
February 6	Hatcher's Run, Va.	H. E. Davies (C)
March 1	Stevenson, Ala.	S. Beatty (A)
March 7	Near Winchester, Va.	W. B. Tibbits (A)
March 25	Fort Stedman, Va.	J. F. Hartranft (W)
March 29	Quaker Road, Va.	J. L. Chamberlain (W)
April 2	Petersburg, Va.	L. A. Grant (W)
		W. H. Penrose (B)
	Ft. Sedgwick, Va.	R. B. Potter (W)
	Selma, Ala.	E. Long (W)
		J. H. Wilson (A)
April 6	Amelia Springs, Va.	G. Mott (W)

DATE	PLACE	NAME
April 7	Farmville, Va.	T. A. Smyth (MW)
April 9	Near Farmville, Va.	T. A. Smyth (D)
April 18	Millwood, Va.	W. B. Tibbits (A)

Glossary

The words included in this glossary were selected from the text in order to provide definitions of medical terms that may not be familiar to the reader, or of terms that over the years have changed meaning. The medical records cited in this work span over a hundred years, during which period concepts of pathophysiology changed and microbiology was introduced. The former names of the infectious diseases that had been described on the basis of signs and symptoms were retained, but once their etiologic agents were identified, their descriptions were more logically defined. The glossary was organized to allow comparison of the older usage of the words with their present meaning. If the definition of the word has not changed essentially then only the recent usage is presented. The older definition, enclosed in square brackets [ ] and following the more modern meaning, is in some cases more of a presentation of the older theories concerning the disease than just a definition. In some instances when a word is no longer in use, only the old definition is supplied.

The 1846 and 1866 editions of *A Dictionary of Medical Science* by Robley Dunglison supplied some of the definitions while Joseph Janvier Woodward, *Outlines of the Chief Camp Diseases of the United States Armies,* was the basis for most of the clinical descriptions. However, in some instances the usage of the words in the present records did not conform to the standard definitions, so the author has tried to present his interpretation.

AFFECTION   [Any mode in which the mind or body is affected or modified.]
AGUE   1. Fever, or any other recurrent symptom resulting from malaria. 2. A chill. [A popular synonym of Intermittent Fever.]
ALBUMINURIA   Presence of albumin in the urine and taken as a reflection of renal disease.
AMAUROSIS   Diminution or complete loss of sight, especially occurring without an apparent lesion of the eye, as from disease of the optic nerve.
AMPUTATION   The removal of a limb or other appendage of the body. CIRCULAR AMPUTATION: Performed by using a single flap and by making a circular cut at a ninety degree angle to the long axis of the limb. PRIMARY AMPUTATION: The

surgery is conducted following the period of shock and before the development of inflammation. [It was believed that when an amputation was required,
there was no period as favorable for the surgery as the first twenty-four hours,
before reaction set in and while the patient had his sensibilities depressed by
shock.] SECONDARY AMPUTATION: [Performed after the onset of suppuration
or to improve a previous circular amputation with open flaps.]

ANASARCA   Accumulation of fluid into the subcutaneous connective tissues, not
limited to a particular locality but becoming more or less generalized.

ANAL FISSURE   A linear ulcer at the edge of the anus.

ANAL FISTULA   An abnormal opening of the skin near the anus, which may or
may not communicate with the rectum. [This was a common affection, particularly among those who frequently rode a horse, caused by an abscess in the
vicinity of the rectum, which, after discharging its purulent contents either into
the rectum or externally, did not heal.]

ANGINA PECTORIS   Paroxysmal pain characterized by a severe crushing or con-
strictive sensation in the chest produced by lack of oxygen to the heart muscles.
The pain frequently radiates to the neck or to the left shoulder and down the
arm. [An affection of the chest, characterized by severe pain, faintness, and anxiety, occurring in paroxysms: connected with disorders of the pneumogastric
and sympathetic nerves and their branches; and frequently associated with organic disease of the heart. Since it appeared to be neuropathic, it was also termed
NEURALGIA OF THE HEART.]

ANKYLOSIS   Immobility or fixation of a joint due to injury, disease, or surgical
procedure.

ANODYNES   Medicine that relieves pain.

APNEA   Cessation of breathing. [Breathlessness, difficulty breathing.]

APOPLEXY   1. A stroke; sudden neurologic impairment due to an intracranial hemorrhage or to cerebrovascular occlusion. 2. Extravasation of blood within any
organ. [It was customary to include among the forms of apoplexy only that
sudden loss of consciousness due to cerebral congestion, and to consider as
apoplectic states only those which resulted from distinct toxemia. The apoplectic conditions were considered due to: (a) the influence upon the brain of a
poison circulating in the blood; (b) a sudden cerebral lesion, such as hemorrhage or vascular obstruction; or (c) a sudden shock or other impression ar-
resting the cerebral functions but causing no visible alteration in the brain.
Also used for every effusion of blood that occurs suddenly into the substance of
organs or tissue, such as apoplexy of the lungs.]

ARTERIOSCLEROSIS   A group of diseases involving the arterial walls and characterized by thickening and loss of elasticity.

ASSIMILATION   The change of food into living tissue after digestion and absorption.

ASTHENIA   Weakness. Lack or loss of energy. [Debility of the whole economy or
diminution of the vital forces.]

ATHEROMA [athroma]   A mass of plaque of degenerated, thickened inner layer of an arterial blood vessel occurring in atherosclerosis.

ATROPHY   A wasting away or a decrease in size.

BILIOUS ATTACK   The term is applied to a group of symptoms consisting of nausea, abdominal distress, headache, and constipation. [One of the most frequent applications of the term was to certain so-called bilious attacks that were commonly attacks of acute dyspepsia or migraine. The term was used when the patient presented a sallow or more or less yellowish tint of the skin but especially if distinctly jaundiced. Bilious diarrhea signified the discharge of a quantity of bile mixed with loose stools. Certain febrile diseases, such as those due to malaria or typhoid, were sometimes designated bilious fever.]

BLACK VOMIT   Vomiting of black material which obtains its color from the action of gastric juice on blood in the stomach. May be present in yellow fever and other conditions in which blood collects in the stomach.

BLUE MASS   Mercury mass. [Also known as the blue pill. It contained 33 parts mercury, 5 liquorice, 25 althaea, 3 glycerine, and 34 of honey of rose. Used for a number of conditions without much rationale.]

BOUGIE   A slender, flexible, cylindrical instrument that may be solid or hollow for introduction into tubular organs or fistulous tracts.

BRAIN, SOFTENING   [A pathological state of brain-tissue, depending commonly on vascular obstruction; attended by diminished consistence which is usually local. Used during life to describe the patient who displays mental, motor, and sensory symptoms which vary according to the seat of the lesion. Many of the present individuals with this diagnosis had unexplained mental changes with occasional paresis.]

BRIGHT'S DISEASE   A general descriptive term used for kidney disease and associated with protein in the urine. [Generic term that included at least three different diseases of the kidney: (1) Inflammatory affection caused by exposure to cold, scarlatina, diphtheria, erysipelas, typhus, ague, acute rheumatism, and pneumonia; (2) Waxy or amyloid affection from constitutional syphilis, tuberculosis, prolonged suppuration, caries, or necrosis of bone; (3) Cirrhotic or gouty affection. The most common cause was considered the abuse of alcohol, particularly in the form of ardent spirits, then gout, lead-poisoning, and unknown causes.]

BRONCHITIS   Inflammation of one or more of the larger air passages of the lungs. [Two causes: (1) Predisposing—age (youngest and oldest), breathing air when many people were present, heated rooms, cold, dampness, and other diseases were all thought to play a role. (2) Exciting causes: transition from cold to heated atmosphere and irritants, such as particles of cotton or pollen.]

CACHEXIA   [A condition in which the body is evidently deprived. A bad habit of body.]

CAMP, STATE   [A term that included various symptoms, such as fever or diarrhea, which occurred among troops crowded together in camp for a long period. In some instances, it was used specifically for the continued fevers, including yellow fever, malarial remittent fever, and typhomalarial fever.]

CARBUNCLE   An infection of the skin and subcutaneous tissue that usually produces localized destruction of tissue and forms a group of boils, due to *Staphylococcus aureus*. [It was considered a constitutional affection, dependent upon conditions of general debility or plethora, and often associated with gouty or diabetic tendencies.]

CARDIAC PARALYSIS   Heart failure or cessation of heart action.

CATARRHUS   Inflammation of the mucous membranes of the air passages of the head and throat, accompanied by a discharge. [Usually restricted to the inflammation of the mucous membrane of the air passages but was extended to that of all mucous membranes. CATARRH GASTRIC: Gastritis. CATARRH INTESTINAL: Diarrhea.] NASALOPHARYNGEAL CATARRUS: Inflammation of the nose and throat.

CELLULITIS   Diffuse inflammation of the soft or connective tissue due to infection.

CEPHALALGIA   Headache.

CEREBRAL HEMORRHAGE   Bleeding into the main portion of the brain occupying the upper part of the cranial cavity.

CEREBRAL HYPEREMIA   Same as cerebral congestion.

CHOLECYSTITIS   Inflammation of the gallbladder.

CHOLERA   An acute infectious disease that is caused by *Vibrio cholerae* and is characterized by severe diarrhea with extreme fluid and electrolyte depletion, producing prostration. The resulting severe dehydration may lead to shock, kidney failure and death. [CHOLERA ASIATIC: A disease characterized by anxiety, griping, spasms in the legs and arms, and vomiting and purging (generally bilious). Vomiting and purging are, indeed, the essential symptoms. Caused by decomposing animal or vegetable substances. Climatic and meteorological influences were thought to materially effect the susceptibility of the human subject to the disease. The malady was apt to prevail as an epidemic in moist or wet seasons of the year. It occurred especially among people whose bodies were predisposed to pass into a diseased condition because they had habitually breathed impure air and consumed unwholesome food and water, or became debilitated from other causes. CHOLERA MORBUS: A milder acute gastroenteritis, with diarrhea, cramps, and vomiting, occurring in summer or autumn, called also summer complaint.]

CICATRIX   Scar.

CLAVICLE   The curved collar bone that joins the sternum and the scapula to form the front of the shoulder.

CLAVUS   A corn.

COLICA   Acute abdominal pain. [Signified an affection or pain in the colon, but it was employed in a more extensive manner to include any acute pain of the abdomen, aggravated at intervals.]

CONCUSSION A severe blow or shock, or the condition which results from such an injury, usually to the brain.

CONGESTION An increase in the accumulation of blood. Results from a decrease or blockage of blood flow from the organ. Also called venous congestion. [It was felt that various organs such as the brain, lung, and liver, for example, became congested or filled with increased amounts of blood, which led to dysfunction of the organ and disease. The concept formed the rationale for depletion therapy.] CONGESTION OF LUNG: Excessive or abnormal accumulation of blood in the lung. [This condition presented with a sudden oppression and dyspnea, intense congestion, and livid blueness of the face and peripheral skin, a high febrile reaction, great prostration, frequently delirium, which was followed by pallor, sinking, apnoea, and death. Physical examination revealed general dullness of the lungs on percussion and moist subcrepitant rales over the lower and posterior portion of the lungs. CONGESTION OF THE BRAIN: Used as a clinical diagnosis when the patient displayed mental symptoms, either unexplained or in association with some disease.]

CONSUMPTION A wasting away of the body. [This was a term for any wasting disease, but it was generally applied to pulmonary phthisis (tuberculosis). Phthisis was used to designate a disease characterized by progressive wasting of the body, persistent cough, and expectoration of opaque matter or sometimes of blood. There was loss of color and strength, shortness of breath, fever, night sweats, and diarrhea. General causes were considered family predisposition, fevers, and exanthemata; syphilis; insufficient food; alcohol; bad ventilation; climatic influences; dampness of soil; and infection.]

CONTUSION [CONTUSIO] A bruise; an injury without a break in the skin.

CYNANCHE Severe sore throat with possible difficulty breathing.

DEBILITY Lack or loss of strength. [The body or any of its organs were considered to be in a state of debility when their vital functions were discharged with less than the normal vigor, being reduced in the amount of activity that they displayed, and of work that they could accomplish. Different than fatigue, which is temporary while debility is generally more permanent.]

DEMENTIA Organic loss of intellectual function. [Insanity. Unsound mind that was characterized by a total loss of the faculty of thought, or by such an imbecility of intellect that the ideas are extremely incoherent, there being at the same time a total loss of the power of reasoning.]

DENGUE "Break bone fever." An infectious, febrile disease, which produces severe pains in the head, eyes, and extremities, that is accompanied by catarrhal symptoms and sometimes a cutaneous eruption. It is caused by a virus and is transmitted by the bite of a mosquito. [Thought to be infectious because of the many cases in which the disease was supposedly conveyed from person to person.]

DIARRHEA An increase in fecal frequency and/or liquidity. [Considered a miasmatic disease. A point of differentiation from dysentery was that diarrhea was not accompanied by painful straining at stool. It was supposed to be caused by food in excess or of improper quality, diseased, decomposed, or imperfectly masticated food; impure water, excessive bile; retained feces, parasites, defective hygiene, and living in dwellings that were damp, cold, dark, and unventilated; foul emanations from decaying animal matter; chills; climatic variations, and nervous disturbances.]

DIPHTHERIA   An acute infectious disease that is produced by the toxic-producing bacteria *Corynebacterium diphtheriae,* affecting primarily the membranes of the nose, throat, or larynx, and is characterized by the presence of a gray-white pseudomembrane. [The diagnosis was based on the presence of a membrane in the oralpharynx. The disease was considered contagious and due to poverty and its concomitants, tuberculous, scarlatina, measles, and whooping-cough.]

DROPSY   Abnormal accumulation of a serous fluid in subcutaneous cellular tissue, or in a body cavity.

DYSENTERY   This includes a number of conditions in conjunction with inflammation of the intestines, particularly involving the colon. There is painful, colicky, abdominal pain, straining at stool, and frequent bowel movements containing blood and mucus. The causative agent may be chemical irritants, bacteria, or parasites. [Considered a miasmatic disease, the chief symptoms of which are fever, more or less inflammatory, with frequent mucous or bloody evacuations, violent colic, and straining at stool. It could sometimes resolve, but frequently terminated in intestinal ulceration. It appeared to exist in direct proportion to the presence of malarious fevers. The belief was that paroxysmal fevers interfered with the nutrition and functions of the digestive organs. Dysentery was considered to be secondary to portal congestion, unwholesome drinking water, bad and unwholesome food, impure air, bile, indigestible articles of diet, and sudden changes in temperature.] DYSENTERY, BILIOUS: Stools have a green, bilious appearance. [This was considered by many as being more severe than other forms of dysentery.]

DYSPEPSIA   The term is often used to describe epigastic discomfort following meals. [A state of the stomach, in which its functions are disturbed. The symptoms are various. Those affecting the stomach itself were considered the loss of appetite, nausea, pain in the epigastrium or hypochondrium, heartburn, sense of fullness or weight in the stomach, acid or fetid eructations, pyrosis, and a sense of fluttering or sinking at the pit of the stomach.]

DYSPNEA   Difficulty breathing.

EDEMA OF LUNGS   The presence of abnormally large amounts of fluid in the spaces between the cells of the lungs.

ENCEPHALITIS   Inflammation of the brain.

ENDOCARDITIS   Inflammation of the lining membranes of the cavities of the heart and the connective tissues around it. It is characterized by the presence of bacterial growths on the surface of the lining of the heart or in the heart muscle itself, and usually involves a heart valve. [Endocarditis was generally considered to occur in association with acute rheumatism and less frequently with other acute specific febrile diseases, such as scarlet fever, measles, erysipelas, pyaemia,and septicemia. On physical examination, the heart's action is visibly increased, easily felt by the examining hand, and at times detects a trembling vibratory motion. Percussion yielded a dull sound over a surface of several inches. On auscultation a bruit is generally heard, and there is a metallic ringing with each systole of the ventricle.]

ENGORGED LIVER   The liver is distended, swollen, or congested with fluid.

ENTERITIS   Inflammation of the small intestine.

EPIDIDYMITIS   Inflammation of the cordlike structure along the posterior border of the testis.

EPITHELIOMA   Any tumor derived from the covering of the internal and external surfaces of the body. [A variety of cancer consisting of essentially epithelial elements.]

ERYSIPELAS   A contagious disease of skin and subcutaneous tissue due to infection with *Streptococcus pyogenes* and is marked by redness and swelling of the affected areas associated with constitutional symptoms. [Considered a miasmatic condition. A disease, so called because it generally extends gradually to the neighboring parts. Superficial inflammation of the skin, with general fever, tension and swelling of the parts, pain but more or less circumscribed. The redness disappears when pressed upon by the finger but returns as soon as the pressure is removed. Frequently small vesicles appear upon the inflamed part. Generally an acute affection with a medium duration of from 10 to 14 days. Many of the infections associated with wounds and called erysipelas were probably more a local cellulitis.]

EXCISION   Removal by cutting. [Removal by excision of a segment of bone, leaving the two remaining ends in place, instead of performing an amputation.]

EXCORIATION [EXCORIATIO]   Loss of superficial skin from scraping or scratching.

EXFOLIATION   [Separation of the dead portions of a bone, tendon, aponeurosis, or cartilage, under the form of lamellae or small scales.]

FATTY DEGENERATION OF THE HEART   Deposition of fat globules in the heart tissue. [The process by which the muscular fibres of the heart are converted into a granular fatty matter. The term was also used to express the state of the heart in which this change has been accomplished. Due primarily to interference with nutrition of the tissue of the heart. The terminal pathologic changes of the heart in individuals who may have died with diseases such as altered coronary circulation, chronic cachectic diseases, acute specific fevers, an enlarged heart, or valvular disease.]

FEBRIS ANOMALUS   [An irregular fever.] FEBRIS COMMINICUS: [A fever that could be communicated from one individual to another.] FEBRIS QUOTIDIAN: A fever recurring every day. FEBRIS REMITTENS: Remittent fever.

FEMUR   The bone that extends from the pelvis to the knee, also called the thigh bone.

FEVER   Elevation of the body temperature above normal. [Derangement of function was attributed to the febrile condition and was considered, in part, independent of the initial cause. It was thought that the fever itself was the chief antagonist with which the physician had to contend.] BILIOUS FEVER: Fever that is accompanied by the vomiting of bile or with yellowing tint of the skin. Usually malaria or typhoid. CAMP FEVER: [A group of conditions that included typhus, typhoid, typhomalaria, common continued fever, remittent fever, and intermittent fever.] CONTINUED FEVER: Persistently elevated body temperature, showing little or no variation and never falling to normal during any 24-hour period. [Three types were recognized: typhus, enteric, and relapsing. They resulted from the introduction into the body of a poison from without and this poison was thought to reproduce in the system. It was noted that the continued fevers rarely affected the same individual twice, and they had a more or less definite duration.] EPHEMERAL FEVER: A fever that rapidly subsides and lasts not more than one day. INTERMITTENT FEVER: Recurring paroxysms of temperature elevations separated by intervals during which the temperature is normal. Usually malarial in origin. [Three forms of ague were recognized, namely the quotidian, in which the fever recurred in twenty-four hours; the tertian fever, which recurred in forty-eight hours; and the quartan, which recurred in seventy-two hours.] RECURRENT FEVER: Relapsing. REMITTENT FEVER: A fever which varies two degrees Fahrenheit or more each day but in which the temperature never reaches a normal level. Also used to mean malaria. TYPHOID FEVER: Infection by *Salmonella typhosa* involving primarily the lymphoid tissue of the distal small intestine. The disease may start suddenly with chills and fever, transient rose spots on the skin, abdominal distension, and an enlarged spleen. [A continued fever of long duration, usually attended with diarrhea and characterized by peculiar intestinal lesions, an eruption of small rose spots, and enlargement of the spleen. In common with other continuous fevers, typhoid fever was considered to be due to the introduction from without of a specific poison into a system more or less predisposed to the disease. There were two views as to the origin of the poison. First, that it was specific in nature and derived only from some preexisting case of the disease. Second, that it could be generated anew by the decomposition of sewage and perhaps of other forms of animal filth. The most common vehicle of the poison was drinking water.] YELLOW FEVER: An acute infectious, viral disease that mosquitoes transmit to man. The patient manifests fever, jaundice, and protein in the urine. [A contagious fever of a continuous and special type that was noted to have two well-defined stages. The first extended from 66 to 150 hours, depending on its severity, and was marked by rapid circulation and elevated temperature. The second was characterized by depression of the nervous and muscular powers, and of the circulation, with slow and often intermittent pulse, jaundice, suppression of urine, protein in the urine, passive bleeding from the mucous surfaces, black vomit, convulsions, delirium, and coma. A certain degree of density of population appeared to be essential to the production of yellow fever, and it was a disease of crowded cities on the shores of the ocean or large rivers, and of ships. It was also the disease of strangers in the warm, moist climates of the islands and tropical parts of America.]

FIBULA   The outer and smaller of the two bones in the lower leg.

FISTULA ANI   An abnormal opening on the cutaneous surface near the anus, which may or may not communicate with the rectum.

FRACTURE   The breaking of a part, especially of a bone. COMMINUTED FRACTURE: The bone is splintered or crushed. COMPOUND FRACTURE: An open fracture.

GASTRALGIA   Cramping pain in the stomach.

GASTRITIS   Inflammation of the inner lining of the stomach. [A disease characterized by pyrexia, great anxiety; heat and pain in the epigastrium; increased by taking anything into the stomach; vomiting and hiccups.]

GOUT   A hereditary form of arthritis associated with an increase of uric acid in the blood and by recurrent attacks of acute arthritis, usually of a single peripheral joint, which is then followed by complete remission. [Inflammation of the fibrous and ligamentous parts of the joints. It almost always attacks first the great toe; whence it passes to the other smaller joints, after having produced, or been attended with various sympathetic effects, particularly in the digestive organs; after this, it may attack the greater articulations.]

HEART PARALYSIS   Heart failure or heart stops.

HEMATEMSIS   Vomiting of blood.

HEMIPLEGIA   Paralysis of motion of one side of the body.

HEMOPTYSIS   Coughing up blood from the lungs.

HEMORRHAGE, SECONDARY   [Any bleeding after forty-eight hours was considered secondary by most surgeons. All injuries to large arteries or any wound that remained unhealed for a long time could produce secondary hemorrhage. Following a wound, suppuration was usually established about the fifth or sixth day. When the walls of blood vessels were involved and the precaution of rest and absolute quiet had not been enforced, secondary hemorrhage occurred. Scurvy was also considered a factor in many cases.]

HEPATITIS   Inflammation of the liver.

HUMERUS   The bone that extends from the shoulder to the elbow. ANATOMICAL NECK OF THE HUMERUS: The slightly narrowed area of the humerus just distal to the head of the bone.

HYDROCELE   A circumcised collection of fluid in the covering of the testicle or along the spermatic cord.

INANITION   A condition usually brought about by weeks to months of very inadequate nutrition. There is extreme weight loss and considerable weakness.

INFERIOR MAXILLA   The bone of the lower jaw.

INFLUENZA (GRIPPE)   An acute viral infection of the respiratory tract. There is inflammation of the mucous membranes of the nasal passages, pharynx, and conjunctiva. Generalized muscle pain, headache, fever, chills, and prostration are usual. [This disease was not regarded as simply an unusually prevalent common catarrh but was considered as a specific affection, which appeared occasionally over wide districts, simultaneously or at about the same time. It was characterized by marked febrile symptoms, often attended by serious complications, and caused great and prolonged prostration of strength.]

IRRITATIO SPINALIS   [Irritation of the spinal cord.]

JAUNDICE   A condition manifest by a yellow color of the skin, mucous membranes, and sclera because of increased bile.

LA GRIPPE   Name for several catarrhal diseases that have reigned epidemically, as influenza.

LUXATION [LUXATIO]   Dislocation. A displacement of a part from its proper situation.

MALARIA   An infectious disease caused by the protozoa of the genus *Plasmodium*, which is parasitic in the red blood cells and transmitted by infected mosquitoes of the genus *Anopheles*. The attacks of chills, fever, and sweating occur at intervals which are determined by the time needed for development of a new generation of parasites. Following recovery from the acute attack, there is a tendency for the disease to become chronic with occasional relapses. [MARSH MIASM: By many, this was considered to be due to an earthborn poison, generated in soils, the energies of which were not expended in the growth and sustenance of healthy vegetation. This poison was supposed to be the cause of all the types of intermittent and remittent fevers, and of the degeneration of the blood and tissues resulting from long residence in places where this poison was generated.]

MALARIAL TOXEMIA   [Poisoning of the blood.] Malaria was considered to produce a poison of some type that poisoned the blood.

MALLEOLUS   The rounded projection on either side of the ankle joint.

MAXILLA, INFERIOR   The bone of the lower jaw.

METACARPALS   The part of the hand between the wrist and fingers, made up of five bones.

MIASMA   A supposed noxious material that is derived from the soil or earth. [The unknown atmospheric influences which could arise either from sources such as vegetable decomposition or from those produced by the decomposition of matters derived from the human body. MIASMATIC DISEASES: In its broadest sense this included a number of conditions such as typhoid fever, yellow fever, remittent fever, intermittent fever, diarrhea, dysentery, erysipelas, hospital gangrene, pyaemia, small pox, measles, mumps, and epidemic catarrh. In it narrowest sense, it included only intermittent and remittent fevers and other malarial diseases.]

MITRAL INSUFFICIENCY   A diseased mitral valve in the heart which allows blood to flow back from the left ventricle into the left atrium.

MORBI   Diseased or unhealthy.

MORBUS VARII. *Morbus* is Latin for disease. When applied to particular diseases, it is associated with a descriptive term that indicates the nature of the disease. No official definition of this term has been found at West Point or in any other army records.

MORTIFICATION   Death, the loss of vitality in part of the body.

MYOCARDITIS   Inflammation of the muscular walls of the heart.

NECROSIS   The combined changes indicative of cell death and caused by the progressive degradative effects of enzymes. [The absolute death of a circumscribed portion of any tissue.]

NEPHRITIS   A general term for inflammation of the kidney. [Characterized by acute pain; burning heat, and a sensation of weight in the region of one or both kidneys; suppression or diminution of urine; fever; dysuria; constipation, more or less obstinate; retraction of the testicle and numbness of the thigh of the same side.] CIRRHOTIC NEPHRITIS: Chronic interstitial nephritis.

NEURALGIA   Paroxysmal pain that extends along the course of one or more nerves. [A generic name for a certain number of diseases, the chief symptom of which is a very acute pain, exacerbating or intermitting, which follows the course of a nervous branch, extends to its ramifications, and seems therefore to be seated in the nerve. Also used to signify pain originating from a specific organ such as the heart or stomach.]

OBSTIPATION [OBSTIPATIO]   Severe constipation.

ODONTALGIA   Toothache.

OPHTHALMIA   Severe inflammation of the eye.

ORCHITIS   Inflammation of the testis.

ORGANIC AFFECTION OF HEART   A general term meaning a diseased state of the heart.

OS CALCIS   The irregular quadrangular bone at the back of the area of articulation between the foot and the leg.

OSTEOMYELITIS   Inflammation of bone that is caused by a pus-producing microorganism. It may remain localized or it may spread throughout the various parts of the bone.

PARALYSIS   Abolition or great diminution of the voluntary motions. INCIPIENT PARALYSIS: The beginning of a paralysis or a stroke.

PARALYSIS AGITANS   Variety of tremor in which the muscles are in a perpetual alternation of contraction and relaxation.

PARESIS   Slight or incomplete paralysis affecting motion, not sensation.

PATELLA   Kneecap.

PERICARDITIS   Inflammation of the sac that surrounds the heart. [Although occasionally idiopathic, more often it was considered to be secondary in its character. Secondary forms could result from wounds, blows, and contusions to the region of the heart, an abscess perforating from the lungs or the liver, or from enteric fever, variola, scarlatina and pyaemia in all forms, and local spread.

Perhaps due to rheumatism or the chronic forms of Bright's disease. By far the larger proportion of cases occurred in connection with the last two named diseases. In rheumatism, pericarditis was thought to occur early, occasionally preceded the joint-affection, and although no period of the disease was regarded as free from the tendency to this complication, it usually affected within the first week of the rheumatic onset.]

PERITONITIS   Inflammation of the internal serous membrane lining the abdominal and pelvic walls.

PHLEGMON   Inflammation of the cellular texture, accompanied with redness, circumscribed swelling, and increased heat and pain, which is at first tensive and lancinating, afterward pulsatory and heavy. Terminates most commonly in suppuration.

PILES   Hemorrhoids.

PILONIDAL CYST   Hair-containing cyst or sinus in the sacrococcygeal area.

PLEURADYNIA   Pain in the chest with respiration.

PLEURISY   Inflammation of the pleural membranes surrounding the lungs and lining the chest cavity, with exudation into its cavity and upon its surface. It may be primary or secondary to disease of a surrounding structure, such as the lung, and is associated with pain during breathing. [An inflammation of the pleura, of whatever nature and extent was considered the most common of the serous inflammations. Of local causes, the chief were wounds or bruises of the chest wall; fracture of the ribs, infections of the spine; escape of irritating matter into the pleural cavity, from the costal side or from the pulmonary side; from disease of the bronchial glands or from the side of the abdomen. Some thought there were grounds for suspecting that a chill alone was a cause of acute pleurisy. It also occurred as a part, or as a complication of other diseases.]

PNEUMONIA   Inflammation of the lungs with consolidation. [Chief symptoms of pneumonia were considered pyrexia, accompanied by pain in some part of the thorax, rapid pulse, pain aggravated by the cough, which with dyspnea exited throughout the disease. At first, the expectoration is difficult and painful, but in the course of a few days it becomes free and gets better.] HYPOSTATIC PNEUMONIA: Pneumonia due to remaining in one position with shallow breathing, such as in the weak or aged. [A class of consolidations of the lung very common in those who were subjects of other diseases, which were, for the most part, noninflammatory in nature. These consolidations were found at the bases and more dependent portions of the lungs, in the course of both chronic and acute diseases, and also in the aged and cachectic. They were the result of weak inspiratory power, feeble circulation, and gravitation. The consolidation thus mechanically induced was increased by more or less exudation of fluid and blood corpuscles into the alveoli.] SENILE PNEUMONIA: Same as hypostatic. TYPHOID PNEUMONIA: Pneumonia associated with typhoid.

PROSTRATION   Extreme exhaustion.

PYELITIS   Inflammation of the pelvis of the kidney.

PYEMIA   A general disease with the presence and persistence of pathogenic microorganisms or their toxins in the blood, with secondary areas of suppuration and formation of multiple abscesses. [A condition of blood-poisoning which gives rise to fever, accompanied either by severe gastroenteritis and visceral congestions, or by certain local lesions, which are chiefly venous thrombosis, embolic abscesses in the viscera, acute suppurations of the serous membranes and joints, multiple abscesses in the connective tissue and eruptions upon the skin. The disease is usually, but not always, sequential to a wound or injury.]

PYROSIS   Heartburn. [Severe spasmodic pain in the epigastrium, frequently attended with feeling of constriction. Relief of the pain sometimes obtained by the rejection of retained fluid.]

QUININE   An alkaloid of *Cinchona*. [Its principal action was in the malarial diseases where it was considered a specific, and was used as a prophylactic for malaria. To control fever, it was used in typhus, typhoid, variola, pneumonia, and acute rheumatism. Neuralgias of malarial origin and neuralgia of the ophthalmic division of the fifth nerve were treated with quinine.]

RADIUS   Bone extending from the elbow to the wrist on the thumb side of the forearm.

RESECTION   Excision. [The term was used by some surgeons for the removal of one end of a bone when the remaining portion was left in place. It was recommended instead of amputation for certain fractures.]

RHEUMATISM   A number of conditions characterized by inflammation, degeneration, or metabolic derangement of the connective tissue structures of the body, especially the joints and related structures, including muscles, bursae, tendons, and fibrous tissue. INFLAMMATORY RHEUMATISM: Rheumatic fever. A febrile disease occurring as a delayed sequel of infections with group A *hemolytic streptococci*. [The disease was considered as having an intimate etiological relation to weather, season, and climate. It was characterized by pyrexia, sweats, and acute shifting inflammation of the joints and other structures. An occasional attack was referred to derangement of digestion and the functions of the liver, or after an injury to a joint. A fatal termination was due to congestion or inflammation of the lungs, and inflammation of the heart and pericardium. The causes of chronic rheumatism were considered to be the same as those of the acute disease.]

SCALED   Material removed from the surface of the bone.

SCAPULA   Flat triangular-shaped bone in the back of the shoulder. The shoulder bone.

SCIATICA   Pain that radiates from the back to the buttock and down into the lower extremity along its posterior or lateral aspect.

SENESCENT   Growing old.

SEPTICEMIA   A systemic disease associated with pathogenic microorganisms or their toxins in the blood stream. [The condition produced by the entrance of putrid matter into the blood. Thought of as two types. First, poisoning by the absorption of the chemical products of putrefaction. Second, cases of general infection from a wound in which no metastatic inflammations are present.]

SETON   A thread that is passed through a sinus, fistula, or open tract to keep the passage open or to act as a guide for later dilatation.

SLOUGHING BONE   Necrotic bone that separates from the viable portions.

STENOSIS   Narrowing or stricture of a duct or canal.

STROKE   A condition with sudden onset. The term is most commonly used to describe an acute vascular lesion of the brain, such as hemorrhage, thrombosis, or ruptured aneurysm.

SUBLUXATION   Incomplete or partial dislocation. Sprain.

SUPPURATION   Formation of pus.

SYNCOPE   A temporary suspension of consciousness due to a generalized decrease in cerebral blood. Faint or swoon. [State of suspended animation, due to a sudden failure of the action of the heart.]

SYNOVITIS, PAROXYSMAL   Inflammation of membrane lining bursa, joint cavity, or tendon sheath. A sudden recurrence or intensification of symptoms.

TENT   A plug of material such as lint or gauze for dilating an opening or for keeping a wound open, so it heals from the bottom.

THROMBUS   A blood clot that frequently causes vascular obstruction at the point of its formation.

TIBIA   The shin bone.

TORPID   [Not acting with normal vigor and function.]

TYPHLITIS   Inflammation of the distal end of the colon, cecum. [Formerly used for the condition now called appendicitis.]

TYPHOMALARIA   [Of malarial origin but with typhoid symptoms.]

UREMIA   The retention of excessive by-products of protein metabolism in the blood and the subsequent toxic condition. It is due to renal dysfunction. [A group of nervous symptoms, which occasionally occurred in the course of acute or chronic Bright's disease, as well as in other maladies, which prevented the secretion or the discharge of the urine. The evidence at the time seemed to point to the probability of the process being due to retention of some material or materials normally excreted.]

ULNA   The bone of the forearm, which is on the side opposite that of the thumb.

VARICOCELE   Varicose condition of the veins that form part of the spermatic cord and produce a wormlike swelling, which is accompanied by a pulling or dull pain in the scrotum.

VULNUS   Wound. VULNUS CONTUSUM: Wound produced by a blunt instrument. VULNUS INCISUM: Cutting wound. VULNUS LACERATUM: Parts lacerated or torn. VULNUS PUNCTUM: Wound made by a pointed object. VULNUS SCLOPETARIUM: Gunshot wound.

Bibliography

MANUSCRIPT SOURCES

Berks County, Historical Society of. Reading, Penn.
  Raphelson, Alfred C. "General Alexander Schimmelfenning's Burial in Reading, Pennsylvania." Typewritten copy.
California State Library, Sacramento, Ca.
  Steamship "Brother Jonathan." Typewritten copy.
Gilcrease Museum. Tulsa, Okla.
  Ethan Allen Hitchcock diaries. Books no. 46, 47, 53, 55, 77.
  Ethan Allen Hitchcock Papers.
Rutherford B. Hayes. Presidential Center, Spiegel Grove, Fremont, Ohio.
  Rutherford B. Hayes Civil War Records. Handwritten list of wounds, by R. B. Hayes.
Iowa, State Historical Society of. Des Moines, Iowa.
  G. M. Dodge Papers.
Missouri Historical Society. St. Louis.
  Daniel Marsh Frost Papers. "Memoirs of Gen. D. M. Frost," 2 vols. Typescript.
National Archives. Washington, D.C.
  Record Group 15. Records of the Veterans Administration.
  Record Group 94. Casualty Lists of Commissioned Officers: Civil War, 1861–65. Entry 655.
  Record Group 94. Letters Received by the Commission Branch of the Adjutant General's Office, 1863–70. M1064. 527 rolls.
  Record Group 94. Letters Received by the Appointment, Commission, and Personal Branch, AGO, 1871–94.
  Record Group 94. New York Hospital Registers. West Point Cadet Hospital Registers. U.S. Military Academy, West Point, N.Y. 14 vols. Entry 544.
  Record Group 94. New York Hospital. Vol. 577. Register of Deaths at Post and General Hospital, Fort Columbia, N.Y. Harbor. May 19 to December 1, 1882.
  Record Group 94. Records of the AGO, 1783–1917, Military Service Records of George A. Custer, 1866–79. Microfilm.
  Record Group 94. Records of the Adjutant General's Office. Compiled Service Records.
  Record Group 94. Records of the Adjutant General's Office. Compiled Service Records. Mexican War.

Record Group 94. Records of the Adjutant General's Office, 1863–70.

Record Group 94. Records of the Adjutant General's Office. Entry 534. Carded medical records, volunteers: Mexican and Civil War, 1846–65.

Record Group 94. Records of the Adjutant General's Office. Entry 623. "File D," 1860s.

Record Group 94. U.S. Army Generals' Reports of Civil War Service, 1864–87. M1098. 8 rolls.

Pennsylvania, Historical Society of. Philadelphia.

"John Buford Memoir." John Gibbon Papers.

U.S. Army Military History Institute. Carlisle Barracks, Pa.

Albert Ames Papers.

George L. Andrews Papers.

Aztec Club Archives Historical Papers.

"Official List of Officers who Marched with the Army under Command of Major General Winfield Scott." Circular. Adjutant General's Office. Mexico. Feb. 7, 1848. American Star Print. Mexico 1848.

Bailey-Stroud Papers.

Henry W. Benham Papers.

David Bell Birney Papers.

Luther P. Bradley Papers.

Henry S. Briggs Papers.

William T. H. Brooks Papers.

Eugene A. Carr Papers.

Civil War Papers Generals.

Crook-Kennon Papers.

Scott Hancock Papers.

Hawkins-Canaby-Speed Papers.

Robert Hubbard Letters.

August Valentine Kautz Papers.

Lewis Leight Collection.

Eli Long Papers.

Nelson A. Miles Papers.

Israel B. Richardson Papers.

David A. Russell Papers.

James Shield Papers.

John Wesley Turner Papers.

E. A. Wild Papers.

West-Stanley-Wright Family.

U.S. Military Academy, West Point, N.Y.

Capt. Henry Brewerton, Superintendent U.S. Military Academy, to Brig. Gen. Joseph G. Totten, U.S. Military Academy, West Point, N.Y., May 30, 1850. Record Group 404. Letters Sent. Vol. 2, July 1, 1849–Feb. 15, 1853; Letters Sent, 1838–40 and 1845–1902. Transcript.

Keogh, Myles W. "Etat de Service of Major Gen. Jno. Buford from his promotion from Brig. Gen'l to his death." Cullum Files. Special Collections.

Record Group 404. National Archives at USMA Archives.

Virginia, University of. Library. Manuscript Division. Special Collections Department. Charlottesville.

Benjamin Huger Papers. No. 9942.
Wisconsin. Milwaukee Public Library.
   Lady Elgin. Ship Information and Data Record.
Wisconsin. State Historical Society of. Archives Division. Madison.
   Fairchild Papers, Correspondence. MSS GC Box 16–18.
Wistar Institute of Anatomy and Biology. Archives of. Philadelphia, Penn.
   Isaac J. Wistar. Last will and testament.
   Isaac J. Wistar Papers.

UNPUBLISHED MATERIALS

Burial, death, and internment records

Illinois
   Springfield. Secretary of Oak Ridge Cemetery Board.
Kansas.
   Stafford. Minnis Funeral Home Records. (Holder of M. S. Barber, undertaker records.)
   Topeka. City clerk.
Michigan
   Ypsilanti. Highland Cemetery Association.
Nebraska
   Omaha. Douglas County. Death Register.
New York
   Buffalo. Register of St. Luke's Church.
   Fishkill. Fishkill Historical Society.
   Westfield. Town Clerk.
Ohio
   Logan County. Probate Court.
   Steubenville. Union Cemetery Allocation.
Rhode Island
   Newport. Death registered in the City of Newport for the year ending December 31, 1894.
South Carolina
   Beaufort. Coroners Inquisitions book, 1888–93.
South Dakota
   Yankton. South Dakota Grave Registration Project. Field data.

Miscellaneous

Pawnee County, Kansas. District Court of. Case no. 2396. Appr. docket no. F, p. 296. Filed April 18, 1892.
Connor to Dr. Edward D. Sabine from Douglas Hospital, Washington, D.C. October 18, 1864. Copy sent to author by David B. Sabine. Hastings-On-Hudson, N.Y., March 21, 1980.
Letter sent to the author from William A. Veitch. Lexington, Ky. June 9, 1990.

Dissertations

Ambrose, Stephen Edward. "Upton and the Army." Ph.D. diss., University of Wisconsin, 1963.

Benson, Harry King. "The Public Career of Adelbert Ames, 1861–1876." Ph.D. diss., University of Virginia, 1975.

Bower, Jerry Lee. "The Civil War Career of Jacob Dolson Cox." Ph.D. diss., Michigan State University, 1970.

Carpenter, John Alcott. "An Account of the Civil War Career of Oliver Otis Howard. Based on his Private Letters." Ph.D. diss., Columbia University, 1954.

Chumney, James Robert, Jr. "Don Carlos Buell, Gentleman General." Ph.D. diss., Rice University, 1964.

Cox, Merlin Gwinn. "John Pope: Fighting General from Illinois." Ph.D. diss., University of Florida, 1956.

Dinges, Bruce Jacob. "The Making of a Cavalryman: Benjamin M. Grierson and the Civil War along the Mississippi, 1861–1865." Ph.D. diss., Rice University, 1987.

Eidson, William Gene. "John Alexander Logan: Hero of the Volunteers." Ph.D. diss., Graduate School of Vanderbilt University, 1967.

Holzman, Robert Stuart. "Benjamin F. Butler: His Public Career." 2 vols. Ph.D. diss., New York University, Graduate School, 1953.

McCoun, Richard Allan. "General George Brinton McClellan; from West Point to the Peninsula; the Education of a Soldier and the Conduct of War." Master's thesis, California State University, Fullerton, 1973.

Marino, Carl William. "General Alfred Howe Terry: Soldier from Connecticut." Ph.D. diss., New York University, 1968.

Merlin, Gwinn Cox. "John Pope, Fighting General from Illinois." Ph.D. diss., University of Florida, 1956.

Nohl, Lessing. "Bad Hand: The Military Career of Ranald Slidell Mackenzie, 1871–1889." Ph.D. diss., University of New Mexico, 1962.

Peskin, Allan Jay. "James A. Garfield, 1831–1863." Ph.D. diss., Western Reserve University, 1965.

Schottenhamel, George Carl. "Lewis Baldwin Parsons and Civil War Transportation." Ph.D. diss., University of Illinois, 1954.

Weigley, Russell F. "M. C. Meigs, Builder of the Capitol and Lincoln's Quartermaster General. A Biography." Ph.D. diss., Graduate School of the University of Pennsylvania, 1956.

Published Materials

Alberts, Don E. Brandy Station to Manila Bay: Biography of General Wesley Merritt. Austin, Tex.: Presidial Press, 1980.

Ames, Blanche Butler, comp. Chronicles from the Nineteenth Century: Family Letters of Blanche Butler and Adelbert Ames. 2 vols. Clinton, Mass.: Colonial Press, 1957.

Anders, Leslie. "Fisticuffs at Headquarters: Sweeny vs. Dodge." Civil War Times Illustrated 15 (Feb. 1977): 8–15.

Andrews, Christopher C. Recollections of Christopher C. Andrews: 1829–1922. Edited by Alice E. Andrews. Cleveland: Arthur H. Clark Co., 1928.

Arnold, Phil, ed. "Grave Matters." Vol. 5, 1995.

Averell, William W. Ten Years in the Saddle: The Memoir of William Woods Averell 1851–1862. Edited by Edward K. Eckert and Nicholas J. Amato. San Rafael, Calif.: Presidio Press, 1978.

Baird, John A., Jr. Profile of a Hero. Philadelphia: Dorrance & Co., 1977.

Bateman, Newton, Paul Selby, A. S. Wilderman, and A. A. Wilderman, eds. *Historical Encyclopedia of Illinois and History of St. Clair County.* Chicago: Munsell Publishing, 1907.

Beatty, John. *The Citizen Soldier: Memoirs of a Volunteer.* Cincinnati: Wilstach, Baldwin & Co., 1879.

Beers, Paul. "A Profile: John W. Geary." *Civil War Times Illustrated* 9 (June 1970): 11–16.

Biographical Encyclopaedia of Maine in the Nineteenth Century. Boston, 1885.

Burgess, Milton V. *David Gregg: Pennsylvania Cavalryman.* State College, Pa.: Nittany Valley Offset, 1984.

Campbell, A. W. *An Interesting Talk with General W. H. Powell.* Chicago: M. Umbdenstock, Printer, 1901.

Cavanagh, Michael. *Memoirs of General Thomas Francis Meagher, Comprising the Leading Events of His Career.* 1892. Reprint. Gaithersburg, Md.: Olde Soldiers Books, 1991.

Chamberlain, Joshua Lawrence. *The Passing of the Armies.* Facsimile 21. Dayton, Ohio: Press of Morningside Bookshop, 1974.

Clark, Walter, ed. *Histories of the Several Regiments and Battalions from North Carolina.* 5 vols. 1901. Reprint. Wendell, N.C.: Broadfoot's Bookmark, 1982.

Cleaves, Freeman. *Rock of Chickamauga, The Life of General George H. Thomas.* Norman: University of Oklahoma Press, 1986.

Cleaves, Freeman. *Meade of Gettysburg.* Dayton: Press of Morningside Bookshop, 1980.

Coco, Gregory A. *A Vast Sea of Misery.* Gettysburg, Pa.: Thomas Publications, 1988.

Commager, Henry Steele, ed. *The Blue and the Gray; the Story of the Civil War as Told by Participants.* 2 vols. Indianapolis: Bobbs-Merrill, 1950.

Confederate Veteran Magazine. 40 vols. 1893–1932. Reprint. Wendell, N.C.: Broadfoot's Bookmark Reprint, n.d.

Conyngham, D. P. *The Irish Brigade and Its Campaigns.* 1869. Reprint. Gaithersburg, Md.: Ron R. Van Sickle Military Books, 1987.

Cox, Jacob Dolson. *Military Reminiscences of the Civil War.* 2 vols. New York: Charles Scribner's Sons, 1900.

Cresap, Bernarr. *Appomattox Commander: The Story of General E. O. C. Ord.* New York: A. S. Barnes & Co., 1981.

Crook, George. *General George Crook: His Autobiography.* Edited by Martin F. Schmitt. Norman: University of Oklahoma Press, 1986.

Daly, Maria Lydig. *Diary of a Union Lady, 1861–1865.* Edited by Harold Earl Hammond. New York: Funk & Wagnalls, 1962.

Davidson, Homer K. *Black Jack Davidson: A Cavalry Commander on the Western Frontier.* Glendale, Calif.: Arthur H. Clark Co., 1974.

Davis, Oliver Wilson. *Life of David Bell Birney: Major-General United States Volunteers.* 1867. Reprint. Gaithersburg, Md.: Ron R. Van Sickle Military Books, 1987.

Dawes, Rufus R. *Service with the Sixth Wisconsin Volunteers.* Dayton, Ohio: Press of Morningside Bookshop, 1985.

Dawson, George Francis. *Life and Services of Gen. John A. Logan.* Chicago: Belford, Clarke & Co., 1887.

Delaney, Norman C. "General Thomas Williams." *Civil War Times Illustrated* 14 (July 1975): 4–9, 36–47.

Dodge, Major General G. M. "General James A. Williams." Des Moines: Register and Leader Co., 1903.

Dunglison, Robley. *A Dictionary of Medical Science.* Philadelphia: Henry C. Lea, 1866.

Engle, Stephen D. *Yankee Dutchman: The Life of Franz Siegel.* Fayetteville: University of Arkansas Press, 1993.

Fish, Stewart A. "The Death of President Garfield." *Bulletin of the History of Medicine* 24 (1950): 378–92.

French, Samuel G. *Two Wars: An Autobiography of General Samuel G. French.* Nashville: Confederate Veteran, 1901.

Fried, Joseph P. "How One Union General Murdered Another." *Civil War Times Illustrated* 1 (June 1962): 14–16.

Gambone, A. M. *Major-General John Frederick Hartranft.* Baltimore, Md.: Butternut and Blue, 1995.

Garfield, James A. *The Wild Life of the Army: Civil War Letters of James A. Garfield.* Edited by Frederick D. Williams. East Lansing: Michigan State University Press, 1964.

Geary, John White. *A Politician Goes to War.* Edited by William Alan Blair. University Park, Pa.: Pennsylvania State University Press, 1995.

Gibbon, John. *Personal Recollections of the Civil War.* 1928. Reprint. Dayton, Ohio: Press of Morningside Bookshop, 1978.

Gordon, John B. *Reminiscences of the Civil War.* 1903. Reprint. New York: Time-Life Books, 1981.

Gould, Edward K. *Major-General Hiram G. Berry.* Rockland, Maine: Press of the Courier-Gazette, 1899.

Grant, Ulysses S. *Personal Memoirs of U. S. Grant.* 2 vols. 1885. Facsimile. New York: Bonanza Books, 1974?

Haskell, John. *The Haskell Memoirs: The Personal Narrative of a Confederate Officer.* Edited by Gilbert E. Govan and James W. Liningood. New York: Van Rees Press, 1960.

Hayes, Rutherford B. *Diary and Letters of Rutherford B. Hayes.* Edited by Charles Richard Williams. Columbus, Ohio: Ohio State Archaeological and Historical Society, 1922–26.

————. *Hayes: The Diary of a President.* Edited by T. Harry Williams. New York: David McKay Co., 1964.

Hazen, William B. *A Narrative of Military Service.* 1885. Reprint. Huntington, W.Va.: Blue Acorn Press, 1993.

Headley, J. T. *Great Riots of New York, 1712–1863.* New York: E. B. Treat, 1873.

Heath, Henry. *The Memoirs of Henry Heath.* Edited by James L. Morrison. Westport, Conn.: Greenwood Press, 1974.

Hebert, Walter H. *Fighting Joe Hooker.* 1944. Reprint. Gaithersburg, Md.: Butternut Press, 1987.

Heitman, Francis B. *Historical Register and Dictionary of the United States Army.* 2 vols. 1903. Reprint. Gaithersburg, Md.: Olde Soldiers Books, 1988.

Heyman, Max L., Jr. *Prudent Soldier: A Biography of Major General E. R. S. Canby, 1817–1873.* Glendale, Calif.: Arthur M. Clark, 1959.

Hirshson, Stanley P. *Grenville M. Dodge: Soldier, Politician, Railroad Pioneer.* Bloomington: Indiana University Press, 1967.

Holt, Daniel M., M.D. *A Surgeon's Civil War.* Edited by James M. Greiner, Janet L. Coryell, and James B. Smither. Kent, Ohio: Kent State University Press, 1994.

Hopkins, Alphonso A. *The Life of Clinton Bowen Fisk.* New York: Funk & Wagnalls, 1910.

Hough, Alfred Lacey. *Soldier in the West: The Civil War Letters of Alfred Lacey Hough.* Edited by Robert G. Athearn. Philadelphia: University of Pennsylvania Press, 1957.

Howard, Oliver Otis. *Autobiography of Oliver Otis Howard.* 2 vols. New York: Baker & Taylor, 1907.

Humphreys, Henry H. *Andrew Atkinson Humphreys.* 1924. Reprint. Gaithersburg, Md.: Ron R. Van Sickle Military Books, 1988.

Hutton, Paul Andrew. *Phil Sheridan and His Army.* Lincoln: University of Nebraska Press, 1985.

Irwin, B. J. D. "Three Cases of Penetrating Gunshot Wound of the Thorax, with Perforation of Lungs; Recovery." *American Journal Medicial Science* NS, 40 (1875): 404–7.

Johnson, J. B., ed. *History of Vernon County Missouri, Past and Present.* Chicago: C. F. Cooper & Co., 1911.

Johnson, Robert U. and Clarence C. Buel, eds. *Battles and Leaders of the Civil War.* 4 vols. New York: Castle Books, 1956.

Jones, James Pickett. *John A. Logan: Stalwart Republican from Illinois.* Tallahassee: University Presses of Florida, 1982.

Jordan, David M. *Winfield Scott Hancock: A Soldier's Life.* Bloomington: Indiana University Press, 1988.

Judson, Amos M. *History of the Eighty-Third Regiment Pennsylvania Volunteers.* 1865. Reprint. Dayton, Ohio: Morningside Bookshop, 1986.

Kearny, Philip. *Letters from the Peninsula: The Civil War Letters of General Philip Kearny.* Edited by William B. Styple. Kearny, N.J.: Belle Grove Publishing, 1988.

Keleher, William A. *Turmoil in New Mexico, 1846–1868.* Santa Fe: Rydal Press, 1952.

King, James T. *War Eagle: A Life of General Eugene A. Carr.* Lincoln: University of Nebraska Press, 1963.

Lane, Phyllis. "Michael Corcoran: Notes Toward a Life." *The Recorder* 3, no. 3 (Summer 1990): 42–54.

Lawler, William T. *The Lawlers, from Ireland to Illinois.* Gallatin, Tenn.: Kirby, 1978.

Leckie, William H., and Shirley A. Leckie. *Unlikely Warriors: General Benjamin Grierson and His Family.* Norman: University of Oklahoma Press, 1984.

Logan, Sheridan A. *Old Saint Jo: Gateway to the West, 1799–1932.* Sublett Logan Foundation, 1979.

Longacre, Edward. "Damable Dan Sickles." *Civil War Times Illustrated* 23 (May 1984): 16–25.

Longacre, Edward G. *From Union Stars to Top Hat.* Harrisburg, Pa.: Stackpole Books, 1972.

———. *The Man Behind the Guns.* Cranbury, N.J.: A. S. Barnes, 1977.

Lymon, Theodore. *Meade's Headquarters, 1863–1865.* Edited by George R. Agassiz. 1922. Reprint. Salem, N.H.: Ayer Co., 1970.

McClellan, George G. *The Civil War Papers of George G. McClellan, selected Correspondence, 1860–1865.* Edited by Stephens W. Sears. New York: Ticknor & Fields, 1989.

McDonough, James L. "John McAllister Schofield." *Civil War Times Illustrated* 13 (August 1974): 10–17.

McFeely, William S. *Grant: A Biography.* New York: W. W. Norton & Co., 1981.

McKee, Irving. *Ben-Hur Wallace.* Berkeley: University of California Press, 1947.

Marszalek, John F. *Sherman: A Soldier's Passion for Order.* New York: Free Press, 1992.

Marvel, William. *Burnside.* Chapel Hill: University of North Carolina Press, 1991.

Marx, Rudolph. *The Health of the Presidents.* New York: G. P. Putnam's Sons, 1960.

Matheny, H. E. *Major General Thomas Maley Harris.* Parsons, W.Va.: McClain Printing, 1963.

Maury, Dabney Herndon. *Recollections of a Virginian in the Mexican, Indian, and Civil Wars.* New York: Charles Scribner's Sons, 1894.

Medical and Surgical History of the War of the Rebellion. 2 vols. Washington, D.C.: GPO, 1870–83.

Michie, Peter S. *The Life and Letters of Emory Upton.* New York: Arno Press, 1979.

Miles, Nelson A. "The Biggest Days of Battle." *Cosmopolitan Magazine* (1911): 408–21.

Miles, Nelson A. *A Documentary Biography of His Military Career, 1861–1903.* Edited by Brian C. Pohanka. Glendale, Calif.: Arthur H. Clark Co., 1985.

Military Order of the Loyal Legion of the United States. 69 vols. 1885–87. Reprint. Wilmington, N.C.: Broadfoot Publishing, 1993.

Miller, David Humphreys. *Custer's Fall: The Indian Side of the Story.* Lincoln: University of Nebraska Press, 1957.

Mogelever, Jacob. *Death to Traitors.* Garden City, N.Y.: Doubleday, 1960.

Monaghan, Jay. *Civil War on the Western Border, 1854–1865.* New York: Bonanza Books, 1954.

Moody, Richard. *The Astor Place Riot.* Bloomington: Indiana University Press, 1958.

Nash, Eugene Arus. *A History of the Forty-Fourth Regiment New York Volunteer Infantry.* Dayton, Ohio: Press of Morningside Bookshop, 1988.

Nash, Howard P., Jr. *Stormy Petrel: The Life and Times of General Benjamin F. Butler, 1818–1893.* Cranbury, N.J.: Associated University Presses, Inc., 1969.

New York Monuments Commission for the Battlefields of Gettysburg and Chattanooga. *Final Report on the Battlefield of Gettysburg.* 3 vols. Albany, N.Y.: J. B. Lyon Co., 1900.

Nichols, Edward J. *Toward Gettysburg: A Biography of General John F. Reynolds.* 1958. Reprint. Gaithersburg, Md.: Butternut Press, 1986.

Norton, O. W. *The Attack and Defense of Little Round Top.* 1913. Reprint. Dayton, Ohio: Press of Morningside Bookshop, 1978.

Ordronaux, John. *Hints on the Preservation of Health in Armies.* Bound with *Manual of Instructions for Military Surgeons.* 1861. Reprint. San Francisco: Norman Publishing, 1990.

Palumbo, Frank A. *George Henry Thomas: The Dependable General.* Dayton, Ohio: Morningside House, 1983.

Peskin, Allan. *Garfield.* Kent, Ohio: Kent State University Press, 1978.

Phillips, Christopher. *Damned Yankee.* Columbia: University of Missouri Press, 1990.

Pitkin, Thomas M. *The Captain Departs: Ulysses S. Grant's Last Campaign.* Carbondale, Ill.: Southern Illinois University Press, 1973.

Porter, Horace. *Campaigning with Grant.* 1897. Reprint. New York: Time-Life Books, 1981.

Pula, James S. *For Liberty and Justice: The Life and Times of Wladimir Krzyzanowski.* Chicago: Polish American Congress Charitable Foundation, 1979.

Reese, John J. "A Review of the Recent Trial of Mrs. Elizabeth G. Wharton on the Charge of Poisoning General W. S. Ketchum." *American Journal of Medical Science* 63 (April 1872): 329–55.

Richardson, H. Edward. *Cassius Marcellus Clay.* Lexington, Ky.: University Press of Kentucky, 1976.

Robinson, Charles M., III. *Bad Hand: A Biography of General Ranald S. Mackenzie.* Austin, Tex.: State House Press, 1993.

Ross, Sam. *The Empty Sleeve: A Biography of Lucius Fairchild.* Madison: State Historical Society of Wisconsin, 1964.

Scanlan, Charles M. *The Lady Elgin Disaster.* Milwaukee: Cannon Printing Co., 1928.

Scharf, J. Thomas. *History of St. Louis City and County.* Philadelphia: Louis H. Everts and Co., 1883.

Schlicke, Carl P. *General George Wright: Guardian of the Pacific Coast.* Norman: University of Oklahoma Press, 1988.

Schofield, John McAllister. *Forty-Six Years in the Army.* New York: Century Co., 1897.

Schutz, Wallace J. *Major General John Pope and the Army of Virginia.* St. Louis Park, Minn.: Gleason Printing Co., 1986.

Sears, Stephen W. *George B. McClellan: The Young Napoleon.* New York: Ticknor & Fields, 1988.

Sherman, William T. *Memoirs of General William T. Sherman.* 2 vols. New York: Da Capo Press, 1984.

Slade, A. D. *A. T. A. Torbert: Southern Gentleman in Union Blue.* Dayton, Ohio: Morningside House, 1992.

———. *That Sterling Soldier: The Life of David A. Russell.* Dayton, Ohio: Morningside House, 1995.

Smith, Arthur D. Howden. *Old Fuss and Feathers: The Life and Exploits of Lt.-General Winfield Scott.* New York: Greystone Press, 1937.

Smith, William F. *Autobiography of Major General William F. Smith, 1861–1864.* Edited by Herbert M. Schiller. Dayton, Ohio: Morningside House, 1990.

Sommers, Richard J. *Richmond Redeemed: Siege at Petersburg.* Garden City, N.Y.: Doubleday & Co., 1981.

Southern Historical Society Papers. 52 vols. 1876–1959. Reprint. Millwood, N.Y.: Kraus Reprint Co., 1979–80.

Stanley, David S. *Personal Memoirs of Major-General D. S. Stanley, U.S.A.* 1917. Reprint. Gaithersburg, Md.: Olde Soldiers Books, 1987.

Steere, Edward. *The Wilderness Campaign.* New York: Bonanza Books, 1960.

Steiner, Paul E. *Disease in the Civil War.* Springfield, Ill.: Charles C. Thomas, 1968.

———. *Medical-Military Portraits of Union and Confederate Generals.* Philadelphia: Whitmore Publishers, 1968.

———. "Medical-Military Studies on the Civil War. No. 1. Lieutenant General Ambrose Powell Hill, C.S.A." *Military Medicine* 130 (1965): 225–28.

———. "Medical-Military Studies on the Civil War. No. 2. Brigadier General William R. Terrill, U.S.A. and Brigadier General James B. Terrill, C.S.A." *Military Medicine* 131 (1966): 178–82.

———. "Medical-Military Studies on the Civil War. No. 3. Major General David Bill Birney, U.S.A." *Military Medicine* 130 (1965): 606–15.

———. *Physician-Generals in the Civil War.* Springfield, Ill.: Charles C. Thomas, 1966.

Stevens, George T. *Three Years in the Sixth Corps.* 1866. Reprint. New York: Time-Life Books, 1984.

Sully, Langdon. *No Tears for the General.* Palo Alto, Calif.: American West Publishing, 1974.

Supplement to the Official Records of the Union and Confederate Armies. 39 vols. to date. Wilmington, N.C.: Broadfoot Publishing, 1994–.

Swanberg, W. A. *Sickles the Incredible.* New York: Charles Scribner's Sons, 1956.

Sweeny, William M. "Brigadier-General Thomas W. Sweeny, United States Army." *Journal of The American Irish Historical Society* 27 (1918): 257–72.

Taylor, Emerson Gifford. *Gouverneur Kemble Warren.* 1932. Reprint. Gaitherburg, Md.: Ron R. Van Sickle Military Books, 1988.

Thompson, Jerry. *Henry Hopkins Sibley: Confederate General of the West.* Natchatoches, La.: Northwestern State University Press, 1987.

Trefousse, Hans L. *Carl Schurz: A Biography.* Knoxville: University of Tennessee Press, 1983.

Trowbridge, Dr. Silas T. "Saving a General." *Civil War Times Illustrated* 11, no. 4 (July 1972): 20–25.

Trulock, Alice Rains. *In the Hands of Providence: Joshua L. Chamberlain and the American Civil War.* Chapel Hill: University of North Carolina Press, 1992.

Tucker, Glenn. *Chickamauga: Bloody Battle in the West.* Dayton, Ohio: Press of Morningside Bookshop, 1976.

Tucker, Glenn. *Hancock the Superb.* Dayton, Ohio: Morningside Bookshop, 1989.

U.S. War Department. *The War of the Rebellion: A Compilation of the Official Records of the Union and Confederate Armies.* 128 vols. Washington D.C.: Government Printing Office, 1880–1900.

Utley, Robert M. *Cavalier in Buckskin.* Norman: University of Oklahoma Press, 1989.

Varley, James F. *Brigham and the Brigadier: General Patrick Connor and His California Volunteers in Utah and Along the Overland Trail.* Tucson, Ariz.: Westernlore Press, 1989.

Wallace, Ernest. *Ranald S. Mackenzie on the Texas Frontier.* College Station, Tex.: Texas A&M University Press, 1993.

Wallace, Willard M. *Soul of the Lion: A Biography of General Joshua L. Chamberlain.* 1960. Reprint. Gaithersburg, Md.: Ron R. Van Sickle Military Books, 1988.

Ward, James A. *That Man Haupt: A Biography of Herman Haupt.* Baton Rouge: Louisiana State University Press, 1973.

Warner, Ezra J. *Generals in Blue: Lives of the Union Commanders.* Baton Rouge: Louisiana State University Press, 1964.

Wellman, Manly Wade. *Giant in Gray.* New York: Charles Scribner's Sons, 1949.

Wiggins, Sarah Woolfolk. "Press Reaction in Alabama to the Attempted Assassination of Judge Richard Busteed." *Alabama Review* (July 1968): 211–19.

West, Richard S., Jr. *Lincoln's Scapegoat General: A Life of Benjamin F. Butler, 1818–1893.* Boston: Houghton Mifflin, 1965.

Wheeler, Richard. *We Knew William Tecumseh Sherman.* New York: Thomas Y. Crowell Co., 1977.

Wilcox, Cadmus M. *History of the Mexican War.* Edited by May R. Wilcox. Washington, D.C.: Church News Publishing Co., 1892.

Williams, Alpheus S. *From the Cannon's Mouth.* Lincoln: University of Nebraska Press, 1995.

Winslow, Richard Elliott, III. *General John Sedgwick.* Novato, Calif.: Presidio Press, 1982.

Wistar, Isaac J. *The Autobiography of General Isaac J. Wistar.* Philadelphia: Wistar Institute of Anatomy and Biology, 1937.

Woodward, Joseph Hanvier. *Outlines of the Chief Camp Diseases of the United States Armies.* 1863. Reprint. San Francisco: Norman Publishing, 1992.

Newspapers

Arizona
  Florence. *The Arizona Enterprise,* October 27, 1892.
  Tucson. *Arizona Daily Star,* April 11, 1884.
California
  San Francisco. *San Francisco Call,* March 6, 1886.
  San Francisco Alta California, January 13, 1868; December 13, 1875.
Florida
  Tallahassee. *Semi-Weekly Floridian,* Sept. 7, 1880.
Illinois
  Galena. *Illinois Weekly Gazette,* December 17, 1867.
  Lincoln. *Lincoln Courier,* April 25, 1899.
Indiana
  Indianapolis. *The Indianapolis Journal,* February 15, 1869.
  New Albany. *Ledger-Standard,* September 28, 1872.
Kansas
  Topeka. *Daily Kansas State Journal,* February 11, 1884.
  St. John. *The St. John Weekly News,* May 26, 1910.
  Topeka. *The Daily Commonwealth,* February 12, 1884.
  Topeka Daily Capital, February 26, 1897.
Kentucky
  Louisville. *Louisville Courier-Journal,* April 25, 1899; July 23, 1903.
  St. John. *The St. John Weekly News,* May 26, 1910.
Louisiana
  New Orleans. *New Orleans Times,* March 15, 1867.
               Daily Picayune, March 15, August 30, 1867.
Maine
  Lewiston. *Lewiston Journal,* Illustrated Magazine Section. N.d.
Massachusetts
  Boston. *Daily Advertiser,* January 12, 1885.
Nebraska
  Omaha. *Morning World Herald,* March 19, 20, 1906.
New Mexico
  Santa Fe. *New Mexico,* December 17, 1867.
New York
  New York. *The New York Times,* February 10, 1886; January 21, 1896; July 25, 1903.
            New York Herald, July 26, 1886.
Ohio
  Napoleon. *The Democratic Northwest,* December 30, 1880; August 16, 1900.
  Fremont. *The Democratic Messenger,* January 26, 1893.
Rhode Island
  Newport. *Herold,* July 25, 1886.
South Dakota
  Scotland. *Scotland Journal,* April 20, 1895.

Tennessee
>   Knoxville. *Daily Press and Herald,* June 18, 1873.
>   *Knoxville Chronicle Daily,* June 18, 1873.
>   Columbia. *Maury Democrat,* March 27, 1890.
Texas
>   San Antonio. *The San Antonio Daily Express,* January 4, 1888.
Wisconsin
>   Fond Du Lac. *The Daily Reporter,* June 20, 1912.
>   Madison. *Wisconsin State Journal,* May, 12, 15, 1882.

MEDICAL HISTORIES OF UNION GENERALS

was composed in 10/12 Minion on a PowerMac 7100/80
by The Kent State University Press;
printed by sheet-fed offset
on Glatfelter 50-pound Supple Opaque Natural stock
(an acid-free recycled paper),
notch bound over binder's boards in Holliston B-grade cloth,
and wrapped with dustjackets printed in three colors
on 100-pound enamel stock
finished with matte film lamination
by Thomson-Shore, Inc.;
designed by Diana Gordy;
and published by
THE KENT STATE UNIVERSITY PRESS
Kent, Ohio 44242